P. J. Frosch, A. Dooms-Goossens,
J.-M. Lachapelle, R. J. G. Rycroft, R. J. Scheper
(Editors)

Current Topics in Contact Dermatitis

On behalf of the European Environmental and Contact Dermatitis Research Group (EECDRG)

K. E. Andersen (Roskilde)
C. Benezra (Strasbourg)
D. Burrows (Belfast)
J. G. Camarasa (Barcelona)
A. Dooms-Goossens (Leuven)
G. Ducombs (Bordeaux)
P. J. Frosch (Heidelberg)
J.-M. Lachapelle (Louvain)
A. Lahti (Oulu)
T. Menné (Copenhagen)
R. J. G. Rycroft (London)
R. J. Scheper (Amsterdam)
I. R. White (London)
J. D. Wilkinson (High Wycombe)

Springer-Verlag Berlin Heidelberg New York
London Paris Tokyo Hong Kong

Editors:

Prof. Dr. med. Peter Frosch
Hautklinik der Universität Heidelberg
Voßstraße 2
6900 Heidelberg 1, FRG

A. Dooms-Goossens, P. Ph., Ph. D.
Department of Medical Research (Dermatology)
Katholieke Universiteit Leuven
3000 Leuven, Belgium

J.-M. Lachapelle, M. D.
Professor of Dermatology
Unit and Laboratory of Occupational and Environmental Dermatology
Catholic University of Louvain
30, Clos Chapelle-aux-Champs, UCL 3033
1200 Brussels, Belgium

Dr. R. J. G. Rycroft
St. John's Hospital for Diseases of the Skin
Lisle Street
London WC2H 7BJ, Great Britain

Dr. R. J. Scheper
Department of Pathology, Free University Hospital
de Boelelaan 1117
1081 HV Amsterdam, The Netherlands

Library of Congress Cataloging in Publication Data.
Current topics in contact dermatitis / P. J. Frosch ... [et al.] (editors). Papers presented at a symposium sponsored by the European Environmental and Contact Dermatitis Research Group, held in Heidelberg, Germany in May 1988.
Bibliography: p. Includes index.
ISBN 978-3-642-74301-6 ISBN 978-3-642-74299-6 (eBook)
DOI 10.1007/978-3-642-74299-6

1. Contact dermatitis–Congresses.
I. Frosch, Peter J. II. European Environmental and Contact Dermatitis Research Group.
RC593.C6C88 1989 616.5'1–dc20 89-6418 CIP

Softcover reprint of the hardcover 1st edition 1989

Typesetting: Appl, Wemding
2127/3145-543210 Printed on acid-free paper

Preface

In recent years the field of contact dermatitis has increased greatly in importance in dermatology. The variety of exogenous, environmentally caused dermatoses has undoubtedly expanded over the past few decades with the increasing number of potentially toxic chemicals, the changes in lifestyle, and the greater life expectancy in industrialized societies.

The value of international cooperation in this field has long been realized and acted upon by the International Contact Dermatitis Research Group (ICDRG). By 1975 the international journal *Contact Dermatitis* had been founded under the editorship of C.D. Calnan. Thanks largely to the ICDRG and *Contact Dermatitis*, there were, by 1986, enough additional dermatologists and scientists with a special interest in this area to form the European Environmental and Contact Dermatitis Research Group (EECDRG). Within 2 years they had instituted the European Society of Contact Dermatitis (ESCD) as an international forum for researchers in the field.

The EECDRG decided to hold a symposium in Heidelberg in May 1988, an initiative supported by the ICDRG, and on this occasion the new ESCD held its inaugural session. The Society already has over 200 members and most national contact dermatitis research groups in Europe are already represented; new members are of course welcome. Subgroups and working committees have been formed to address various topics including the standardization of patch testing, photodermatology, and bioengineering.

The symposium included a large number of presentations covering virtually all aspects of contact dermatitis of current interest. This book contains almost all these papers and thus reflects the multiple facets of research activity in the field of contact dermatitis today. To speed publication, the papers have not been reviewed in detail. However, before acceptance for the symposium all abstracts submitted were reviewed by a committee of five members of the EECDRG.

We hope that this volume will prove to be a valuable source of reference and stimulate further research. The next symposium of the ESCD will be held in Brussels in 1992.

January 1989 The Editors

Table of Contents

Part 1
The Basics (Immunological Aspects)

Part 2
Morphological Aspects

Part 3
Current Contact Allergens

Epidemiology

Antimicrobials and Preservatives

Part 5
Contact Urticaria

Part 6
Photosensitizers

Part 7
Diagnostic Methods

Patch Testing

Part 1

The Basics (Immunological Aspects)

Allergic Contact Dermatitis: Carrier Proteins for Nickel

T. Chu, M. Shaw, J. Elliot, and A. Dash

Summary

In this study we examined nickel binding to serum proteins. In animal studies, immobilised metal ion affinity chromatography (IMAC) and sodium dodecylsulphate polyacylamide gel electrophoresis (SDS-PAGE) of the IMAC elution peaks was used to examine nickel binding to sera of rabbits, guinea pigs and mice. Elution profiles from the IMAC columns were comparable in all species. SDS-PAGE analysis showed only minor differences between the species.

In human studies, no differences were seen in the IMAC elution profiles between nickel sensitive and non-sensitive individuals, with major peaks eluting at pH 6 and pH 5 in all individuals and a minor peak eluting at pH 4 in two nickel sensitive and one nickel-non-sensitive individuals. SDS-PAGE analysis showed no consistent differences between the nickel sensitive and non-sensitive individuals. Ouchterlony analysis of the IMAC elution peaks showed albumin to be present in the pH 6 elution peak and C3, IgG, Clq, immunoglobulin and α_1-antitrypsin to be present in various fractions of the pH 5 elution peaks, but there were no consistent differences between nickel sensitive and nickel non-sensitive individuals.

Functional assays using lymphocytes from nickel sensitive and nickel non-sensitive individuals and IMAC fractions preincubated with nickel showed that cells from non-sensitive individuals did not respond to nickel-protein complexes. Cells from nickel sensitive patients responded to whole homologous serum and in two individuals responded to homologous serum and IMAC fractions from nickel sensitive individuals but not to IMAC fractions from nickel non-sensitive individuals.

This study suggest that nickel binds to a large number of different serum proteins and that different complexes are antigenic in different individuals. No single protein acts as the major or sole carrier of nickel in induced contact sensitivity.

Key words:

Carrier proteins - Nickel

Introduction

Allergic contact dermatitis to metals is a complex reaction involving the binding or haptenising of the metal to a native protein to produce an antigen and then a type IV reaction by the body's cellular immune system against the altered protein-metal complex. The importance and identity of the carrier proteins have been contentious issues that are only now being elucidated. The new techniques of T-cell cloning will undoubtedly tell us a lot about the importance of such carrier proteins.

When the metal ions bind to native proteins they cause a change in the protein so that the metal-protein complex is recognised by the body's immune system as being foreign. The fate of the newly formed antigen will depend on the type of antigen that has been formed [1]. Certain antigens have sufficient conformational mobility to allow the expression of both the agretope, which binds to the HLA DR or class II molecule of the antigen-presenting cell, and the epitope, which is the part of the antigen that binds to the receptor of the antigen-specific T-cell. Such antigens are called type I antigens. Type II antigens require denaturing of the protein before the agretope and the epitope can be expressed and type III antigens require enzymatic digestion of the molecule before the agretope and the epitope can be expressed. Therefore, depending on the type of antigen that is formed the antigen will need either processing by antigen-presenting cells or, if it is type I, the antigen will bind directly to the class II molecule on the surface of the antigen-presenting cell and be presented directly to the sensitized T-cell.

T-cell specificity depends on the T-cell receptor, which determines the antigenic specificity of that particular T-cell and its resulting clonal progeny. Enormous advances have been made in understanding the nature of the T-cell receptor and current understanding is that the T-cell receptor is composed of two chains, an alpha and a beta chain, which are linked by disulphide bonds. These chains carry both fixed and variable portions. The antigenic specificity is determined by the variable portion of the alpha and beta chains. The alpha and beta chains are linked to the CD3 complex on the T-cell which allows triggering of the T-cell proliferative response following binding of the antigen to the T-cell receptor [9, 10].

Nickel acts as a hapten and following penetration of the stratum corneum binds to tissue or serum proteins to produce an antigen that the T-cells respond to. The nature and importance of the carrier protein for nickel is both speculative and controversial. Initial studies suggested that nickel was preferentially haptenised to albumin [8]. In solution, 95% of nickel bound to serum proteins is found to be bound to albumin, but the affinity of albumin for nickel is low ($K = 10^2–10^3$) and the nickel-albumin complex is thus reasonably unstable. In type I reactions to nickel in the lung, the binding of nickel to the copper binding site of human serum albumin has been shown to be the stimulus for the production of anti-nickel/albumin complex IgE which initiates the reaction [6]. The importance of albumin in contact allergic reactions has not been demonstrated. Nickel in neutral solutions preferentially ligands to sulphur and nitrogen in cysteine and histidine residues and to a minor extent to amino and tryptophan indole groups [2]. Nickel thus binds to a large number of different proteins in serum. The purpose of the present study was to ascertain the importance to different nickel-protein complexes in inducing an immunological response. We also examined interspecies differences in nickel binding to serum protein and the specificity of serum protein binding in nickel sensitive individuals as compared to nickel non-reactive individuals to see whether there was a recognisable difference. Serum proteins were used, partly because of their accessibility and partly because of the similarity of serum proteins and tissue proteins.

Material and Methods

Patients. Three nickel sensitive individuals who had been shown to be nickel sensitive on standard patch testing (J.W., L.B. and J.E.) and three healthy controls who were found to be non-sensitive on nickel patch testing (F.A., B.H. and T.C.) were studied. Blood was taken from these patients; part was stored in glass bottles and allowed to clot and serum separated; part was taken in heparinised tubes and peripheral blood mononuclear cells were separated by Ficoll/Hypaque velocity sedimentation.

Animals. Sera from rabbits, mice and guinea pigs were examined to see whether we could identify differences in nickel binding to serum proteins between these species. Guinea pigs are relatively easy to sensitise to nickel, rabbits are very difficult to sensitise to nickel and there is no evidence that mice can be sensitised to nickel [5, 12]. Finding a detectable difference in the binding pattern of serum proteins to nickel in these three species would give us some indication of the importance of different proteins in haptenising nickel and producing an antigen that the animal responds to.

Immobilised Metal Ion Affinity Chromatography (IMAC). Chelating Sepharose B (Pharmacia) was used as a solid support for nickel ion affinity chromatography [7]. Chelating sepharose (10 ml) was washed in distilled water and packed vertically into a 10-ml plastic syringe plugged with nylon wool. The column was washed several times and then loaded with 10 ml 15 m*M* nickel chloride aqueous solution. As nickel ions bound to the Sepharose it could be seen to turn green. The column was then washed several times with distilled water until no further nickel could be seen to be eluted. The column was then equilibrated using 0.05 *M* phosphate buffer containing 1 *M* sodium chloride (pH 8).

Serum samples collected from nickel sensitive and non-sensitive patients were dialysed overnight against the running buffer and 1 ml samples were applied to the charged column. The column was washed with running buffer until the optimal density of the eluent at 280 nm was zero. The material that bound to the column was then eluted by stepwise reduction in pH using 0.5 *M* sodium acetate containing 1 *M* sodium chloride (pH 6, pH 5 and pH 4). Fractions of 2 ml were collected at each pH until the optical density at 280 nm of the eluent was zero. After each experiment the column was stripped of chelated metal ions by the passage of two columns' worth of 0.5 *M* EDTA containing 1 *M* sodium chloride. The column was then recharged as previously described before application of the next serum sample.

SDS Polyacrylamide Gel Electrophoresis (SDS-PAGE). SDS-PAGE gels were prepared according to Laemmli [4]. Samples from the stepwise pH elution of the serum components were examined using molecular weight markers of 17, 30, 45, 67 and 190 kDa to calibrate the gels. Gels were stained with Coomassie Blue and destained with a mixture of 80% distilled water, 15% ethanol and 5% glacial acetic acid.

Ouchterlony Analysis. Ouchterlony analysis of the elution peaks of pH 4, pH 5 and pH 6 was done using antihuman albumin, IgG, Clq, C3, antihuman immunoglobulin and α_1-antitrypsin. The gels were developed for 16 h and stained with Coomassie Blue.

Bioassay of Fractions Prepared by IMAC. Selected fractions from the optical density peaks were dialysed overnight against phosphate-buffered saline. Fractions were filter sterilised using 0.2 μ*M* Millipore filters and then incubated with an equal volume of 2% stock solution of nickel sulphate for 1 h at room temperature. Fractions were incubated with peripheral blood mononuclear cells from both nickel sensitive and non-sensitive subjects using a 96-well plate assay and a standard 6-day incubation. Activation was detected by thymidine uptake and the stimulation index calculated from the maximal counts with nickel divided by background counts. A stimulation index of >3 was considered significant.

Results

Animal Studies

IMAC (Fig. 1). Elution profiles on IMAC were very similar in rabbit, guinea pig and mouse, with elution peaks being identified at pH 6, pH 5 and pH 4. No major differences were observed.

SDS-PAGE. The major protein peaks on IMAC eluted at pH 5 and the largest number of different protein bands was seen with elution at pH 5. A very similar pattern was seen in all animals, with the heaviest protein bands at 45 and 62 kDa (Table 1).

Table 1. SDS-PAGE analysis

Species	pH 6 elution (kDa)	pH 5 elution (kDa)	pH 4 elution (kDa)	Comment
Guinea pig	45	45, 46, 47, 62, 76, 95, 144, >200	49	10
Mouse	45	41, 45, 49, 62, 66, 76, >200	49	9
Rabbit	45	45, 49, 62, 66, 76, >200	45, 49	9

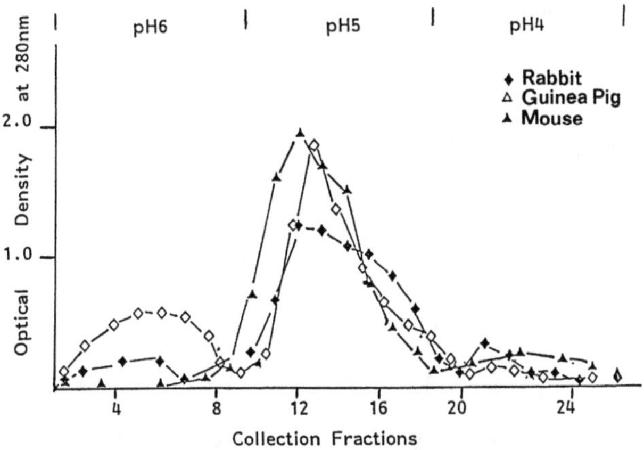

Fig. 1. Elution curves at pH 6, pH 5 and pH 4 from IMAC column using sera from guinea pig, rabbit and mouse

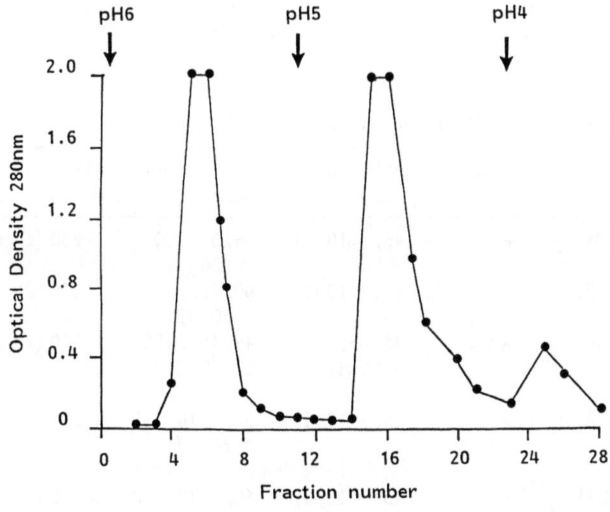

Fig. 2. IMAC elution profiles from J.E. (nickel sensitive) and B.H. and T.C. (nickel non-sensitive) showing peaks eluting at pH 6 and pH 5

Human Studies

IMAC. The results of IMAC are shown in Figs. 2 and 3. All subjects showed distinctive protein peaks eluting at pH 6 and pH 5. All samples gave highly reproducible elution profiles at pH 6 and pH 5 and no difference could be seen between the behaviour of nickel positive and nickel negative sera (Fig. 1). However, in three of the six sera examined, a further smaller protein peak also eluted at pH 4. This peak was found to be present in two of the three samples from nickel sensitive subjects and in one of the nickel negative sera.

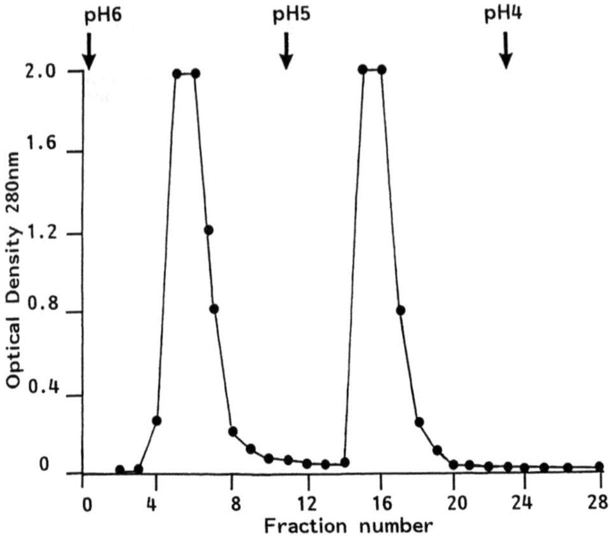

Fig. 3. IMAC elution profiles from J.W. and L.B. (nickel sensitive) and F.A. (nickel non-sensitive) showing peaks eluting at pH 6, pH 5 and pH 4

Table 2. SDS-PAGE gel analysis

Patients	Ni status	pH 6 elution (kDa)	pH 5 elution (kDa)	pH 4 elution (kDa)	Comments
J.W.	+	45, <10 (2)	59, 53, 200, >200 (2)	>200 (2)	10
L.B.	+	45, <10 (1)	60, 200, >200 (2)	>200 (2)	8, strong low molecular weight
J.E.	+	45, 65, <10 (1)	49, 150, 100, >200 (5)	>200 (1)	12, large no. of high molecular weight bands
F.A.	–	45, <10 (2)	55, <10, 150 >200 (1)	>200 (2)	9, very strong low molecular weight bands
B.H.	–	45, <10 (1) faint	60, <10, 150 >200 (1)	>200 (2)	8
T.C.	–	50, <10 (1)	55, 59, 63, >200 (3)	–	8

SDS-PAGE (Table 2). Proteins eluted from the columns at pH 6 appeared to be highly comparable, with all samples showing a strong band of protein at around 45 kDa. In addition to this major component all samples eluted at least one, if not two, low molecular weight fractions of <10 kDa, and in two samples (one from a nickel sensitive subject and one from a control) bands were identified at around 65 kDa, in the region of albumin. The pH 5 eluates showed major bands between 55 and 60 kDa in all cases. High molecular weight components of >200 kDa were identified in all six sera and protein bands at around 150 kDa (in the region of IgG)

Table 3. Results of ouchterlony analysis

Subject	Ni status	pH 6	pH 5				
		Albumin	C3	IgG	Clq	Ig	α_1-antitrypsin
B.H.	−	+	−	−	−	−	−
F.A.	−	+	+	−	+	−	−
T.C.	−	+	+	+	−	+	+
L.B.	+	+	−	+	−	+	−
J.W.	+	+	+	+	−	+	+
J.M.	+	+	−	−	−	−	−

were seen in three sera. In two subjects in the control group low molecular weight bands in the region of 10 kDa were also identified.

When pH 4 eluates were examined at least one high molecular weight band was seen in all six sera. This was despite the absence of peaks as demonstrated by optical density assessment. This presumably relates to the low concentration of these proteins within the eluates. In addition, three subjects (two nickel sensitive and one nickel non-sensitive) showed a further high molecular weight band.

Ouchterlony. Albumin was identified in all sera eluted at pH 6. It was not seen in any samples eluted at pH 5 or pH 4. Eluates at pH 5 contained variable amounts of C3, IgG, Clq, immunoglobulins, and α_1 antitrypsin (see Table 3).

Assessment of Biological Activity of the IMAC Fractions by Lymphocyte Transformation

When peripheral blood mononuclear cells from nickel non-sensitive subjects was used, no stimulation was seen when neat serum from nickel negative or nickel sensitive subjects was used. These lymphocytes also failed to respond to any of the IMAC fractions. When lymphocytes from nickel sensitive subjects were used, stimulation was seen with their autologous serum and to different fractions from the eluates. Two subjects responded to fractions from pH 5 and pH 4 eluates, while one subject responded only to proteins from the pH 6 eluate. When tested against serum from nickel negative subjects, in two nickel sensitive patients there was no response to whole serum or to the individual pH eluates from the IMAC column.

Conclusions

The conclusions from this study is therefore that although nickel binds to albumin, this is certainly not the only protein that it binds to and in the majority of patients it does not seem to be a significant carrier protein for nickel in producing an antigen. In different subjects it binds to different serum components to produce an antigen that they respond to.

Although this study was very small, the finding that in two subjects nickel sensitive lymphocytes responded to homologous serum but not to serum from nickel negative subjects is of great interest. This would suggest that a factor is present in nickel sensitive patients to which nickel binds and with which lymphocytes preferentially react. The nature of this protein remains to be elucidated. One could speculate that it may be an immunoglobulin, which would explain its presence in nickel sensitive but not in nickel negative subjects. It is obvious from clone studies that nickel binds to various proteins that are recognised by individual clones [3, 11]. There is some suggestion that nickel may bind to the class II molecule of antigen-presenting cells and may stimulate T-cells directly without haptenising to proteins. Further studies using T-cell clones will obviously show us the diversity of serum proteins to which nickel binds and the importance of these in initiating contact allergic dermatitis to nickel.

Acknowledgements. Tony Chu is a Wellcome Senior Research Fellow. This work was supported by grants from the Wellcome Trust and the Welton Foundation.

References

1. Allen PA (1987) Antigen processing at the molecular level. Immunol Today 8: 270–273
2. Glennon JD, Sarkar B (1982) Nickel (II) transport in human blood serum. Biochem J 203: 15–23
3. Kapsenberg ML, Res P, Bos JD, Schootemijer A, Teunissen MBM, van Schooten W (1987) Nickel-specific T lymphocyte clones derived from allergic nickel-contact dermatitis lesions in man: heterogeneity based on requirement of dendritic antigen presenting cell subsets. Eur J Immunol 1987: 17,861–865
4. Laemmli UK (1970) Cleavage of structural proteins during the assembly of the head of bacteriophage T4. Nature 227: 680–685
5. Lammintausta K, Kalimo K, Jansen CT (1985) Experimental nickel sensitization in the guinea pig; comparison of different protocols. Contact Dermatitis 12: 258–262
6. Niebaer E, Evans SL, Dolovich J (1984) Occupational asthma from nickel sensitivity: 11 factors influencing the interaction of Ni^{2+}, HSA and serum antibodies with nickel related specificity. Br J Ind Med 41: 56–63
7. Porath J, Olin B (1983) Immobilized metal ion affinity absorption and immobilized metal ion affinity chromatography of biomaterials. Serum protein affinities for gel immobilized ion and nickel ions. Biochemistry 22: 1621–1636
8. Rao MSN, Lal H (1958) Metal protein interactions in buffer solutions. Part III. Interaction of Ca^{11}, Zn^{11}, Cd^{11}, Co^{11} and Ni^{11} with native and modified bovine serum albumins. J Am Chem Soc 80: 3226–3235
9. Robertson M (1984a) Receptor gene rearrangement and ontogeny of T lymphocytes. Nature 311: 305
10. Robertson M (1984b) T cell antigen receptor – The Capture of the Snark. Nature 312: 16
11. Sinigaglia F, Schneidegger D, Garotta G, Scheper R, Pletscher M, Lanzavecchia A (1985) Isolation and characterisation of Ni-specific T cell clones from patients with Ni-contact dermatitis. J Immunol 135: 3929–3932
12. Spiechowicz E, Nyquist G, Goliszewska E, Chmielewski W (1983) Experimental investigation on sensitivity to nickel present in alloys used in dentistry carried out on guinea pigs previously sensitised to this metal. Swed Dent J 7: 39–43

Addresses

T. Chu
Unit of Dermatology, Royal Postgraduate Medical School, Hammersmith Hospital, Du Cane Road, London W12 ONN, UK

M. Shaw
Unit of Dermatology, Royal Postgraduate Medical School, Hammersmith Hospital, Du Cane Road, London W12 ONN, UK

J. Elliot
Unit of Dermatology, Royal Postgraduate Medical School, Hammersmith Hospital, Du Cane Road, London W12 ONN, UK

A. Dash
Unit of Renal Medicine, Royal Postgraduate Medical School, Hammersmith Hospital, Du Cane Road, London W12 ONN, UK

Allergic Contact Dermatitis: T-Cell Receptors and Migration

R. J. Scheper and B. M. E. von Blomberg

Summary

T cells mediating allergic contact dermatitis (ACD) are tentatively defined as recently activated, CD3+4+8− cells producing interferon-gamma and interleukin-2. These cells recognize allergen-modified class II molecules on specialized allergen-presenting cells, e.g. Langerhans' cells, and on other skin cells including vascular endothelial cells, fibroblasts and keratinocytes. Such interactions contribute to considerable specificity of the T-cell infiltrate in contact-sensitivity lesions. T-cell receptor-mediated binding is facilitated by additional sets of non-specific intercellular adhesion molecules. Expression of these adhesion molecules is augmented by inflammatory mediators, in particular T-cell-derived interferon-gamma.

Key words:

Contact dermatitis - Allergy - T-cell receptor - Adhesion molecules - Allergen presentation

Introduction

Understanding of the immunological basis of allergic contact dermatitis (ACD) grew in the 1960s. The mechanistic models proposed by Turk [1] and Polak [2] still provide the framework of our current thinking. It has been suggested that one must distinguish between afferent and efferent phases in the development of allergic contact dermatitis (ACD). The afferent phase includes the events following a first contact with the allergen and is completed when the individual is sensitized and capable of giving a positive elicitation reaction, namely the efferent phase. The entire process of the afferent phase takes from at least 3 days to several weeks, whereas full development of the elicitation reaction only requires 24–48 h.

In the past two decades several holes in the framework have been filled. Our knowledge about the basic mechanisms underlying induction, expression and regulation of ACD has considerably increased.

Highlights from this period are the identification of the Langerhans' cells (LCs) as allergen-presenting cells (APCs) and the characterization of thymus-derived lymphocytes as the primary cells mediating ACD. In the present review we describe recent discoveries with regard to T-cell function in ACD, with particular discussion of receptors and migration.

T-Cell Receptors

In contrast to the specific B-cell receptor (surface-membrane-bound immunoglobulin), which may have a strong antigen-binding capacity in its own right, the specific T-cell receptor (TCR) only displays weak antigen binding. For this reason identification of antigen-specific T cells in inflammatory infiltrates, e.g. by appropriate cytochemical assays, has not been possible. This has also retarded molecular characterization of the T-cell receptor, until more advanced molecular biological tools have recently helped to solve the issue. It is now clear that the T cell's antigen receptor has structural homologies with immunoglobulin domains. It also has a V region and a C region, but it is encoded by genes which are wholly separate from the immunoglobulin genes. Antigenic fragments or allergens are only recognized if they are presented together with MHC-encoded products: class II molecules for T cells of the helper/inducer type (CD3+4+8−) and class I molecules for the cytotoxic/suppressor type (CD3+4−8+). In both of these T-cell subsets, which form the large majority of mature circulating T cells, the receptor is composed of an alpha and a beta chain. Another subset of T cells (CD3+4−8−) can be found in the thymus, as well as in small numbers in the circulation, possessing gamma-delta chain receptors able to recognize class I MHC gene products. Although the latter cells have special affinity to epithelia, where they reside in the spaces between epithelial cells [3], and T-cytotoxic cells may be capable of mediating skin inflammatory reactions with a delayed time course [4], it is the T-helper/-inducer cell type which is assumed to be the primary subset mediating ACD.

The CD3+4+8− cells are not all equally capable of mediating allergic skin reactivity: apparently those clones with highest interferon-gamma (INF-γ) and interleukin-2 (IL-2) production upon antigenic stimulation are most active in generating an inflammatory response [5]. Moreover, to enter inflammatory skin sites from the circulation, optimal migratory capacity is required as found in the recent progeny of dividing cell clones [6]. Possibly activation markers, as detected by recently developed monoclonal antibodies on T cells present in skin infiltrates (4B4, WR19) relate to this migratory capacity [7]. At this stage, therefore, T cells mediating ACD can be tentatively defined as recently activated, CD3+4+8− cells producing INF-γ and IL-2 (Fig. 1). These cells are stimulated by antigen upon binding to the TCR, and subsequent perturbation of CD3 molecules closely associated with the TCR causing intracellular activation.

How allergen associates with class II molecules to provide a full antigenic stimulatory complex is still unclear. Three possibilities may be considered: (a) direct bind-

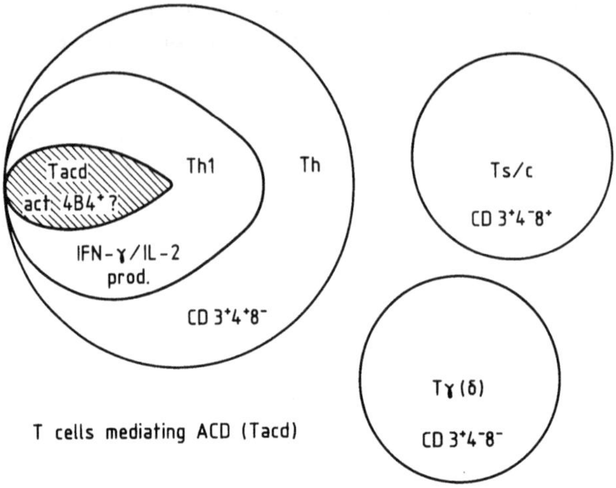

Fig. 1. A subset *(hatched area)* of one of the three major T-cell populations mediates allergic contact dermatitis (ACD). This subset can be tentatively defined as recently activated CD 3+4+8− T cells producing INF-γ and IL-2 (see text)

ing to class II molecules; (b) binding to other cell-membrane-associated molecules located in the close vicinity of class II molecules; or (c) binding to soluble carrier-molecules, that after uptake and degradation by APC are exposed at the cell surface close to class II molecules.

Recently reported data favour the view that direct allergen modification of class II molecules (a) is of major importance. Nickel-specific T-cell clones, derived from nickel-hypersensitive individuals, could be fully activated to proliferate and produce lymphokines in vitro in the absence of skin constituents, only if class II molecules were present [8]. Moreover, such in vitro stimulation could be obtained with serum-free culture media and chloroquin-treated APC, i.e. in the absence of intracellular uptake and degradation of allergen-protein complexes [9]. In line with this view it has recently been suggested that one of the major nickel-binding proteins isolated from mononuclear cells in the beta-chain of the class II molecule [10].

However, presentation of allergen by class II molecules does not provide sufficient binding. Additional sets of cellular-interaction molecules have been recently defined, that together facilitate full activation of T cells. Three of these sets deserve mention here. First, the CD4 molecule bears affinity to a constant region of the class II molecule, providing additional binding stability in T-cell/APC interaction. Second, the "integrin" family of cell-surface receptors plays an important role: leukocyte-function-associated antigen LFA-1 (a 180/95 kDa two-chain cell-surface molecule) is abundantly present on T cells and is known to bind to counter-structures found on APC, e.g. ICAM-1 (intercellular adhesion molecule 1, a single-chain 90 kDa molecule) [11–13]. Interestingly, CD2 (T 11; known from its binding to sheep red blood cells), also has its counter-structure: the 25–29 kDa molecule LFA-3, anchored in the plasma membrane of APC. In particular LFA-3/CD2 interaction may provide a signal that synergizes with the TCR+CD3-mediated signal [14]. All together these sets of interaction molecules resemble a delicate zipper which has to be closed for turning on T cells (see Fig. 2).

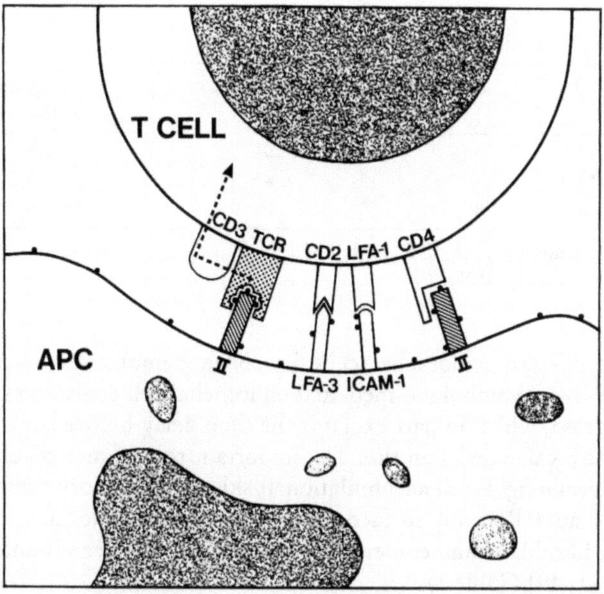

Fig. 2. Intermolecular interactions during cell-cell contact between an allergen *(small black dots)* -presenting cell *(APC)* and a specific CD 3+4+8− T cell. The T-cell receptor *(TCR)* recognizes a modified class II molecule, thereby allowing a receptor-associated CD 3 molecule to provide a signal for cellular activation (---→). Additional binding and signals result from CD 4/class II, CD 2/LFA-3, and LFA-1/ICAM-1 interactions

T-Cell Migration

In a non-allergic individual the frequency of T cells possessing specific receptors for a given allergen is low (supposedly between $1:10^5$ to 10^4). After sensitization, the frequency of such specific T cells in the circulation, as well as in peripheral tissues, will be persistently increased. Upon a repeated skin challenge with the allergen, therefore, allergen-bearing LCs are likely to locally encounter such specific cells: actually, one specific T cell is sufficient to set off a macroscopically detectable inflammatory reaction [15]. The impressive amplification of events during the development of a delayed hypersensitivity reaction is mediated by lymphokines, in particular INF-γ [16].

An active role for vascular endothelial cells at the onset of inflammatory and immunological responses, including adhesion of circulating leukocytes, stimulation of intravascular coagulation, and presentation of antigen to T cells, is now supported by considerable evidence. Interestingly, all zipper elements described above play a crucial role in facilitating T-cell migration into inflammatory sites of the skin. Vascular endothelial cells in unaffected skin bear low, but significant amounts of adhesion molecules as found on APC: ICAM-1 and LFA-3, as well as class II molecules. Both INF-γ and the macrophage-derived mediators IL-1 and TNF, as well as the microbial product LPS, readily augment the production and cell-surface-membrane expression of adhesion molecules on endothelial cells. Increased adhesion of T cells

Table 1. Enhanced expression of non-specific interaction molecules on (epi-)dermal cells facilitating T-cell infiltration and activation

Ligand	Endothelium	Fibroblasts	Langerhans' cells	Keratinocytes
Class II	+[a]	+[a]	++[b]	+[b]
ICAM-1	+[a]	+[a]	++[b]	+[b]
LFA-3	+	+	+	+

[a] Induction by TNF, LPS, IL-1, and IFN-γ
[b] Induction by IFN-γ

to activated endothelial cells has been demonstrated both in vitro and in vivo [16–18]. Lymphokine-mediated endothelial cell activation may take several hours to develop, which in part explains the time delay before large numbers of T cells infiltrate a callenged skin site. The important role of intercellular adhesion molecules in determining T-cell accumulation at skin inflammatory sites has only begun to be appreciated. Recently surface expression of these molecules on many skin cells, including fibroblasts and epidermal keratinocytes, has been found to be inducible by INF-γ [11, 19] (Table 1).

From the early 1960s [20] to now [16] research groups have promoted the concept that migration of T cells is not governed by the specificity of these cells. Data obtained by us and other groups make clear, however, that various factors may contribute to preferential accumulation of allergen-specific T cells at a contact-reaction site. First, on top of the persistent systemic increase of specific cells after sensitization, the frequency of these cells within the circulation shows transient peaks shortly after the first and every further contact with the allergen. Moreover, as mentioned above, recently activated T cells possess a uniquely high migratory capacity [6, 21]. An inflammatory reaction, therefore, when elicited within a few weeks after sensitization or boosting, will contain an increased frequency of allergen-specific T cells. At the skin level, selective accumulation of allergen-specific T cells at challenged skin sites may be further enhanced by preferential adhesion of specific T cells to allergen-presenting endothelial cells. All molecular elements required for such binding are provided by endothelial cells, even more upon local lymphokine release. Using radiolabelled DNCB-specific guinea pig T-cell lines we were able to show strong preferential recruitment at DNCB skin reaction sites [22]. Trapping at the DNCB-contact reaction site was found to depend primarily on the amount of hapten locally presented, rather than on the intensity of the allergic reaction. This indicates that a minimum dose of hapten is required at vascular endothelial surfaces for preferential adherence and entry of specific T cells. In support of this view Kapsenberg et al. [23] demonstrated that approximately 10% of the T cells present at 48 h in nickel-induced contact skin lesions were nickel-specific. In this study inflammatory T cells were cloned with a 100% cloning efficiency, thereby providing a full reflection of the T-cell repertoire within the lesional infiltrates.

Accumulation of allergen-specific T cells may be further promoted by local retention through haptenized, adhesion-molecule-bearing dermal cells, followed by one or more cell divisions. This mechanism will gradually increase the frequency of allergen-specific T cells at a skin reaction site, particularly during the first week following the peak reaction. It should be emphasized that the local frequency of specific T cells may considerably increase despite a large fall in absolute numbers of residual T cells. Thus, various mechanisms may contribute to increase specificity of T-lymphoid cellular infiltrates in contact-sensitivity lesions. These mechanisms explain the marked specificity observed in contact-allergen-induced retest and flare-up reactions [24, 25].

Conclusion

The mechanisms of specific recognition, and non-specific receptor-ligand interactions determining inflammatory cell migration are now being unravelled. The important contribution of T cell-derived mediators (lymphokines) to the development of delayed hypersensitivity reactions has been highlighted by the interaction-promoting activity of both INF-γ and IL-2. Better understanding of these primary mechanisms in ACD provide a basis for further studies on the regulatory mechanisms involved. Such studies should facilitate the design of preventive and therapeutic intervention procedures.

Acknowledgements. We are grateful to Drs S. T. Pals and H. Bril for valuable discussions during preparation of this manuscript

References

1. Turk JL (1980) Delayed hypersensitivity, 3rd ed. North-Holland, Amsterdam Oxford
2. Polak L (1980) Immunological aspects of contact hypersensitivity. Karger, Basel (Monographs in allergy, vol 15)
3. Janeway CA, Jones B, Hayday A (1988) Specificity and function of T cells bearing gamma-delta receptors. Immunol Today 9: 73–75
4. Shimada S, Katz SI (1985) TNP-specific Lyt-2+ cytolytic T cell clones preferentially respond to TNP-conjugated epidermal cells. J Immunol 135: 1558–1563
5. Mosmann TR, Cherwinski H, Bond MW, Giedlin MA, Coffman RL (1986) Two types of murine helper T cell clones. I. Definition according to profiles of lymphokine activities and secreted proteins. J Immunol 136: 2348–2357
6. Van Dinther-Janssen ACHM, Van Maarsseveen ACMT, Groot J, Scheper RJ (1983) Comparative migration of T and B lymphocyte subpopulations into skin inflammatory sites. Immunology 48: 519–527
7. Moore K, Nesbitt AM (1987) Functional heterogeneity of CD4+ T lymphocytes: two subpopulations with counteracting immunoregulatory functions identified with the monoclonal antibodies WR16 and WR19. Immunology 61: 159–165
8. Sinigaglia F, Scheidegger D, Garotta G, Scheper RJ, Pletscher M, Lanzavecchia A (1985) Isolation and characterization of Ni-specific T cell clones from patients with Ni-contact dermatitis. J Immunol 135: 3929–3935
9. Kapsenberg ML, van der Pouw-Kraan T, Stiekema FEM, Schootemeijer A, Bos JD (1988) Direct and indirect nickel-specific stimulation of T lymphocytes from patients with allergic contact dermatitis to nickel. Eur J Immunol 18: 977–982

10. Silvennoinen-Kassinen S, Jakkula H, Karvonen J (1987) Binding of nickel to the mononuclear cells and in the serum of nickel-sensitive and healthy subjects. Clin Exp Dermatol 12: 265–272
11. Dustin ML, Rothlein R, Bhan AK, Dinarello CA, Springer TA (1986) Induction by IL-1 and interferon-gamma: tissue distribution, biochemistry, and function of a natural adherence molecule (ICAM-1). J Immunol 137: 245–254
12. Ruoslahti E, Pierschbacher MD (1987) New perspectives in cell adhesion: RGD and integrins. Science 238: 491–497
13. Pals ST, den Otter A, Miedema F, Kabel P, Keizer GD, Scheper RJ, Meijer CJLM (1988) Evidence that leukocyte function-associated antigen-1 is involved in recirculation and homing of human lymphocytes via high endothelial venules. J Immunol 140: 1851–1853
14. Breitmayer JB (1987) Lymphocyte activation: how T cells communicate. Nature 329: 760–761
15. Marchal G, Seman M, Milon G, Truffa-Bachi P, Zilberfarb V (1982) Local adoptive transfer of skin delayed type hypersensitivity initiated by a single T lymphocyte. J Immunol 129: 954–958
16. Issekutz TB, Stoltz JM, von der Meide P (1988) Lymphocyte recruitment in delayed hypersensitivity; the role of interferon-gamma. J Immunol 140: 2989–2993
17. Messadi DV, Pober JS, Fiers W, Gimbrone MA, Murphy GF (1987) Induction of an activation antigen on postcapillary venular endothelium in human skin organ culture. J Immunol 139: 1557–1562
18. Haskard DO, Druie Cavender D, Fleck RM, Sontheimer R, Ziff M (1987) Human dermal microvascular endothelial cells behave like umbilical vein endothelial cells in T cell adhesion studies. J Invest Dermatol 88: 340–344
19. Dustin ML, Singer KH, Tuck DT, Springer TA (1988) Adhesion of T lymphoblasts to epidermal keratinocytes is regulated by interferon-gamma and is mediated by intercellular adhesion molecule 1 (ICAM-1). J Exp Med 167: 1323–1340
20. McCluskey RT, Benacerraf B, McCluskey JW (1963) Studies on the specificity of the cellular infiltrate in delayed hypersensitivity reactions. J Immunol 90: 466–474
21. Scheper RJ, von Blomberg M, Boerrigter GH, Bruynzeel D, van Dinther A, Vos A (1983) Induction of local memory in the skin. Role of local T cell retention. Clin Exp Immunol 51: 141–151
22. Scheper RJ, van Dinther-Janssen ACHM, Polak L (1985) Specific accumulation of hapten-reactive T cells in contact sensitivity reaction sites. J Immunol 134: 1333–1336
23. Kapsenberg ML, Res P, Bos JD, Teunissen MBM, Schooten W (1987) Nickel-specific T lymphocyte clones derived from nickel-contact dermatitic lesions in man: 1. Heterogeneity based on requirement of dendritic cell subsets. Eur J Immunol 17: 861–865
24. Nakagawa S, Fukushiru S, Gotoh M, Kohda M, Namba M, Tanioky K (1978) Studies on the retest reaction in contact sensitivity to DNCB. Dermatologica 157: 13–21
25. Christensen OB, Lindstrom C, Lofberg H, Moller H (1981) Micromorphology and specificity or orally induced flare-up reactions in nickel-sensitive patients. Acta Derm Venerol (Stockh) 61: 505–512

Addresses

R. J. Scheper
Department of Pathology, Free University Hospital, Amsterdam, The Netherlands

B. M. E. von Blomberg
Department of Pathology, Free University Hospital, Amsterdam, The Netherlands

Epidermal Mediators for Lymphocytes in Contact Eczema

C. G. Larsen, T. Ternowitz, and K. Thestrup-Pedersen

Summary

A total of 56 persons were studied for the presence of epidermal mediators in tuberculin skin tests, allergic patch tests, or irritant reactions from sodium lauryl sulphate (SLS) 3%. Epidermis was obtained with the suction blister technique, homogenized, dialysed, and ultrafiltered, leaving substances larger than 3 kDa for further studies. The epidermal homogenate was assayed for interleukin-1 (IL-1) activity and for the presence of epidermal lymphocyte chemotactic factor (ELCF). Our results show that simple occlusion of the skin in non-eczematous persons does not induce any significant amount of mediators. However, if the person in question suffers from irritant eczema, then occlusion per se will induce a significant amount of ELCF, but not IL-1. Both mediators are induced following a cell-mediated immune reaction in the skin irrespective of the presence of eczema. In patients with cutaneous allergy, the mediators are expressed in normal-looking, non-tested skin, when an allergic patch test is applied elsewhere. This may in part explain the excited skin syndrome.

Key words:

Chemotactic factors - Eczema - Epidermis - Interleukin-1 - Lymphocytes

Introduction

Contact eczema is a lymphocyte-mediated inflammation of the skin, affecting 1%–2% of the general population and up to 10% of the work force in certain industrial branches. The eczema may be due to allergy towards various compounds as diagnosed through patch testing, or it may be regarded as toxic or irritant, if cutaneous allergy is not found.

Recent studies have shown that many cells can secrete mediators, which in various in vitro assays enhance the immunological reactivity of lymphocytes. Thus, fibroblasts, keratinocytes, and cells in the early inflammatory response (monocytes) secrete peptides which can augment the in vitro reactivity of thymocytes from young mice [interleukin-1 (IL-1) activity] and increase the motility of T lymphocytes [epidermal lymphocyte chemotactic factor (ELCF) activity]. Such amplifying mediators could be of importance for the development of eczematous changes following an allergic or toxic/irritant impact to the skin. We have therefore studied the presence of such mediators in epidermal tissue under various experimental conditions.

Participants and Methods

Participants. A total of 56 persons were studied, either patients in our department or volunteers without skin disorders. A more detailed description of their age and sex is given in the reports of the various studies [1–3, 6].

Patch Testing. Using Finn chambers with a diameter of 10 mm, patch testing was applied for 48 h on the volar aspect of the lower arm. Allergens were chosen from the European Standard Series according to knowledge of previous allergy [2]. Irritant patch tests used sodium lauryl sulphate (SLS) 3%, and occlusion was studied using petrolatum alone [3]. Readings were done according to international guidelines. Tuberculin skin tests (2 tuberculin units) were applied to the lower abdominal wall [2, 6].

Epidermal Homogenates. Only epidermis was used in all investigations. Suction blisters were induced over the patch tests, tuberculin tests, irritant tests, and "control skin", which was clinically normal skin. Following blister formation, epidermis was removed, rinsed in medium, homogenized, filtered, dialysed to remove small-molecular-weight substances, and finally ultrafiltered with a cut-off at 3 kDa to any suitable volume [1–3, 6].

Interleukin-1 Assay. Epidermal thymocyte-activating factor (ETAF), which exhibits IL-1-like activity [4], was assayed in a conventional in vitro assay by studying the enhancing effect of epidermal homogenate on phytohaemagglutinin-induced proliferation of murine thymocytes from 6- to 8-week-old female C3H mice. The activity was compared with that of a standard IL-1 preparation and calculated as described elsewhere [4].

Lymphocyte Chemotaxis. Using a ^{51}Cr assay, lymphocyte chemotaxis was measured: radioactively labelled T lymphocytes were applied to a Boyden chamber with an upper polycarbonate filter (pore size 5 μm) and a lower nitrocellulose filter of similar pore size. The epidermal homogenate was placed in the lower chamber. The chemotactic activity was expressed as a chemotactic index (CI), being the ratio of active migration in the presence of chemotactic stimulus to random migration in the presence of medium alone. The incubation period was 1 h. A $CI > 1.20$ was considered positive [6].

Results

Interleukin-1 Activity. Table 1 shows a summary of our results from studying non-eczematous persons with a cutaneous cell-mediated reaction (tuberculin study), persons with or without eczema in whom an irritant patch test was performed (irritant study), and persons with known cutaneous allergy (allergic study). IL-1 activity was observed in normal epidermis, and its activity increased significantly in tuberculin tests and positive patch test, whereas an irritant stimulus with SLS 3% did not induce any change, irrespective of whether there was a clinical reaction or not.

Chemotactic Activity. Table 2 summarizes our findings of ELCF in similar experimental conditions. Simple occlusion did not induce ELCF, except in four persons who had eczema or were known to have cutaneous allergy. A positive tuberculin skin test induced ELCF in the test areas, similar to the observation with SLS 3% in patients with or without eczema. There was a significant tendency for patients with

Table 1. Interleukin-1 (IL-1) activity in epidermal homogenate during allergic or irritant skin reactions

Study	(*n*)	IL-1 activity[a]		
		Before test	48 h after test	
			Non-tested skin	Tested skin
Tuberculin [1]	8	n.d.	204	380[b]
Irritant [3]	15	193	172	200
Allergic [2]	13	296	571	836[b]

n.d., not determined
[a] Given in arbitrary units per square centimetre of epidermis.
[b] Statistically significant difference (non-parametric Wilcoxon test).

Table 2. Epidermal lymphocyte chemotactic factor(s) (ELCF) in epidermal homogenate during irritant or allergic skin reactions

Study	(*n*)	Chemotactic index		
		Before test	48 h after test	
			Non-tested skin	Tested skin
Occlusion [3]				
– Eczema	5	n.d.	1.15	1.10
+ Eczema	4	n.d.	1.07	1.52
Tuberculin [1]	19	n.d.	1.18	1.52
Irritant [3]				
– Eczema	8	1.12	1.21	1.80
+ Eczema	7	1.15	1.23	2.17
Allergic [6]	13	1.26	1.51	2.31

A chemotactic index > 1.20 is regarded as a positive response (presence of ELCF).
n.d., not determined

present eczema to have higher ELCF activity in test area epidermis following an irritant patch test. When patients with cutaneous allergy were tested, ELCF was found in tested skin, but also to a significant degree in non-tested, normal-looking epidermis, even before the patch test was applied. Similar significant amounts of IL-1 were also found (see Table 1). Preliminary data (to be published) suggest that the increase of mediators in patients with cutaneous allergy occurs before the clinical reaction takes place.

Discussion

The lymphocyte-mediated immune inflammation of contact eczema is apparently similar in allergic and toxic/irritant cases of eczema, as judged by clinical and immunohistological criteria. Epidermis carries a potential for "stimulating" an immune inflammation in both conditions, a clinical observation which Bruno Bloch in 1922 termed *Überempfindlichkeit* (hypersensitivity) of epidermis, and which has later been termed the angry back or excited skin syndrome [5]. From our present knowledge of the immune mechanisms in allergic eczema, it is difficult to explain toxic eczema. Our studies indicate that damage to epidermis with ensuing epidermal repair mechanisms in persons with present eczema or known cutaneous allergy can lead to the release of factors carrying activity towards T lymphocytes. ELCF seems to be the "first" signal of epidermal damage, and its early appearance may be due to its release from the membrane of keratinocytes in a pre-existing form, whereas IL-1 is only induced following a type IV immune reaction. One could also speculate whether ELCF is mainly derived from keratinocytes, and IL-1 from Langerhans' cells. The presence of increased IL-1 and ELCF in non-tested skin of persons exhibiting a positive patch test indicates that these mediators are not merely limited to the reaction area but also occur in remote areas of the skin, thereby supporting our clinical knowledge of excited skin. Further studies are needed for a biochemical characterization of both epidermal activities.

References

1. Larsen CG, Ternowitz T, Larsen FG, Thestrup-Pedersen K (1988) Epidermis and lymphocyte interactions during a tuberculin skin reaction. I. Increased ETAF/IL-1 like activity, expression of tissue antigens and mixed skin lymphocyte reactivity. Arch Dermatol Res 280: 83–9
2. Larsen CG, Ternowitz T, Larsen FG, Thestrup-Pedersen K (1988) Epidermis and lymphocyte interactions during an allergic patch test reaction. Increased activity of ETAF/IL-1, epidermal derived lymphocyte chemotactic factor and mixed skin lymphocyte reactivity in persons with type IV allergy. J Invest Dermatol 90: 230–3
3. Larsen CG, Ternowitz T, Larsen FG, Zachariae C, Thestrup-Pedersen K (1988) ETAF/Interleukin-1 and epidermal lymphocyte chemotactic factor in epidermis overlying an irritant patch test. Submitted for publication.

4. Luger TA, Stadler BM, Luger BM, Sztein MB, Schmidt JA, Hawley-Nelson P, Grabner G, Oppenheim JJ (1983) Characteristics of an epidermal cell thymocyte-activating factor (ETAF) produced by human epidermal cells and a human squamous cell carcinoma cell line. J Invest Dermatol 81: 187–93
5. Mitchell JC (1975) The angry back syndrome: eczema creates eczema. Contact Dermatitis 1: 193
6. Ternowitz T, Thestrup-Pedersen K (1986) Epidermis and lymphocyte interactions during a tuberculin skin reaction. II. Epidermis contains specific lymphocyte chemotactic factors. J Invest Dermatol 87: 613–6

Addresses

C. G. Larsen
Department of Dermatology, University of Aarhus, Marselisborg Hospital, 8000 Aarhus C., Denmark

T. Ternowitz
Department of Dermatology, University of Aarhus, Marselisborg Hospital, 8000 Aarhus C., Denmark

K. Thestrup-Pedersen
Department of Dermatology, University of Aarhus, Marselisborg Hospital, 8000 Aarhus C., Denmark

Evidence for the Existence of Prohapten-Activating Enzyme in the Skin: Induction of Contact Sensitivity to Monocrotaline in Mice*

R. J. Schmidt and L. Khan

Summary

Many contact sensitizers do not appear to be sufficiently reactive with protein to behave as haptens. It has therefore been presumed that they are prohaptens, which become activated in or on the skin to form suitably reactive haptens. This contribution is the first to provide compelling evidence for the occurrence of this phenomenon of prohapten activation in the skin. Epicutaneous experiments were carried out in mice, using 3-methylcholanthrene (3-MC) as a known inducer of mixed function oxidase activity, piperonyl butoxide (PBO) as a known inhibitor of this activity, and monocrotaline – a pyrrolizidine alkaloid – as a presumed prohapten. The mice could be sensitized to monocrotaline after pretreatment with 3-MC, but not after pretreatment with 3-MC followed by PBO or after no pretreatment. PBO was also found to inhibit elicitation of the contact allergic reaction to monocrotaline in monocrotaline-sensitized mice. The monocrotaline is believed to have become converted into a reactive pyrrolic ester through dehydrogenation by an induced mixed function oxidase in the skin.

Key words:

Prohapten activation - 3-Methylcholanthrene - Piperonyl butoxide - Monocrotaline - Contact sensitization

* L. K. is grateful to the British Council for financial support. The work was made possible by a grant from the Welsh Scheme for the Development of Health and Social Research.

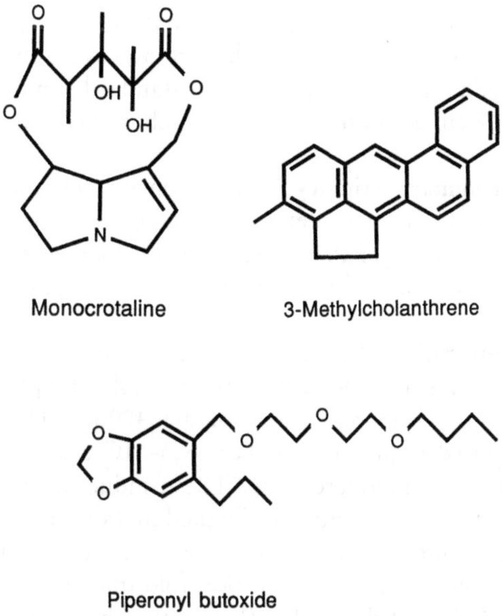

Fig. 1. Structures of monocrotaline, piperonyl butoxide, and 3-methylcholanthrene

Introduction

It has long been accepted that contact allergens are not themselves allergenic, but are able to bind covalently (or otherwise) with protein(s) in the skin to produce altered protein(s) which the body then regards as 'foreign'. This would normally result in the elicitation of a type IV or cell-mediated immune response. Such contact allergens have therefore been described as haptens or incomplete allergens. However, it is apparent that very many known contact allergens lack the necessary reactivity with protein. This has led to the suggestion that such compounds become activated by some process either in or on the skin, and hence they have been described as prohaptens. Dupuis and Benezra [1] provide a theoretical discussion of the likely modes of activation of prohaptens, but experimental evidence for the occurrence of prohapten activation in skin is conspicuously absent from the literature. In order to investigate the concept of prohapten activation, we chose monocrotaline as a presumed prohapten, 3-methylcholanthrene (3-MC) as a known inducer of mixed function oxidase (MFO) activity in the skin (see [13, 14, 3]), and piperonyl butoxide (PBO) as a known inhibitor of MFO (see [11, 5]), on the basis that MFO is very likely to be a prohapten-activating enzyme (PAE). The structures of 3-MC, PBO, and monocrotaline are presented in Fig. 1.

Materials and Methods

Materials. Monocrotaline and 3-MC were obtained from Sigma Chemical Company. PBO was obtained from the Aldrich Chemical Company.

Animals. An in-house strain (WSP) of 10-week-old male white mice was used. Ten mice were housed in each cage and were maintained under normal animal house conditions with free access to standard food pellets and water. Before treatment, a 2 × 2 cm area on the back of each mouse was shaved with electric clippers.

Preliminary Irritancy Assays. Non-irritant concentrations of all materials tested were used. These were determined using a standard mouse ear irritancy assay described elsewhere [2]. Ethanol was used as solvent both in the preliminary irritancy determinations and in the sensitization procedures described below.

Sensitization Procedures. Initially, the individuals in each cage of ten mice were treated epicutaneously with ethanol (400 μl), 3-MC (2 mg/400 μl), PBO (2 mg/400 μl), or monocrotaline (2 mg/400 μl). The individuals in two further cages were exposed sequentially either to 3-MC and then monocrotaline or to 3-MC, PBO, and then monocrotaline. These induction phase procedures were carried out on days 1, 3, 5, 7, and 9 as detailed in Table 1. A visual assessment of the skin reactions was made on day 10. Reactions were categorized as being either positive or negative, in conjunction with skin fold thickness measurements of the treated sites using an Oditest ODI 20 RK/K gauge. The animals were then allowed to recover until day 24, when they were all challenged with an epicutaneous application of monocrotaline (3 mg/400 μl). On day 26, a visual assessment of the skin reactions at the test sites was again made, as were skin thickness measurements.

Inhibition Procedures. The individuals in four cages of ten mice were treated epicutaneously either with ethanol or with 3-MC and then monocrotaline as before (for details see Table 2). On day 24, all were challenged with monocrotaline, and a visual assessment of the test site, together with skin thickness measurements, was again

Table 1. Results of sensitization procedures

Test substance[a]	Treatment days	Day 10 results: Skin reactions (n) +	–	Skin thickness[b] (mm)	Results of challenge[c]: Skin reactions (n) +	–	Thickness[b] (mm)
Ethanol	1, 3, 5, 7, 9	0	10	0.8	0	10	0.8
3-MC	1, 3, 5, 7, 9	7	3	1.4	0	10	0.9
PBO	1, 3, 5, 7, 9	0	10	0.8	0	10	0.8
Monocrotaline	1, 3, 5, 7, 9	0	10	0.8	0	10	0.8
3-MC Monocrotaline	1, 3 5, 7, 9	8	2	1.9	8	2	1.8; 0.8
3-MC PBO Monocrotaline	1 3 5, 7, 9	0	10	0.8	0	10	0.8

[a] Induction doses: ethanol 400 μl, 3-MC 2 mg/400 μl, PBO 2 mg/400 μl, monocrotaline 2 mg/400 μl.
[b] Mean results of skinfold thickness measurements (Oditest).
[c] Monocrotaline challenge (3 mg/400 μl) on day 24; results read on day 26.

Table 2. Results of inhibition procedures

Test substance[a]	Treatment days	Results of 1st challenge[b]			Test substance[a]	Treatment days	Results of 2nd challenge[d]		
		Skin reactions (n)		Thickness[c] (mm)			Skin reactions (n)		Thickness[c] (mm)
		+	−				+	−	
Ethanol	1, 3, 5, 7, 9	0	10	0.8	Ethanol	27, 29	0	10	0.8
3-MC Monocrotaline	1, 3 5, 7, 9	8	2	1.8; 0.8	Ethanol	27, 29	8	0	1.8
3-MC Monocrotaline	1, 3 5, 7, 9	7	3	1.8; 0.8	PBO	27, 29	1	6	1.0; 0.8
3-MC Monocrotaline	1, 3 5, 7, 9	8	2	1.8; 0.8	PBO	27, 29	1	7	1.0; 0.8

[a] Induction doses: ethanol 400 µl, 3-MC 2 mg/400 µl, monocrotaline 2 mg/400 µl, PBO 2 mg/400 µl.
[b] Monocrotaline challenge (3 mg/400 µl) on day 24; results read on day 26.
[c] Mean results of skinfold thickness measurements (Oditest).
[d] Monocrotaline challenge (3 mg/400 µl) on day 31; results read on day 33.

made on day 26. Mice found to have become sensitized to monocrotaline were then treated epicutaneously on days 27 and 29 either with ethanol or with PBO. On day 31 (when visible skin reactions had subsided), the mice were again challenged with monocrotaline (see Table 2). The responses to this second challenge were read on day 33.

Results

Results of the sensitization procedures are recorded in Table 1; results of the inhibition procedures are recorded in Table 2. It is clear from the results presented in Table 1 that monocrotaline can exhibit contact-sensitizing activity when applied to an area of mouse skin previously treated with 3-MC, a known inducer of MFO activity in the skin. Also, it would appear that PBO application after 3-MC application can effectively inhibit or reverse the effects of 3-MC. The observation regarding the activation of monocrotaline by 3-MC was confirmed in the inhibition experiments recorded in Table 2. The inhibition experiments also demonstrated that PBO was capable of inhibiting or reversing the effects of 3-MC in monocrotaline-sensitized mice challenged with monocrotaline.

Discussion

Although there is no doubt that the skin can display metabolic activity, generally only low levels of potentially relevant activities such as mixed function oxidation can be demonstrated in skin. However, MFO activity in the skin is readily induced by topical applications of many of the agents known to induce hepatic metabolism (see [8]). In the case of skin application of a prohapten, it may therefore be presumed that there will normally be insufficient hapten produced to elicit a clinical response. Therefore, the hypothesis may be developed that highly active presumed prohaptens, such as the urushiols of poison ivy (see [1]), have the ability to induce the expression of an appropriate PAE, through the action of which a hapten (thought to be a quinone in the case of the urushiols; see [4]) is produced. Conversely, weakly allergenic prohaptens may be supposed not to induce appropriate PAE activity. If this hypothesis is to be tested, it has to be assumed that induction of an appropriate PAE is a necessary event before induction of contact sensitization to weakly active prohaptens can occur. Hence, a known inducer of such an enzyme needs to be selected. Perhaps the only suitable compounds for this purpose at present are the polycyclic hydrocarbons, such as 7,12-dimethylbenz(a)anthracene (DMBA) and 3-MC.

These compounds have been well studied as potent carcinogens [13, 14, 3], and the events leading to carcinogenesis are now well documented. Briefly, 3-MC, for example, can induce MFO activity for which it can act as substrate. The product formed first is thought to be an epoxide, which then serves as a substrate for another induced enzyme, namely epoxide hydrase (EH). EH then opens the epoxide ring and forms a dihydrodiol. Further cycling of this metabolite results in a second epoxidation event, by which the 7,8-epoxide-9,10-dihydrodiol of 3-MC is produced. This is believed to be the ultimate carcinogen [13]. The structures of these two metabolites of 3-MC are presented in Fig. 2. 3-MC also exhibits contact allergenic activity in guinea pigs [12], presumably through a similar mechanism, except that skin protein(s) rather than DNA become(s) altered. We believe therefore that the carcinogenic activity of 3-MC does not preclude its use in our experiments and indeed may be an inevitable consequence of its profound ability (or that of its metabolites) to bind covalently with protein and/or DNA. During the course of our own work (unpublished), we were able to confirm the contact-sensitizing properties of 3-MC in mice. Consequently, 3-MC should also be regarded as a PAE-activatable prohapten.

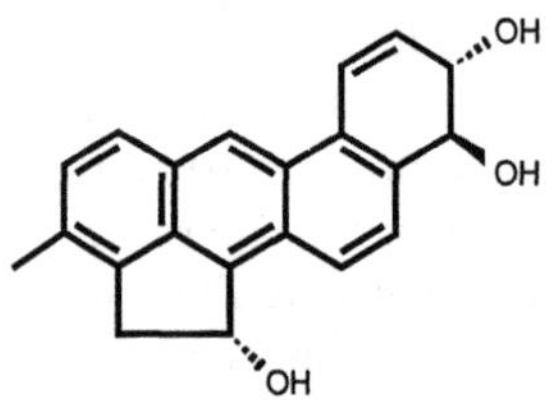

1-Hydroxy-3-methylcholanthrene-9,10-dihydrodiol

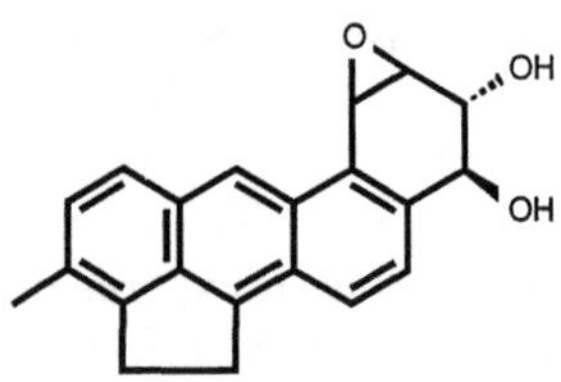

3-Methylcholanthrene-7,8-epoxide-9,10-dihydrodiol

Fig. 2. Carcinogenic metabolites of 3-methylcholanthrene

It is interesting to note that Pohl et al. [9] observed that 3-MC caused only a slight increase in cutaneous cytochrome P-450 levels in mouse skin after topical application, and that these returned to control levels within 72 h. Our results suggest that one or two applications of 3-MC can result in the induction of PAE which lasts at least 30 days, an observation that appears to suggest that PAE is not a cytochrome P-450-dependent MFO. Further experiments to investigate this are being planned.

Having found a likely PAE inducer in 3-MC, a suitable prohapten had to be selected. Ideally, the chosen compound should be only a weakly active contact allergen with the ability to act as substrate for the induced PAE. 3-MC is known to induce MFO; a well-studied family of compounds with proven ability to act as MFO substrates are the pyrrolizidine alkaloids [6, 7]. More importantly, the products of such metabolic alteration of pyrrolizidine alkaloids are known to be highly reactive pyrrolic esters (see Fig. 3), which would be expected to behave as potent haptens. Thus, the compound chosen, monocrotaline, was considered to be the ideal model prohapten. The suitability of this compound for this role is further enhanced by a lack of evidence in the literature that it may act as a contact allergen.

Having chosen a suitable PAE inducer and substrate, there remained the need to provide evidence that the substrate was being altered by the induced enzyme in the expected manner. This was achieved by treating 3-MC-pretreated mice with PBO. This compound is a known inhibitor of MFO activity (see [11]) and is used commercially for this purpose to prevent enzymic degradation of pyrethrins being used as insecticides (see [5]). There is evidence that insect MFOs are similar to those found in animals [10]. Mice treated with 3-MC and then PBO subsequently failed either to become sensitized to monocrotaline or to respond to monocrotaline once sensitized.

We believe that the results presented, though only of a preliminary nature in mice, open up the possibility that PAE inhibitors could be developed for prophylaxis of

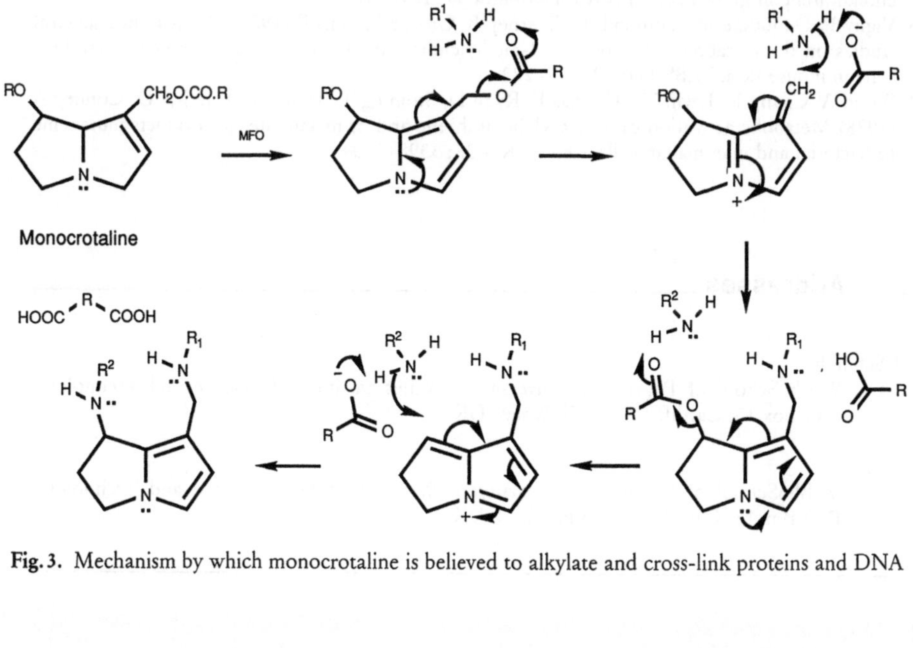

Fig. 3. Mechanism by which monocrotaline is believed to alkylate and cross-link proteins and DNA

certain types of allergic contact dermatitis. The experimental procedure will certainly facilitate the identification of further PAE-activatable prohaptens and also other PAE inducers and inhibitors.

References

1. Dupuis G, Benezra C (1982) Allergic contact dermatitis to simple chemicals. A molecular approach. Dekker, New York
2. Evans FJ, Schmidt RJ (1979) An assay procedure for the comparative irritancy testing of esters in the tigliane and daphnane series. Inflammation 3: 215–223
3. Levin W, Buening MK, Wood A, Chang R, Thakker D, Jerina D, Conney A (1979) Tumorigenic activity of 3-methylcholanthrene metabolites on mouse skin and in newborn mice. Cancer Res 39: 3549–3553
4. Liberato DJ, Byers VS, Dennick RG, Castagnoli N (1981) Regiospecific attack of nitrogen and sulfur nucleophiles on quinones derived from poison oak/ivy catechols (urushiols) and analogues as models for urushiol-protein conjugate formation. J Med Chem 24: 28–33
5. Matsumara F (1985) Toxicology of insecticides, 2nd edn. Plenum, New York
6. Mattocks AR (1973) Mechanisms of pyrrolizidine alkaloid toxicity. Proc 5th Internat Congr Pharmacol, San Francisco, 1972, vol 2, pp 114–123
7. Mattocks AR (1968) Toxicity of pyrrolizidine alkaloids. Nature 217: 723–729
8. Noonan PK, Wester RC (1985) Cutaneous metabolism of xenobiotics. In: Bronaugh RL, Maibach HI (eds) Percutaneous absorption. Dekker, New York, pp 65–85
9. Pohl R, Philpot R, Fouts J (1976) Cytochrome P-450 content and mixed function oxidase activity in microsomes isolated from mouse skin. Drug Metab Dispos 4: 442–450
10. Rivière J-L, Cabanne F (1987) Animal and plant cytochrome P-450 systems. Biochimie 69: 743–752
11. Snyder R, Remmer H (1979) Classes of hepatic microsomal mixed function oxidase inducers. Pharmacol Ther 7: 203–244
12. Sulzberger MB, Sherwin RW, Herrmann F (1962) Delayed contact-type sensitization to methylcholanthrene in guinea pigs. J Invest Dermatol 39: 179–181
13. Vigny P, Duquesne M, Coulomb H, Tierney B, Grover P, Sims P (1977) Fluorescence spectral studies on the metabolic activation of 3-methylcholanthrene and 7,12-dimethylbenz(a)anthracene in mouse skin. FEBS Lett 82: 278–282
14. Wood A, Chang R, Levin W, Thomas P, Ryan D, Stoming T, Thakker D, Jerina D, Conney A (1978) Metabolic activation of 3-methylcholanthrene and its metabolites to products mutagenic to bacterial and mammalian cells. Cancer Res 38: 3398–3404

Addresses

R.J. Schmidt

Welsh School of Pharmacy, University of Wales Institute of Science and Technology, P.O. Box 13, Cardiff CF1 3XF, Wales, UK

L. Khan

Welsh School of Pharmacy, University of Wales Institute of Science and Technology, P.O. Box 13, Cardiff CF1 3XF, Wales, UK

Part 2

Morphological Aspects

Light- and Electron-Microscopic Morphology of Contact Urticaria

J. Daróczy and E. Temesvári

Summary

We observed contact urticarial lesions not combined with late appearance of delayed type eczema response. The biopsy material, taken from the wheals within 40 min after epicutaneous testing, was studied light- and electron-microscopically. In these cases, we were able to demonstrate in the epidermis and in the perivascular infiltrate the cellular components of the delayed eczematic reaction pattern.

Key words:

Contact urticaria - Immediate cellular reaction - Delayed cellular reaction - Electron microscopy

Introduction

The pathogenic mechanisms of contact urticaria (CU) have not yet been clarified [1, 7, 8]. Different mechanisms are discussed: nonimmunologically based for release of vasoactive mediators; immunologically based for increased amount of IgE, IgG, and IgM [11]; and the CU syndrome of unknown mechanism [8–10]. The existence of CU followed by delayed eczematous reaction (for different chemicals and food proteins) has become well known, and the rapid reaction pattern (within 30 min) of eczematous lesion could be proved histologically [8]. In our present cases, we observed CU lesions not combined with later eczematic dermatitis, but the rapid occurrence of cellular response was demonstrated.

Materials and Methods

From 1977 to 1986, 720 cases of CU were diagnosed. Biopsy materials were taken from seven female patients and one male patient. The average age was 43 years 2 months. In four cases, CU was elicited by one substance (balsam of Peru, benzoic acid), in three cases by two substances (balsam of Peru and $HgCl_2$, balsam of Peru and benzoic acid, balsam of Peru and turpentine), and in one case by four substances (balsam of Peru, benzoic acid, cinnamon, vanillin). The specimens were prepared for light- and electron-microscopic studies.

Results

The perivascular infiltrate consists of mastocytes, lymphocytes, and mononuclear macrophages. In the spongiotic basal layer of the epidermis, mononuclear cells appeared (Fig. 1). The subepidermal dermis was edemic, the blood vessels and lymphatic capillaries being dilated. The complicated luminal labyrinth of the small lymphatics was dissected by narrow connective tissue bridges, and large gaps appeared between the endothelial processes (Fig. 2). The granulous substance of the connective tissue increased around the vessels, and the basal laminae of the blood capillaries seemed to be multiplied. Mastocytes, lymphocytes, and mononuclear macrophages were revealed around the blood vessels (Fig. 3). Lymphocytes, intermediary type of dendritic cells, and Langerhans' cells were observed in the intercellular spaces of the spongiotic epidermis (Fig. 4).

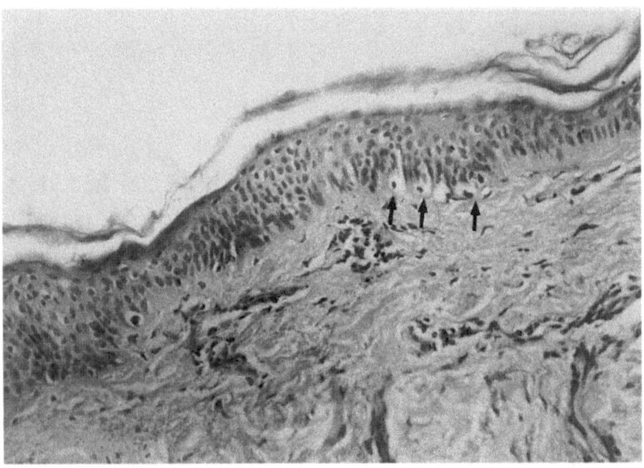

Fig. 1. Mild perivascular infiltrate is seen around the dermal blood capillaries. Mononuclear cells *(arrow)* appeared in the spongiotic basal epidermal layer. H & E, ×200

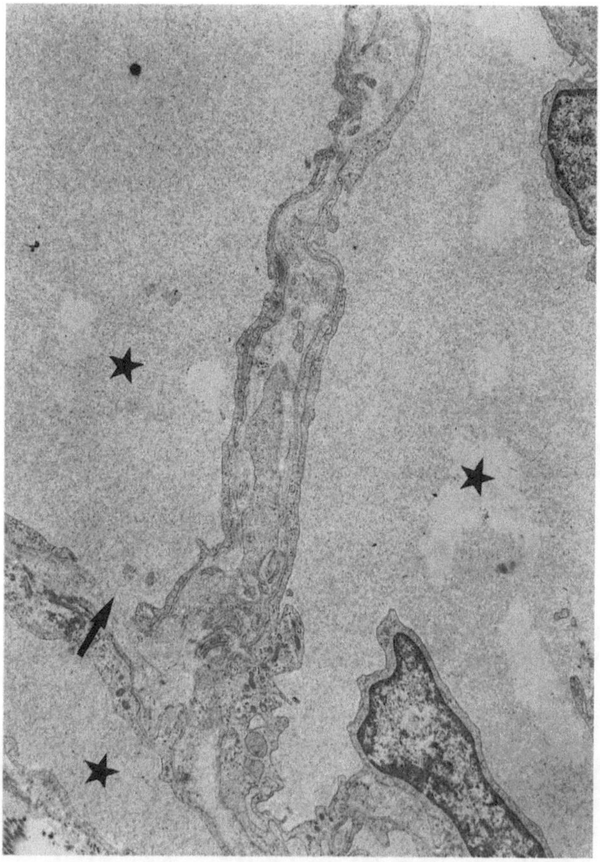

Fig. 2. A complicated labyrinth is produced by the wide lumina *(stars)* of the dilated lymphatic capillaries. Large gap *(arrow)* is seen between the endothelial processes. ×8200

Discussion

Authors studying CU in biopsy material have described unremarkable epidermal changes, dermal edema, and a mild perivascular lymphohistiocytic infiltrate [2, 3, 5]. In cases of combined occurrence of CU and delayed eczematic response, spongiotic epidermis and lymphocytic epidermal infiltrate have been observed [4, 6]. In our present cases, we observed CU not combined with later eczematic dermatitis. The contact wheals disappeared in 60–80 min. In the dermis and in the spongiotic epidermis, we were able to demonstrate the cellular components of the immunologic reaction [12].

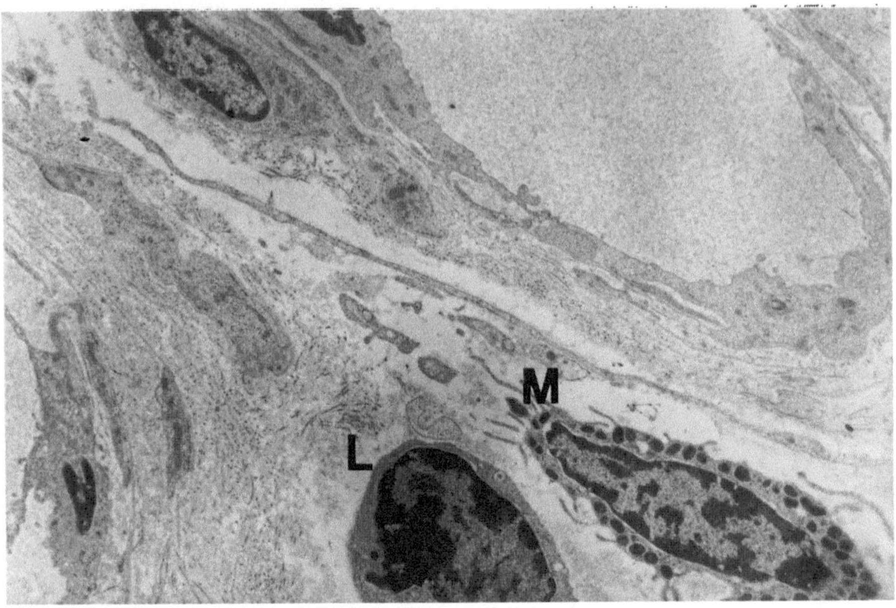

Fig. 3. The multiplied basal laminae of the blood vessels and a mastocyte *(M)* and lymphocyte *(L)* are embedded in the increased amount of perivascular granular substance. × 8200

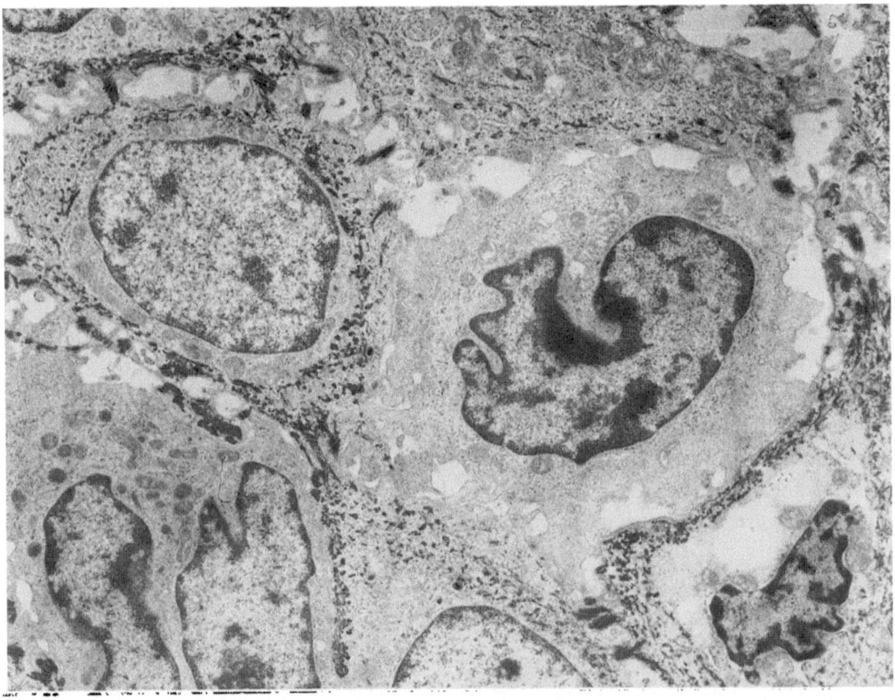

Fig. 4. Intermediary type of epidermal dendritic cells (characterized by lobulated nuclei and large, dendritic cytoplasms) are seen in the spongiotic epidermis. × 8200

References

1. Boonk WJ, van Ketel WG (1981) Skin testing in chronic urticaria. Dermatologica 163: 151–159
2. Edwards EK, Kowalczyk AP (1986) Contact urticaria and allergic contact dermatitis the Saddleback caterpillar with histologic correlation. Int J Dermatol 25: 467–468
3. Fischer AA (1982) Allergic contact urticaria to raw beef: histopathology of the specific wheal reaction at the scratch test site. Contact Dermatitis 8: 425–426
4. Hjorth N, Roed-Petersen J (1978) Occupational protein contact dermatitis in food handlers. Contact Dermatitis 2: 28–42
5. Hunziker N, Brun R (1978) Contact urticaria and dermatitis to citraconic anhydride in guinea pigs. Contact Dermatitis 4: 236–238
6. Krook G (1977) Occupational dermatitis from Lactura sativa (lettuce) and Chicorium (endive). Contact Dermatitis 3: 27–36
7. Krogh G, et al. (1981) The contact urticaria syndrome: an updated review. J Am Acad Dermatol 5: 328–342
8. Lahti A, Krogh G, Maibach HI (1985) Contact urticaria syndrome. In: Stone J (ed) Dermatologic Immunology and Allergy. Mosby, St. Louis, pp 379–390
9. Odom BR, Maibach HI (1976) Contact urticaria: a different contact dermatitis. Cutis 18: 672–676
10. Reitano C, et al. (1981) Allergic and toxic contact dermatitis: inflammatory cell subtypes in epicutaneous test reactions. Br J Dermatol 105: 521–527
11. Temesvári E, Jobbágy A (1985) Serum proteins and immunoglobulins in contact urticaria. Contact Dermatitis 13: 197–198
12. Daróczy J, Temesvári E (1988) Light and electron microscopic examination of contact urticaria. Contact Dermatitis 19: 156–158

Addresses

J. Daróczy

Dermatology and Venereology Clinic of Semmelweis, Medical University, Budapest, Hungary

E. Temesvári

Dermatology and Venereology Clinic of Semmelweis, Medical University, Budapest, Hungary

The Occurrence of Different Morphological Parameters in Allergic and Irritant Patch Test Reactions

C. Avnstorp, E. Balslev, and H. K. Thomsen

Summary

Skin-punch biopsies from 16 allergic and 13 irritant patch test reactions were evaluated in blind studies using a semiquantitative and qualitative histological registration of individual morphological parameters. Focal extension of inflammatory cells in allergic reactions was found to be statistically significantly different from diffuse extension in irritant reactions, while epidermal necrosis was found to be more pronounced in irritant reactions. Other variables which had a high value in histopathological diagnosis of allergic patch test reactions were the presence of oedema, lymphocytes and spongiosis; the presence of dermal and epidermal neutrophilic granulocytes was of value in the diagnosis of irritant patch test reactions.

Statistical analysis by correlation of 17 selected variables gave a diagnostic specificity of 87% and a sensitivity of 81% for allergic reactions. In irritant reactions, the specificity was 100% and the sensitivity 46%. By multiple regression analysis, an index could be calculated ($4 \times$ necrosis $- 3 \times$ oedema $- 2 \rightarrow \geq 0$ = irritant reaction and ≤ 0 = allergic reaction) for differentiation of allergic and irritant reactions. If this index was used in cases of allergic patch test reactions, all would be reported as allergic reactions while half of the irritant reactions would be reported as allergic. The semiquantitative and qualitative registration of histopathological parameters has shed light on the problem of histological differentiation of allergic and irritant contact dermatitis.

Key words:

Allergic - Irritant - Microscopy - Morphology - Patch testing

Introduction

The reading of patch test reactions may be difficult even for experienced readers due to false-positive reactions and angry back or excited skin syndromes. In the differentiation and diagnosis of doubtful test reactions, some specific histopathological parameters could be helpful.

The aims of the present study were (a) to investigate whether, in the light microscope, a semiquantitative and qualitative registration of the individual morphological parameters of the lesions would permit differentiation of allergic and irritant patch test reactions and (b) to determine the diagnostic value of the individual features or combinations there of.

Materials and Methods

Of the 22 volunteers who participated in the study, 16 had a well-known delayed type of hypersensitivity, while 6 did not suffer from any delayed-type hypersensitivity and were selected solely for patch tests with irritants.

Patch-testing and reading was done in accordance with internationally accepted recommendations [1]. The allergens were nickel sulphate 5% in petrolatum, formaldehyde 1% in water, thiuram mix 1% in petrolatum, chlorhexidine gluconate 1% in water, fragrance mix 8% in petrolatum (European Standard Series, Hermal Chemie, FRG), Tansy 10% in alcohol (oleoresin, Professor Hausen, FRG) and Amercol (International Contact Dermatitis Research Group). The irritants were croton oil 1% in petrolatum and Sodium lauryl sulphate 5% in water.

At biopsy, 4-mm skin-punch samples were taken, 48 h after application. Sections were stained with haematoxylin and eosin, PAS, van Gieson Hansen and Alcian blue. Qualitative and semiquantitative morphological parameters were registered, and a histopathological diagnosis was reported for each case. The histopathological parameters were evaluated in blind studies by two of the investigators.

For the statistical analysis, non-parametric statistics were done with Fisher's test. Multivariate analysis was used in the calculation of correlation coefficients and as a multiple regression analysis. The diagnostic specificity and sensitivity was calculated.

Results

The allergic reactions were found to be characterized by a focal distribution of the inflammatory cells in epidermis (10/16; $P<0.01$, Fisher's test), spongiosis sometimes with vesicles (13/16; NS), dermal infiltration of lymphocytes (16/16; NS) and dermal oedema (4/16; $P<0.05$, multivariate analysis). The irritant reactions were characterized by a diffuse distribution of the inflammatory cells in epidermis (7/13; $P<0.01$, Fisher's test), epidermal necrosis (6/13; $P<0.05$, multivariate analysis; $P<0.01$, Fisher's test) and dermal infiltration of neutrophilic granulocytes (11/13; $P<0.05$, multivariate analysis).

Table 1. Histopathological diagnosis compared with the two kinds of patch test reactions

	Patch test reactions	
	Allergic	Irritant
Total	16	13
Histology (n)		
ACD	13	2
ICD	0	6
Allergic dermal reaction	2	0
Minimal dermal changes	1	3
Seborrhoeic dermatitis	0	1
ACD and ICD	0	1

The histopathological diagnosis was compared with the two kinds of patch test reactions (Table 1). In 13 of 16 allergic reactions, the diagnosis was allergic contact dermatitis (ACD). In two biopsy samples, an allergic dermal reaction was reported, and one showed only minimal dermal changes. In 6 of 13 irritant reactions, the histopathological diagnosis was irritant contact dermatitis (ICD). Two were reported as ACD, one as ACD and ICD, and one as seborrhoeic dermatitis, while three showed minimal changes. The specificity and sensitivity of the diagnosis of allergic reactions were 87% and 81%, respectively, while the values for the irritant reactions were 100% and 46%.

In the multivariate analysis excluding non-significant parameters at a significance level of 5%, a diagnostic index was calculated: $4 \times$ necrosis $- 3 \times$ oedema $- 2$. Values $\geqslant 0$ indicate a diagnosis of ICD, and values < 0 one of ACD. Using this index on the present material, all allergic reactions would be reported as ACD, but only 6 of 13 irritant reactions would be reported as ICD, and the rest as ACD. The reproducibility of the histopathological diagnosis was found to be 97% ($R^2 = 0.97$, $P < 0.01$).

Discussion

Previous studies on the discrimination of allergic and irritant patch test reactions in human skin have been contradictory. Some authors have found doubtful differences [2], and others no differences [3–5]. In guinea pigs, some differences have been found [6–9], especially the presence of polymorphonuclear leucocytes in irritant reactions [7–9]. In the present study, a focal distribution of the inflammatory cells within epidermis was significant in allergic reactions, in contrast to a diffuse distribution in irritant reactions.

The significance of the finding of dermal oedema in allergic reactions has not been described previously; however, registration of oedema may be a problem, as variations in the preparation technique may influence the water content of the tissue. Necrosis was a significant parameter in the diagnosis of irritant reactions, as was the finding of neutrophilic granulocytes infiltrating the dermal stroma. In agreement with the variability of the clinical responses in irritant patch test reactions, histopathological diagnosis was more difficult, with sensitivity of 46%.

It seems that the computerized calculations have given some new views on the value of the individual histopathological parameters, but is has also been shown that more than two parameters are needed in the discrimination of allergic and irritant patch test reactions.

References

1. Fregert S (1981) Manual of contact dermatitis, 2nd edn. Munksgaard, Copenhagen
2. Wilhelm E, Sarkany I, Calnan CD (1958) Studies in contact dermatitis. Trans St. John's Hosp Dermatol Soc 41: 31–37
3. Nater JP, Hoedemaeker PHJ (1976) Histological differences between irritant and allergic patch test reactions in man. Contact Dermatitis 2: 247–253
4. Hartman A, Hoedemaeker PHJ, Nater JP (1976) Histological aspects of DNCB sensitization and challenge test. Br J Dermatol 94: 407–416
5. Willis CM, Young E, Brandon DR, Wilkinson JD (1986) Immunopathological and ultrastructural findings in human allergic and irritant contact dermatitis. Br J Dermatol 115: 305–316
6. Baer RL, Rosenthal SA, Sims CF (1957) The allergic eczema-like reaction and primary irritant reaction. AMA Arch Dermatol 76: 549–560
7. Medemica M, Rostenberg A (1971) A comparative light and electron microscopic study of primary irritant contact dermatitis and allergic contact dermatitis. J Invest Dermatol 56: 259–271
8. Jidoi J, Kitano M, Urabe Y (1974) A comparative study of primary irritant and allergic contact dermatitis in guinea pigs. Hiroshima J Med Sci 23: 115–125
9. Kerl H, Burg G, Braun-Falco O (1974) Quantitative and qualitative dynamics of the epidermal and cellular inflammatory reaction in primary toxic and allergic dinitrochlorobenzene contact dermatitis in guinea pigs. Arch Dermatol Forsch 249: 207–226

Addresses

C. Avnstorp
Departments of Dermatology, Gentofte Hospital, and Bispebjerg Hospital, University of Copenhagen, DK-2900 Hellerup, Denmark

E. Balslev
Department of Pathology, Bispebjerg Hospital, University of Copenhagen, Denmark

H. K. Thomsen
Department of Pathology, Bispebjerg Hospital, University of Copenhagen, Denmark

Preliminary Findings on the Patterns of Epidermal Damage Induced by Irritants in Man

C. M. Willis, C. J. M. Stephens, and J. D. Wilkinson

Summary

The histopathology of the primary irritant reactions induced after 48 h in human volunteers by benzalkonium chloride, sodium lauryl sulphate, croton oil, nonanoic acid, dithranol, and propylene glycol has been investigated. Patterns of epidermal damage were identified for each irritant, reflecting their differing chemical interactions with the cellular components of the skin.

Key words:

Irritant contact dermatitis - Histopathology

Introduction

Whilst much interest has been shown in allergic contact dermatitis in recent years, irritant contact dermatitis has been largely ignored, despite the fact that it is a much more common disease. The results of those studies which have been performed, have often been contradictory, particularly with respect to the responding cell populations. A major problem when attempting to evaluate these results is the variation in both the irritants tested and the animal species used. As chemically unrelated irritants interact with the components of the skin in differing ways, it is likely that this will be reflected in the inflammatory responses seen. We therefore decided to systematically investigate the effects of a range of different irritants on human skin. Our preliminary results concerning the patterns of cellular damage induced in the epidermis, as judged by light microscopy, are presented in this paper.

Method

Subjects. A panel of healthy, non-atopic male volunteers with no past or present history of skin disease participated in the study. Their ages ranged from 18 to 61 years, with a mean age of 35 years. Approval for the study was obtained from the Wycombe Ethical Research Committee and all patients gave informed, written consent.

Irritants. The following irritants were tested (ten biopsies per irritant): 0.5% aqueous benzalkonium chloride, 5% aqueous sodium lauryl sulphate, 0.8% croton oil in yellow soft paraffin, 80% nonanoic acid in propan-1-ol, 100% propylene glycol, and 0.02% dithranol in yellow soft paraffin. Controls of distilled water, yellow soft paraffin, propan-1-ol and occlusion only were also included (five biopsies/control). In addition, samples of normal skin, removed from areas adjacent to the patch test sites, were taken from all volunteers.

Patch Testing. Test substances were applied to the volar aspect of the forearm, using 8-mm Finn chambers (Epitest Ltd., Oy, Helsinki, Finland) secured by Scanpore tape. Those in solution were placed on filter-paper discs inserted into the chamber, using 15 μl/Finn chamber. Samples in yellow soft paraffin were applied directly to the chamber surface, using 25 mg/Finn chamber. After 48 h the patch tests were removed and 1 h later 4-mm punch biopsies were taken, using 2% lignocaine as local anaesthetic. The skin samples were immediately bisected and prepared for microscopy.

Histology. One-half of each biopsy was snap frozen in liquid nitrogen. Cryostat sections (4 μm) were cut and stained with haematoxylin and eosin. The remaining samples were fixed in 3% glutaraldehyde and processed into Araldite resin as described previously [4]. Semi-thin sections (1 μm) were cut and stained with toluidine blue.

Results

The major histopathological features of epidermal damage induced by each irritant are outlined in Table 1. Also included is the variability of response between individuals, judged clinically by the presence of erythema, vesiculation, etc.

All controls were negative by visual assessment and, with the exception of two yellow soft paraffin and one distilled water patch tests which had occasional small areas of mild spongiosis, there were no pathological changes on histological examination.

Discussion

The objective of this study was to systematically investigate the action of a range of irritants on human skin. As is frequently observed with such experimentally induced irritant reactions, there was considerable variation in the degree of response between

Table 1. Results

Irritant	Clinical evaluation of response	Major histopathological features of epidermis
Dithranol	Mild→moderate	Hydropic swelling of cells in upper stratum spinosum, with basally located spongiosis in moderate reactions. Patchy areas of spongiosis with exocytosis in mild reactions.
Croton oil	Mild→moderate (2 severe)	Spongiosis with frequent microvesiculation in the upper stratum spinosum. Extensive exocytosis of predominantly mononuclear cells. In the severe reactions, formation of bullae with infiltration of polymorphonuclear leucocytes
Sodium lauryl sulphate	Mild→moderate (1 severe)	Parakeratosis. Mild spongiosis and exocytosis. Detachment of epidermis and infiltration of polymorphonuclear leucocytes in the severe reaction.
Benzalkonium chloride	Negative→mild	Mild, patchy spongiosis with accompanying exocytosis of predominantly mononuclear cells. Spotty areas of necrosis in upper stratum spinosum.
Nonanoic acid	Mild→moderate	"Tongues" of dyskeratotic/necrotic cells extending down into the stratum spinosum.
Propylene glycol	Negative	"Basketweave" appearance to stratum corneum.

individuals. This was apparent both visually and in the inflammatory changes, including the cellular infiltration, observed histologically. The three severe reactions elicited by croton oil and sodium lauryl sulphate caused the influx of significant numbers of polymorphonuclear leucocytes into the epidermis as well as the dermis, whilst mild to moderate reactions induced a predominantly mononuclear cell response only.

Of particular interest in this study were the patterns of epidermal cell damage observed with each irritant. The majority of dithranol reactions were characterized by hydropic swelling of cells in the upper stratum spinosum, a feature similar to that seen in cutaneous viral infections, and one which may be due to the interference in mitochondrial function known to occur on exposure to this drug [3].

Reactions to croton oil exhibited the greatest degree of spongiosis and exocytosis and, except where pustulation occurred, closely resembled allergic contact dermatitis reactions.

The major response to the anionic detergent sodium lauryl sulphate was parakeratosis, indicating increased epidermal cell turnover, whilst benzalkonium chloride, a cationic detergent, caused a different type of reaction, that of spongiosis and exocytosis with spotty necrotic damage, similar to that described by Gisslén and Magnusson [2].

Reactions to nonanoic acid were generally fairly mild and failed to induce the marked necrolytic changes observed by Dowd et al. [1]. However, unusual dyskeratotic cells, similar to those seen in early toxic epidermal necrolysis (E. Wilson Jones, personal communication), were evident in the majority of biopsies.

Propylene glycol, an agent with hygroscopic properties, induced little inflammatory change but produced a 'basketweave' appearance to the stratum corneum caused by hydration of the corneal cells.

In conclusion, our preliminary findings demonstrate the diversity of histopathological changes produced by irritants as a consequence of their differing chemical interactions with the skin. Further work is now in progress to examine these changes at the ultrastructural level.

References

1. Dowd PM et al. (1985) Cutaneous responses to 12 hydroxy – 5, 8, 10, 14 eicosatetraenoic acid (12 HETE) J Invest Dermatol 84: 537–541
2. Gisslén H, Magnusson B (1966) Effects of detergents on guinea pig skin. Acta Derm Venereol 46: 269–274
3. Swanbeck G, Liden S (1966) The inhibitary effect of dithranol (anthralin) on DNA synthesis. Acta Derm Venereol 46: 228
4. Willis CM et al. (1986) Immunopathological and ultrastructural findings in human allergic and irritant contact dermatitis. Br J Dermatol 115: 305–316

Addresses

C. M. Willis
Department of Dermatology, Wycombe General Hospital, High Wycombe, Buckinghamshire HP11 2TT, UK

C. J. M. Stephens
Department of Dermatology, Wycombe General Hospital, High Wycombe, Buckinghamshire HP11 2TT, UK

J. D. Wilkinson
Department of Dermatology, Wycombe General Hospital, High Wycombe, Buckinghamshire HP11 2TT, UK

Part 3

Current Contact Allergens

Epidemiology

Contact Dermatitis 1988: Historical Reflections and Current Problems in Patch-Testing

J. M. Lachapelle

Historical Reflections

A remarkable history of epicutaneous testing was written in 1984 by Foussereau [6]. Among the scientists who have undoubtedly used epicutaneous testing to repeat – experimentally – their clinical observations, two names are traditionally quoted as the real pioneers in the field: the dermatologist Jadassohn and the entomologist Fabre.

By applying chemicals (on a piece of blotting paper) to the skin, Jadassohn [9, 12] was able to reproduce the clinical picture of contact dermatitis to iodoform or to mercury salts in patients suffering from skin intolerance to those substances. He suspected the specific significance of such tests ("specific intolerance") at a time when the term "allergy" had not yet been created and defined. As judiciously pointed out by Foussereau, Jadassohn most probably applied and expanded – in a practical way – Neisser's observations (and interpretations) already made in 1884 [17]. The tests were performed at the University of Breslau, a city that – in those days – was a part of Germany (now Wroclaw in Poland). The room where Jadassohn most probably applied the first patch tests has not been altered, but its vocation has changed since it is nowadays transformed into a tiny museum devoted to dermatology (Fig. 1). An interesting survey of Jadassohn's life and work has been made by Sulzberger [19].

At the same period, the entomologist Fabre [3] (Fig. 2), who worked – alone – at Serignan-du-Comtat near Orange in Provence (France), reported in 1897 in the sixth volume of his *Souvenirs entomologiques* that he had studied the effect of processionary caterpillars on his own skin: A square of blotting paper, a novel kind of plaster, was covered by a rubber sheet and held in place with a bandage. The paper used was a slip of four-folded blotting paper previously dipped into an extract of caterpillar hair, so as to form a square with one inch sides. The paper was applied to the volar aspect of the forearm. The next day, i.e. 24 hours later, the plaster was removed. A red mark, slightly swollen and very clearly outlined, occupied the square which had been covered by the poisoned paper.

In these experiments and in further ones, he dissected various anatomical parts of the insects in order to isolate noxious ones, i.e. those which provoked burning and/ or itching sensations. Rostenberg and Solomon [18] have emphasized the importance to dermatology of Fabre's methodology, so often used in the past decades by dermatoallergologists.

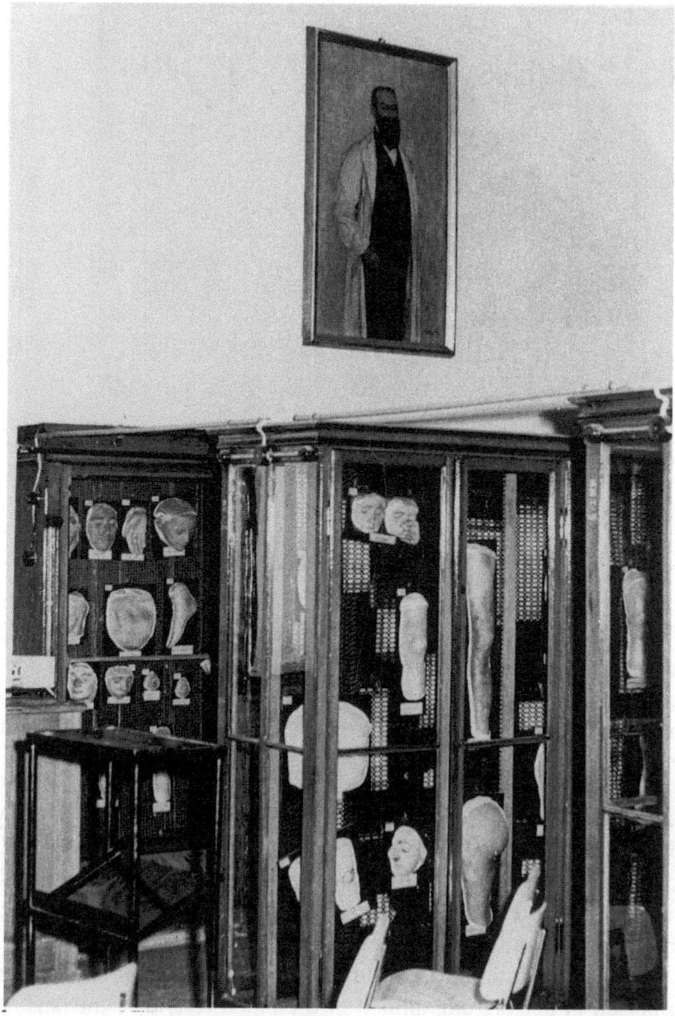

Fig. 1. Dermatology clinic at Breslau University (now Wroclaw in Poland), where Jadassohn performed his famous patch tests to iodoform and mercury salts. The painting represents Neisser

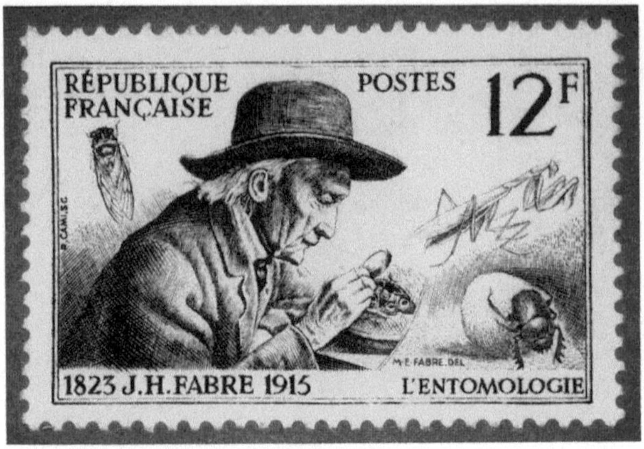

Fig. 2. The French entomologist Fabre. Due to his experiments, he is (unbeknown to him!) one of the pioneers of patch-testing in dermatology

Current Problems in Patch-Testing

Ninety years later, it is puzzling that so many problems are still partly unsolved in the practice of testing patients at the dermatological clinic. I would like to consider some of those technical or practical difficulties encountered in routine and/or clinical research work. Considerations will be limited to the investigation of type IV reactions.

Patch Test Material. It is surprising that standardization has not yet been reached in 1988 at the European level. Various patch test materials are still in use; they differ considerably with regard to the size of the patch test surface and the physicochemical nature of the support. In European clinics, the most commonly used materials are Al-Test, Finn Chamber, Leukotest, Silver Patch and Square Chamber Interderm. Whatever the material used, differences are presumed in the quantities of allergens dispersed in petrolatum applied in the patch tests by clinicians. We recently demonstrated [1] that the quantities of petrolatum applied in the patch test Leukotest (Beiersdorf) by different dermatologists varied considerably between them. Moreover, we showed that for a given dermatologist there were differences from day to day. Practical implications of such differences in terms of patch test reading were not evaluated; nevertheless, potential discrepancies regarding the intensity of positive patch test results can be anticipated from this study.

The development of the Epiquick patch test (Hermal) avoids such variations: in this new, ready-for-use system, strips of 5 Finn Chambers are mounted on Scanpore tape; each Finn Chamber contains 18 µl of the test substance dispersed in petrolatum. A recent study conducted in our department emphasizes the good reproducibility of the patch test results obtained by this new system [11].

True Test System. The True Test Pharmacia is a new system for patch-testing, which is easy to handle and carefully standardized. The allergen is incorporated into a gel, which is printed onto a plastic sheet, dried and cut into 0.81-mm^2 patches. The patches of different allergens are attached to a tape, forming a test kit [4, 5].

The True Test has been evaluated by a European multicenter study conducted on 698 consecutive patients with suspected contact dermatitis [12]. The patients were tested with 12 different allergens. Simultaneously, the same 12 allergens in petrolatum (Trolab) were applied symmetrically to the opposite side of the upper back using the conventional Finn Chamber technique. There were positive test reactions to all 12 allergens tested in the patient group. The concordance of positive reactions between the True Test and the Finn Chamber test was 67%; 13% of all positive reactions were recorded only for the True Test, and 20% only for the Finn Chamber method. The frequency of questionable and irritant reactions was of the same low order of magnitude for both test methods; such reactions were recorded in around 2% of all patches. Further studies are needed to confirm these promising results.

Standard Series with Common Allergens. In 1938, a list of the most common allergens used routinely at the patch test clinic was proposed by Bonnevie and published in his famous textbook of environmental dermatology [2]. The list (Table 1) can be considered as the first version of the "standard" series of patch tests. It was built on the experience gained at the Finsen Institute in Copenhagen regarding the occurrence of positive reactions to various chemicals among patch-tested patients. It is remarkable that the list was used in Copenhagen without any change from 1938 till 1955; this allowed Marcussen to publish in 1962 [15] a most impressive epidemiological survey concerning time fluctuations in the relative occurrence of contact al-

Table 1. The standard series proposed by Bonnevie (1939)

Allergen	Concentration (%)	Vehicle
Turpentine	50	Olive oil
Colophony	10	Olive oil
Balsam of Peru	25	Lanolin
Salicylic acid	5	Lanolin
Formaldehyde	4	Water
Mercuric chloride	0.1	Water
Potassium dichromate	0.5	Water
Silver nitrate	2	Water
Nickel sulphate	5	Water
Resorcinol	5	Water
Primula obconica	As is	
Sodium perborate	10	Water
Brown soap	As is	
Coal tar	Pure	
Wood tars	Pure	
Quinine chlorhydrate	1	Water
Iodine	0.5	Ethanol
Pyrogallol	5	Petrolatum
Paraphenylenediamine	2	Petrolatum
Paraaminophenol	2	Petrolatum
Adhesive plaster	As is	

lergies to the different chemicals. It is noteworthy that 7 of the 21 allergens proposed in Bonnevie's list are still present in the series used throughout the world in 1988.

In the late 1960s the standard series was remodelled by the International Contact Dermatitis Research Group (ICDRG) and (from time to time) adapted to the changes occurring in our daily environment. Some changes (regarding in particular concentrations of allergens) were dictated by the discussion of results collected in joint studies. It was decided during the meeting of the European Contact Dermatitis Society in Heidelberg in 1988 that further changes in the standard series (including reasons why such changes occur) will be jointly published in the journal *Contact Dermatitis* by the ICDRG and the European and Environmental Contact Dermatitis Research Group (EECDRG).

As regards the introduction of new allergens into the standard series, it is logical to include for instance the mixture of isothiazolinones (usually quoted by one of its trade names, Kathon CG) since it is widely used as a biocide in our daily life.

Patch Test Reading. In many patients, patch test reading gives clear-cut results; nonetheless, in a small number of cases, it still remains a difficult issue. Differentiating between irritant and allergic positive patch test reactions can be problematic, especially when chemicals sharing irritant and allergenic properties are considered. In this respect, histological examination of doubtful positive patch test reactions is of minor help, and more sophisticated techniques, such as cell immunotyping of the infiltrate, have led to inconclusive results.

The excited skin syndrome (angry back) that has been recognized in recent years [16, 14] is another pitfall for the reliability of patch test reading. It relates to two or more positives occurring in battery testing, which, on repetition one by one, reveals some to be non-reproducible. Until more is known about the mechanisms and biology involved, the patch tester can only be warned to seek clinical relevance in testing; awareness of the excited skin syndrome prevents many misinterpretations. Assessing the relevance (or otherwise) of a positive patch test reaction is a primordial task for each clinician. It may be useful to distinguish between "old" relevance and "current" relevance. Additional means for relevance assessment are urgently needed.

Revival of Open Test. One of the means for refining relevance assessment is most probably widespread use of repeated open tests with the incriminated allergen ("in use" tests). The Repeated Open Application Test (ROAT; [8]) is a good approach to the problem. It is under current evaluation in many clinics throughout Europe and the United States. A good example of its use in clinical practice is presented in Table 2.

Uncommon and/or "New" Allergens. When uncommon or "new" (i.e. unreported) allergens are concerned, it is of great importance to deal with chemicals of analytical grade (*pro analysi*, i.e. devoid of any impurities, which could possibly be the real allergen!). Such discipline precludes false interpretation of patch test results. As emphasized by Fregert [7], "Just as we have had to master histological examination, it may become necessary to gain ready access to thin-layer chromatography and high-pressure liquid chromatography."

Table 2. Patch-testing and Repeated Open Application Test in three patients with suspected allergy to minoxidil

	Results		
	Patient 1	Patient 2	Patient 3
Patch test[a]			
Regaine as is	++	++	++
Minoxidil 2% in petrolatum	–	–	–
Minoxidil 2% in ethanol	–	–	–
Minoxidil 2% in 20% aqueous solution of propylene glycol	++	++	++
Propylene glycol 20% in water	–	–	++
Repeated Open Application Test			
Minoxidil in 20% aqueous solution of propylene glycol	+ (after 3 applications)	+ (after 2 applications)	+ (after 4 applications)

[a] Results read at 72 h.

Testing patients suspected of being allergic to minoxidil is a good illustration of this policy. The chemical purity of minoxidil to be used for patch- and open-testing is carefully checked before use [13]. Results collected in Table 2 can therefore be considered as reflecting a true allergy to minoxidil in two of the three patients tested, and possibly also a concomitant allergy to minoxidil and to propylene glycol in patient 3.

Conclusions

The following conclusions may be drawn:

1. Standardization of patch- and open-testing is still imperfect. Improvements are accelerating since many teams of research workers are now facing the current problems.
2. Epicutaneous testing needs constant adaptation and flexibility to environmental changes.

References

1. Antoine JL, Lachapelle JM (1988) Variations in the quantities of petrolatum applied in patch testing. Derm Beruf Umwelt (in press)
2. Bonnevie P (1939) Aetiologie und Pathogenese der Ekzemkrankheiten. Klinische Studien über die Ursachen der Ekzeme unter besonderer Berücksichtigung des Diagnostischen Wertes der Ekzemproben. Busch Copenhagen and Barth Leipzig
3. Fabre JH (1897) Souvenirs entomologiques (sixième série). Etudes sur l'instinct et les moeurs des insectes. Delagrave, Paris, pp 378–401

4. Fischer T, Maibach HI (1985) The thin layer rapid use epicutaneous test (TRUE-test), a new patch test method with high accuracy. Br J Dermatol 12: 63–68
5. Fischer T, Maibach HI (1987) Patch testing in allergic contact dermatitis: an update. In: Maibach HI (ed) Occupational and industrial dermatology. Year Book, Chicago, pp 190–210
6. Foussereau J (1984) History of epicutaneous testing: the blotting-paper and other methods. Contact Dermatitis 11: 219–223
7. Fregert S (1988) Physicochemical methods for detection of contact allergens. Dermatol Clin 6: 97–104
8. Hannuksela M, Salo H (1986) The repeated open application test (ROAT). Contact Dermatitis 14: 221–227
9. Jadassohn J (1896 a) Zur Kenntnis der Arzneiexantheme. Arch Dermatol Forsch 34: 103
10. Jadassohn J (1896 b) Zur Kenntnis der medicamentösen Dermatosen. Verhandlungen der Deutschen Dermatologischen Gesellschaft, V Congress, Wien (1895) Braumüller, Wien, pp 103–129
11. Lachapelle JM (1988 a) A left/right side comparative study of Epiquick patch test among 100 consecutive patients. Contact Dermatitis (in press)
12. Lachapelle JM, Bruynzeel DP, Ducombs G, Hannuksela M, Ring J, White IR, Wilkinson J, Fischer T, Billberg K (1988 b) European multicenter study of the TRUE test. Contact Dermatitis 19: 91–97
13. Lachapelle JM, Tennstedt D, Leroy B, van den Haute V, Naert F (1989) Patch testing procedures in patients suffering from suspected allergic contact dermatitis to minoxidil. In: Van Neste D, Lachapelle JM, Antoine JL (eds) Trends in human hair growth research. MTP, Lancaster, (in press)
14. Maibach HI, Fregert S, Magnusson B, Pirila V, Hjorth N, Wilkinson D, Malten K, Meneghini C, Lachapelle JM, Calnan C, Cronin E (1982) Quantification of the excited skin syndrome (the "angry back"). Retesting one patch at a time. Contact Dermatitis 8: 78
15. Marcussen PV (1962) Variations in the incidence of contact hypersensitivities. Trans St. John's Hosp Dermatol Soc 48: 40–48
16. Mitchell J (1977) Multiple concomitant positive patch test reactions. Contact Dermatitis 3: 315–320
17. Neisser A (1884) Ueber Jodoform-Exantheme. Dtsch Med Wochenschr 30: 467
18. Rostenberg A, Solomon LM (1968) Jean Henri Fabre and the patch-test. Arch Dermatol 98: 188–190
19. Sulzberger MD (1936) Josef Jadassohn (1863–1936) Arch Dermatol 33: 1063

Addresses

J. M. Lachapelle
Unit and Laboratory of Occupational and Environmental Dermatology, Louvain University, 30, Clos Chapelle-aux-Champs, UCL 3033, B-1200 Brussels, Belgium

Epidemiology of Contact Allergic Dermatitis in Croatia

J. Lipozenčić, A. Kansky, Z. Periš, and A. Wolf

Summary

The first attempt to carry out an epidemiological study of contact allergic dermatitis (CAD) in Croatia (Yugoslavia) was made during the 5-year period from 1980 to 1984 [14]. The data were obtained from Departments of Allergy in Zagreb and Rijeka, as well as from some other Dermatology Centres in Dubrovnik, Split, Pula, Slavonski Brod and Osijek [14]. In this period, 2280 cases of CAD were verified; of these, 1412 cases (Zagreb and Rijeka) were analysed in detail [14]. The analysis showed that there were twice as many positive reactions to chromium, nickel and formaldehyde as to other allergens. Similar epidemiological studies of CAD have already been performed in many countries [1–7, 11–14]. Efforts were made to obtain the data on the frequency of CAD in Zagreb and Rijeka in the 7-year period 1980–1986. In this period, 2020 cases of CAD were analysed. The results obtained in our studies were compared with findings of the above-mentioned studies.

Key words:

Contact allergy - Patch testing - Trend analysis - Chromate nickel - Formaldehyde - Epidemiology of contact allergic dermatitis

Materials and Methods

In Zagreb and Rijeka during the 7-year period 1980–1986, 2020 persons were tested. The testing was carried out partly with the standard series of allergens of Hermal (Trolab) and partly with allergens of the same concentration made according to the method of the Central Pharmacy of the University Hospital Centre of Zagreb.

by patches to the selected persons with suspected CAD. The tests were read 48 and 72 h after applications and evaluated according to the generally accepted criteria [9, 10].

Results

On the basis of the available documentation, 2020 patients (1211 women and 809 men) were confirmed to have CAD during the 1980–1986 period in Zagreb and Rijeka. In all cases, the clinical diagnosis was substantiated by patch-testing. From 1984 to 1987 in Zagreb, 953 CAD cases were proved, as illustrated in Table 1.

In order to gain insight into which groups and categories of inhabitants were most affected by CAD, the patients with positive patch tests were divided into 10-year age groups. The data show that the greatest number of patients with CAD belonged to the age groups 21–30 (Zagreb 20.34% of women and 14.76% of men; Rijeka 18.27% of women and 11.32% of men) and 31–40 (Zagreb 15.74% of women and 11.35% of men; Rijeka 19.94% of women and 10.07% of men). As a category, the workers showed the highest incidence of CAD. Of all CAD patients in Zagreb, 57.90% were female and 42.10% male; in Rijeka, 62.20% were female and 37.80% male.

Detailed analysis of 2388 positive patch tests recorded at the Dermatology Clinic of the Medical School of Zagreb [1429 (59.84%) in women and 959 (40.16%) in men] showed that there were 1057 CAD patients. The most frequent allergens were

Table 1. Incidence of positive patch tests during the 1984–1987 period

Allergen	Positive patch tests							
	1984		1985		1986		1987	
	n	%	*n*	%	*n*	%	*n*	%
Potassium dichromate	37	23.27	21	9.33	30	10.07	29	10.70
Chromium nitrate	18	11.32	34	15.11	42	14.09	39	14.39
Cobalt nitrate	23	14.46	31	13.78	32	10.74	44	16.23
Nickel sulphate	28	17.61	62	27.56	69	23.15	63	23.24
White precipitate	4	2.51	15	6.67	19	6.37	7	2.58
p-Phenylenediamine	11	6.92	14	6.22	23	7.72	15	5.53
Formaldehyde	22	13.84	31	13.78	42	14.09	41	15.12
Rubber mixture	1	0.63	1	0.44	4	1.34	5	1.84
Colophony	0	0	2	0.89	5	1.68	6	2.21
Turpentine	0	0	0	0	12	4.03	5	1.84
Epoxy resin	2	1.26	1	0.44	3	1.01	3	1.10
Paraben mixture	0	0	0	0	1	0.34	2	0.73
Balsam of Peru	13	8.18	13	5.78	16	5.37	12	4.42
Total	159	100.00	225	100.00	298	100.00	271	100.00
Total no. of examinees		3672		3949		4021		4413
Incidence of CAD (%)		4.33		5.70		7.41		6.14

Data were obtained from the Department of Allergy, Dermatology Clinic, Medical Faculty, University of Zagreb chromium (321, 13.44%), nickel (273, 11.43%), detergents (257, 10.76%), cobalt (151, 6.32%) and formaldehyde (135, 5.65%). In Rijeka, there were 963 CAD patients with 2373 positive patch tests [1414 (59.59%) in women and 959 (40.41%) in men]. The most frequent allergens were detergents (338, 14.24%), chromium (315, 13.27%), soaps (271, 11.42%) and nickel (225, 9.48%). Other frequent allergens were tars (151, 6.36%), cobalt (143, 6.03%) and formaldehyde (88, 3.71%). During the 1984–1987 period in Zagreb, there were 953 CAD patients, with a yearly incidence of 4.33%–7.41%. Chromium, nickel, cobalt and formaldehyde are still the most frequent allergens. Further details are presented in Table 1.

Discussion

The data presented in this paper reveal that the greatest percentage of CAD patients are sensitive to chromium in both Zagreb and Rijeka [3, 4, 8, 13, 14]. Chromates are the essential ingredients in different materials used in the building industry and in the production of building materials. Evidently, the exposure to chromates is considerable because of outdated technology, an essential amount of work still being done by hand in our country. CAD will be found to be prevalent in certain occupational settings, such as the bricklaying and the metal industry [14, 15]. The incidence of sensitization to nickel could be explained by the presence of nickel products used in everyday life. Similar results were described in a similar study in North America [2] and in papers by some other authors [8, 13, 14]. Formaldehyde is widely used in everyday life. Cobalt is frequently present together with nickel and six-valent chromium in different metal products, mineral oils, food additives, rubber, synthetic resins and other materials. It is interesting to compare our data with those from the above-mentioned studies. Due to the improved technology, the number of sensitized persons in developed countries was decreased.

Conclusions

Epidemiologic data on the incidence of CAD in Zagreb and Rijeka during 1980–1986 period were collected. In this period, 2020 CAD patients were detected. The most frequent allergens were chromium, nickel, detergents and formaldehyde. On the basis of the results of our studies, it is necessary to consider making improvements in technology processes of work, especially in the building industry, and improving the conditions of work by regular use of protective gloves and clothes [12]. The aim of this survey was to stimulate further studies in the field of CAD.

References

1. Fregert S, Hjorth N, Magnuson B et al. (1969) Epidemiology of contact dermatitis. Trans St. John's Hosp Dermatol Soc 55: 17–35
2. Rudner EJ, Clendenning WR, Epstein E, Jillson OF, Jordan WP, Fisher AA, Kanof N, Larsen W, Maibach H, Mitchell JC, O'Quinn SE, Schorr WF, Sulzberger MB (1973) Epidemiology of contact dermatitis in North America 1972. Arch Dermatol, vol 108, no 4, 537–540
3. Breit R, Türk RBM (1976) The medical and social fate of the dichromate allergy patient. Review article. Br J Dermatol 94, no 3, 349–351
4. Calas A, Castelain PY, Piriou A (1978) Épidémiologe des Dermatoses de Contact à Marseille. Ann Dermatol Venereol, vol 105, no 3, 345–347
5. Baer LR, Gigli I (1979) Allergic eczematous contact dermatitis. In: Fitzpatrick TB (ed) Dermatology in general medicine. McGraw-Hill, New York, pp 512–519
6. Lämmer D (1979) Testergebnisse von 1008 Patienten mit Kontaktallergie. Z Hautkr 54 (12): 571–579
7. Hjorth N (1980) Contact dermatitis. Br J Dermatol 103: 19–20
8. Dooms-Goossens A, Ceuterick A, Vanmaele N, Degreef H (1980) Follow-Up study of patients with contact dermatitis caused by chromates, nickel and cobalt. Dermatologica 160: 249–260
9. Bandmann HJ, Agathos M (1981) Topography of contact dermatitis and patch testing. In: Ring J, Burg G (eds) New Trends in allergy. Springer, Berlin Heidelberg New York, pp 200–207
10. Zečević J, Kansky A (1983) Dijagnostičko značenje i klinička interpretacija epikutanog testa. U: Standardizacija dijagnostičkih postupaka u alergiji i kliničkoj imunologiji. SAKI, Zbor liječnika Hrvatske, pp 75–87
11. Keil JE, Shmunes E (1984) Epidemiology of work-related skin disease in South Carolina. Arch Dermatol 119: 650–654
12. Emmett EA (1985) Contact dermatitis. In: Provost, Farmer (eds) Current therapy in dermatology. Decker, Philadelphia, pp 26–29
13. Laubstein H, Mönnich HT (1985) Zur Epidemiologie der Berufsdermatosen (IV). Dermatol Monatsschr 171: 2–13
14. Wolf A, Periš Z, Zečević J, Kansky A (1986) Epidemiology of contact allergic dermatitis in croatia. In: Kansky A (ed) Dermatologic lesions of palms and soles. School of Medicine University, Zagreb, pp 61–67
15. Coenraads PJ, Nater JP (1987) Some general epidemiological and statistical considerations in the design of studies on dermatitis in selected occupational populations. Bolletino di Dermatologia Allergologica e professionale Dermatiti da Contollo e Ambienti 2: 105–116

Addresses

J. Lipozenčić
Clinic of Dermatology, Medical School, University of Zagreb, Zagreb, Šalata 4, Yugoslavia

A. Kansky
Clinic of Dermatology, Medical School, University of Zagreb, Zagreb, Šalata 4, Yugoslavia

Z. Periš
Clinic of Dermatology, Medical School, University of Rijeka, Rijeka, Yugoslavia

A. Wolf
Clinic of Dermatology, Medical School, University of Rijeka, Rijeka, Yugoslavia

Patch Tests in Mycosis Fungoides

V. Ziegler, E. Temesvari, C. Quednow, G. Richter, U. Nagel, K. Schlenzka, and N. Berowa

Summary

In a multicenter study, 116 patients with mycosis fungoides (MF; stages I and II according to [1]) were tested with the standard series of the "CDRG in CMEA Countries". The results were compared with those of two control groups (9477 patients attending patch test clinics and 147 people without any allergological symptoms). Exact occupational histories were also noted.

The numbers of positive patch tests in patients with MF and in those attending patch test clinics were not different. The number of positive reactions to metals was significantly higher in the mf group than in both control groups. Patients with MF were more often employed in metal and construction industries than people in the control groups. The results from the different centers were not uniform.

Further coordinated epidemiological and experimental studies are required to clarify the remaining problems of the relation between MF and contact sensitization.

Introduction

The etiology and pathogenesis of mycosis fungoides (MF) is not known. At present, most research workers favor viral etiology, but some authors stress the role of contact sensitivity in the pathogenesis of the disease. Tan et al. and Schuppli et al. [6–8] believe that chronic antigen stimulation may be the underlying cause of this T-cell lymphoma. Schuppli in particular emphasizes the role of metal allergens. In a case-controlled study evaluating occupational factors, Cohen et al. [2] determined that patients with MF who were employed in manufacturing or construction industries were at significantly increased risk for the development of MF, and that once they developed MF, their survival time was considerably reduced. A shorter survival time was also described by McFadden [3]. In 1985, Shupp and Winkelmann [5] reported their results from patch-testing 34 patients with Sézary syndrome or MF. Of these patients, 82% reacted positively, nearly 50% being positive to metals. Schlenzka and Quednow have reported comparable results [4].

Material and Methods

A multicenter study was instigated by the Contact Dermatitis Research Group (CRDG) in socialist countries to evaluate this problem. In Budapest, Magdeburg, Leipzig, and Dresden, all MF patients (stages I and II according to Burg and Braun-Falco [1], including cases of dermatopathic lymphadenopathy) were tested with standard allergens and other suspected substances. Control groups included patients without MF attending the patch test clinics; in addition, as a case-controlled study, each MF patient was matched with three persons of the same age, sex, and county who were without any allergic symptomatology. Additionally, detailed occupational history was obtained from 84 MF patients and from 252 persons of the same age, sex, and county. Only occupations with a duration of 2 years or longer were recorded.

Results

The results of the study are summarized in Tables 1–8. In Table 1, the departments and the number of patients participating in this multicenter study are listed. In Table 2, the number of patients with positive patch tests in each group is given. There is no statistically significant difference between the two groups in Table 2. It appears that MF patients have the same incidence of positive reactions to patch test allergens as routine patients without MF attending the patch test clinics with allergological delayed-type hypersensitivity problems. The number of reactions per MF patient was 1.7, and the number per patch test clinic patient was 2.0. As an additional control, 147 persons of the same age, sex, and county without any allergic

Table 1. Departments and patients taking part in the multicenter study

Department	No. of patients	
	MF	Patch test clinic
Budapest	48	2687
Magdeburg	31	4265
Leipzig	27	1445
Dresden	10	1080
Total	116	9477

Table 2. Patients with positive patch tests to standard allergens

Patients	Positive/total no.	Positive (%)
MF	53/ 116	46
Patch test clinic	3770/9477	40

signs were patch-tested (Table 3). As expected, the difference between the two groups of patients in Table 3 is statistically significant ($\beta < 0.01$).

The results concerning the incidence of positive reactions to the metals potassium dichromate, nickel II sulfate, and cobalt chloride are impressive (Tables 4–6). In each case, the difference between the MF group and the control group is statistically significant ($P < 0.01$). Tables 4–6 thus demonstrate that in accordance with the results of Schuppli [6], Schlenzka et al. [4], and Shupp and Winkelmann [5], the number of patients with positive patch tests to metals and the number of positive reactions (independent of the number of patients) are significantly higher in the MF group than in both control groups.

In Table 7, all patients with positive patch tests to standard allergens excluding metals are summarized. The difference between the two groups in Table 7 is not statistically significant.

There were also differences noted between the MF group and a control group (1 MF patient: 3 controls) with regard to occupational history (Table 8). The difference between the two groups in Table 8 is statistically significant ($\beta < 0.01$). Our da-

Table 3. Patients in Magdeburg und Leipzig with positive patch tests to standard allergens

Patients	Positive/total no.	Positive (%)
MF	28/ 58	48
Control	26/147	18

Table 4. Patients in Magdeburg, Leipzig, and Dresden with positive patch tests to metals

Patients	Positive/total no.	Positive (%)
MF	23/ 68	34
Patch test clinic	1176/6790	17

Table 5. Patients in Magdeburg and Leipzig with positive patch tests to metals

Patients	Positive/total no.	Positive (%)
MF	21/ 58	36
Control	13/147	9

Table 6. Patients in Budapest, Magdeburg, Dresden, and Leipzig with positive patch tests to metals

Patients	Positive/total no.	Positive (%)
MF	54/ 89	61
Patch test clinic	2659/7448	36

Table 7. Patients in Magdeburg, Leipzig, and Dresden with positive patch tests to standard allergens excluding metals

Patients	Positive/total no.	Positive (%)
MF	8/ 68	12
Patch test clinic	1267/6790	19

Table 8. Number of patients working in metal or construction industries (MCI) in Budapest, Leipzig, and Dresden

Patients	MCI/total no.	MCI (%)
MF	36/ 84	43
Control	47/252	19

ta show that patients with MF are more often employed in metal and construction industries than persons not suffering from this disease. Our results are comparable to the findings of Cohen et al. [2], who also described an increased risk for the development of T-cell lymphoma in metal workers.

The results may be summarized as follows:

1. Patients with MF (stages I and II) have a higher incidence of positive patch test reactions to metals than either control persons of the same age, sex, and county or routine patients attending patch test clinics.
2. The total number of positive patch test reactions is similar between MF patients and routine patients attending patch test clinics.
3. Patients with MF give a history of working in metal and construction industries more often than persons of control populations.

Conclusions

Future research endeavors should include more coordinated multicenter studies evaluating occupational factors and patch tests in MF and non-MF patients. Furthermore, animal experiments (simulating a chronic antigenic stimulation) and a search for metal traces in the skin of MF patients should be performed. We are ready to take part in such research.

References

1. Burg G, Braun-Falco O (1983) Cutaneous lymphomas – pseudolymphomas and related disorders. Springer, Berlin Heidelberg New York, p 104
2. Cohen SR, Stenn KS, Braverman IM, Beck GJ (1978) Mycosis fungoides: a retrospective study with observations on occupation as a new prognostic factor. J Invest Dermatol 70: 221
3. McFadden N, Nyfors A, Tanum G, Granholt A, Helme P, Kavli G (1983) Mycosis fungoides in Norway 1960–80 (a retrospective study). Acta Dermatol Venerol [Suppl] 109: 4–13
4. Schlenzka K, Quednow C (1983) Prevalence of nickel and other contact allergies among patients with mycosis fungoides. 7th international symposium in contact dermatitis, Erfurt, GDR, 3–5 June 1983
5. Shupp DL, Winkelmann RK (1985) Patch tests in Sezary syndrome and mycosis fungoides. Contact Dermatitis 13: 180–185
6. Schuppli R (1976) Is mycosis an "immunoma" (editorial). Dermatologica 153: 1–6
7. Schuppli R (1980) Immunom, ein neuer pathogenetischer Begriff. Z. Hautkr 55: 1372–1377
8. Tan RSH, Butterworth CM, McLaughlin H, Malka S, Samman P (1974) Mycosis fungoides – a disease of antigen persistence. Br J Dermatol 91: 607–616

Addresses

V. Ziegler
Department of Dermatology, Karl-Marx-University, Liebigstr. 21, 7010 Leibzig, GDR

U. Nagel
Department of Dermatology, Karl-Marx-University, Liebigstr. 21, 7010 Leipzig, GDR

E. Temesvari
Department of Dermatology, Semmelweis-University, Mária ut. 41, 1085 Budapest, Hungary

C. Quednow
Department of Dermatology, Medical Academy Magdeburg, Leipziger Str. 44, 3090 Magdeburg, GDR

K. Schlenzka
Department of Dermatology, Medical Academy Magdeburg, Leipziger Str. 44, 3090 Magdeburg, GDR

G. Richter
Department of Dermatology, Medical Academy "Carl Gustav Carus", Fetscherstr. 74, 7019 Dresden, GDR

N. Berowa
Department of Dermatology, University Sofia, Georgi Sofiiskystr. 1, Sofia, Bulgaria

Lymphomatoid Contact Dermatitis

A. Alomar, R. M. Pujol, A. Tuneu, and A. Moreno

Summary

A 62-year-old man was seen with a generalized pruritic eczematous eruption of 2 months' duration. The eruption initially appeared on the legs, becoming generalized and involving the hands, face, and trunk. A cutaneous lymphoma was suspected and a skin biopsy was performed. Histopathologic features were considered compatible with mycosis fungoides. In the meantime, 7 days of prednisone (30 mg orally) had cleared the eruption. The patient relapsed after wearing a pair of brown trousers again. Physical examination and a complete screening to rule out a cutaneous lymphoma were negative. Patch tests were positive to azo dyes and trouser cloth. Skin biopsies from positive patch tests showed a similar histologic pattern to that of spontaneous dermatitis. A diagnosis of lymphomatoid contact dermatitis was made. The clinicopathologic features and diagnostic criteria of lymphomatoid contact dermatitis are reviewed.

Key words:

Lymphomatoid contact dermatitis - Azo dyes

Introduction

In 1976, Gómez Orbaneja et al. [6] reported a group of patients with contact dermatitis showing a histopathologic picture indistinguishable from mycosis fungoides. The diagnosis was established on the basis of a clinical suspicion and after a careful and prolonged follow-up. Positive patch tests to suspected allergens are a basic tool to confirm the diagnosis. Removal of the incriminated antigen often leads to total remission of the disease.

A case of lymphomatoid contact dermatitis (LCD) to azo dyes is reported below. The histopathologic findings of sequential positive patch tests suggest that LCD may represent a transient event in an otherwise standard contact dermatitis.

Case Report

A 62-year-old man presented an eczematous eruption of 2 months' duration that began on the lower extremities and gradually became generalized. The patient came to our Department in October 1986 for evaluation of a new flare of his cutaneous eruption. Physical examination revealed a healthy obese man with a generalized erythroderma. The skin also showed slight thickening, involving the face, trunk, and extremities. The palms and soles were hyperkeratotic. Small, 1- to 2-cm, axillary, inguinal, and cervical lymph nodes were palpated. The size of the liver and spleen was normal.

Routine blood test disclosed the following: erythrocyte sedimentation rate 11 mm/h; hemoglobin level 14.1 g/dl; white blood cell count 7220 per cubic millimeter, with 52% neutrophils, 38% lymphocytes, 7% monocytes, and 1% eosinophils; and platelets 282000 per cubic millimeter. Rare Sézary cells (approx. 2%) were seen on the peripheral blood smear. Blood electrolytes, protides, hemostasis, urinalysis, and liver and renal function test were normal, except for alkaline phosphatase

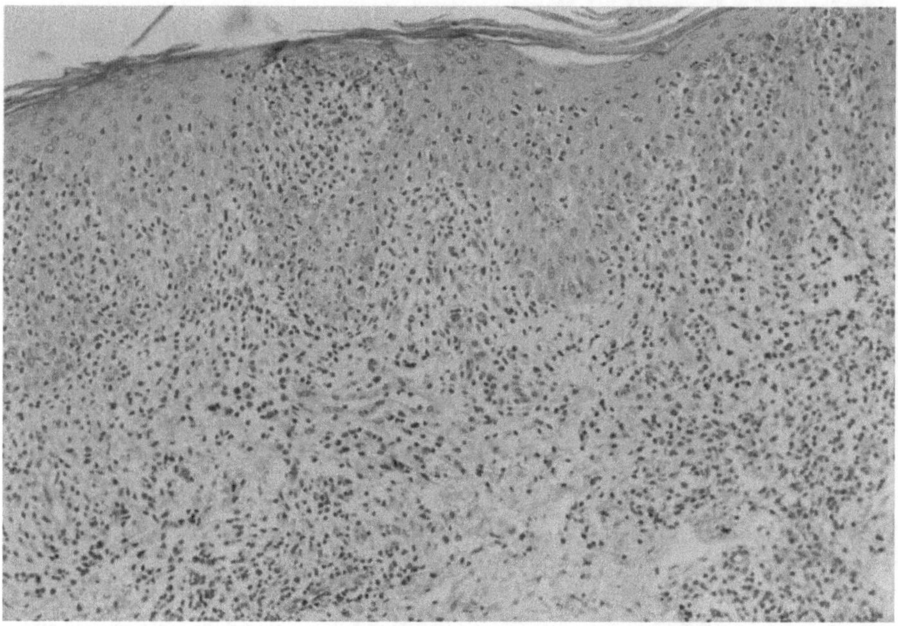

Fig. 1. Spontaneous lesions: superficial parakeratosis, irregular epidermal hyperplasia, and bandlike superficial lymphocytic infiltrate with slight atypia. Exocytosis with occasional microabscesses. H & E, × 100

level that was elevated at 780 units/liter (normal value 90–279 units/liter). The following values were either normal or negative: serum protein electrophoresis, antinuclear factor, complement, rheumatoid factor, and antibodies against smooth muscle and mitochondria. Values for monoclonal reagents were as follows: OKT3 (peripheral blood T cells) 70%, OKT4 (helper-induced T subset) 58%, OKT8 (suppressor-cytotoxic T subset) 2%, B1 (peripheral blood B cells) 12%. X-ray of the skull and pelvic bones revealed absence of striations adopting a mosaic pattern of Paget's disease of bone. Abdominal and thoracic computerized tomography did not reveal abnormalities.

Two punch biopsies revealed similar morphologic changes: superficial parakeratosis, irregular epidermal hyperplasia, and a dense bandlike lymphocytic infiltrate in the papillary dermis. The lymphocyte showed slight atypia and intense exocytosis, with occasional microabscesses. The histopathologic picture observed suggested the diagnosis of mycosis fungoides (Fig. 1). Immunohistochemical studies of the lymphocytic infiltrate showed that cells expressing the phenotype of T cytotoxic-suppressor lymphocytes (T8) predominated over T helper-inducer cells (T4).

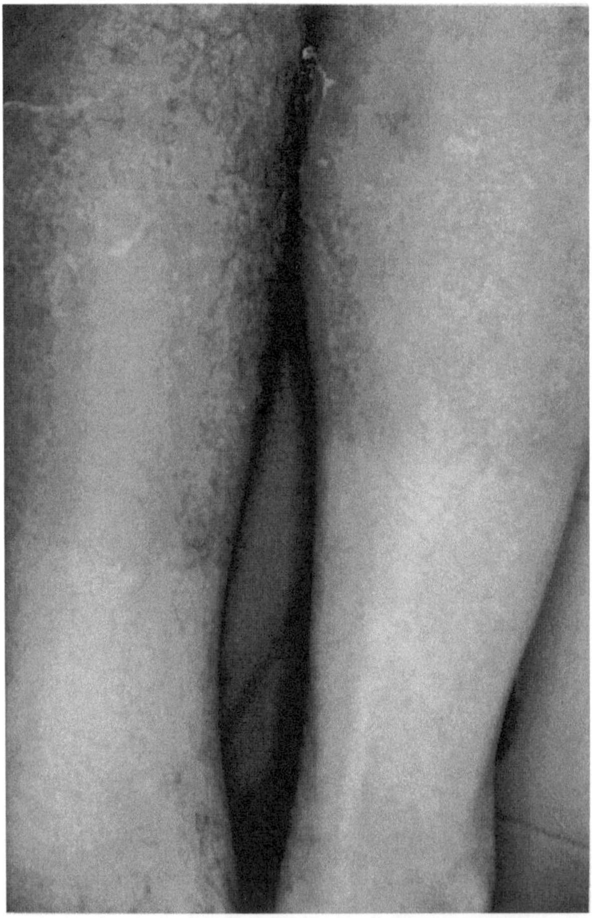

Fig. 2. Clinical features: erythematous eruption that spared the areas covered by the socks. Note the sharp line dividing involved and noninvolved skin

Treatment with orally administered corticosteroid (prednisone 30 mg/day) was prescribed. The cutaneous skin rash and lymphadenopathy resolved in a period of 7 days.

The patient presented a relapse of cutaneous lesions 1 month later. However, the eruption spared the socks and underwear areas, with a clear-cut line between involved and uninvolved skin (Fig. 2). The diagnosis of allergic contact dermatitis was suspected. After a careful clinical history, the patient associated the skin flares with wearing a pair of dark brown trousers.

After clearing the skin rash, patch tests were carried out with the contact allergen series of the Spanish Contact Dermatitis Group, as well as dyes and textile batteries. Positive results were obtained with purified protein derivative (PPD) 1% (+ +), PPD mix (+ + +), IPPD 0.1% (+ + +), *p*-aminoazobenzene 0.25% (+ +), Disperse Orange 3 1% (+ +), and Disperse Blue 106 1% (+). A strong positivity (+ +) was also obtained after patch-testing a small piece of trouser cloth. IPPD-positive patch test without treatment remained erythematous for a month. Skin biopsies from a positive patch test were performed at 96 h and 21 days after testing. Microscopic examination revealed a morphological pattern similar to the spontaneous lesions (Fig. 3).

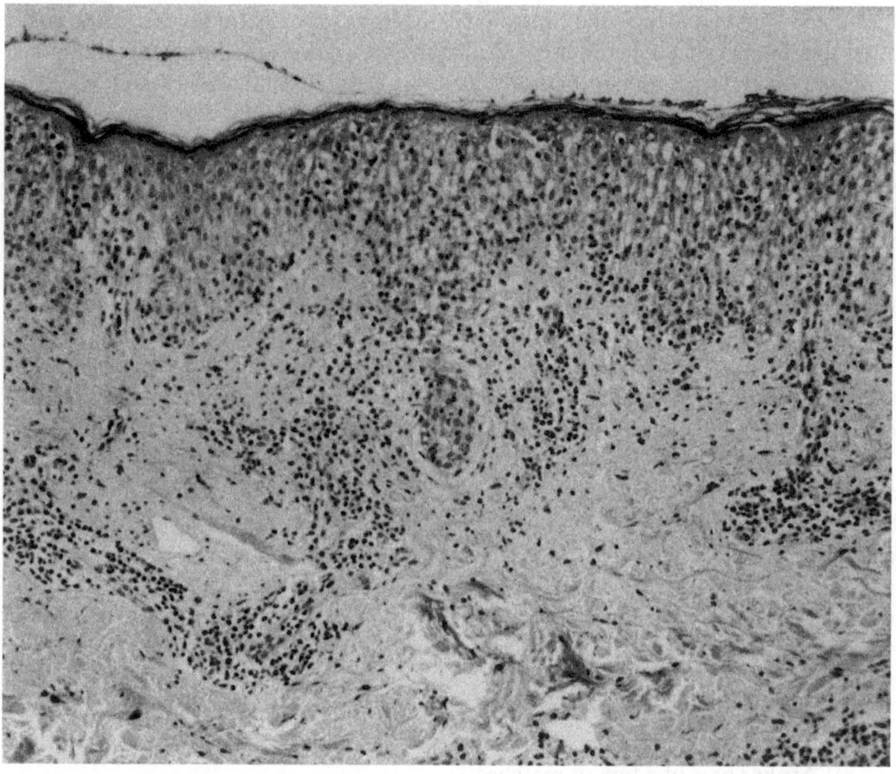

Fig. 3. Patch test reaction. Acute phase: diffuse spongiosis without vesicles, exocytosis of lymphocytes in a pattern similar to that of the spontaneous lesions. H & E, × 100

Thin-layer chromatography from a piece of trouser cloth revealed an unidentified Disperse dye in the Orange group, and other in the Blue group, that seems to correspond to Disperse Blue 35. There had been no recurrence of the lesions after avoiding further contact with the causative agent (brown trousers).

In January 1988, a new IPPD patch test was performed with a similar positive result. A 4-mm punch biopsy was performed 96 h after testing. Histopathologic examination revealed a dense perivascular and diffuse inflammatory infiltrate without either epidermotropism or epidermal spongiosis. This pattern was considered consistent with a dermal contact hypersensivity reaction.

Discussion

The term "lymphomatoid contact dermatitis" (LCD) was coined by Gomez Orbaneja et al. [6] to describe lesions of allergic contact dermatitis mimicking histopathologically a cutaneous T-cell lymphoma (CTCL). The term LCD should be reserved for cases in which the lymphomatoid reaction appears in areas of contact dermatitis, clearing with avoidance of the allergen.

Ackerman et al. [1] referred to allergic contact dermatitis as lesions that sometimes could not be distinguished histologically from mycosis fungoides. They suggested that in allergic contact dermatitis, antigen-recognizing lymphocytes might be stimulated to undergo transformation into blast cells. In 1981, Ecker and Winkelmann [3] reviewed five new cases of LCD, in which the clinical and histologic features were quite different to those previously described: in their cases, the patients had generalized, erythrodermic eruptions that did not clear upon avoidance of contact with the chemicals responsible for the positive patch test. Besides, in three of their patients, Sézary cell blood count was 1%–2%. The authors interpreted these cases as a potential pre-Sézary state and included LCD within the spectrum of disorders evolving into CTCL. Nevertheless, to the best of our knowledge, cases of LCD evolving into CTCL have not been reported.

Wall et al. [7] described a case of LCD to ethylenediamine dihydrochloride. The authors suggested that in any contact reaction a lymphoblastic reaction may be expected when the allergenic stimulus is prolonged and repetitive.

After reviewing the literature [1–7], two clinical forms of LCD may be (a) localized type, presenting as one or few infiltrated erythematous plaques resembling chronic eczema, and (b) generalized type, characterized by an erythrodermic or generalized eruption in which transient circulating Sézary cells could be detected. In these forms of LCD, the differential diagnosis should be established with other causes of generalized erythroderma, and with contact dermatitis in a patient with mycosis fungoides. Allergens incriminated in the two types of LCD are as follows:

1. Localized
   a) Striker part of a box of matches
   b) Mercaptobenzothiazole
   c) Ethylenediamine dihydrochloride

2. Generalized
   a) Formalin
   b) Glutaraldehyde
   c) Fig tree sawdust
   d) Phosphorus sesquisulfide
   e) Ragweed
   f) Potassium dichromate
   g) Tetramethylthiram
   h) Gold
   i) Azo dyes

Since LCD could not be differentiated from mycosis fungoides by histology alone, a careful clinical review and follow-up seems advisable. In our case, the diagnosis of LCD was established on the basis of the clinical picture and the evolutive course.

Histopathologic examination of the initial positive patch tests showed a picture similar to those of spontaneous lesions. Nevertheless, these changes were transient, and 1 year later, a skin biopsy performed from a new positive patch test showed histopathologic features of dermal contact dermatitis without epidermotropism and cellular atypia. These findings support the idea that the "lymphomatoid" pattern may be a transient event in an otherwise standard contact dermatitis.

In summary, diagnostic criteria of LCD should include:

1. A localized or generalized eruption in which the clinical history and physical examination suggest contact dermatitis
2. Mycosis fungoides-like histopathologic findings
3. Positive patch test
4. Clearing of the lesions after corticosteroid therapy and total avoidance of the allergen

Acknowledgements. We are grateful to Drs. F. Menezes Brandao and Luis Conde for the thin-layer chromatography studies.

References

1. Ackerman AB, Breza TS, Capland L (1974). Spongiotic simulants of mycosis fungoides. Arch Dermatol 109: 218–220
2. Ayala F, Blato N, Nappa P, De Rosa G lembo G (1987) Lymphomatoid contact dermatitis. Contact Dermatitis 13: 311–313
3. Ecker RI, Winkelmann RK (1981) Lymphomatoid contact dermatitis. Contact Dermatitis 7: 84–93
4. Fisher AA (1987) Chronic allergic contact dermatitis simulating mycosis fungoides. Boll Dermatol Allergol Profession 2: 13–16
5. Fisher AA (1987) Allergic contact dermatitis mimicking mycosis fungoides. Cutis 40: 19–21
6. Gomez Orbaneja J, Iglesias Díaz L, Sánchez Lozano JL, Conde Salazar L (1976) Lymphomatoid contact dermatitis. A syndrome produced by epicutaneous hypersensitivity with clinical features and histopathologic picture similar to that of mycosis fungoides. Contact Dermatitis 2: 139–143
7. Wall LM (1982) Lymphomatoid contact dermatitis due to ethylenediamine dihydrochloride. Contact Dermatitis 8: 51–54

Addresses

A. Alomar
Department of Dermatology, Hospital de la Santa Creu i Sant Pau, Avd. Sant Antoni M. Claret 167, 08025 Barcelona, Spain

R. M. Pujol
Department of Dermatology, Hospital de la Santa Creu i Sant Pau, Avd. Sant Antoni M. Claret 167, 08025 Barcelona, Spain

A. Tuneu
Department of Dermatology, Hospital de la Santa Creu i Sant Pau, Avd. Sant Antoni M. Claret 167, 08025 Barcelona, Spain

A. Moreno
Department of Pathology, Hospital de la Santa Creu i Sant Pau, Avd. Sant Antoni M. Claret 167, 08025 Barcelona, Spain

Patch Testing in Children

N. Balato, G. Lembo, C. Patruno, and F. Ayala

Summary

Over a 3-year period, 533 children aged between 4 months and 14 years were patch-tested with a "pediatric" series of haptens. The children were affected with various types of eczema or with psoriasis of the hands ($n = 31$). In 78 positive children, there were 112 positive test reactions to various allergens. Nickel, cobalt, ethylenediamine, and potassium dichromate were the most frequent sensitizers. Positive reactions were relevant in 52 (67%) of 78 positive children.

Key words:

Patch test - Children - Eczema - Relevance

Introduction

Varying points of view have been expressed about patch testing in children. Even if previous opinions were often consistent with a relatively low susceptibility of the immune system to contact allergy in children, it is now accepted that contact sensitization can occur spontaneously [6, 8–11, 13], besides experimental induction [3, 7, 12], in neonates and more generally in children. Nevertheless, allergic contact dermatitis (ACD) is infrequently diagnosed in infants. Due to both the conflicting results and the limited number of reports on the subject, the aim of the present study was to evaluate the incidence of positive patch test reactions in children affected with various types of eczema.

Material and Methods

Over a 3-year period, 533 consecutive patients (249 males and 284 females) aged from 4 months to 14 years were studied. Table 1 summarizes the clinical diagnoses. In addition to patients with eczema, children with psoriasis of the hands were tested, provided that fissures and/or moderate pruritus had been present for at least 4 months. The hapten series used is reported in Table 2. During the last 6 months, four haptens (propylene glycol, sulfanilamide, chloramphenicol and penicillin) which always gave negative results have been replaced by other haptens (resorcin, Bronopol, merbromin, thimerosal, and Kathon CG).

The patch test concentration was not adjusted according to the age of the child. Finn chambers on Scanpor were employed, with the exception of mercury compounds, which were tested by means of Al-test. The patch tests were routinely applied on disease-free skin of the back and were read after 48 h and 72 h. The parents were told to examine the dorsum once a day during the following 4 days in order to detect any positivity.

Difficulties were rarely encountered in the classification of allergic or irritant patch test results. Vesicular patch tests spreading beyond the site of application of the test substance were considered positive. Weakly positive (+), doubtful, and irritant reactions were not considered significant. When possible, retesting was performed in these cases. As regards relevance, positive reactions were recorded as (a) present, (b) past, or (c) unexplained. Of the 78 positive children, 35 (45%) had a personal or family history of atopy.

Results

In 78 positive children, there were 112 positive test reactions to various allergens (Table 3). The commonest positive hapten was nickel sulphate, followed by cobalt chloride, ethylenediamine, and potassium dichromate (Table 4). The most frequent false-positive results were noted with nickel, mercury compounds, and wood tars. The youngest patient with sensitivity was a 1-year-old atopic child who reacted positively to neomycin. In this case, the reaction was relevant, being caused by topical application of a cream containing the antibiotic. The youngest patient with nickel

Table 1. Clinical diagnosis in 533 patch-tested children

Diagnosis	No. of cases
Atopic dermatitis	286
Contact dermatitis (irritant + allergic)	92
Dyshidrosis	74
Psoriasis of the hands	31
Perioral dermatitis	23
Juvenile plantar dermatosis	16
Lichenoid frictional eruption	11

Table 2. Pediatric hapten series used for patch testing

Hapten	Concentration (%)	Vehicle
Petrolatum	100	
Thiram mix	1	Pet
Potassium dichromate	0.5	Pet
Balsam of Peru	25	Pet
PPD mix	0.6	Pet
Quaternium 15	1	Pet
Carba mix	3	Pet
PPD dichlorhydrate	0.5	Pet
Wool alcohols	30	Pet
Colophony	20	Pet
Neomycin	20	Pet
Imidazolidinylurea	2	Pet
Ethylenediamine	1	Pet
Epoxy resin	1	Pet
Cobalt chloride	1	Pet
Quinoline mix	6	Pet
Formaldehyde	1	Aq
Benzocaine	5	Pet
Mercapto mix	2	Pet
Nickel sulphate	5	Pet
Mercaptobenzothiazole	1	Pet
Parabens	15	Pet
Fragrance mix	8	Pet
Diaminodiphenylmethane	1	Pet
Ammoniated mercury	1	Pet
Propylene glycol[a]	5	Aq
Sulfanilamide[a]	5	Pet
Lanolin	30	Pet
Chloramphenicol[a]	2	Pet
Penicillin[a]	10000 IU/g	Pet
Promethazine HCl	2.5	Pet
Wood tars	12	Pet

PPD, paraphenylenediamine; Pet, petrolatum; Aq, water

[a] During the last 6 months, four haptens have been replaced by resorcin 1% pet, Bronopol 0.2% pet, merbromin 0.1% aq, thimerosal 0.1% pet, and Kathon CG 100 ppm aq.

Table 3. Number of positive patch test reactions in children

Clinical diagnosis	Positive patients/ total no. (%)	Positive Reactions (*n*)
Atopic dermatitis	31/286 (10.8)	39
Contact dermatitis	36/92 (39.1)	62
Dyshidrosis	5/74 (6.8)	5
Psoriasis of the hands	2/31 (6.5)	2
Perioral dermatitis	3/23 (13.0)	3
Juvenile plantar dermatosis	0/16 –	0
Lichenoid frictional eruption	1/11 (9.0)	1
Total	78/533 (14.6)	112

Table 4. Number of positive reactions to the individual haptens

Hapten	No. of reactions
Nickel sulphate	20
Cobalt chloride	13
Ethylenediamine	11
Potassium dichromate	10
Ammoniated mercury	9
Mercaptobenzothiazole	9
Neomycin	8
Mercapto mix	4
Carba mix	3
Fragrance mix	3
Quinoline mix	3
Epoxy resin	3
Balsam of Peru	2
Colophony	2
Imidazolidinylurea	2
Promethazine HCl	2
Thiram mix	2
Diaminodiphenylmethane	1
Lanolin	1
Merbromin	1
Thimerosal	1
Wood tars	1
Wool alcohols	1

sensitivity was a 3-year-old girl who had pierced ears. This patient was also sensitive to neomycin. Eczema of the earlobes was not present at the time of testing, probably due to the use of gold earrings. Of the 20 positive reactions to nickel sulphate, 14 were observed in young females (mean age 9.3 years) who had their ears pierced in early childhood.

Generally, the positive tests were relevant to the current disease in 26 (33%) of the 78 children. Moreover, relevance to a preceding bout of dermatitis was evident in 18 (23%) of the 78 children. Doubtful relevance was found in 8 children, while 26 (33%) of the children reacted positively to some of the allergens, but no relevance was found at all. Thus, 52 (67%) of the 78 positive children had at least one possibly relevant reaction. If one considers the total number of positive reactions, 74 (66%) of 112 were relevant or probably so.

In addition, we noted that the frequency of multiple sensitizations increased slightly with the child's age (Fig. 1). No cases of excited skin syndrome were observed, even if irritant reactions to adhesives, lasting from 24 to 48 h, were sometimes registered in children aged less than 1 year.

Positivity towards cobalt chloride was associated in about half the cases to positive patch test reactions to nickel or potassium dichromate. As far as mercury is concerned, a past history of exposure to various mercury salts (mercury oxide, merbromin, mercury bichloride) was found in only some children with positive test reactions to mercury. Nevertheless, Mercurochrome (merbromin) is most widely used as a topical disinfectant in our country, thus causing a relatively high incidence

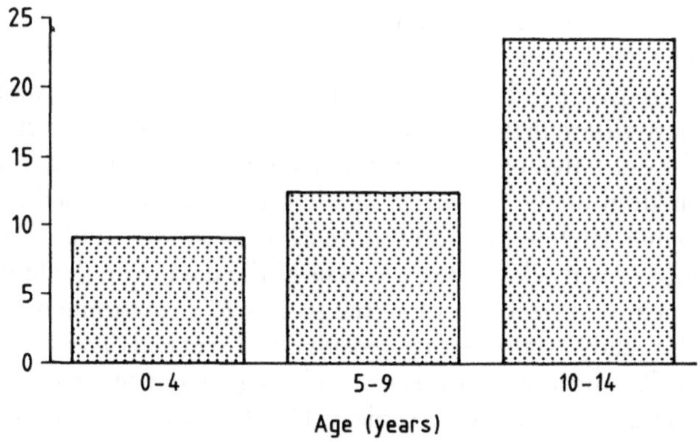

Fig. 1. Percentage of children showing multiple positive reactions according to age

of contact allergy to mercurials. Even at birth, umbilical cord is frequently treated by Mercurochrome. In one of our patients, a probably ACD had occurred in the umbilical area when the infant was 2 weeks old.

Among topics, ethylenediamine (EDA), neomycin, and fragrances were the most frequent sensitizers. EDA is an excipient found in widely used medicaments in Italy. It accounts for about 12% of the sensitivities in all the ACD patients seen in our department, regardless of the age considered. Of 78 positive children, 11 were sensitive to EDA. In all of them, a past history of contact with topics containing EDA was found. In 5 of the 11 sensitized children, it was the only hapten that gave a positive reaction, whereas in 6 (54%) of them other haptens were also positive.

Involvement of the dorsum of the foot and poor tolerance of shoes was seen in 34 children. Leather was the most frequent cause of shoe dermatitis, as potassium dichromate was positive in seven children (age 3–13 years). In three of them, cobalt sensitization coexisted, while mercaptobenzothiazole (MBT) was positive in one. MBT was the only sensitizer in four patients, thus confirming that rubber chemicals are less important than leather components in Italy [1]. Moreover, in Italy many shoes have nickel ornaments, especially buckles. In two children with patches of dermatitis on the feet, nickel sulphate was the only positive hapten. Finally, in five children with a clinical picture of shoe dermatitis, we found that ammoniated mercury ($n=3$) and cobalt chloride ($n=2$) were positive; in these cases, however, relevance to the current dermatitis was doubtful. In the group of patients with juvenile plantar dermatosis, none reacted positively. These results are in agreement with the data reported in the literature [2], where little evidence exists on the relationship between contact allergy and the materials used in the manufacture of socks and shoes in the pathogenesis of the disorder.

Discussion

At present, patch testing in children is undoubtedly performed in most dermatology centers. However, clinicians are reluctant to patch-test all children with eczema because of a supposedly infrequent exposure to potential allergens in the first years of life. Furthermore, the problem of patches detaching from the back before 48 h in a mobile child undoubtedly lowers the propensity to test haptens in infants.

Moreover, patch testing in children has not yet been standardized. Some authors suggest differentiating the concentration of allergens for children [4, 6], while others prefer one patch test series for all patients. Using one-half of the adult concentration in children under 5 years of age has also been proposed [5]. In our study, we used the same patch test concentration as that used for adults. The special pediatric series employed was selected on the basis of the data from the literature; the most frequent potential sensitizers encountered in a child's environment were added.

Our study confirms that sensitivity to metals is not infrequent in nonatopic children. We did not find a statistically higher incidence of nickel sensitivity in atopic (6/31) than in nonatopic subjects (12/47). Moreover, personal history of atopy did not affect the frequency of positivity to other haptens. Our data confirm that EDA sensitization frequently occurs because of topical remedies employed in the treatment of eczematous conditions. As is widely known, topical medicament allergy may be so subtly superimposed on another dermatitis that the existence of a contact dermatitis to topical medicaments is not suspected. Therefore, patch testing of children can also reveal a present or previous sensitization to medicaments, thus helping to prevent widespread reactions to other chemically related drugs after parenteral administration.

In conclusion, it is our impression that patch testing during childhood must be performed in eczematous conditions, especially when the dermatitis is long lasting or in the case of previous recurrent, unexplained exacerbations of the disease.

References

1. Angelini G, Vena GA, Meneghini CL (1980) Shoe contact dermatitis. Contact Dermatitis 6: 279–283
2. Ashton RE, Griffiths WAD (1986) Juvenile plantar dermatosis – atopy or footwear? Clin Exp Dermatol 11: 529–534
3. Epstein WL (1961) Contact type delayed hypersensitivity in infants and children. Induction of rhus sensitivity. Pediatrics 27: 51–53
4. Fisher AA (1975) Childhood allergic contact dermatitis. Cutis 15: 635–642
5. Fisher AA (1986) Contact Dermatitis, 3rd edn. Lea and Febiger, Philadelphia
6. Hjorth N (1981) Contact dermatitis in children. Acta Derm Venereol [Suppl] 95: 36–39
7. Hobley SL, Hansmann HC (1974) Current status of skin testing in children with contact dermatitis. Cutis 13: 995–1000
8. Levy A, Hanau D, Fousserau J (1980) Contact dermatitis in children. Contact Dermatitis 6: 260–262
9. Pevny I, Brennenstuhl M, Razinkas G (1984) Patch testing in children (I). Collective test results; skin testability in children. Contact Dermatitis 11: 201–206
10. Pevny I, Brennenstuhl M, Razinskas G (1984) Patch testing in children (II). Results and case reports. Contact Dermatitis 11: 302–310
11. Romaguera C, Alomar A, Camarasa JMG, Garcia Bravo B, Garcia Perez A, Grimalt F, Guerra P, Lopez Gorretcher B, Martin Pascual A, Miranda A, Moran M, Pena ML (1985) Contact dermatitis in children. Contact Dermatitis 12: 283–284
12. Straus HW (1931) Artificial sensitization of infants to poison ivy. J Allergy 1: 137–144
13. Veien NK, Hattel T, Justensen O, Norholm A (1982) Contact dermatitis in children. Contact Dermatitis 8: 373–375

Addresses

N. Balato
Clinica Dermatologica, II Facoltà di Medicina e Chirurgia, via Pansini, 5, I-80131 Napoli, Italy

G. Lembo
Clinica Dermatologica, II Facoltà di Medicina e Chirurgia, via Pansini, 5, I-80131 Napoli, Italy

C. Patruno
Clinica Dermatologica, II Facoltà di Medicina e Chirurgia, via Pansini, 5, I-80131 Napoli, Italy

F. Ayala
Clinica Dermatologica, II Facoltà di Medicina e Chirurgia, via Pansini, 5, I-80131 Napoli, Italy

Contact Dermatitis with Multiple Sensitization in an 8-Year-Old Child

M. A. Barros, A. Baptista, and F. Amado

Summary

We present a case of multiple sensitization in an 8-year-old child who had a serious hand eczema.

Key words:

Contact dermatitis - Child - Multiple sensitization

Case Report

An 8-year-old girl had developed erythema, scaling, and fissuration with intense itching on both palms when she was 3 years old (Fig. 1). The lesions persisted for 5 years with alternating periods of improvement and worsening. During this time, she was treated with a great number of topicals, which were never able to clear the lesions. She often played with perfumes and cosmetics easily available at her home, using them profusely on her hands. She also helped her mother doing housework and thus contacted detergents and soaps.

Patch Testing

Patch tests with the GPEDC standard series, as well as the detergents (Super Pop limão), perfumes (Flor de País), and deodorant (Lander), produced the following results:

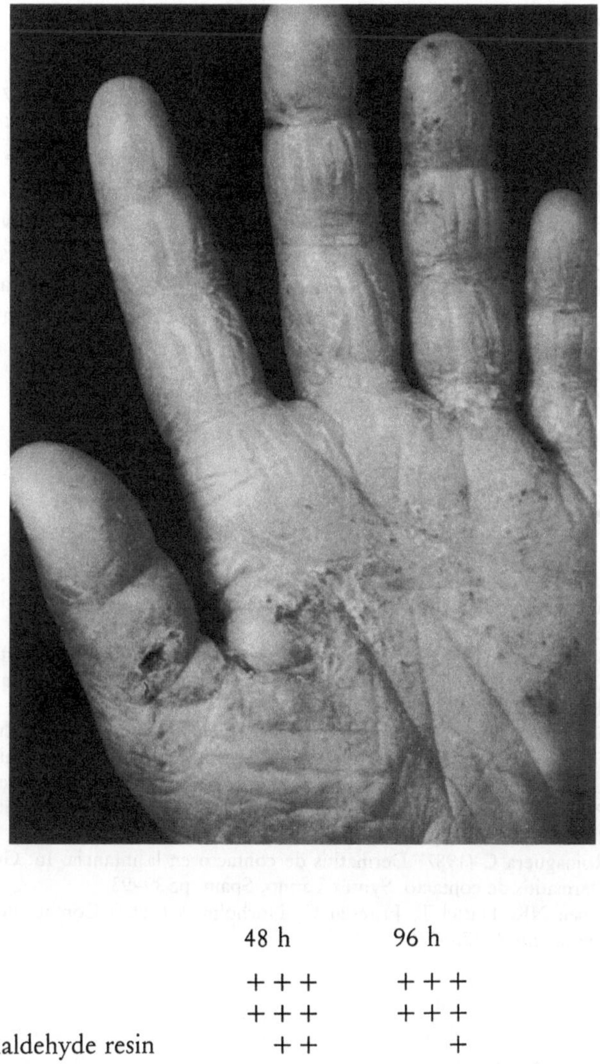

Fig. 1. Left hand showing erythema and fissuration

	48 h	96 h
Caine mix	+ + +	+ + +
Parabens	+ + +	+ + +
p-ter-Butylphenol formaldehyde resin	+ +	+
Fragance mix	+ + +	+ + +

We also tested the preservatives, antimicrobials, perfumes, vehicles, and emulsifiers series, and each of the separate components of paraben and caine mix. We found positive (+ + +) reactions at both 48 h and 96 h to:

1. Butylated hydroxyanisole
2. Sorbic acid
3. Methylparaben
4. Ethylparaben
5. Propylparaben
6. Isoeugenol
7. Benzocaine

Discussion

Contact dermatitis is not frequently seen in children [1–3, 7, 9]; a rare finding in the first 4 years of life, its incidence increases subsequently [1]. Monosensitization is more frequent than multiple sensitization in children, the latter increasing in frequency after the 10th year [6]. According to Epstein [4], the most frequent causative agents of contact dermatitis in children are plants, followed by drugs (neomycin, ethylenediamine, and thiomerosal), metals, and cosmetics. Children may become sensitized by contacting cosmetics used by their mothers and other relatives, using them for play [5, 8]. In our patient, the lesions were present from quite an early age (3 years). We found an impressive number of sensitizers, a finding we think is not very common in children.

References

1. Angelini G, Meneghini CL (1977) Contact and bacterial allergy in children with atopic dermatitis. Contact Dermatitis 3: 163–174
2. Brandão FM (1982) Eczema de contacto na infância. Trab Soc Port Derm Venereol 50: 119–123
3. Camarasa JMG, Aspiolea F, Alomar A (1982) Sensibilización a metales en niños. Med Cutan Ibero Lat Am 10: 183–186
4. Epstein E (1971) Contact dermatitis in children. Pediatr Clin North Am 18: 839–852
5. Fisher AA (1986) Contact dermatitis, 3rd edn. Lea and Febiger, Philadelphia, pp 49–76
6. Gonçalo S, Sousa I, Freitas JD (1984) Eczema de contacto na criança. Acta Med Port 5: 87–90
7. Pevny I, Brennenstuhl M, Razinskas G (1984) Patch testing in children. Contact Dermatitis 11: 201–206
8. Romaguera C (1987) Dermatitis de contacto en la infancia. In: Grimalt F, Romaguera C (eds) Dermatitis de contacto. Syntex Latino, Spain, pp 89–93
9. Veien NK, Hattel T, Justesen O, Norholm A (1982) Contact dermatitis in children. Contact Dermatitis 8: 373–375

Addresses

M. A. Barros
Department of Dermatology and Venereology, S. João Hospital, Alameda Prof. Hernâni Monteiro, 4200 Porto, Portugal

A. Baptista
Department of Dermatology and Venereology, S. João Hospital, Alameda Prof. Hernâni Monteiro, 4200 Porto, Portugal

F. Amado
Department of Dermatology and Venereology, S. João Hospital, Alameda Prof. Hernâni Monteiro, 4200 Porto, Portugal

Antimicrobials and Preservatives

Contact Allergy to Preservatives

K. E. Andersen

Preservatives may be defined as chemicals added to topical drugs, cosmetics, toiletries, household products, and aqueous and emulsion systems in industry to prevent them from spoiling. They may act by interfering with certain chemical reactions or with the growth of molds, fungi, bacteria or parasites. The use concentration in the finished products is generally in the range of 0.01% to 1%. Owing to their inherent reactivity, many of these chemicals can induce allergic contact dermatitis (ACD). An overwhelming number of preservative formulations are marketed under various trade names and their synonyms. Unfortunately, there is no single source of information regarding the production, import and use of the different preservatives. The present paper focuses on four issues related to contact allergy to preservatives.

Relationship Between Predictive Test Results in Animals and Man and Clinical Experience

Chlorocresol is known to be a strong sensitizer in the guinea pig maximization test, with a frequency of positive reactions ranging from 15% to 84% of the animals tested, depending on the concentration used for induction. Interestingly, the use of chlorocresol as a preservative in topical corticosteroids is extensive, and in spite of that, clinical chlorocresol allergy occurs only sporadically [1].

Cytox 3522, containing 10% methylene-*bis*-thiocyanate, and equivalent products are used as biocides in industrial water systems. Cytox 3522 sensitized all animals in the guinea pig maximization test. In spite of that, human sensitization has not yet been reported. Exposed workers in a Finnish paper-manufacturing plant have been tested with a negative result [1]. The company uses about 25 tons per year of chemicals containing methylene-*bis*-thiocyanate. These two chemicals represent examples of strong experimental allergens used in the environment with a resulting low incidence of clinical contact allergy.

The parabens are moderate to weak experimental sensitizers. They are widely used and about 6000 of the 19000 or so cosmetic formulas in the United States are preserved with parabens. Paraben allergy occurs with a frequency of around 1% in patch-test materials, which justifies the parabens being included in the standard series for patch testing. Among 8000 patients tested at Gentofte from 1971 to 1986,

0.8% of females and 1.2% of males were paraben-sensitive [16]. Earlier, when parabens were used in higher concentrations as antifungal agents, paraben sensitivity was more frequent.

Edman and Möller [8] and Gollhausen and co-workers [9] both found an increasing frequency of paraben sensitivity over the years among their eczema patients subjected to patch testing.

Animal data with the parabens show a low sensitization rate. Goodwin [10] did not sensitize with ethyl-paraben using the guinea pig maximization test. Maurer [15] used the optimization test and sensitized 3–4 of 20 guinea pigs to methyl-paraben and none of 20 to propyl-paraben using epicutaneous challenge, while 10 of 20 reacted following intradermal challenge.

The predictive test data cannot stand alone but must be evaluated in relation to diagnostic patch tests and the exposure situation. There are examples of biocides with a strong allergenic potential in animal tests, but giving a low incidence of allergic contact dermatitis during practical use. There are biocides with a lower sensitizing potential which provoke a significant number of contact allergies, probably due to a widespread use often in higher concentrations.

We know from experimental and clinical data that allergic sensitization is dose-dependent. Therefore, it might be a good idea to also include dose-response determinations in standard predictive tests [1].

Routine Patch Testing with Preservatives - Ingredient Labelling

The Danish contact dermatitis research group tested a number of biocides on consecutive eczema patients in 1983–1984 [2]. Some positive reactions were found, but they were of limited clinical value because the results were frequently unexplainable. In most cases it was not possible to trace the exposure to the biocides in question. This is an argument for the demand on labelling of biocide content in all products, in order to make it easier to choose the appropriate biocides for testing of the patients.

Kathon CG

Kathon CG is of course very much in focus, due to its widespread use and the prevalence of contact allergy to it. De Groot and Weyland [11] have recently published a comprehensive review on Kathon CG. The literature contains pros and cons. The active ingredients in Kathon CG, methylchloroisothiazolinone and methylisothiazolinone are strong sensitizers in guinea pig allergy tests [4, 5]. A number of reports have documented a varying and in some countries an increasing incidence of allergic contact dermatitis to these chemicals [6, 11], which justifies the inclusion of Kathon CG in the standard series.

The patch test concentration is currently 100 ppm in aqueous solution. This is a compromise, as higher concentrations (200–300 ppm) may produce irritation and patch test sensitization [3, 14]. In some cases, Kathon CG 100 ppm may give false-negative test results on normal back skin in patients with an isothiazolinone-induced aggravation of a hand dermatitis. Further studies are needed to substantiate the choice of patch-test concentration.

The Kathon story is still dynamic and more details are to be expected. The controversies include: patch-test concentration, the risk of sensitization related to use on healthy versus diseased skin, and the use in stay-on and rinse-off products. There are a multitude of trade names for chloromethyl-isothiazolinones. It is appropriate to choose another name for the compound in order to focus on all exposure possibilities – Cl + me-isothiazolinone is a suggestion.

Changes in the Industry's Choice of Preservatives

The choice of preservatives in the cosmetic industry is interesting to follow. New preservatives bring along new reports on allergic contact dermatitis. Unfortunately, the figures are published with a considerable delay; the latest figures are from 1984 [7]. Besides Kathon CG, Germall 2 and DMDM hydantoin are used in increasing amounts and subsequently reports on contact allergy to these new preservatives appear in the literature [12, 13].

In conclusion a better understanding of preservative contact allergy requires: (a) a balanced view on predictive allergy test results and dose-response determinations; (b) information about biocide consumption and distribution; and (c) labelling of biocide content in products. The quotation from Theophrastus Paracelsus remains pertinent:

Alle Ding sind Gift
und nichts ohn' Gift.
Allein die Dosis macht,
daß ein Ding kein Gift ist.

References

1. Andersen KE (1986) Contact allergy to chlorocresol, formaldehyde and other biocides. Guinea pig tests and clinical studies. Acta Derm Venereol (Stockh) [Suppl 125] 66
2. Andersen KE, Veien N (1985) Biocide patch tests. Contact Dermatitis 12: 99–103
3. Björkner B, Bruze M, Dahlquist I, Fregert S, Gruvberger B, Persson K (1986) Contact allergy to the preservative Kathon CG. Contact Dermatitis 14: 85–90
4. Bruze M, Dahlquist I, Fregert S, Gruvberger B, Persson K (1987) Contact allergy to the active ingredients of Kathon CG. Contact Dermatitis 16: 183–188
5. Chan PK, Baldwin RC, Parsons RD, et al. (1983) Kathon biocide: manifestation of delayed

contact dermatitis in guinea pigs is dependent on the concentration for induction and challenge. J Invest Dermatol 81: 409–411
6. Cronin E, Hannuksela M, Lachapelle J-M, Maibach HI, Malten KE, Meneghini CL (1988) Frequency of sensitization to the preservative Kathon CG. Contact Dermatitis 18: 274–279
7. Decker RL Jr (1985) Frequency of preservative use in cosmetic formulas as disclosed to FDA – 1984. Cosmetics Toiletries 100: 65–68
8. Edman B, Möller H (1982) Trends and forecasts for standard allergens in a 12-year patch test material. Contact Dermatitis 8: 95–104
9. Gollhausen R, et al. (1988) Trends in allergic contact sensitization. Contact Dermatitis 18: 147–154
10. Goodwin BFJ, Johnson AW (1985) Single injection adjuvant test. Curr Probl Dermatol 14: 201–207
11. de Groot AC, Weyland JW (1988) Kathon CG: a review. J Am Acad Dermatol 18: 350–358
12. de Groot AC, van Joost T, Bos JD, van der Meeren HLM, Weyland JW (1988) Patch test reactivity to DMDM hydantoin. Relationship to formaldehyde allergy. Contact Dermatitis 18: 197–201
13. de Groot AC, Bruynzeel DP, Jagtman BA, Weyland JW (1988) Contact allergy to diazolidinyl urea (Germall II). Contact Dermatitis 18: 202–205
14. Maibach HI (1985) Diagnostic patch test concentration for Kathon CG. Contact Dermatitis 13: 242–245
15. Maurer Th (1985) The optimization test. Curr Probl Dermatol 14: 114–151
16. Menné T, Hjorth N (1988) Routine patch testing with paraben esters. Contact Dermatitis 19: 189–191

Addresses

K. E. Andersen
Dermatology Clinic, Algade 33, DK-4000 Roskilde, Denmark

Occupational Skin Sensitization to the Antimicrobials *ortho*-Benzyl *para*-Chlorophenol and Ampholyte 103 G

T. Estlander, L. Kanerva, and R. Jolanki

Key words:

Contact dermatitis - Allergy - Dodecyl-di-(aminoethyl)glycine - disinfectants - Dental personnel

Introduction

Many antimicrobials contained in commercial disinfectant and antiseptic detergents are allergens and irritants. Allergic dermatitis from dodecyl-di-(aminoethyl)glycine (DDG), glutaraldehyde, and quaternary ammonium compounds is common [2, 4, 6–8, 16, 20]. The sensitization capacity of different phenol derivates varies. Rather a lot of reports show delayed and even immediate allergy to *p*-chlorometacresol (pCmC) [3, 9, 10], whereas few reports on contact sensitivity to *ortho*-benzyl *para*-chlorophenol (oBpCP) and *o*-phenylphenol have been published [1, 11, 19]. oBpCP has also been reported to be a skin irritant and a depigmenting agent [11]. A patient who became sensitized to oBpCP after allergic dermatitis from Desimex-I is presented here.

Case Report

The patient is a 55-year-old woman, neither herself atopic nor with a family history of atopy. She has been working as an instrument caretaker in a dental care unit for 19 years, and in spite of appropriate hand protection, she has had hand dermatitis connected with her work for 10 years. Desimex-I (Orion Corporation, Finland), containing 15% DDG as Ampholyte 103 G in a 1%–2% water solution (pH 8.0), was used up to 1981, and thereafter Phenosol-I (Oy Rohto Ab, Finland), containing 3% oBpCP and 23% pCmC in a 2%–3% water solution (pH 10.3) has been used to disinfect instruments. The patient's dermatitis has been followed for 7 years; patch tests have been performed on three occasions. The tests have been done using Finn chambers on the patient's back and read three times as previously reported [15]. The initial testing with suspected Desimex-I solution gave a positive result (Table 1). In a rubber series (Trolab, Denmark), 4,4-dihydroxydiphenyl (DOD) gave a positive (+ + +) reaction, but tests with two rubber glove materials were negative. An International Contact Dermatitis Research Group (ICDRG) standard series (Epicon Oy, Finland), a series of antimicrobials (Trolab, Denmark), a series of cosmetics and local medicaments (Epicon Oy, Finland), and a fragrance series (Trolab, Denmark) were all negative. A new disinfectant, Phenosol-I, and polyvinylchloride (PVC) gloves were taken into use. However, 3 years later her hand dermatitis relapsed, and patch testing with Phenosol-I solution was positive (Table 2). Testing with individual components showed a positive reaction to oBpCP only (Table 3); 20 control tests with oBpCP showed mild irritation to 2% (w/w) petrolatum, but not to 0.5% (w/w) petrolatum. A series of antimicrobials (Trolab, Denmark), a fragrance series, and tests with two PVC gloves were negative. The employer refused to change the disinfectant, and the patient continued working despite almost constant hand dermatitis. No leukoderma developed. Retesting 4 years later using a dilution series was positive with oBpCP (Table 2) and Ampholyte 103 G (Table 1), which is the allergen in Desimex-I [20]. An ICDRG standard series (Chemotechnique, Sweden) and a series of antimicrobials excluding oBpCP (Chemotechnique, Sweden) were negative.

Table 1. Results of patch tests with Desimex-I and its allergenic constituent dodecyl-di-(aminoethyl)glycine as Ampholyte 103 G

Year	Substance	Vehicle	Results according to concentration[c]			
			1%	0.5%	0.33%	0.1%
1981	Desimex-I[a]	Petrolatum	+ +	+	NT	NT
1988	Ampholyte 103 G[b]	Petrolatum	+ + +	NT	+ + +	+
1988	Ampholyte 103 G[b]	Aqua	+ + +	NT	+ + +	+ +

NT, not tested
[a] Occlusion time 24 h; readings 24, 48, 120 h.
[b] Occlusion time 48 h; readings 48, 72, 96 h.
[c] Weight ratio.

Table 2. Results of patch tests with Phenosol-I and its allergenic constituent *ortho*-Benzyl *para*-Chlorophenol (oBpCP)

Year	Substance	Vehicle	Results according to concentration[c]					
			5%	2%	1%	0.5%	0.33%	0.1%
1984	Phenosol-I[a]	Petrolatum	+ +	+ +	+ ?	NT	NT	NT
1984	oBpCP[a]	Petrolatum	NT	+ + +	NT	+ +	NT	NT
1988	oBpCP[b]	Petrolatum	NT	NT	+ + +	NT	+	–

NT, not tested
[a] Occlusion time 24 h; readings 24, 48, 120 h.
[b] Occlusion time 48 h; readings 48, 72, 96 h.
[c] Weight ratio.

Table 3. Results of patch tests with the constituents of Phenosol-I

Constituent	Concentration[a] (%)	Result
ortho-Benzyl *para*-Chlorophenol	2	+++
p-Chlorometacresol	2	–
3 others	1–10	–
NaOH	NT	

NT, not tested
[a] Weight ratio; petrolatum vehicle.

Discussion

Disinfectants, detergents, and cleansers are potential causes of occupational hand dermatitis among dental care personnel [5, 17, 18]. The sensitization of workers may differ from one country to another, depending on the products used, as has been stated previously [17]. DDG containing four active ingredients and sold under several trade names (e.g., Ampholyt G, Tego 103 G, and Ampholyte 103 G) has been known to be a contact allergen for at least 20 years [2, 4, 7, 8, 12–14, 16, 20]. A dilution series with Ampholyte 103 G (DDG) in petrolatum and aqua confirmed the sensitization of our patient. No other difference between the test results could be found, but the reactions produced by DDG in aqua were more pronounced than those in petrolatum. Ampholyte 103 G is sold in Finland in two formulations, one for disinfection and the other as an antiseptic detergent, under the trade name Desimex. It is probably the most common antimicrobial causing occupational allergic dermatitis among dental care personnel in Finland [12–14, 20]. Ampholyte 103 G will be included in our series of antimicrobials (1% aqua).

Allergic eczema from oBpCP has been described in two previous reports, one published in 1970 and dealing with hospital antiseptic detergents, the other in 1986 and dealing with a detergent for drinking glasses [11, 20]. Patch testing with a dilution series using oBpCP and negative control tests confirmed the allergic nature of our patient's test reactions. Wet work, the alkaline pH of the disinfectant solution, and previous allergic dermatitis may have promoted the development of allergy to oBpCP. Despite the regular use of protective gloves, contact with the allergen may occur in many ways, e.g., through unnoticeable punctures in the gloves caused by sharp instruments and through handling contaminated instruments or surfaces, thereby causing continuous hand dermatitis problems. oBpCP is sold in Finland in seven formulations, all for the same purposes as DDG. It has been included in our series of antimicrobials (1% petrolatum) for 4 years, but no other cases of allergy have been found.

To summarize, oBpCP should be borne in mind as a rare allergen contained in disinfectant and antiseptic detergents. Ampholyte 103 G is probably the most common antimicrobial sensitizing dental care personnel in Finland. The use of protective gloves does not always solve occupationally induced allergic hand dermatitis problems. The allergen(s) should be totally removed from the workplace.

References

1. Adams RM (1970) Allergic contact dermatitis due to o-phenylphenol. Contact Dermatitis 7: 332
2. Bowers RE (1986) Tego (dodecylic aminoethyl glycine hydrochloride). Contact Dermatitis Newsletter 4: 76
3. Burry JN, Kirk J, Reid JG, Turner T (1975) Chlorocresol sensitivity. Contact Dermatitis 1: 41–42
4. Calnan CD (1974) Tego dermatitis (telephone cleaner). Contact Dermatitis Newsletter 8: 439
5. Calnan CD, Stevenson CJ (1963) Studies in contact dermatitis XV. – Dental materials. Trans St. John's Hosp Dermatol Soc 49: 9–26
6. Fisher AA (1986) Contact Dermatitis, 3rd edn. Lea and Febiger, Philadelphia, pp 515–530
7. Foussereau J, Samsoen M, Hecht MTh (1983) Occupational dermatitis to Ampholyt G in hospital personnel. Contact Dermatitis 9: 233–234
8. Fregert S, Dahlquist I (1969) Allergic dermatitis from Tego (dodecylic aminoethyl glycine hydrochloride). Contact Dermatitis Newsletter 5: 103
9. Freitas JP, Brandao FM (1986) Contact urticaria to chlorocresol. Contact Dermatitis 15: 252
10. Goncalo M, Goncalo S, Moreno A (1987) Immediate and delayed allergy to chlorocresol. Contact Dermatitis 17: 46–47
11. Kahn G (1970) Depigmentation caused by phenolic detergent germicides. Arch Dermatol 102: 177–178
12. Kanerva L, Jolanki R, Estlander T (1986) Occupational dermatitis due to an epoxy acrylate. Contact Dermatitis 14: 80–84
13. Kanerva L, Estlander T, Jolanki R (1988) Occupational skin disease in Finland. An analysis of 10 years statistics from an occupational dermatology clinic. Int Arch Occup Environ Health 60: 89–94
14. Kanerva L, Estlander T, Jolanki R (1988) Allergic contact dermatitis from dental composite resins due to aromatic epoxy acrylates and aliphatic acrylates. Contact Dermatitis (in press)
15. Kanerva L, Estlander T, Jolanki R (1988) Sensitization to patch test acrylates. Contact Dermatitis 18: 10–15
16. Lachapelle JM, Reginster JP (1977) Occupational contact dermatitis from an ampholytic soap (TEGO). Contact Dermatitis 3: 211–212
17. Rudzki E (1979) Occupational dermatitis among health service workers. Derm Beruf Umwelt 27: 112–115
18. Samitz MH, Shmunes E (1969) Occupational dermatoses in dentists and allied personnel. Cutis 5: 180–184
19. Sonnex TS, Rycroft RJG (1986) Allergic contact dermatitis from orthobenzyl parachlorophenol in a drinking glass cleaner. Contact Dermatitis 14: 247–248
20. Suhonen R (1980) Contact allergy to dodecyl-di-(aminoethyl)glycine (Desimex i). Contact Dermatitis 6: 290–291

Addresses

T. Estlander

Section of Dermatology, Institute of Occupational Health, Topeliuksenkatu 41 a A, SF-00250 Helsinki, Finland

L. Kanerva

Section of Dermatology, Institute of Occupational Health, Topeliuksenkatu 41 a A, SF-00250 Helsinki, Finland

R. Jolanki

Section of Dermatology, Institute of Occupational Health, Topeliuksenkatu 41 a A, SF-00250 Helsinki, Finland

Contact Sensitivity to Diazolidinylurea (Germall II)

C. M. Perret and R. Happle

Summary

Diazolidinylurea (DU; Germall II) is a new broad-spectrum preservative. From July 1984 to February 1988, we tested 2142 consecutive patients suffering from eczemas of suspected allergic origin with the European standard series (Trolab) and our additional standard series including DU 2% in water. We found the following:

1. Sensitization to DU was seen in 12 patients (0.6%).
2. Of 12 patients, 7 reacted to DU, but not to formaldehyde or formaldehyde releasers. In these patients, the reaction can be attributed to sensitivity to DU itself.
3. Of 12 patients, 5 reacted to DU, formaldehyde, and all formaldehyde releasers tested. In these patients, the reaction to DU is probably to be attributed to released formaldehyde; therefore, DU should be added to the list of formaldehyde releasers.
4. In some of the patients, concomitant sensitizations to strong and/or ubiquitous allergens (nickel, cobalt, chromate), or a long history of skin disease could be found; therefore, it seems reasonable to assume that in these cases sensitization to DU occurred secondarily on eczematous skin with reduced barrier function.

Key words:

Contact sensitivity - Contact allergy - Diazolidinylurea - Formaldehyde releasers

Introduction

In water-containing cosmetics, an effective preservative is needed to prevent the unwanted growth of microorganisms. The most commonly used preservatives are the parabens, followed by imidazolidinylurea, known as Germall 115. Recently, a new cosmetic preservative with structural similarities to imidazolidinylurea, diazolidinylurea (*N*-[1,3-bis(hydroxymethyl)-2,5-dioxo-4-imidazolidinyl]-*N,N'*-bis(hydroxymethyl)-urea) (DU; Germall II), has been introduced. We analyzed the sensitization to DU in a group of more than 2100 patients.

Patients and Methods

From July 1984 to February 1988, we tested 2142 consecutive patients referred to our allergy department with eczemas of suspected allergic origin. The patients were tested with the European standard series (Trolab) and our additional standard series including DU 2% in water. All patients sensitive to DU were tested additionally with a panel of substances known to release formaldehyde (FA): ureum formaldehyde (8% aqua), glyoxal ureum (10% aqua), quaternium 15 (1% petrolatum), and dimethyloldimethyl-hydantoin (3% aqua).

Results

The following results were obtained:

1. Testing of 2142 consecutive patients with eczemas of suspected allergic origin revealed sensitization to DU in 12 patients (0.6%).
2. Of 12 patients, 7 reacted to DU, but not to FA or FA releasers. In these patients, the reaction can be attributed to sensitivity to DU itself.
3. Of 12 patients, 5 reacted to DU, FA, and all FA releasers tested. In these patients, the reaction to DU is probably due to released FA.
4. In 2 of 12 patients, DU was the only allergen giving a positive patch test reaction. In some of the other patients, concomitant sensitizations to strong and/or ubiquitous allergens (nickel, chromate, cobalt), or a long history of skin disease could be found. This indicates that reduced barrier function, due, for example, to eczematous skin, and thus enhanced penetration of the allergen may often be a prerequisite for the induction of sensitization to DU.

Discussion

DU is a potent new preservative. In 1985, Kantor et al. reported the first case of acute allergic contact dermatitis from DU in a hair gel [2]. Maximization tests done by Stephens [4] in guinea pigs indicate that DU is a mild sensitizer (grade 2, using the allergenicity rating scale of Magnusson and Kligman [3]). Our results – a sensitization rate of 0.6% in more than 2100 patients with eczemas of suspected allergic origin – support this view. Some of the positive patch test results are in fact cross-reactions due to released FA. This can be concluded from the fact that in 5 of our 12 DU-positive patients, positive reactions could also be found to FA and a panel of known FA releasers. These cross-reactions were also reported by Zaugg and Hunziker [5] and recently by de Groot et al., who described four patients sensitive to DU, two of them being reactive to FA as well [1]. Therefore, DU should be added to the list of FA releasers.

At present, it does not seem reasonable to include DU in the standard series. On the other hand, DU should be added to series of preservatives. Testing in water at a concentration of 2% seems appropriate. Moreover, patients reacting to FA should be advised to avoid the use of cosmetics containing DU as a preservative.

References

1. De Groot AC, Bruynzeel DP, Jagtman BA, Weyland JW (1988) Contact allergy to diazolidinyl urea (Germall II). Contact Dermatitis 18: 202–205
2. Kantor GR, Taylor JS, Ratz JL, Evey PL (1985) Acute allergic contact dermatitis from diazolidinyl urea (Germall II) in a hair gel. J Am Acad Dermatol 13: 116–119
3. Magnusson B, Kligman AM (1969) The identification of contact allergens by animal assay. The guinea pig maximization test. J Invest Dermatol 52: 268–276
4. Stephens TS, Drake KD, Drotman RB (1987) Experimental delayed contact sensitization to diazolidinylurea (Germall II) in guinea pigs. Contact Dermatitis 16: 164–168
5. Zaugg T, Hunziker T (1987) Germall II and Triclosan. Contact Dermatitis 17: 262

Addresses

C. M. Perret
Department of Dermatology, University of Nijmegen, Javastraat 104, NL-6524 MJ Nijmegen, The Netherlands

R. Happle
Department of Dermatology, University of Nijmegen, Javastraat 104, NL-6524 MJ Nijmegen, The Netherlands

Occupational Contact Dermatitis from Glutaraldehyde Used as a Cold Sterilizing Agent

M. Nelis and J. Oleffe

Summary

We present a report on three patients who had allergic contact dermatitis from glutaraldehyde used professionally as a cold sterilizing agent. The dermatitis improved during weekends and holidays. The diagnosis of allergy was confirmed by positive patch test reactions to working solutions and to glutaraldehyde incorporated therein.

Key words:

Glutaraldehyde - Cold sterilizing agent - Contact dermatitis

Introduction

Glutaraldehyde (1,5-pentanedial-OCH-$(CH_2)_3CHO$) is mostly used in a 2% water solution as a cold sterilizing agent in hospital and dental clinics (for disinfection and sterilization of endoscopes and surgical instruments and of floors). We report three cases of glutaraldehyde contact dermatitis related to its use.

Case Reports

Case 1. A 25-year-old patient, a nurse in the Department of Endoscopy, developed allergic contact dermatitis to Aldosan (used for disinfection of endoscopic instruments). Aldosan is mainly composed of glutaraldehyde, formaldehyde, and quaternium 12. Examination revealed eczema with redness, peeling, and fissures in the fingers of both hands, and nummular eczema on the wrists. The dermatitis improved during weekends and disappeared during holidays. Patch tests (with pharmaceutical/cosmetic/standard Belgian tri-contact patch series, gloves, and components of Aldosan) showed positive reactions to Aldosan (2% aqua) and glutaraldehyde (1% aqua).

Case 2. A 44-year-old woman working in the intensive care unit of the hospital developed dermatitis of the eyelids and generalized pruritus. She used gloves and hence showed no eczema on the hands. There was no personal or family history of atopy. Patch tests (with pharmaceutical/cosmetic/standard Belgian tri-contact patch series, gloves, and working solutions, as well as their isolated components) were positive to Melsitt (2% aqua), quaternium 12 (0,1% aqua), and glutaraldehyde (1% aqua). Melsitt, used for hospital disinfection, is mainly made of glutaraldehyde, formaldehyde, and dimethyldidecylammonium chloride. The dermatitis is probably maintained and/or heightened by daily contact with Melsitt carried by hands when scratching.

Case 3. A 27-year-old cleaning woman working in the intensive care unit of the hospital developed eczema of the hands and of the feet (she used to work barefooted, only wearing sandals). The dermatitis improved during weekends and disappeared during holidays. She used gloves after the eczema appeared. There was no personal or family history of atopy. Patch tests (with pharmaceutical/cosmetic/standard Belgian tri-contact patch series, gloves, and working solutions) were positive to Melsitt and glutaraldehyde (1% aqua).

Discussion

There are several reports about nurses who acquired allergic glutaraldehyde contact dermatitis after handlung instruments sterilized with this compound (Cidex, Alhydex, or Korsolin) [1, 7–9]. During a study of 541 cleaning women working in a hospital, the incidence of occupational dermatitis was found to be 15.3%; 21% of the women had allergic contact dermatitis, only one case being caused by glutaraldehyde [3].

Cases of sensitization to glutaraldehyde have been reported in various settings [2]:

1. Exposure to glutaraldehyde in medical and allied professions
   a) Cold sterilizing agent [buffered (Cidex), renal dialysis, pulmonary apparatus]
   b) Embalming
   c) Tissue fixative
   d) X-ray film solution
2. Therapeutic uses of glutaraldehyde
   a) Antifungal agent
   b) Bullous diseases

  c) Hyperhidrosis
  d) Warts
3. Industrial exposure to glutaraldehyde
  a) Clothing
  b) Hardening of photographic gelatin
  c) Increase in water resistance of wallpaper
  d) Intermediate in resin and dyes
  e) Liquid fabric softener
  f) Tanning of leather

However, sensitization to glutaraldehyde mainly occurs through its use as a cold sterilizing agent.

Glutaraldehyde is a moderately irritant agent and a weak allergen. Solutions of more than 20% concentration are strongly irritant to skin, and those of more than 1% have the same effect on ocular membranes [4]. The glutaraldehyde vapors may provoke irritation of the upper respiratory apparatus, and repetitive exposure could produce symptoms suggestive of allergic reactions [2]. Glutaraldehyde contact dermatitis is usually localized to the back of the hands. Cases of pulpitis have also been reported [8]. Cross-reactions between glutaraldehyde and formaldehyde do not occur. Maibach [5] found that 20 patients showing sensitization to glutaraldehyde (1% aqua) did not react to formaldehyde (2% aqua).

As glutaraldehyde is more and more being used as a disinfectant, an increase in contact dermatitis from this compound may be expected. Rubber gloves can be penetrated by glutaraldehyde and as such are not to be considered as a safe protection [6]. Sterilized instruments should also be thoroughly rinsed before use. The use of alternative, safer products for hospital disinfection should be considered in the near future.

References

1. Fisher AA (1981) Reactions to glutaraldehyde with particular reference to radiologist and X-ray technicians. Cutis 29: 113
2. Fisher AA (1986) Contact Dermatitis, 3rd edn. Lea and Febiger, Philadelphia
3. Hansen KS (1983) Occupational dermatoses in hospital cleaning women. Contact Dermatitis 9: 343–351
4. Institut National de recherche et de sécurité. Supplément aux cahiers de notes, no 126, fiche toxicologique no 171
5. Maibach H (1975) Glutaraldehyde: cross-rections to formaldehyde? Contact Dermatitis 1: 326–327
6. Moursiden HT, Faber O (1973) Penetration of protective gloves by allergens and irritants. Trans St. Johns Hosp Dermatol Soc 59: 230–234
7. Neering H, Van Ketel WG (1974) Glutaraldehyde and formaldehyde contact allergy. Contact Dermatitis Newsletter 16: 518
8. Sandersen KV, Cronin E (1968) Glutaraldehyde and contact dermatitis. Br Med J 3: 802
9. Zach RG (1980) How prevalent is glutaraldehyde sensitivity? Consultant 6: 116

Addresses

M. Nelis

Clinique Dermatologique, Université Libre de Bruxelles, Hôpital Erasme, Route de Lennik, 808, 1070 Bruxelles, Belgium

J. Oleffe

Clinique Dermatologique, Université Libre de Bruxelles, Hôpital Erasme, Route de Lennik, 808, 1070 Bruxelles, Belgium

Anaphylactic Allergy to Chlorhexidine Cream

P. Susitaival and L. Häkkinen

Summary

A female patient with atopic dermatitis was examined intravaginally by a gynaecologist using obstetric cream with 1% chlorhexidine digluconate as a lubricant. Urticaria and wheezing appeared within 5 min of the examination. Open application tests made 1 month later with 5% chlorhexidine digluconate in water and with the obstretic cream as is were clearly positive. Skin tests were repeated 1 year later with positive results. In a passive cutaneous anaphylaxis test, a 2-mm reaction (+) was achieved.

Key words:

Chlorhexidine - Contact urticaria - Anaphylaxis

Introduction

Chlorhexidine has been widely used as a skin antiseptic all over the world for about 25 years. It is used not only against skin and mucous membrane infections but also for disinfection before examinations, operations, etc.

Delayed contact allergy to chlorhexidine is unusual, but we encounter it every now and then in dermatology clinics. On the other hand, immediate anaphylactic allergy to chlorhexidine is obviously extremely rare. Six cases have been reported from Japan [3–5], one from Australia [2], and one quite recent case from Sweden [1]. We report here one further case of immediate-type allergy to chlorhexidine.

Case Report

An 18-year-old white woman had suffered from mild atopic dermatitis since childhood. She had earlier used a cream containing chlorhexidine, but not for several months. In September 1986, she was examined intravaginally by a gynaecologist who used a 1% chlorhexidine obstetric cream (Hibitane, ICI Pharmaceuticals, England) as a lubricant. Within 5 min, urticaria started spreading all over her skin, her lips and eyelids swelled, and she started wheezing and coughing. The symptoms subsided rapidly after 0.3 ml Adrenalin (1/1000) was given intravenously.

Table 1. Results of open application test made on the volar forearm in November 1986

Test substance	Results	
	15 min	30 min
Hibitane obstetric cream as is	Wheal (5 × 6 mm)	Wheal (7 × 8 mm) flare (15 × 40 mm)
Chlorhexidine digluconate 5% in water	Wheal (2 × 3 mm) flare (15 × 20 mm)	Urticaria larger than treated area

Table 2. Results of skin tests made on the volar forearm in December 1987

Test	Results		
	15 min	30 min	1 h
Open application			
Hibitane obstretic cream as is	Flare	Flare	Flare with wheal (1 × 1 cm)
Chlorhexidine digluconate			
1% in water	Negative	Negative	Negative
5% in water	Wheal (5 × 4 mm), some flare	Urticaria on test area (2.5 × 5 cm)	
Skin-prick			
Chlorhexidine digluconate 1% in water	Wheal (9 mm)[a]		
Control	Negative		
Histamine dihydrochloride (3 mg/ml)	Wheal (5 mm)[a]		

[a] Mean of the longest diameter and the diameter perpendicular to it.

Table 3. Results of passive cutaneous anaphylaxis test

Test substance	Results at 15 min
Chlorhexidine digluconate 1% in water	
Test site	Wheal (2 mm)[a]
Control site	Negative
Water	Negative
Histamine dihydrochloride (3 mg/ml)	Wheal (6 mm)[a]

[a] Mean of the longest diameter and the diameter perpendicular to it.

Table 4. Details of eight cases of immediate allergy to chlorhexidine reported in the literature and the present case

Case no.	Age (years)	Sex	Indicaton and site of chlorhexidine use	Immediate reaction	Chlorhexidine skin test results	Other test results	Reference
1	9	M	Preoperative, genital area	Wheezing, urticaria, eyelid oedema	Open patch test and scratch test positive		[4]
2	15	M	Traumatic wound, forehead	Wheezing, facial oedema	Intradermal test positive		[4]
3	9	M	Traumatic wound, upper lip	Generalized urticaria	Intradermal test positive		[4]
4	26	M	Preoperative, genital area	Generalized urticaria	Intradermal test positive		[4]
5[a]	9	M	Preoperative[b]	Anaphylaxis	Open patch test and prick test positive	P-K test and histamine release test positive	[3]
6	64	M	Preoperative + chlorhexidine-containing wound dressing, leg	Erythema and shock. Blood pressure 60/40	Intradermal test positive		[2]
7	24	M	Traumatic wound, elbow	Generalized urticaria, anaphylaxis, loss of consciousness		P-K test and RAST positive	[5]
8	66	M	Preoperative, genital area + intraurethral anaesthetic gel	Urticaria from genital area to trunk and lower extremities	Open test and scratch chamber test positive	Scratch chamber tests with Hibiscrub sponge as is and Citanest gel as is positive	[1]
9	18	F	Gynaecological examination, intravaginal	Wheezing, generalized urticaria, oedema in eyelids and lips	Open application test and prick test positive	Open application test with Hibitane obstetric cream as is positive	Present study

RAST, radioallergosorbent test; P-K, Prausnitz-Küstner
[a] Probably the same case as no. 1.
[b] Area not indicated.

Test Results

In November 1986, open application tests were made on the volar aspects of the patient's forearms with Hibitane obstetric cream as is and chlorhexidine digluconate 5% in water. Both tests were positive (Table 1). An open application test with chlorhexidine digluconate 5% in water and a skin-prick test with chlorhexidine digluconate 1% in water were positive in December 1987 (Table 2).

Serum was taken from the patient in November 1986 for a passive cutaneous anaphylaxis test. This was carried out later on a volunteer non-atopic nurse by injecting 0.15 ml of the patient's serum intradermally on the volar aspect of the volunteer's forearm. A prick test was made 48 h later with chlorhexidine digluconate 1% in water on the injection site and on the other forearm. Chlorhexidine digluconate produced a positive reaction (+) on the site where the patient's serum was injected (Table 3).

Discussion

Chlorhexidine is an antiseptic that has been commonly used over the past 10–15 years in Finland in topical preparations, e.g. for atopic dermatitis. A lubricant cream with chlorhexidine for examinations and a skin disinfectant with chlorhexidine are found in almost every physician's office and operating room. This patient had been in contact with chlorhexidine several times without any adverse effects.

According to Ohtoshi et al. [5], there have been more than 30 registered cases of shock reaction following chlorhexidine application in Japan. Table 4 summarizes the eight cases of immediate allergy to chlorhexidine reported in the literature together with the present case. It thus seems that immediate hypersensitivity to chlorhexidine is an uncommon adverse reaction, but there might be some racial differences in the development of this type of allergy.

References

1. Bergqvist-Karlsson A (1988) Delayed and immediate type hypersensitivity to chlorhexidine. Contact Dermatitis 18: 84–88
2. Cheung J, O'Leary JJ (1985) Allergic reaction to chlorhexidine in an anaesthetised patient. Anaesth Intensive Care 13: 429–430
3. Nishioka K, Doi T, Katayama I (1984) Histamine release in contact urticaria. Contact Dermatitis 11: 191
4. Nomura M, Okano M, Okada N et al. (1983) Four cases with anaphylaxis induced by chlorhexidine (in Japanese). Skin Res 25: 306
5. Ohtoshi T, Yamauchi N, Tadokoro K, Miyachi S, Suzuki S, Miyamoto T, Muranaka M (1986) IgE antibody-mediated shock reaction caused by topical application of chlorhexidine. Clin Allergy 16: 155–161

Addresses

P. Susitaival
Dermatology Department, Central Hospital of North Carelia, 80210 Joensuu, Finland

L. Häkkinen
Gynecology Department, Central Hospital of North Carelia, 80210 Joensuu, Finland

Contact Sensitivity to Nonoxynols: A Cause of Intolerance to Antiseptic Preparations

A. Dooms-Goossens, A. Gidi de Alam, and H. Degreef

Key words:

Nonoxynol - Contact allergy - Antiseptics

Seven cases of allergic contact dermatitis to antiseptic preparations are presented in which the reactions were caused not by active principles, but rather by nonoxynols used in the offending substances as nonionic surface-active agents.

Nonoxynols are ethoxylated alkyl phenols or nonylphenylethers that conform in general to the formula $C_9H_{19}C_6H_4(OCH_2CH_2)_nOH$. Nonoxynols are indicated by a number *n*, which is the approximate number of ethylene oxide groups in the polyoxyethylene chain [1].

Nonoxynols have emulsifying, wetting, foaming, and solubilizing properties, and they are used in a large number of industrial, household, agricultural, cosmetic, and pharmaceutical products. They are also used as spermicides [2].

The clinical data and associated positive tests in the nonoxynol-sensitive patients are given in Table 1. Figure 1 shows a positive test reaction to nonoxynol-9 (2% aqua) observed in case 1 (96 h). The ingredients of the commercial products mentioned are as follows:

1. Hibitane solution (ICI)
   a) Chlorhexidine digluconate
   b) Amaranth
   c) Gluconolactone
   d) Isopropyl alcohol
   e) Linalyl acetate
   f) Water
   g) Nonoxynol-"8.3"
2. Isobetadine dermicum solution (Belgana)
   a) Povidone iodine
   b) Glycerol

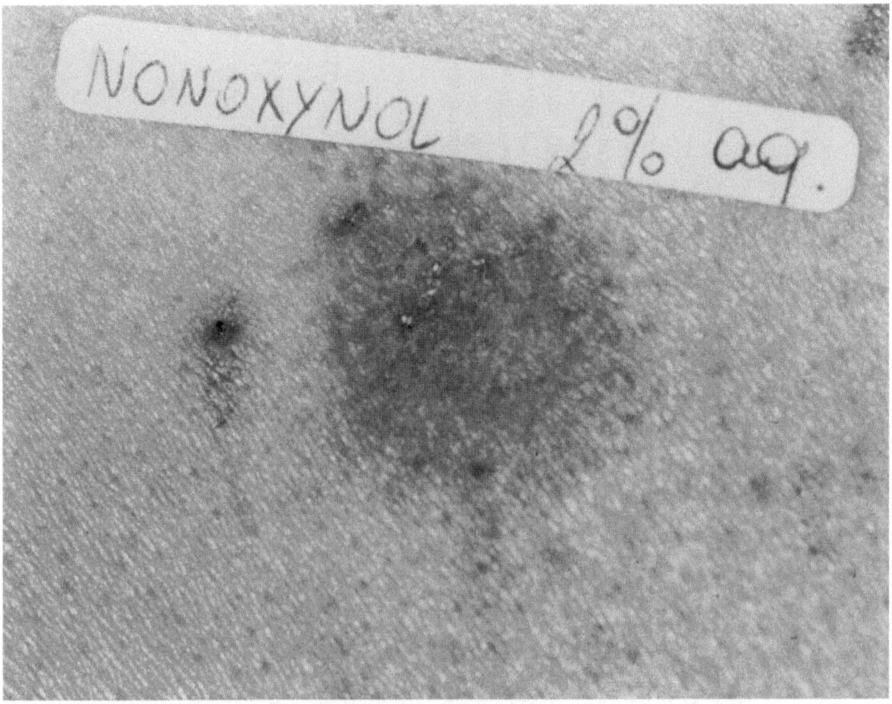

Fig. 1. A positive test reaction to nonoxynol-9 (2% aqua), observed in case 1 (96 h)

c) Nonoxynol-9
d) Citric acid
e) Sodium hydroxide
f) Sodium phosphate
g) Water

3. Hexomedine ointment (Specia)
   a) Hexamidine isethionate
   b) Nonoxynol-9
   c) Cholesterol
   d) Wool fat
   e) Liquid paraffin
   f) Petrolatum

There are only a few reports in the literature of skin problems due to nonoxynols [3, 4].

Table 1. Clinical data and associated positive tests in the nonoxynol-sensitive patients

Case no.	Age (years)	Sex	Atopy	Indication for antiseptic preparation	Nonoxynol-containing products used	Nonoxynols initially tested[a]	Other allergens
1	62	F	No	Varicose leg ulcers	Isobetadine dermicum, Hibitane	Nonoxynol-9, Nonoxynol-"8.3"	Wool alcohols, parabens, balsam of Peru, cetyl alcohol (20% petrolatum), chinoform
2	72	F	Yes	Arterial leg ulcers	Isobetadine dermicum, Hibitane	Nonoxynol-9	Wool alcohols, cetyl alcohol (20% petrolatum), propylene glycol (5% aqua), cetrimide (0.1% aqua)
3	75	F	No	Post-traumatic leg ulcer	Hibitane	Nonoxynol-10	Wool alcohols, asiaticoside (5% petrolatum)
4	57	F	No	Arterial leg ulcer	Isobetadine dermicum	Nonoxynol-9	Wool alcohols, eucerin (as is), iodine (0.5% aqua)
5	73	M	No	Traumatic injury (forearm)	Isobetadine dermicum	Nonoxynol-9	None
6	58	M	No	Ulcer on right foot (diabetic)	Isobetadine dermicum	Nonoxynol-9	Neomycin, chloramine (0.1% aqua)
7	63	M	No	Venous leg ulcer	Isobetadine dermicum, Hexomedine ointment	Nonoxynol-9	Wool alcohols, aftershave lotion

[a] All tested in 2% aqua.

References

1. CTFA (1982) Cosmetic Ingredient Dictionary, 3rd edn. Cosmetic, Toiletry and Fragrance Association, Washington DC, pp 181–184, 187–188
2. Martindale, The Extra Pharmacopoeia (1982) 28th edn. The Pharmaceutical Press, London, pp 373–374
3. Meding B (1985) Occupational contact dermatitis from nonylphenolpoly-glycolether. Contact Dermatitis 13: 122–123
4. Nethercott JR, Laurence MJ (1984) Allergic contact dermatitis due to nonylphenol ethoxylate (nonoxynol-6). Contact Dermatitis 10: 235–239

Addresses

A. Dooms-Goossens
Department of Medical Research (Dermatology), Katholieke Universiteit Leuven, B-3000 Leuven, Belgium

A. Gidi de Alam
Department of Medical Research (Dermatology), Katholieke Universiteit Leuven, B-3000 Leuven, Belgium

H. Degreef
Department of Medical Research (Dermatology), Katholieke Universiteit Leuven, B-3000 Leuven, Belgium

Preservatives in Geneva

F. Pasche and N. Hunziker

Summary

Between January 1984 and September 1986, we conducted epicutaneous testing on 1000 patients with suspected allergic contact dermatitis, and between October 1986 and December 1987 on 800 patients. The number of positive reactions to formaldehyde, parabens, and mercury seemed high to us compared with what was published by certain authors. This is due to the still widespread use of formaldehyde and parabens in the environment, and to the presence in Swiss homes and hospitals of mercury-containing products. Among the 800 patients tested between October 1986 and December 1987, we observed 29 positive reactions to Kathon CG (3.6%). The increased use of this preservative in cosmetics since the 1970s may possibly explain the high sensitization rate observed.

Key words:

Mercury - Patch testing - Formaldehyde - Kathon CG - Parabens

Introduction

Between January 1984 and September 1986, we conducted epicutaneous testing on 1000 patients with suspected allergic contact dermatitis (group 1); between October 1986 and December 1987, we conducted a second set of tests on 800 patients (group 2). Our tests focused on the positive reactions to the preservatives formaldehyde, parabens, and mercury. For the second set of tests, we also studied Kathon CG sensitization. In this study, we compare our sensitization rates with results from other countries, previously published, and discuss some possible sources of sensitization.

Material and Methods

All our patients were routinely patch-tested with our standard series of epicutaneous tests (Hermal-Chemie, FRG), to which we added Kathon CG at 100 ppm in aqua (prepared by W. Griffith, Pharmacie Centrale, Hôpital Cantonal Universitaire). The patch system was Finn Chamber, and patch testing was carried out according to International Contact Dermatitis Research Group (ICDRG) recommendations.

Results

The number of positive reactions to each preservative and the sensitization rates are all given in Table 1. We added together all the observed positive reactions to preservatives and compared the total with the positive reactions to nickel sulfate 5% (Table 2). The sensitization rates for both groups are within the same range. For nickel, 80% of the positive reactions were encountered in women, whereas we found an equal number of men and women with positive reactions to preservatives. In Table 3, our test results are compared with those of studies carried out since 1970 in other European countries and in the United States.

Table 1. Results of patch tests with preservatives

Preservative	Positive reactions			
	Group 1[a]		Group 2[b]	
	n	%	*n*	%
Mercury 1%	173	18.0	68	8.5
Formaldehyde 1%	140	14.6	47	5.9
Paraben mix 15%	51	5.3	21	2.6
Kathon CG 100 ppm	–	–	29	3.6
Total	364	36.4	165	20.6

[a] $n=1000$.
[b] $n=800$.

Table 2. Results of patch tests with nickel

	Positive reactions			
	Group 1[a]		Group 2[b]	
	n	%	*n*	%
Nickel sulfate 5%	240	25	127	16

[a] $n=1000$.
[b] $n=420$.

Table 3. Results of patch tests with preservatives compared with those obtained in other studies

Reference	Study period	No. of patients	Positive reactions (%)			
			Formaldehyde	Paraben mix 15%	Ammoniated mercury 1%	Kathon CG 100 ppm
[8]	1970–1972	1200	4[a]	3	5	–
[8]	1972–1974	3000	3.4[a]	3.5	4.6	–
[8]	1974–1975	1900	5[a]	3.7	4.1	–
[8]	1975–1976	900–2000	3.8[a]	2.7	3.6	–
[4]	1973–1977	3225	2.5[a]	1.1	2.7	–
[7]	1973–1977	4600	2.5[a]	1.1	3.1	–
[6]	0000–0000	465	4.7[a]	1.9	3.8	–
[1]	1985	627	3.3[b]	0.3	–	–
[2]	1985	505	2[b]	0.2	–	1.4
[5]	1984	260	–	–	–	1.2
[5]	1985–1986	1034	–	–	–	2.9
[3]	1985–1986	243	–	–	–	3.3
Present study	1984–1986	1000	14.6[b]	5.3	18	–
Present study	1986–1987	800	5.9[b]	2.6	8.5	3.6

[a] Formaldehyde 2% in aqua.
[b] Formaldehyde 1% in aqua.

Discussion

We have found high sensitization rates to some preservatives in Geneva, especially as compared with what was published by certain authors [1, 2]; however, a definite decrease is observed from October 1986 on. For parabens and formaldehyde sensitization, our results are closer to some older studies, as published by Rudner [8] for the North American Contact Dermatitis Group (NACDG; see Table 3). For mercury, however, we obtained high rates of relevant positive reactions. This may be due to the wide use in households and hospitals of popular mercury-containing products, in particular an ointment and disinfectants produced and distributed by Swiss pharmaceutical firm from the area.

If the sensitization rates obtained between January 1984 and September 1986 are so elevated, it might be because they correspond to a time when we were very restrictive in selecting patients for patch testing. However, the second set of tests were conducted after the opening of our environmental center, from which time the restrictive patch-testing policy was modified.

Kathon CG is found in many cosmetics but is also encountered in industry in cooling-tower water, paper mills, latex emulsions, glues, and cutting oils. In Geneva, however, we could not trace any industrial sensitization. All the relevant cases came from the use of cosmetics, especially leave-on products. Kathon CG sensitization rates seem to be increasing in some European countries [2, 3, 5], and our results are comparable to the most recent publications.

References

1. De Groot AC, Weyland JW, Bos JD, Jagtman BA (1986) Contact allergy to preservatives (I). Contact Dermatitis 14: 120–122
2. De Groot AC, Bos JD, Jagtman BA, Bruynzeel DP, van Joost T, Weyland JW (1986) Contact allergy to preservatives - II. Contact Dermatitis 15: 218–222
3. De Groot AC (1987) Isothiazolinone preservative as important contact allergen in cosmetics. Derm Beruf Umwelt 35: 169–173
4. Hammershoy O (1980) Standard patch test results in 3,225 consecutive Danish patients from 1973 to 1977. Contact Dermatitis 6: 263–268
5. Hannuksela M (1986) Rapid increase in contact allergy to Kathon CG in Finland. Contact Dermatitis 15: 211–214
6. Meynadier J-M, Meynadier J, Colmas A, Castelain P-Y, Ducombs G, Chabeau G, Lacroix M, Martin P, Ngangu Z (1982) Allergie aux conservateurs. Ann Dermatol Venereol 109: 1017-1023
7. Romaguera C, Grimalt F (1980) Statistical and comparative study of 4,600 patients tested in Barcelona (1973–1977). Contact Dermatitis 6: 309–315
8. Rudner EJ (1977) North American Group Results. Contact Dermatitis 3: 208–209

Addresses

F. Pasche
Clinique de Dermatologie, Hôpital Cantonal Universitaire, 1211 Genève 4, Switzerland

N. Hunziker
Clinique de Dermatologie, Hôpital Cantonal Universitaire, 1211 Genève 4, Switzerland

Industrial Dermatitis Due to Kathon CG and 1-Chloro-Hydroxy-3:6:8:11:14 Pentaoxahexadecane (Acticide BG)

T. P. Kingston, R. J. G. Chalmers, and M. H. Beck

Summary

Industrial dermatitis due to sensitisation by Kathon CG and 1-chloro-hydroxy-3:6:8:11:14 pentaoxahexadecane (Acticide BG) occurred in two production line workers assembling cardboard box files. The source of sensitisation to these two biocides was a water-based paste adhesive. The sensitisation was independent and sequential. Sensitisation to Kathon CG from this source and to Acticide BG has not been previously reported.

Key words:

Kathon CG - Acticide BG - 1-chloro-hydroxy-3:6:8:11:14 pentaoxahexadecane - Industrial dermatitis

Introduction

Industrial dermatitis is a recognised hazard for workers who use adhesives. They may suffer from irritant and/or allergic contact dermatitis to one or more constituents of the adhesive. We describe two patients employed in the manufacture of box files who became sensitised to two biocides, Kathon CG and Acticide BG. These biocides were present in a water-based paste adhesive, which was used to attach a paper lining to a cardboard box frame.

Table 1. Results of patch testing at 96 h

Sustance	Reaction	
	Case 1	Case 2
ICDRG series	−	−
Other adhesive ingredients	−	−
Kathon CG 0.01% aqua	++	++
Acticide BG		
2.0% aqua	++	NT
1.0% aqua	+	NT
0.5% aqua	+	+++
2.0% petrolatum	+	NT
1.0% petrolatum	+	NT
0.5% petrolatum	±	++
0.1% petrolatum	−	++

NT, not tested.

Case Reports

Manufacturing Process. In this process, hard paper-lined and paper-covered cardboard box files are produced from a cardboard skeleton. Paper strips and squares of appropriate size are passed by hand over electrically operated rollers, which pick up a paste adhesive from a small trough. The coated papers are then pasted down into the appropriate place on the cardboard box file and smoothed down by hand. During this process, the hands of the paster are inevitably covered with the adhesive. Once the box files have been lined and covered, a metal ring is inserted into the spine, and a large clip is fixed inside by a different worker.

Case 1. A 31-year-old woman with no past history of skin disease, who was employed for 9 years as a box file coverer, developed recurrent dermatitis affecting the fingers, wrists and forearms over a period of 16 months. The dermatitis resolved when she stopped working on the production line.

Case 2. A 34-year-old woman with a past history of mild irritant hand dermatitis, who worked as a box file coverer for 11 years, developed recurrent dermatitis affecting the fingers, wrists and forearm over a period of 6 months. The dermatitis resolved when she stopped working as a coverer but returned when she worked inserting rings into box files.

Patch Testing. Both patients were tested to the International Contact Dermatitis Research Group (ICDRG) standard series and the adhesive constituents (Table 1).

Discussion

Both patients showed strongly positive reactions to two different biocides when tested at concentrations similar to those found in the adhesives to which they were exposed. Thirty control subjects showed negative reactions when tested to Acticide BG, confirming that the reactions in the two affected workers were truly allergic. Kathon CG 0.01% aqua has been included in our standard battery, as suggested by De Groot [1]; it has since been tested in over 3000 subjects at a 0.01% aqueous dilution, and a low rate of sensitisation has been found. Both patients were thus allergic to Kathon CG and Acticide BG. Subsequent enquiry revealed that the biocide used in the paste adhesive initially contained Kathon CG but was later changed by the supplier to the biocide Acticide BG, a mixture of halogenated formals and hemiformals normally used at a concentration of 0.2%–0.6% net weight. Chemical analysis of Acticide BG revealed that it is chemically unrelated to and does not contain Kathon CG.

The two patients' dermatitis resolved when they stopped working with the paste adhesive. Their sensitisation to the two biocides was independent and sequential, and their exposure to Acticide BG was relatively short (10 months and 3 months, respectively), which suggests that Acticide BG may be a potent sensitiser. In these cases, the positive reactions to Kathon CG are of direct relevance to their employment. We are not aware of any previous reports of sensitisation to Kathon CG from this source, an additive to a paste adhesive, or of allergic sensitisation to Acticide BG.

Acknowledgements. Chemical analysis of Acticide BG was kindly carried out by Prof. Sigfrid Fregert of the Department of Occupational Dermatology, University Hospital, Lund, Sweden.

References

1. De Groot A, Bos JD, Jagtman BA, Bruynzeel DP, Van Joost T, Willem Weyland J (1986) Contact allergy to preservatives – II. Contact Dermatitis 15: 218–222

Addresses

T. P. Kingston
The Skin Hospital, Quay Street, Manchester M3 3HL, UK

R. J. G. Chalmers
The Skin Hospital, Quay Street, Manchester M3 3HL, UK

M. H. Beck
The Skin Hospital, Quay Street, Manchester M3 3HL, UK

Sensitization to Kathon CG in Switzerland: Report of the Swiss Contact Dermatitis Research Group

N. Hunziker, F. Pasche, L. Bruckner-Tuderman, D. Perrenoud, R. Rufli, A. Bircher, H. Suter, and W. Thürliman

Summary

In 1987, the rate of sensitization to Kathon CG in the six main Swiss Dermatology Clinics was 3.5% (87 positive reactions in 2491 patients). In 1005 tested men, 30 positive reactions were observed (3%), and in 1486 tested women, 57 positive reactions (3.8%). In about one-third of our patients, relevance could be confirmed clinically by the disappearance of dermatitis when the use of Kathon-containing creams was discontinued, by a positive patch test reaction with the Kathon-containing cosmetic, or (in Geneva) by threshold patch testing.

Key words:

Kathon CG - Isothiazolinones - Preservative - Patch test - Cosmetics

Introduction

Since Kathon, an isothiazolinone biocide, has been widely used for several years as a preservative (industrially and in cosmetics) at levels of 7–22 ppm, we introduced Kathon CG at 15 ppm in water into our standard International Contact Dermatitis Research Group (ICDRG) patch test series in Geneva in 1984. Between 1984 and 1986, we observed 11 positive reactions in 625 patients. The rate of positive reactions (1.76%) seemed quite high to us [9]. After 1986, according to the ICDRG [10], we decided to introduce Kathon CG at 100 ppm in water (i.e., 100 ppm of active ingredient) into our standard series. As we expected, the rate of positive reactions rose to 5.5% (23 positive reactions in 420 tested patients) [11]. In order to have a comparison with what was happening in other parts of Switzerland, we enlarged our study of the incidence of sensitization to Kathon CG (100 ppm) to include the participating clinics of the Swiss Contact Dermatitis Research Group.

Material and Methods

In 1987, six University Dermatology Departments (Geneva, Lausanne, Basel, Bern, and Zürich Stadtpoliklinik and Universitätsklinik) participated in the study. Of the 2491 patients referred for patch testing, most had suspected contact dermatitis. A patch test with Kathon CG at 100 ppm in water was included in the standard series. The reactions were observed after 48 and 72 h and scored by dermatologists according to international criteria. Kathon CG was supplied by Rohm and Haas (Deutschland GmbH). The solutions of active ingredients were prepared by W. Griffiths (pharmacy, Geneva University Hospital) [4]. In Geneva, among the patients presenting with positive reactions to Kathon CG (100 ppm in water), we tested 15 patients with serial dilutions (50, 25, 15, and 7 ppm) and with the Trolab-Hermal Kathon CG test solution containing 0.01% of active ingredients in water (corresponding to 100 ppm in water).

Results

The incidence of sensitization to Kathon CG in Geneva, Lausanne, Basel, Bern, and Zürich is reported for the year 1987 in Table 1: in 2491 tested patients, 87 positive reactions were observed. The mean rate was 3.5%, the rate of positive reactions varying from 2.5% (Zürich Universitätskinik) to 6.2% (Zürich Stadtpoliklinik). We observed 30 positive reactions in 1005 tested men (rate 3%) and 57 positive reactions in 1486 tested women (rate 3.8%) (Table 2). The difference is not statistically significant. However, more women than men presented a positive reaction to Kathon CG in Lausanne, Zürich (Universitätsklinik), and Geneva (Table 2).

Most of the patients with a positive reaction to Kathon CG had eczema of the hand and/or face. In Lausanne, the source of exposure was ascertained in two of five patients, with a positive reaction to Kathon CG and probably ascertained in the other three patients. In Basel, 2 of 17 positive reactions to Kathon CG were relevant, and 4 of 17 were possibly relevant. In Bern, two of five patients with a positive reaction to Kathon CG had a positive reaction to two different leave-on creams, probably containing Kathon CG. In Zürich (Stadtpoliklinik), three of six patients

Table 1. Incidence of sensitization to Kathon CG (100 ppm in water) in six Swiss Clinics

Clinic	No. of patients	Positive reactions	
		n	%
Geneva	726	25	3.4
Lausanne	176	5	2.8
Basel	368	17	4.6
Bern	182	10	5.5
Zürich (Stadtpoliklinik)	97	6	6.2
Zürich (Universitätsklinik)	942	24	2.5
Total/overall	2491	87	3.5

Table 2. Incidence of sensitization to Kathon CG in men and women

Clinic	Men			Women		
	No. of patients	Positive reactions		No. of patients	Positive reactions	
		n	%		*n*	%
Geneva	326	9	2.8	400	16	4
Lausanne	65	1	1.5	111	4	3.6
Basel	153	7	4.6	215	10	4.5
Bern	81	6	7.4	101	4	3.4
Zürich (Stadtpoliklinik)	54	3	5.8	43	3	6.9
Zürich (Universitätsklinik)	326	4	1.2	616	20	3.3
Total/overall	1005	30	3.0	1486	57	3.8

Table 3. Results of patch tests with decreasing concentrations of Kathon CG

Case no.	Sex	Age (years)	Results according to concentration					
			Trolab 0.01%	100 ppm	50 ppm	25 ppm	15 ppm	7 ppm
1	F	48	+	+	+	+	+	−
2	M	30	++	++	+	+	+	+
3	F	79	++	++	++	+	+	+?
4	M	38	+++	++	++	++	+	−
5	F	28	++	++	++	+	+	+?
6	F	47	+++	++	+	+	+?	+?
7	F	52	++	+	+	+	−	−
8	F	63	++	++	+	−	−	−
9	M	55	+	+	+	+	+	+
10	F	28	+	+	+	+	+?	+
11	F	31	++	++	++	+	+	−
12	F	18	++	++	+?	+?	+	−
13	F	38	++	++	++	++	+	+?
14	M	23	++	++	++	+	+?	+?
15	F	70	++	++	++	+	−	−

with positive reactions to Kathon CG used a lot of cosmetics; exposure to Kathon CG was therefore possible. No observation about the relevance of the reaction was reported in Zürich (Universitätsklinik).

In Geneva, it was possible to test 15 of 25 patients who showed a positive reaction to Kathon CG with decreasing concentrations of this preservative (50, 25, 15, and 7 ppm of active ingredients). All patients were still strongly positive with 50 ppm, most of them with 25 ppm, and 8 with 15 ppm; with 7 ppm, 3 were positive and 5 even presented a weak reaction. In the 15 patients, we observed a reaction with Kathon CG 0.01% (Trolab) not significantly different from the reactions produced by the solution of Kathon CG (100 ppm in water) used in this study (Table 3). In five patients, patch tests were positive with their leave-on creams containing Kathon CG, and in one patient with a shampoo containing the same preservative.

Discussion

In 1987, the mean rate of sensitization was 3.5% in Switzerland, if we accept that this Swiss multicenter study is representative of the entire country. However, the rate of positive reactions in one and the same city (Zürich) varied from 2.5% (Universitätsklinik) to 6.2% (Stadtpoliklinik). This difference could depend on the recruitment of the patients for patch testing and/or the interpretation of the reactions. In other countries, rates of positive reactions to Kathon CG 100 ppm varied: 0.5% (ICDRG) [10], 0.8% (Denmark) [8], 0.8%–0.9% (England) [12, 13], 1.9% (Sweden) [1], 3.4% (FRG) [6], and 6.1% (Italy) [14]. Shuster and Spiro [13] testing patients between 1985 and 1987 observed a low stable incidence of Kathon CG sensitivity between 0.8% and 1.1%. Nevertheless, Hannuksela [7] (1983–1986) and de Groot et al. [2, 3] (1985–1987) observed a progressive rate of sensitization to Kathon CG.

In our study, the incidence of sensitization to Kathon CG was consistently higher for women than for men in three clinics (Zürich Universitätsklinik, Lausanne, and Geneva). In two other clinics (Basel and Zürich Stadtpoliklinik), almost no difference between men and women was observed, and in Bern the incidence of sensitization to Kathon CG was higher for men than for women (Table 2). However, if we consider the Swiss Clinics overall, the incidence of sensitization, was essentially the same for women and men: 3.8% (57) of 1486 women and 3% (30) of 1005 men. We could not confirm the preponderance of women observed in other studies [6–8].

The rate of sensitization to Kathon CG in men could not be explained by any industrial exposure to the preservative (Geneva, Lausanne, Basel, Bern, Zürich Stadtpoliklinik). Most of them were using different cosmetic products. In some patients, relevance was confirmed by positive reactions after patch tests with the suspected cosmetic and by clinical observation of the disappearance of dermatitis when the use of the Kathon-containing cosmetic was discontinued. In the tracing of sensitization, we did not find any popular cosmetic containing Kathon CG to be the only cause of Kathon allergy as was observed in Finland [7], where two-thirds of the cases were attributed to the use of a popular moisturizing cream containing 19 ppm isothiazolinone.

In Geneva, threshold patch testing in 15 patients revealed positive reactions at 25, 15, and even 7 ppm (Fig. 1). These observations confirm our first study on Kathon CG (15 ppm in water), where we obtained 11 positive reactions in 625 tested patients. The relevance of these positive reactions seems obvious since Kathon CG is used in cosmetics and household products in the range of 7–25 ppm [the maximum concentration of 30 ppm active ingredient has been approved for use as a cosmetic and toiletry preservative in the European Economic Community (1976)] [6]. Our observations did not confirm that there is a practical threshold level for contact sensitization to Kathon CG situated around 25 ppm [15].

In conclusion, after the first report on cosmetic allergy to Kathon CG by Foussereau et al. [5], many reports were published about sensitization to this preservative. The rate of sensitization is 3.5% in Switzerland. This is high in comparison to other countries [1, 8, 10, 12, 13]. However, about the same rate was observed in Holland [3] and in Heidelberg [6]. We therefore have to be aware of the risk of sensitization to the isothiazolinones and have to help our patients with precise diagnostic proce-

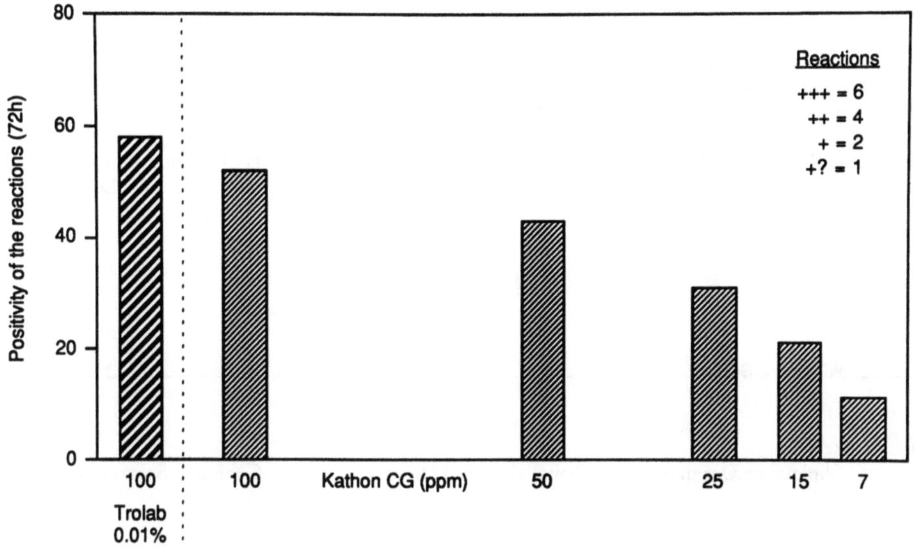

Fig. 1. Results of threshold patch testing with Kathon CG in 15 sensitized patients. The total positivity was calculated by assigning a numerical value *(top right)* to each reaction

dures and the identification of the causative agent in cosmetics and toiletries. The labelling of the ingredients and preservatives in cosmetics would be of great help.

References

1. Björkner B, Bruze M, Dahlquist I, Fregert S, Gruvberger B, Persson K (1986) Contact allergy to the preservative Kathon CG. Contact Dermatitis 14: 85–90
2. De Groot AC, Bos JD, Jagtman BA, Bruynzeel DP, Van Joost T, Weyland JW (1986) Contact allergy to preservatives – II. Contact Dermatitis 15: 218–222
3. De Groot J, Weyland W (1988) Kathon CG: a review. J Am Acad Dermatol 18: 350–358
4. Favet J, Griffiths W, Hunziker N, Amacker P-A, Schorer E (1987) Sensibilité aux tests épicutanés pour le Kathon CG et le Germal II. Pharm Acta Helv 62: 282–286
5. Foussereau J, Brandle I, Boujnah-Khouadja A (1984) Allergisches Kontaktekzem durch Isothiazolin-3-on-Derivate. Dermatosen 32: 208–211
6. Frosch PJ, Schulze-Dirks A (1987) Kontaktallergie auf Kathon CG. Hautarzt 38: 422–425
7. Hannuksela M (1986) Rapid increase in contact allergy to Kathon CG in Finland. Contact Dermatitis 15: 211–214
8. Hjorth N, Roed-Petersen J (1986) Patch test sensitivity to Kathon CG. Contact Dermatitis 14: 155–157
9. Hunziker N, Favet J, Griffiths W (1987) Contact sensitization to Kathon CG in Geneva. Boll Dermatol Allergol Profession 2: 145–148
10. Lewis PG (1986) Contact allergy to the preservative Kathon CG. Contact Dermatitis 14: 198–200
11. Pasche F, Hunziker N (1989) Sensitization to Kathon CG in Geneva and Switzerland. Contact Dermatitis (in press)

12. Shaw S, Wilkinson JD (1986) Kathon CG – A perspective. 8th international symposium on contact dermatitis, Cambridge
13. Shuster S, Spiro J (1987) Measurement of risk of sensitisation and its application to Kathon. Contact Dermatitis 17: 299–302
14. Tosti A, Manuzzi P, de Padova MP (1986) Contact dermatitis to Kathon CG. Contact Dermatitis 14:326–327
15. Weaver JE, Cardin CW, Maibach HI (1985) Dose-response assessments of Kathon Biocide. (I). Diagnostic use and diagnostic threshold patch testing with sensitized humans. Contact Dermatitis 12: 141–145

Addresses

N. Hunziker
Clinique de Dermatologie, Hôpital Cantonal Universitaire, 1211 Geneva 4, Switzerland

F. Pasche
Clinique de Dermatologie, Hôpital Cantonal Universitaire, 1211 Geneva 4, Switzerland

L. Bruckner-Tuderman
Dermatologische Klinik, Universitätsspital, 8091 Zürich, Switzerland

D. Perrenoud
Policlinique de Dermatologie, CHUV, 1001 Lausanne, Switzerland

R. Rufli
Dermatologische Universitätsklinik, Kantonsspital, 4031 Basel, Switzerland

A. Bircher
Dermatologische Universitätsklinik, Kantonsspital, 4031 Basel, Switzerland

H. Suter
Dermatologische Universitätsklinik, Inselspital, 3010 Bern, Switzerland

W. Thürliman
Dermatologische Stadtpoliklinik, 8004 Zürich, Switzerland

Fragrances

Summary

[illegible]

IFRA relies on data provided by industry and other sources, especially the Research Institute for Fragrance Materials Inc. (RIFM), which carries out research on fragrance ingredients for the sole purpose of establishing fragrance safety. The work of IFRA and RIFM is detailed and co-ordinated through a Joint Advisory Committee (JAC). We describe here the workings of these groups and consider the [illegible] bases available and future approaches to safety.

Fragrances are [illegible] a long history of [illegible] and are subjected to [illegible] prior to introduction. [illegible] chemical composition and the degree

Data Generation for Perfume Ingredient Safety Evaluation

M. A. Cooke, P. A. Cadby, and R. G. Harrison

Summary

There is minimal legislation referring to perfumes as such, but regulations concerning chemicals in general and cosmetics and toiletries in particular contain many items which may be referable to perfumes. In addition, the fragrance industry has established a system of industry self-regulation. This is based on the International Fragrance Association (IFRA), an association of national associations, whose Technical Advisory Committee (TAC) issues a Code of Practice for the industry and Industry Guidelines on ingredient usage.

IFRA relies on data provided by industry and other sources, especially the Research Institute for Fragrance Materials Inc. (RIFM), which carries out research on fragrance ingredients for the sole purpose of establishing fragrance safety. The work of IFRA and RIFM is detailed and co-ordinated through a Joint Advisory Committee (JAC). We describe here the workings of these groups and consider the data banks available and future approaches to safety.

Key words:

IFRA - RIFM - Perfumes - Safety

Introduction

Fragrances are, by nature and design, relatively innocuous products. Most ingredients have a long history of use, are chosen carefully and are subjected to rigorous screening prior to introduction. Even so, the chemical composition and the degree

Estimation of Exposure

Factors influencing exposure to a fragrance ingredient are as follows:

1. Its typical concentration in different types of perfumed products
2. The amount used of each type of perfumed product containing it
3. The likely extent of exposure (skin retention, penetration, etc.) resulting from normal use of each type of perfumed product containing it

A data bank of such exposure may be developed from (a) industry sales data and (b) consumer surveys.

Industry Sales Data. Fragrance sales are divided by the total population; for example, for aerosols in the United Kingdom in 1985, total units sold =697 million, total fragrance =1020 tonnes, fragrance per capita =18 g (data from British Aerosol Manufacturers). To take another example, for soaps and detergents in 1985, total tonnage =1.3 million, total fragrance =3512 tonnes, fragrance per capita =60 g (data from Soap and Detergents Industry).

However, per capita statistics suffer from several defects:

1. Non-consumers introduce a bias.
2. No idea is given of exposure in excessive users (the section of the community most at risk).
3. There is no indication of how individual ingredients which may be used selectively in certain types of products behave.

Consumer Surveys. For each type of perfumed product, the average and upper 90th precentile frequency of use in consumers can be estimated. Estimates are then needed for (a) how much of each product is used per application, (b) typical concentration of ingredient in each type of product and (c) skin retention factor for each type of product.

Typical estimates of daily skin surface retention are as follows:

	Average consumer	Excessive consumer
d-Limonene	2.5 mg	35 mg
Phenylethyl alcohol	1.5 mg	28 mg

Organisations

The Research Institute for Fragrance Materials Inc. (RIFM) was formed in the United States in 1966 to carry out definitive research on fragrance ingredients for the sole purpose of establishing fragrance safety. RIFM has compiled a computer bank of data on the majority of fragrance ingredients currently in use. The results of RIFM findings are presented as ingredient monographs published in *Food and*

Chemical Toxicology. To date, some 1500 monographs on the most frequently used fragrance materials have been prepared. Routine toxicological tests for the ingredient monograph include: (a) acute oral toxicity (rat LD_{50} or limit test), (b) acute dermal toxicity (rabbit LD_{50} or limit test), (c) dermal irritation (rabbit and human), (d) dermal sensitisation (guinea pig and human) and (e) dermal phototoxicity (photoirritation and photosensitisation).

RIFM compiles and evaluates all available data and test results but does not issue guidance on safe levels. Such interpretation is left to member companies and to the International Fragrance Association (IFRA). IFRA, with headquarters in Geneva,

Table 1. Examples of controlled materials

Potential sensitisers	
	Acetyl isovaleryl, allantroot oil, benzylidene acetone, cinnamic alcohol, cinnamic aldehyde[a], citral[a], isoeugenol, costus root oil, balsam of Peru, phenylacetaldehyde[a], verbena oil
Dermotoxic agent	
	Nitrobenzene
Potential photoallergens	
	6- and 7-Methylcoumarin, 7-methoxycoumarin, 4-methyl-7-ethoxycoumarin, musk ambrette
Phototoxic agents	
	Bergamot expressed, cumin oil, lemon oil, orange bitter oil
Neurotoxic agent	
	Acetylethyltetramethyltetralin
Depigmenting allergen	
	p-tert-butylphenol

[a] Studies by RIFM indicate that certain potential sensitisers can be quenched by other fragrance ingredients, e.g. cinnamic aldehyde by *d*-limonene. The mechanism of this is not known.

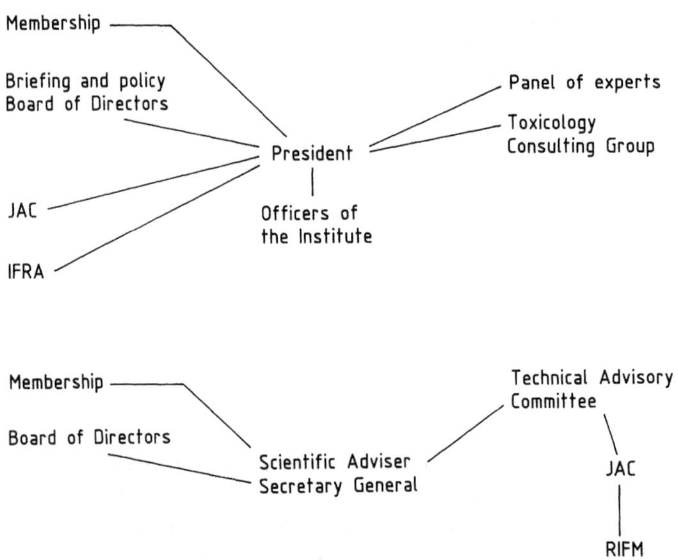

Fig. 1 a, b. Organisation charts of **a** RIFM and **b** IFRA. For abbreviations see text was formed in 1973 to ensure safety in the use of fragrance materials by promoting industry compliance with internationally agreed regulations and standards for the use of fragrances in consumer products. Membership comprises 14 national Industry Associations. IFRA has produced an Industry Code of Practice and circulates Guidelines on specific fragrance materials, limiting or prohibiting their use in response to adverse scientific evidence from RIFM or other sources. Some examples of controlled materials are given in Table 1. RIFM and IFRA interact via a Joint Advisory Committee (JAC) established in 1978 (Fig. 1).

IFRA Code of Practice. The Code of Practice issued by IFRA is a loose-leaf folder, which is periodically updated in the light of new scientific data relating to fragrance materials. It makes recommendations on the limitation or non-use of certain materials, i.e. a restricted/negative list. It also defines the Industry Code of Practice covering aspects such as definitions, good manufacturing practice and use of fragrance materials. The Code also outlines a minimum base set of toxicity tests which should be completed satisfactorily before introduction of a new fragrance chemical.

Safety

Fragrance House Controls. Fragrance creation is based on good creative practice in compliance with:

1. IFRA Code of Practice and Guidelines
2. Client-specific requirements
3. National and international legislation
   a) Toxic Substances Control Act (TOSCA, USA)
   b) Cosmetics directive (EEC)
   c) Cosmetics products (safety) regulations
   d) Regulations on notification of new chemical substances
   e) Regulations concerning classification, packaging and labelling
   f) Regulations concerning worker safety
   g) Regulations concerning animals and scientific procedures
   h) Regulations on product liability

Future Approaches. The following are examples of future approaches to safety:

1. Predictive assessment of acute toxicity of finished fragrances by modelling based on the toxicity of individual ingredients
2. Predictive assessment of dermal irritation of finished fragrances based on the irritant potential of individual ingredients
3. Estimation of the degree to which different sections of the consumer population are exposed to each fragrance ingredient
4. Establishment of data bases identifying, for all fragrance ingredients, their chemical composition, toxicological test data and any other available data of relevance to their safe use

5. Predictive safety evaluation, e.g. quantitative structure-activity relationships (QSARs; 'judgemental toxicology')
6. Reduction in animal testing (in vitro evaluation of fragrance toxicity, e.g. tissue and cell culture systems)

Addresses

M.A. Cooke
Health and Safety Unit, Department of Mechanical and Production Engineering, Aston University, Birmingham, B4 7ET, UK

P.A. Cadby
Department of Product Safety and Regulatory Affaires, Firmenich SA, Case Postale 239, CH-1211 Geneva 8, Switzerland

R.G. Harrison
Firmenich UK Limited, Hayes Road, Southhall, Middlesex UB2 5NN, UK

Preliminary Results on the Effectiveness of Two Forms of Fragrance Mix as Screening Agents for Fragrance Sensitivity

J. D. Wilkinson, K. Andersen, J. Camarasa, G. Ducombs, P. Frosch, A. Lahti, T. Menné, R. J. G. Rycroft, and I. White*

Summary

2455 consecutive patch test patients were tested to two separate fragrance mixes: one the standard 8% Hermal/Larsen fragrance mix and the other a new 9.5% Hausen mix containing dihydrocoumarin and citral but excluding oak moss and amyl cinnamaldehyde. The overall incidences of allergy to fragrance materials as measured by these mixes were 7.8% and 6.7%, respectively. There was relatively poor concordance between the mixes which could not be explained only by their different composition. False-positive reactions and false-negative reactions occurred with both types of mix. The 9.5% Hausen mix gave rather more unexplained positive results but both dihydrocoumarin and citral were found to give significant numbers of positive reactions.

Key words:

Contact dermatitis - Fragrance

Introduction

Fragrances are now ubiquitous and any individual fragrance may contain many different fragrance chemicals. Screening for fragrance sensitivity is therefore difficult and most physicians will initially usually test with one or two fragrance "markers" or "mixes" as well as individual cosmetic product as is. Balsam of Peru and wood tars are the two most widely used "markers" of fragrance sensitivity and the Larsen [2]

* members of European Environmental Contact Dermatitis Research Group

fragrance mix is nowadays included in most standard batteries. Since there are several thousand individual fragrance chemicals and since several hundred have been shown to be either actual or potential sensitisers [1, 3], it is impractical to consider screening all fragrances singly.

This study was designed to assess the frequency of fragrance sensitivity in Europe and to compare the current standard of fragrance mix (Larsen) with a new experimental fragrance mix that had been proposed by Hausen (containing citral and dihydrocoumarin but excluding oak moss and amylcinnemaldehyde) and to check the reliability of both these mixes by also testing positive reactors with the individual fragrances.

Method

The two fragrance mixes studied were (a) the Hermal (Larsen) 8% fragrance mix and (b) a 9.5% (Hausen) fragrance mix. The Hermal 8% Mix consists of cinnamyl alcohol 1%, cinnamaldehyde 1%, eugenol 1%, amyl cinnamaldehyde 1%, hydroxycitronellal 1%, geraniol 1%, isoeugenol 1% and oak moss absolute 1% with sorbitan sesquioleate as emulsifier. The Hausen 9.5% Mix contained cinnamyl alcohol 0.5%, cinnamaldehyde 0.5%, isoeugenol 1%, eugenol 1%, dihydrocoumarin 2.5%, hydroxycitronellal 2.5%, geraniol 0.5% and citral 1%.

2455 consecutive patients attending patch test clinics in England, Denmark, Spain, France, Federal Republic of Germany and Finland were, wherever possible, tested to both fragrance mixes and, when one or other of these was positive, to all the individual fragrance compounds contained in both mixes. Patch test technique and readings were as recommended by the International Contact Dermatitis Research Group and, for positive results, an assessment of clinical relevance was also made.

Results

The overall incidence of fragrance sensitivity, as measured in eight European patch test centres, was 7.8% using the Hermal/Larsen mix and 6.7% with the Hausen mix, confirming fragrances to be some of our most important environmental allergens.

In 146 patients a direct comparison of the two fragrance mixes could be made. In 32 of these the reactions were marginal or weak (± or ?+); in 114 the reactions were 1+ or greater. Marginal reactions occurred with equal frequency with both mixes (Table 1), 20 with the 8% Hermal/Larsen mix and 19 with the 9.5% Hausen mix. Of these "marginal" reactions, 25 were regarded as being irritant, 10 having been tested and found negative to individual fragrances. Seven individuals with only marginal reactions to a fragrance mix were, however, found to be positive to one or other fragrance material. Of these, three only gave marginal reactions but four gave solid positive reactions: one to eugenol (current relevance), two to geraniol and citral (past relevance) and one to isoeugenol (relevance unknown). Among the 114 patients with solid reactions to one or other fragrance mix, 78 were tested to in-

Table 1. Fragrance study of the European Environmental Contact Dermatitis Research Group: marginal reactions

32 "marginal" reactions < 20 to 8% mix; 19 to 9.5% mix

15 not tested: irritant
10 negative to individual fragrances: irritant
7 *positive* to individual fragrances:
- 3 "marginal": 1ir, 1 ir/ad, 1ao (oak moss)
- 4 "positives": 1ac (eugenol)
  2ao (geraniol and citral)
  1ad (isoeugenol)

ir, irritant reaction; ac, current relevance; ao, past relevance; ad, relevance unknown; 8% mix, Hermal/Larsen 8% mix; 9.5% mix, Hausen 9.5% fragrance mix

Table 2. Fragrance study: reactions to individual fragrances: positive reactions

53 positive to individual fragrances	8% mix' +ve/9.5%-ve: 12(5ac,1ao, 4ad/ir) Both mixes positive: 29 9.5% mix +ve/8% mix-ve: 12(8ac,1ao, 3ad)

Abbreviations, see Table 1

Table 3. Frequence of positive reactions to individual fragrance substances

Ingredient	No. of positive reactions
Isoeugenol 2% pet.	16
Citral 2% pet.	13
Dihydrocoumarin 5% pet.	11
Cinnemaldehyde 1% pet.	10
Eugenol 2% pet.	8
Hydroxycitronellal 5% pet.	7
Oak moss absolute 2% pet.	6
Cinnamylalcohol 1% pet.	5
Geraniol 1% pet.	4
Amylcinnamaldehyde 2% pet.	2
Sorbitan sesquioleate 2% pet.	2

dividual fragrance materials. Fifty-three were positive to one or more individual fragrance ingredients; 25 were negative. Of these 25 that were positive to a mix but negative to individual fragrances, 11 had shown positive reactions to both mixes, four were positive only to the 8% Hermal/Larsen mix and ten were positive only to the 9.5% Hausen mix. It is presumed that the majority of these were false-positive reactions, although the possibility of compound allergy in some cases cannot be ruled out. Of the 53 individuals found to be allergic to one or more individual fragrance chemical, 29 had been positive with both mixes and the number of false-positive and false-negative results appeared to be the same with both types of mix (Table 2).

The results of testing with individual fragrance chemicals is given in Table 3. In comparing the two mixes, discordant results (95) were as frequent as concordant (96) and a positive reaction to an individual fragrance was nearly as common in discordant (39%) as in concordant (43%) results.

Discussion

Fragrance remains an important sensitiser in both men and women. Screening with individual fragrances is both time-consuming and impractical and may give rise to multiple positive reactions and excited skin syndrome. The development of a fragrance mix [2] has made the screening of such patients much easier but there remains some anxiety over the irritant potential of such mixes and a suspicion that not all fragrant-sensitive patients will be detected by this method. The present investigation was conducted to establish the frequency of positive reactions to fragrance throughout Europe and to correlate fragrance mix positive results with the results of testing to individual fragrances.

There were frequent discordant reactions between both types of fragrance mix. This can only partially be explained by the presence of dihydrocoumarin and citral in the 9.5% Hausen mix and the presence of oak moss, sorbitan sesquioleate and amyl cinnamaldehyde in the 8% Hermal/Larsen mix.

Marginal and irritant reactions were seen with both types of mix but our study shows that not all marginal reactions can be dismissed as being irritant since some patients were found to have significant and clinically relevant sensitivities when tested to individual fragrance materials. In some cases fragrance sensitivity was detected with one mix and not the other, even when the sensitising components were present in both. Missed sensitivities may therefore be just as important as false-positive reactions when testing with either of these mixes. Although the number of marginal/irritant reactions and the "pick-up" rate were approximately equal with both types of mix, there were more unsubstantiated positive reactions with the 9.5% Hausen mix, suggesting that this may be somewhat irritant in some individuals. Citral and dihydrocoumarin, however, would both appear to be important fragrance allergens which are missed with the current Hermal/Larsen mix.

Fragrance mixes remain imperfect detectors of fragrance allergy. Both false-positive and false-negative reactions are quite common. Although imperfect, they remain, however, the best method we have to screen for fragrance sensitivity. Much work, however, remains to be done to improve the quality and reproducibility of these mixes.

References

1. Fisher AA (1975) Patch testing with perfume ingredients. Contact Dermatitis 1: 166–168
2. Larsen WG (1977) Perfume dermatitis. A study of 20 patients. Arch Dermatol 113: 623–626
3. Opdyke DL (1975) The safety of fragrance ingredients. Br J Dermatol 93: 351

Addresses

J. D. Wilkinson
Department of Dermatology, Wycombe General Hospital, High Wycombe, Buckinghamshire HP11 2TT, UK

K. Andersen
Department of Dermatology, Algade 33, DK-4000 Roskilde, Denmark

J. Camarasa
Department of Dermatology, Hospital de N. S. del Mar, Paseo Maritimo S/n, 08003 Barcelona, Spain

G. Ducombs
Service de Dermatologie, Hopital Pellegrin, Place Amélie Raba-Leon 33076, Bordeaux Cedex, France

P. Frosch
Abteilung Dermatologie, Ruprecht-Karls-Universität Heidelberg, Voßstraße 2, D-6900 Heidelberg 1, West Germany

A. Lahti
Department of Dermatology, University of Oulu, SF-90220 Oulu 22, Finland

T. Menné
Department of Dermatology, Kas-Gentofte, N. Andersenvej, 63, DK-2900 Hellerup, Denmark

R. J. G. Rycroft
St. John's Hospital for Diseases of the Skin, 5 Lisle Street, London WC2H 7BJ, UK

I. White
St. John's Hospital for Diseases of the Skin, 5 Lisle Street, London WC2H 7BJ, UK

Rubber

Condoms and Rubber Allergy: A Preliminary Report of a New "Hypoallergenic" Condom

M. Rademaker and A. Forsyth

Summary

Contact dermatitis to rubber condoms is well recognised. In an attempt to develop a rubber condom suitable for use by rubber-sensitive individuals, a "hypoallergenic" condom was manufactured. This condom was washed in ammonia to reduce the residues of rubber accelerators. Twenty-one rubber-sensitive patients were patch-tested with the washed condom, as were a similar number of non-rubber-sensitive controls. Of the 21 rubber-sensitive patients, 6 (29%) had a positive reaction to the new rubber condom; none of the control patients had a positive reaction. Washing rubber condoms in ammonia does not appear to reduce the residues of rubber accelerators sufficiently for their use by rubber-sensitive individuals. A "non-allergenic" condom is required.

Key words:

Contact dermatitis - Condoms - Rubber sensitivity

Introduction

With the increasing public awareness of the human immunodeficiency virus, AIDS, and the various high-profile campaigns for safer sex, the use of rubber condoms has increased over the last 2 years. As contact dermatitis to rubber accounts for 5%–10% of patients patch-tested [1–4], it is likely that there will be a similar increase in the incidence of contact dermatitis to rubber condoms. The need for the development of a non- or hypoallergenic condom is therefore obvious. We have assessed a new, hypoallergenic, rubber condom in a group of rubber-sensitive patients.

Materials and Methods

The hypoallergenic condom was manufactured in identical fashion to, and from the same raw ingredients as, ordinary condoms; only at the end of the manufacturing process was the handling different. The hypoallergenic condom was washed in a 5% aqueous solution of ammonia for 24 h in an attempt to leach out any known sensitisers and then repeatedly rinsed in water.

We patch-tested known rubber-sensitive individuals (positive patch tests and relevant history) and a group of non-rubber-sensitive controls (negative patch tests and no suggestive history) both to the inner and outer surface of the washed condom (without lubricant) and to the inner and outer surface of an ordinary, non-washed, condom.

Twenty-one rubber-sensitive patients (14 female, 7 male; age 45 years, range 16–67 years) were studied. Most (13/21) had a hand eczema secondary to rubber gloves, although some (6/21) had a rubber footwear dermatitis. Of the 21 patients, 16 were allergic to thiram mix, 6 to mercapto mix and 6 to carba mix. The same number of patients undergoing routine patch testing, who had no history suggestive of rubber allergy and who had negative rubber patch tests, were used as controls.

Results

In total, nine of the rubber-sensitive patients reacted to the condoms (three to the new condom only, three to the ordinary condom only and three to both). Of the six patients who reacted to the new (washed) rubber sheath, three reacted to the outer surface, one to the inner surface and the remaining two to both surfaces. Similarly, of the six patients who reacted to the ordinary (non-washed) condom, three did so to the outer surface, one to the inner surface and two to both surfaces. Of these nine rubber-sensitive patients, six were allergic to thiuram mix only, one to thiuram mix and mercapto mix, one to thiuram mix and carba mix, and one to mercapto mix only. None of the 21 controls reacted to either the new (washed) condom or the ordinary (non-washed) condom.

Discussion

Contact dermatitis to rubber is a substantial clinical problem, with 5%–10% [1–4] of all patients patch-tested being allergic to rubber compounds. The incidence of contact dermatitis to rubber condoms [5, 6] is less well established, although Hindson reported 43 cases over a 10-year period at St John's Hospital, in London [6]. The sensitisers were tetramethylthiuram disulphide (28/38), mercaptobenzothiazole (6/38) and zinc dithiocarbamate (6/19).

Currently, thiuram is no longer used as an accelerator in rubber used for condom manufacture, although it is usually added as a preservative (0.05% concentration) at the point of extraction of the rubber latex. Condoms manufactured in this country have low residues of carbamates (ZBUD 0.20%–0.25% and zinc dithiocarbamate 0.12%–0.15%), although they can still give rise to problems. In an attempt to reduce these residues even further, the manufacturers have washed the finished condom in a 5% ammonia solution for 24 h. This has the drawback of reducing the shelf life of the sheath from 5 years to 18 months. From the results of this study, however, it is obvious that washing the sheath in ammonia is insufficient for those individuals who have already been sensitised to the rubber accelerators. Whether the washed condom is less likely to cause primary sensitisation to rubber accelerators remains to be seen, but this would seem likely.

What alternatives does the socially conscious rubber-sensitive patient have? Non-rubber condoms (e.g. sheep gut) do exist, but there is concern as to how impervious they are to viral particles. We can therefore only hope that the industry becomes aware of the need for a non-allergenic condom.

Acknowledgements. We are grateful to the London Rubber Company for supplying the condoms.

References

1. Nurse DS (1979) Rubber sensitivity. Aust J Dermatol 20: 31–33
2. North American Contact Dermatitis Group (Rudner EJ et al.) (1973) Epidemiology of contact dermatitis in North America: 1972. Arch Dermatol 108: 537–540
3. Cronin E (1980) Contact Dermatitis. Churchill Livingston, Edinburgh, pp 714–770
4. Taylor JS (1986) Rubber. In: Fisher AA (ed) Contact Dermatitis, 3rd edn. Lea and Febiger, Philadelphia, pp 603–643
5. Wilson HTH (1969) Rubber dermatitis. An investigation of 106 cases of contact dermatitis caused by rubber. Br J Dermatol 81: 175–179
6. Hindson TC (1966) Studies in contact dermatitis. xvi Contraceptives. Trans St John's Hosp Dermatol Soc 52: 1–9

Addresses

M. Rademaker
Contact Dermatitis Investigation Unit, Belvidere Hospital, Glasgow, Scotland, UK

A. Forsyth
Contact Dermatitis Investigation Unit, Belvidere Hospital, Glasgow, Scotland, UK

Carba Mix: A Useful Indicator of Rubber Sensitivity

M. Rademaker and A. Forsyth

Summary

The value of carba mix as a contact allergen in the European standard battery of allergens has come under question. A retrospective analysis of data from 5986 patients undergoing patch testing revealed that, had carba mix been excluded from the standard battery, 84 cases of contact dermatitis to rubber compounds would have been missed (i.e. 1.3% of all patients patch-tested). However, during the same period there were 83 false-positive reactions to carba mix (i.e. 1.3% of all patients patch-tested). Carba mix is therefore a useful indicator of rubber sensitivity, although the high false-positive rate underlines the need for a degree of expertise and experience in reading patch tests.

Key words:

Contact dermatitis - Carba mix - Rubber sensitivity - European standard battery

Introduction

The allergens in the European standard battery of contact allergens are under regular review, and recently discussion has taken place as to the continued inclusion of carba mix in the battery. Carba mix is a known frequent irritant, and some individuals go so far as to consider that carba mix is only useful for discriminating between contact dermatitis investigators of ability (i.e. those who record carba mix reactions as irritants) and those without ability (i.e. those who record carba mix reactions as positives). We have therefore analysed the results of 7 years of patch testing to determine whether carba mix was of value as an indicator of rubber sensitivity.

Materials and Methods

The data from 5986 patients patch-tested between 1981 and 1987 at the regional contact dermatitis investigation unit, Belvidere Hospital, Glasgow, were analysed retrospectively. Following an in-depth questionnaire administered by nursing staff and a shorter interview by a dermatologist, each patient, had the current European standard battery applied, in addition to any other batteries considered relevant. The patch tests were read at 48 and 96 h; further test batteries and break-downs were applied at 48 h if indicated. Reactions were graded according to the International Contact Dermatitis Research Group (ICDRG) recommendations. The relevance of each positive reaction was determined by the appearance of the reaction, the appropriateness of the positive reaction to the presenting clinical history, and flaring of the patient's dermatosis during the patch-testing procedure.

The case notes of all patients who had a positive (i.e. +, + + or + + +) or irritant (i) reaction to carba mix at 96 h were analysed. The following information was extracted for each patient: demographic details, site of dermatosis, referral diagnosis, patch test results, relevance and the likely responsible contact item.

Results

Table 1 indicates the total number of patients who gave a positive or irritant reaction to the three rubber mixes in the European battery. Of the 324 patients who were carba mix positive at 96 h, 200 had an additional positive reaction to thiuram and/or mercapto mix at either 48 or 96 h. In other words, in 124 patients the only evidence of possible rubber sensitivity was a positive carba mix reaction at 96 h. Similarly, 21 of the 64 patients who had an irritant reaction to carba mix at 96 h were thiuram and/or mercapto mix positive as well (i.e. only 43 patients had solely carba mix irritant reactions). These 124 patients with carba-mix-positive and 43 with irritant reactions made up the study population (94 men and 73 women; mean age 45 years, range 13–87 years). The carba mix break-down was applied to 108 of the 124 patients in the carba-mix-positive group and to 36 of the 43 in the carba mix irritant group (Table 2).

Of the 124 carba-mix-positive reactions, 58 were considered relevant, 25 probably relevant and 10 not relevant, and in the remaining 31 patients the relevance could

Table 1. Rubber-mix-positive and irritant reactions ($n=5986$)

Rubber mix	Reaction			Total	
	Positive		Irritants (*n*)	*n*	%
	n	%			
Thiuram mix	383	6.4	14	397	6.6
Mercapto mix	162	2.7	14	176	2.9
Carba mix	324	5.4	64	388	6.5
Carba mix only	124	2.1	43	167	2.8

Table 2. Results of carba mix break-down applied to patients with carba mix-positive or irritant reactions

Substance	Reaction	Group (*n*)	
		Positive	Irritant
DPG 1%	ND	16	7
	−	13	20
	+	87	4
	i	8	12
ZDC 1%	ND	16	7
	−	96	35
	+	12	1
	i	0	0
ZBC 1%	ND	16	7
	−	95	36
	+	12	0
	i	1	0

DPG, 1,3-diphenylguanidine; ZDC, bis(diethyldithiocarbamato) zinc; ZBC, bis(dibutyldithiocarbamato) zinc; ND, not done; −, negative; +, positive; i, irritant

Table 3. Site of primary dermatosis in patients with carba mix-positive ($n = 124$)

Site	Group				Reaction[a]			
	Positive		Irritant		True-positive		False-positive	
	n	%	*n*	%	*n*	%	*n*	%
Hands	43	35	16	37	32	39	27	32
Feet	17	14	5	12	13	16	9	11
Legs	8	6	1	2	7	8	2	2
Arms	5	4	3	7	3	4	5	6
Limbs	12	10	0	0	9	11	3	4
Trunk	17	14	8	19	15	18	10	12
Generalised	25	20	9	21	12	14	22	26
Face	20	16	10	23	14	17	16	19
Head	11	9	1	2	5	6	7	8
Other	6	5	0	0	1	1	5	6

[a] There were 84 true-positive and 83 false-positive reactions.

not be established. In the carba mix irritant group, only 1 of the 43 patients was considered to have a possible rubber sensitivity, the remainder all being not relevant. Thus, in total, there were 84 cases (58 relevant + 25 probable + 1 with irritant reaction) of contact dermatitis to rubber which would have been missed had carba mix been excluded from the European battery (i.e. 1.3% of all cases patch-tested). During the same period, there were 83 cases (10 not relevant + 31 unknown + 42 with irritant reaction) where the carba mix reaction was potentially misleading (i.e. 1.3% of all cases patch-tested). On comparing the two groups, relevant (true-positive) against misleading (false-positive) carba mix reactions, there was no significant difference with respect to sex of the patient, age, occupation or site of dermatosis, except for the combination of relevance and site of dermatosis in women (χ^2 test $P=0.03$). Table 3 summarises the primary site of the dermatosis in both groups.

Discussion

Although the carbamates are frequently present in domestic rubber such as gloves, clothing and bedding, there have been few reports of carba-mix-only positive reactions [1, 2]. Cronin [1] found 31 cases of isolated carba mix reaction compared with 154 patients who were carba mix and thiuram mix positive. She thought that this was due to the similar chemical structure of the two groups of chemicals. Cronin further points out that the sensitiser in the carba mix-only positive patient was usually diphenylguanidine, which our results certainly confirm. Carba mix is well recognised as a frequent irritant (the irritant component of the mix being the 1% diphenylguanidine), and the routine use of the carba mix break-down battery may be helpful in distinguishing true-positive from irritant reactions.

Despite the high level of false-positive reactions, we feel that carba mix is invaluable as a general indicator of rubber sensitivity. In particular, had carba mix been excluded from the standard battery, 84 cases (1.3% of all patients patch-tested) of contact dermatitis to rubber would have been missed. We therefore feel that carba mix should remain in the European standard battery of allergens.

References

1. Cronin E (1980) Contact Dermatitis. Churchill Livingston, Edinburgh, pp 714–770
2. Taylor JS (1986) Rubber. In: Fisher AA (ed) Contact dermatitis, 3rd edn. Lea and Febiger, Philadelphia, pp 603–643

Addresses

M. Rademaker
Contact Dermatitis Investigation Unit, Belvidere Hospital, Glasgow, Scotland, UK

A. Forsyth
Contact Dermatitis Investigation Unit, Belvidere Hospital, Glasgow, Scotland, UK

Plants

Contact Sensitivity to *Anthemis* Plants

L. Fernández de Corres, I. Leanizbarrutia, and D. Muñoz

Summary

Among 12 patients with contact dermatitis from Compositae, only 3 were sensitised to *Anthemis* plants. These patients were tested with extracts from *Anthemis arvensis*, *A. cotula* and *Anthemis* mix (a mixture of both genera). The *Anthemis* mix extract at 5% produced an irritant reaction in 9 (18%) of the 50 controls; hence, we established the concentration 1% as non-irritant and suitable for testing. The skin reactions with plants gathered in spring were more intense than those with plants gathered in autumn. Extracts from the flowers produced stronger reactions than the ones obtained from the stems and the leaves, which were similar. *Anthemis arvensis* and *A. cotula* extracts lose their reactivity after reduction; hence, the allergen responsible has an aldehyde or cetonic function. On the other hand, the acetylation process elicited no change; from this we can conclude that the allergen has no alcoholic group. In thin-layer chromatography, the *Anthemis* extracts produced from plants gathered in spring show more intense and numerous spots than extracts from plants picked in autumn. The spots obtained from flowers are the most numerous and colourful. The stem has fewer fractions than the leaf.

Key words:

Allergic contact dermatitis - *Anthemis arvensis* - *Anthemis cotula*

Introduction

Allergic contact dermatitis (CD) from Compositae plants is well known, but few cases due to the *Anthemis* genus (Compositae family) have been reported. Fivoli [1] and Moslein [2] reported cases of allergic CD from *Anthemis arvensis.* L. The irritant capacity of *Anthemis cotula* L. was pointed out by several authors, although Mackoff and Dahl have reported an allergenic capacity of this plant [3]. Among our 12 patients with CD from Compositae, only 3 were sensitised to *Anthemis* plants [4].

Material and Methods

The three patients were tested with ether extracts from *A. arvensis, A. cotula* and *Anthemis* mix (a mixture of both genera) obtained according to the rapid method reported by Hausen [5]. We also tested *Anthemis* mix extracts separately from flowers, leaves and stems, and from plants gathered in spring and in autumn. The irritant threshold of *Anthemis* mix whole extracts was established by means of testing several progressive concentrations from 1% to 50% on 50 volunteers. After reduction and acetylation, extracts were also tested following Foussereau's recommendations [6]. We also studied fractions separated by thin-layer chromatography (TLC). We used silica gel 60 Merck plates and a solvent system composed of cyclohexane, chloroform and ethyl acetate (2.5:7:0.5). The spots were developed and the fractions obtained according to Hausen [7].

Results

The *Anthemis* mix extract at 5% produced an irritant reaction in 9 (18%) of 50 controls, while no reaction was observed with 1% concentration. In Table 1, it can be observed that the patch tests with *A. arvensis* and *A. cotula* extracts elicited reactions except in one case (no reaction with *A. cotula*). The skin reactions with plants gathered in spring were more intense than those with plants gathered in autumn. Extracts from flowers produced stronger reactions than the ones obtained from stems and leaves, which were similar to each other. No reaction was elicited with extracts after reduction. On the other hand, the acetylation process elicited no change.

The fractions separated by TLC are shown in Fig. 1. Few differences are observed between TLC with *A. cotula* and *A. arvensis. Anthemis* mix extracts produced from

Table 1. Patch test results (96-h readings) obtained with *Anthemis* plants (P) and extracts (E)

Allergen	Case no. 1	2	3
Anthemis mix E	++	+++	++
Spring	+++	+++	+++
Autumn	+	+++	++
Stems	++	+	++
Leaves	++	+	++
Flowers	+++	++	+++
A. arvensis P	++	+++	++
A. cotula P	–	++	++

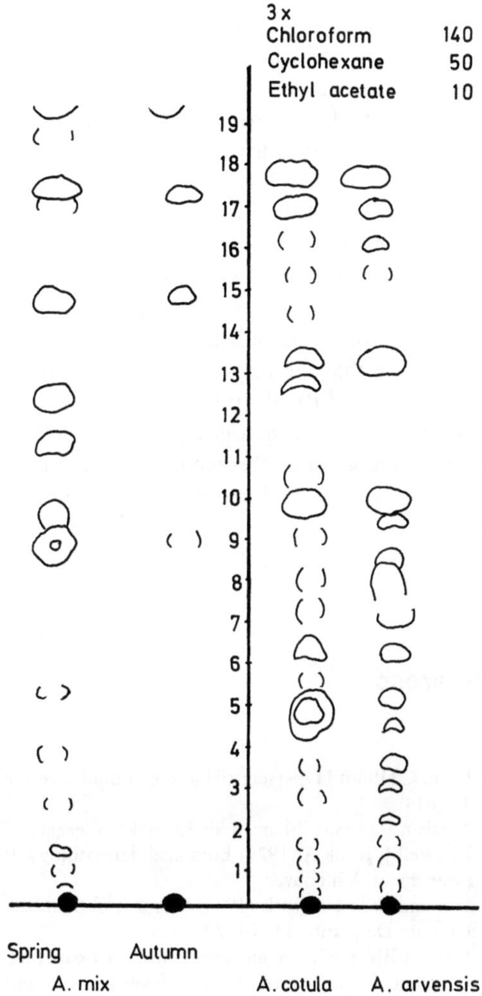

Fig. 1. Thin-layer chromatogram from *Anthemis* mix; extracts from plants gathered in spring and autumn. *Anthemis* cotula and *Anthemis* arvensis

plants gathered in spring show more intense and numerous spots than extracts from plants gathered in autumn. There are also differences between the extracts obtained from flowers, leaves and stems. The stems have fewer fractions than the leaves. The spots obtained from flowers are the most numerous and colourful.

Discussion

An *Anthemis* mix extract concentration higher than 5% is irritant (as with the helenin extract), while 1% is the suitable concentration for patch tests. The difference between patch tests with *Anthemis* plants gathered in spring and in autumn is due to the smaller concentration of antigens in the extract obtained in plants collected in autumn. Hjort [8] reported negative patch tests with *Primula obconica* gathered in winter in patients with strong sensitisation against this plant. The patch test reactions with extracts from the *Anthemis* flowers are stronger than those elicited by the leaf and stem extracts. Fivoli [1] reported positive patch tests with the leaves in sensitised patients with *A. arvensis.* Moslein [2] found similar reactions with *Anthemis* flowers and leaves. Two of our three patients have positive patch tests with *Matricaria chamomilla* [4]. Moslein [2] found positive reactions with this plant among 50% of his patients sensitised with *A. arvensis.*

As Foussereau [6] observed in *Laurus nobilis* cases, the *A. arvensis* and *A. cotula* extracts do not elicit a reaction after being treated by a reduction process. This fact suggests that the allergen responsible for the reaction is an aldehydic or cetonic group. However, after being acetylated, the extracts remained reactive; hence, we can deduce that the responsible allergen has an alcoholic function or that the alcoholic group is difficult to esterify.

While TLC chromatograms from *A. arvensis* and *A. cotula* are very similar, very clear differences are observed among the extracts produced from plants gathered in different seasons and from different parts of the plant (the flowers, leaves and stems).

References

1. Fivoli C (1936) Hypersensitivity to camomile: dermatitis and general symptoms. Dermosifilografo 11: 614
2. Moslein P (1963) Pflanzen als Kontakt-Allergene. Berufs – Dermatosen 11: 24–32
3. Mitchell J, Rook A (1979) Botanical dermatology. Plants and plant products injurious to the skin. Greengrass, Vancouver
4. Fernández de Corres L (1984) Contact dermatitis from Frullania, Compositae and other plants. Contact Dermatitis 11: 74–79
5. Hausen BM (1977) A simple method for extracting crude sesquiterpene lactones from Compositae plants for skin tests, chemical investigations and sensitizing experiments in guinea pigs. Contact Dermatitis 3: 58–60
6. Foussereau J, Benezra C, Ourisson G (1967) Contact dermatitis from Laurel. II. Chemical aspects. Trans St John's Hosp Dermatol Soc 53: 147–153
7. Hausen BM, Schulz KH (1976) Chrysanthemum allergy. III Identification of the allergens. Arch Dermatol Res 255: 111–121
8. Hjorth N (1967) Seasonal variations in contact dermatitis. Acta Dermatol Venereol 47: 409–418

Addresses

L. Fernández de Corres
Servicio de Alergología, Hospital Santiago Apostol, Olaguibel, 29, Vitoria-Gasteiz 01004, Spain

I. Leanizbarrutia
Servicio de Alergología, Hospital Santiago Apostol, Olaguibel, 29, Vitoria-Gasteiz 01004, Spain

D. Muñoz
Servicio de Alergología, Hospital Santiago Apostol, Olaguibel, 29, Vitoria-Gasteiz 01004, Spain

Allergic Contact Dermatitis from Silver Birch Pollen

G. M. Murphy and R. J. G. Rycroft

Key words:

Allergic contact dermatitis - Silver birch pollen

A 32-year-old housewife and schoolteacher presented annually from 1983 to 1986 with a seasonal April-to-September dermatitis of the exposed skin of her face, neck, and limbs, with extreme swelling of the eyelids. Her dermatitis was most severe at home, where it was not prevented by staying inside. It was improved by continuous rain, holidays by the sea, holidays abroad, and systemic steroids. She had a past history of earring dermatitis, but otherwise a completely negative personal and family history of eczema, asthma, or hay fever. She was a keen gardener.

During 1983–1986, she was admitted to hospital with severe dermatitis on three occasions; patch-tested three times and prick-tested, the tests including samples of garden plants, open tests with plant oleoresins (Hollister-Stier Laboratories), and both a patch test and a prick test with a standard birch pollen prick test solution (Bencard M2716); photopatch-tested twice; monochromator light-tested twice; biopsied; and blood-tested. The only positive or abnormal results of all these tests were positive patch tests to nickel, cobalt, and neomycin; these could not account for her seasonal dermatitis. Biopsy, late in the summer, showed chronic eczema. Her serum IgE level was normal (93 units/ml).

In February 1987, she was reviewed as an out-patient. She was depressed, despairing, and dreading the prospect of another summer. We arranged to visit her home that April, when, using the patient's own excellent botanical knowledge, we documented 67 different species of plants in her garden. There were two silver birch trees (*Betula pendula* L.). There were also silver birch trees in neighbouring gardens. Her car, parked in the driveway outside her house, was visibly coated in pollen. We arranged that she should reattend with pollen-bearing plant samples for further patch testing. Samples of her plants had already been patch-tested, but not specifically their pollens.

In May 1987, repeatedly positive open and closed patch tests with silver birch pollen (as is) were elicited at 2 and 4 days. A 20-min open patch test and a prick test with the same pollen were negative. A prick test with the same standard pollen solution was again negative. All other patch tests were negative.

The patient acquired a pollen-filtering helmet designed to protect hay fever sufferers (Hincherton Hayfever Helmet, R.H.Hinchcliffe and Sons Ltd., Pershore, Worcestershire, UK). She wore this "bubble" helmet for several hours a day during the rest of the summer, and it appeared to control her symptoms.

The patient was most recently reviewed again as an out-patient in May 1988. She had so far found it impractical to wear the helmet for longer than 3–4 h each day. She was achieving partial control of her symptoms but had required some low-dose systemic steroid therapy in addition.

Allergic contact dermatitis from primula and, more controversially, Compositae pollen has been reported before [2]. Birch pollen is familiar as a cause, via type I sensitivity, of asthma and rhinoconjunctivitis [5], as well as contact urticaria [4]. There is an association here, particularly in atopics, with type I sensitivity to apple, hazelnut, and potato [1]. Birch wood has been reported as a cause of contact dermatitis [3]. In 17 patients with atopic eczema, 6 positive patch test reactions to birch pollen have been reported, with 1 such positive reaction in 13 patients with allergic rhinitis without eczema, but no such reactions in 10 controls [7].

What has not been reported before is a case such as ours of allergic contact dermatitis from birch pollen in a non-atopic, with no evidence of type I sensitivity to birch pollen or to any other common type I allergens. Pollens may have two distinct antigens: a protein fraction causing type I sensitivity and an oleoresin causing type IV sensitivity. Like our patient, most individuals with ragweed oil dermatitis are not atopic and do not have ragweed rhinitis or asthma [6]. It is still too soon to know how effective a pollen-filtering helmet is going to be in controlling the patient's symptoms. Other preventive strategies may yet be required.

References

1. Andersen KE, Löwenstein H (1978) An investigation of the possible immunological relationship between allergen extracts from birch pollen, hazelnut, potato and apple. Contact Dermatitis 4: 73–79
2. Arlette J, Mitchell JC (1981) Compositae dermatitis. Current aspects. Contact Dermatitis 7: 129–136
3. Hausen BM (1981) Woods injurious to human health. A manual. de Gruyter, Berlin
4. Lahti A, Hannuksela M (1980) Immediate contact allergy to birch leaves and sap. Contact Dermatitis 6: 464–465
5. Larko Ö, Lindstedt G, Lundberg P-A, Mobacken H (1983) Biochemical and clinical studies in a case of contact urticaria to potato. Contact Dermatitis 9: 108–114
6. Mitchell JC, Fisher AA (1986) Dermatitis due to plants and spices. In: Contact dermatitis, 3rd edn. Lea and Febiger, Philadelphia, pp 426–427
7. Reitamo S, Visa K, Kähönen K, Käyhkö K, Stubb S, Salo OP (1986) Eczematous reactions in atopic patients caused by epicutaneous testing with inhalant allergens. Br J Dermatol 114: 303–309

Addresses

G. M. Murphy
St John's Hospital for Diseases of the Skin, 5 Lisle Street, Leicester Square, London WC2H 7BJ, UK

R. J. G. Rycroft
St John's Hospital for Diseases of the Skin, 5 Lisle Street, Leicester Square, London WC2H 7BJ, UK

Occupational Contact Dermatitis Due to *Codiaeum Variegatum* L., *Chrysanthemum indicum* L., *Chrysanthemum* x *hortorum* and *Frullania dilatata* L.

M.-B. Cleenewerck and P. Martin

Summary

This report describes a case of contact eczema in a driver-deliverer of plants and flowers. The evolution of his dermatitis was closely connected with this work. Patch tests showed positive reactions to *Codiaeum variegatum* (L.) A. Juss. var. *pictum* (Lodd.) Müll. Arg., cultivars Excellent, Mrs Iceton and Norma, to *Chrysanthemum indicum* L., *Chrysanthemum* x *hortorum*, *Frullania dilatata* L. and to balsam of Peru. Patch test results were also positive to water, methanol and ethyl acetate extracts of the leaves of the cultivar Excellent but negative to a hexane extract. Therefore, hypersensitivity included some plants that belong to three different families: Euphorbiaceae, Compositae and Hepaticae. Contact allergy to *Chrysanthemum* and to *Frullania* is well known. A few cases of allergic contact dermatitis due to *Codiaeum variegatum* have been described in the literature. This plant, often called florists croton, should not be confused with *Croton tiglium* L., or croton oil plant, which is a strong irritant to the skin. This case focused our attention on the difficulty of skin protection and the serious problem concerning the patient's occupational future.

Key words:

Occupational plant dermatitis - *Codiaeum* allergy - *Chrysanthemum* allergy - *Frullania dilatata* allergy - Plant extracts

Case Report

In December 1987 we observed a 54-year-old patient who had been working as a driver-deliverer of plants and flowers for 2 years. Two months before our examination, he developed eczema on his hands with fissured lesions of the fingertips. The eczema spread over the forearms, arms, abdomen, and thighs. The skin was erythematous, papular and intensely itchy, so he took sick leave. He had no personal or family history of atopy. The patient transported and delivered a great variety of plants and flowers without any protection for his hands. He used some sprays to keep the plants sparkling. He also worked in his own garden, which meant he had much contact with plants even outside his work.

Patch tests (for methods, see below) were performed using Finn Chambers on Scanpor tape applied for 48 h. Results are shown in Table 1.

Patch testing with other plants *(Microlepia, Dieffenbachia, Ficus, Philodendron, Nephrolepsis, Solanum, Kalanchoe, Phoenix, Yucca, Spathiphyllum, Adiantum, Schefflera, Geranium* and *Syngonium)* was negative at 48 and 72 h, and also with a shining product for green plants (Algobril), a product for protection of plants and a house cleaner (Soleil). There was a strong focal reaction when the patient underwent the tests with the plant samples.

He was seen again in May 1988. In February he had tried to resume work. A sudden relapse happened and he was forced to stop working only 4 days after starting. Once again, patch tests were carried out (Table 2).

Similar results to those of the first patch testing were obtained with *Frullania, Chrysanthemum indicum* and *Chrysanthemum* x *hortorum* Tokyo. Once again, there was a strong focal reaction on the neck, fingers and forearms (Figs. 1, 2).

Patch tests were also performed with extracts of the leaves of the cultivar Excellent. After evaporation to dryness, the aqueous extract was dissolved in water, and

Table 1. Results of skin tests

	48 h	72 h
1. ICDRG standard series Trolab Hermal Chemie completed by GERDA[a]:		
Balsam of Peru	+	++
Frullania dilatata (L.) Dum.	++	++
2. Samples of plants frequently handled by the patient		
Codiaeum variegatum (L.) A. Juss. var. *pictum* (Lodd.) Müll. Arg. cultivar Excellent (leaf)	+++	+++
Chrysanthemum indicum (L.) (leaf)	++	++
Chrysanthemum x *hortorum* Tokyo (leaf)[b]		++
(flower)[b]		++

[a] The allergens added by GERDA are: mercury, thiomersal, and *Frullania dilatata* (L.) Dum.
[b] Read at 72 h only.

Table 2. Results of the second patch testing

	48 h	72 h
Codiaeum variegatum (L.) A. Juss. var. *pictum* (Lodd.) Müll. Arg.		
cultivar Excellent (leaf)	+++	+++
cultivar Norma (leaf)	+++	+++
cultivar Mrs Iceton (leaf)	?+	+
Primula obconica Hance (leaf)	–	–
Alantolactone	–	–

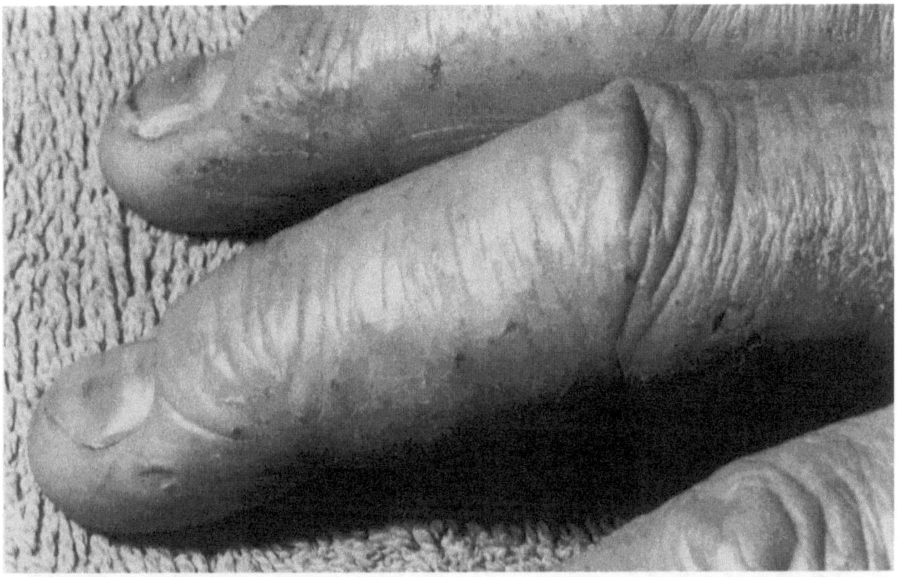

Fig. 1. Focal reaction to patch testing on the fingers

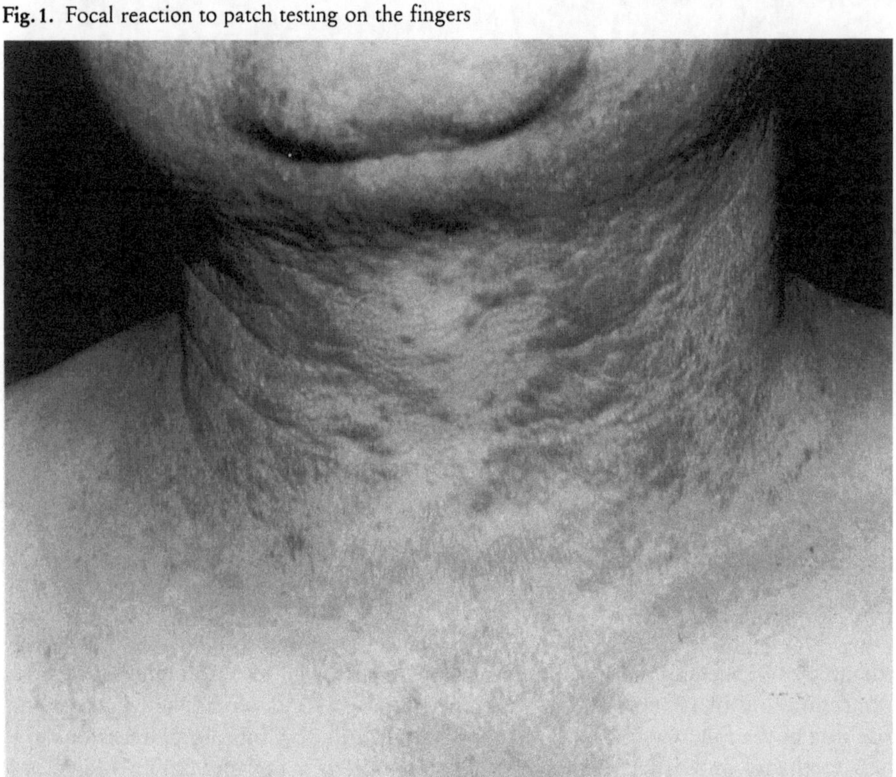

Fig. 2. Focal reaction to patch testing on the neck

Table 3. Patch test results with various extracts of leaves of *Codiaeum variegatum* (L.) A. Juss. var. *pictum* (Lodd.) Müll. Arg., cultivar Excellent

Extract		48 h	72 h
Water	10 mg/l	++	+++
	50 mg/l	++	+++
Methanol	10 mg/l	+++	+++
	50 mg/l	+++	+++
Ethyl acetate	10 mg/l	++	++
	50 mg/l	++	++
Hexane	10 mg/l	–	?+
	50 mg/l	–	–

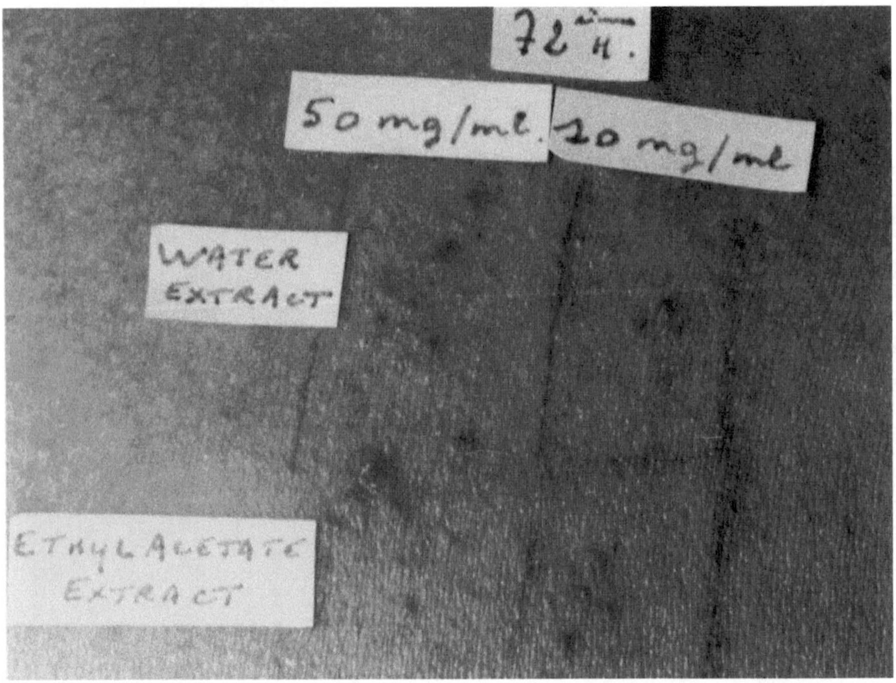

Fig. 3. Reactions after 72 h to water and ethyl acetate extracts of *Codiaeum variegatum* cultivar Excellent

methanol, ethyl acetate and hexane extracts were dissolved in absolute ethanol, all at concentrations of 10 mg/l and 50 mg/l. A volume of 20 µl was applied to the cellulose disc of the Finn Chambers on Scanpor. At 48 and 72 h there were reactions to water, methanol and ethyl acetate extracts, but not to a hexane extract (Table 3, Figs. 3, 4).

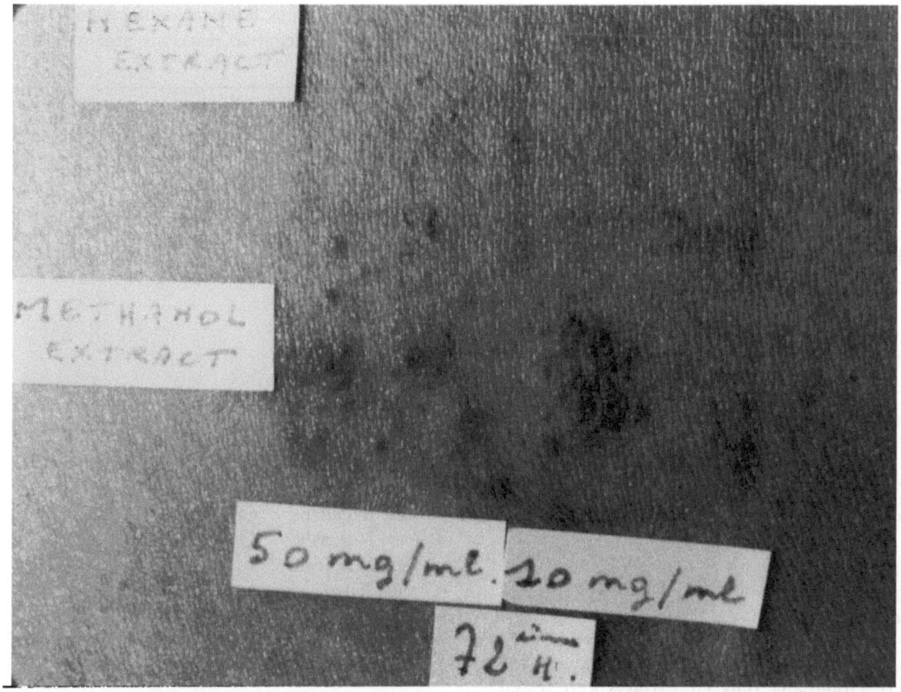

Fig. 4. Reactions after 72 h to hexane and methanol extracts of *Codiaeum* variegatum cultivar Excellent

Discussion

The results showed that the patient was allergic to *Codiaeum variegatum* L. cultivars Excellent, Norma and Mrs Iceton and to water, methanol and ethyl acetate extracts of the leaves of cultivar Excellent, but not to the hexane extract. He was also sensitive to *Chrysanthemum indicum* L., *Chrysanthemum* x *hortorum* Tokyo, *Frullania dilatata* L. and balsam of Peru. He was thus hypersensitive to plants belonging to three different families: Euphorbiaceae, Compositae (Asteraceae) and Hepaticae.

Which parts were affected (hands, forearms and arms) can be explained by his daily contact with the plants. The lesions on the abdomen resulted from his holding the plants against his body while transporting them. On the other hand, since his neck was affected but the skin under his chin, which was protected from the sun, was not, it is possible that there was also a photosensitivity reaction.

Hypersensitivity to *Chrysanthemum* and to *Frullania* is well known, and there may be cross-sensitivity to both of them [4]. The lack of reaction in the patch test with alantolactone confirms the idea of Hjorth [8]: alantolactone is unsatisfactory in routine screening tests as a test substance for Compositae allergy. Nevertheless, patch testing revealed a positive reaction to balsam of Peru, which contains the allergen farnesol [7], a precursor of sesquiterpene lactones [6]. A few cases of sensitization by *Codiaeum variegatum* have been reported in the literature (Table 4). Commonly

Table 4. Positive patch test reactions to leaves and/or stems of *Codiaeum variegatum* (L). A. Juss. var. *pictum* (Lodd.) Müll. Arg. mentioned in the literature; negative reactions obtained in control subjects

Study	No. of cases	Occupation of the patient	Plants tested	Negative control test
Agrup [1]	1	housewife	*Codiaeum variegatum*	
Tafelkruyer and van Ketel [11]	1	flower-grower	*Codiaeum variegatum*[LS]	5
Schmidt and Ølholm-Larsen [10]	4	gardeners	cv. Geduldig cv. Bravo cv. Hollufiana[a]	
Hausen and Schulz [5]	1	nursery gardener	cv. Geduldig[L] cv. Pucciana[L] cv. Florida[L]	10
Van Ketel [12]	3	flower-growers	cv. Hollufiana[LS] cv. Aucubufolia[LS] cv. Geduldig[LS] cv. Norma[LS]	3
Present study	1	driver-deliverer	cv. Excellent[L] cv. Norma[L] cv. Mrs Iceton[L]	1
Lynne-Davies and Mitchell [9]	0		*Codiaeum variegatum*[L]	2

cv., cultivar; L, leaves; S, stems.

[a] For Hollufiana, only sap extracts were tested.

[b] For Hollufiana, only the aqueous extract was positive. Patch testing with leaves and stems was negative.

called florists' croton, this popular potted plant belongs to the family Euphorbiaceae (Fig. 5). It is a beautiful tropical shrub, 0.5–2.5 m high, with highly ornamental alternate and petiolate leaves which are thick, leathery, glabrous and varied in colour, the green and yellows of the young leaves often changing later to shades of red [2]. Many cultivars[1] are available (Fig. 6). Like all Euphorbiaceae, *Codiaeum* produces a somewhat milky latex. It should not be confused with the true croton, the croton oil plant or purging croton (*Croton tiglium* L.), which is an evergreen shrub or small tree with yellowish-green leaves and small flowers. Its seeds can be used to extract croton oil which contains a toxic, vesicant, strongly irritant resin. The irritating agents of the true croton are not only present in the seeds but also in the leaves and stems [3].

Several authors have also tested extracts of *Codiaeum variegatum* (Table 5). Results of patch tests show that the unknown sensitizer is soluble in water, methanol and ethyl acetate, but insoluble in ether and hexane. Schmidt and Ølholm-Larsen

[1] The terms "cultivar" and "hybrid" should not be confused. A hybrid is the product of crossing two different species of plants which belong to the same genus or two varieties of the same species. The hybrid has the properties of the parent plants. A cultivar or clone is a variety of a plant which is obtained by cultivating slips or cells of this plant under particular conditions. In this way, one obtains, through genic or chromosomal mutations, plants with new characteristics which differ from the original plant.

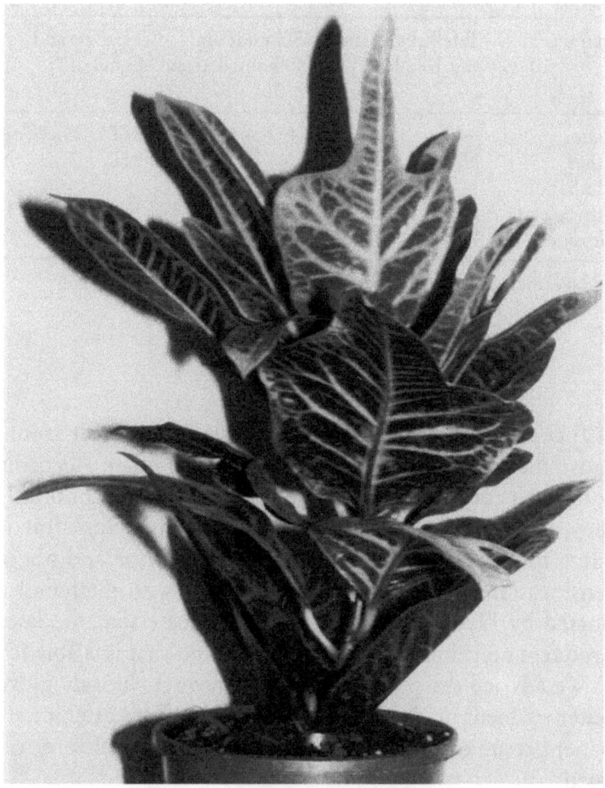

Fig. 5. *Codiaeum variegatum*

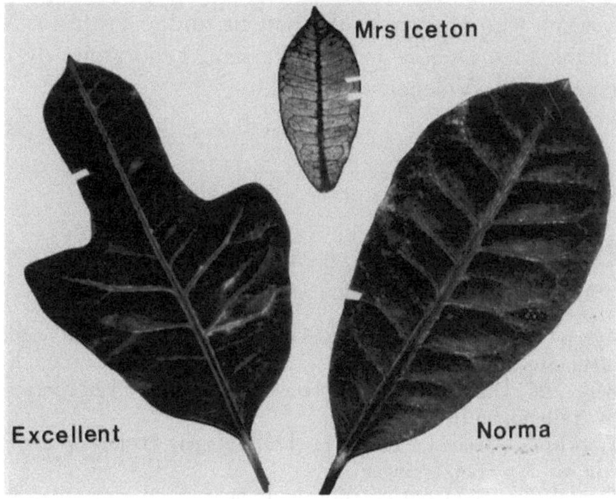

Fig. 6. Leaves of cultivars of *Codiaeum variegatum*

Table 5. Patch test results with various extracts of *Codiaeum variegatum* L.

Extract	Tafelkruyer and van Ketel [11]	Schmidt and Ølholm-Larsen [10]	Hausen and Schulz [5]	van Ketel [12]	Present study
Water	++	+++	NT	++[a]	+++
Ether	NT	–	NT	NT	NT
Methanol	–	NT	++[b]	NT	+++
Ethylacetate	NT	NT	NT	NT	++
Hexane	NT	NT	NT	NT	–

[a] Nevertheless, several negative reactions.
[b] Sensitization experiments in guinea pigs.
NT, Not tested

[10] consider that the allergenic substance(s) differ from the croton oil irritants because they are soluble in water but not in ether. According to R. Schmidt (personal communication, 1988), if there are some irritant phorbol-type esters in the extracts, they should be in the ethyl acetate and methanol fractions only. In any case, the patch test reactions in our patient were allergic and not irritant. On the other hand, sensitization experiments in guinea pigs with methanol extracts of the leaves conducted by Hausen and Schulz [5], indicate that the latex of *Codiaeum variegatum* produces no primary irritant reaction and that it is able to induce contact allergy.

We advised the patient to wear polyvinyl chloride gloves with long sleeves and an outer garment made of fine polyethylene. This attempt at protection failed when the patient resumed work. His future as a driver-deliverer of plants seems to be threatened.

Acknowledgements. We express our sincere thanks to Richard J. Schmidt and Claude Benezra for the extracts that they prepared, to Dr. Rouzé, occupational physician, who referred us this patient, and to Professor Mizon. We would like also to thank Mrs. Dubois and Mr. Vasseur, Laboratoire de Physiologie végétale, Université de Lille-Villeneuve d'Ascq.

References

1. Agrup G (1969) Hand eczema and other hand dermatoses in South Sweden. Acta Derm Venereol 49 (Suppl 61): 57
2. Benezra C, Ducombs G, Sell Y, Foussereau J (1985) Plant contact dermatitis. Decker and Mosby, Toronto, pp 162–163
3. Frerichs G, Arends G, Zörnig H (1938) Hagers Handbuch der Pharmazeutischen Praxis, 2nd edn, vol 2, p 1124. Springer
4. Gonçalo S (1987) Contact sensitivity to lichens and compositae in Frullania dermatitis. Contact Dermatitis 16: 84–86
5. Hausen BM, Schulz KH (1977) Occupational contact dermatitis due to Croton (*Codiaeum variegatum* (L.) A.Juss.var. *pictum* (Lodd.) Muell. Arg.). Contact Dermatitis 3: 289–292

6. Hendrickson JB (1959) Stereochemical implications in sesquiterpene biogenesis. Tetrahedron 7: 82–89
7. Hjorth N (1961) Eczematous allergy to balsams. Munksgaard, Copenhagen
8. Hjorth N (1970) Active sensitisation with alantolactone. Contact Dermatitis Newsletter 8: 175
9. Lynne-Davies G, Mitchell JC (1974) Patch tests for irritancy – some common house plants. Contact Dermatitis Newsletter 16: 501–502
10. Schmidt H, Ølholm-Larsen P (1977) Allergic contact dermatitis from Croton *(Codiaeum)*. Contact Dermatitis 3: 100
11. Tafelkruyer J, Van Ketel WG (1976) Sensitivity to *Codiaeum variegatum*. Contact Dermatitis 2: 288
12. Van Ketel WG (1979) Occupational contact dermatitis due to *Codiaeum variegatum* and possibly to *Aeschynantus Pulcher*. Derm Beruf Umwelt 27: 141–142

Addresses

M.-B. Cleenewerck
Comité pour le Développement de la Médecine du Travail, B.P. 1365 Lille R.P, 59015 Lille Cedex, France

P. Martin
Clinique Dermatologique C.H.R., Hôpital Claude Huriez, 59037 Lille Cedex, France

Allergic Contact Dermatitis to *Ginkgo biloba* L.: Relationship with Urushiol

J.-P. Lepoittevin, C. Benezra, and Y. Asakawa

Summary

A *Ginkgo biloba* L. fruit extract was prepared and purified. Three groups of guinea pigs were sensitized to the crude extract, anacardic acids and cardanols respectively, using Freund's complete adjuvant test (FCAT) and the fourth group to urushiol by the epicutaneous route. Each group was tested to the primary sensitizer and to the different main aromatic compounds isolated from Ginkgo fruits. Anacardic acids were found to be good sensitizers, while cardanols failed to induce allergic contact dermatitis (ACD). No cross reactions were observed among the compounds tested.

Key words:

Ginkgo biloba L. - Delayed hypersensitivity - Urushiol - Anacardic acids - Cardanols - Cardols

In our study of allergic contact dermatitis (ACD) to natural long-chain alkyl compounds we were interested in ACD to *Ginkgo biloba* L. and its related relations with urushiol. The main aromatic components of ginkgo fruits have been identified as anacardic acids, cardanols and cardols [1]. Each group consists of a complex mixture of homologues with alk(en)yl chains containing from 13 to 19 carbons and from 0 to 2 double bonds (see Fig. 1).

The close structure between ginkgolic acids and components of urushiol (the allergen of poison ivy), and cross reactions reported in the literature, have led some authors [2, 3] to suggest that alkylcatechols, resulting from in vivo biotransformation of anacardic acids in the skin could be the "actual" allergen of *Ginkgo biloba* L. (Fig. 2).

If the first step occurs spontaneously in solution (anacardic acids have been demonstrated to be the precursors of cardanols in the plant), the direct oxidation of

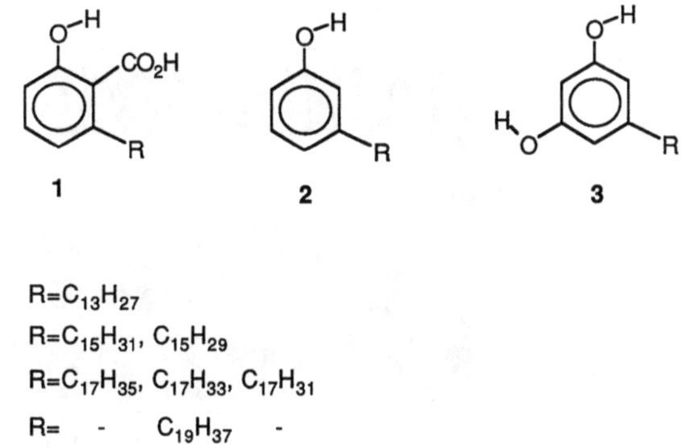

Fig. 1. Main aromatic compounds from *Ginkgo biloba* L.

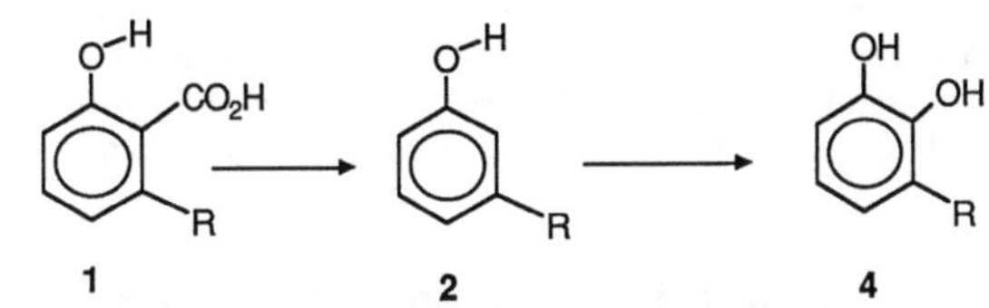

Fig. 2. Possible biotransformation of anacardic acids

cardanols to urushiol which has recently been achieved chemically (J. P. Lepoittevin, Y. Asakawa, unpublished results), is still the subject of speculation as an in vivo process.

In an attempt to determine the true structure of ginkgo allergen(s) and test the hypothesis of an in vivo biotransformation of 1, we now report the first animal sensitization studies on *Ginkgo biloba* L. components.

Material and Methods

Chemicals. The crude extract of *Ginkgo biloba* L. fruits, collected in the Tokushima area (Japan) in autumn 1984, was prepared and purified as previously reported [1].

Animal Sensitization. Female Himalayan spotted guinea pigs (Füllingsdorf, Switzerland), weighing 250–350 g, were used. Sensitization induction treatment to the crude extract, to anacardic acids and cardanols product was achieved using Freund's complete adjuvant test (FCAT); groups of eight animals were used. Guinea pigs were sensitized to urushiol epicutaneously.

Skin Testing. Skin testing was carried out as previously reported [4].

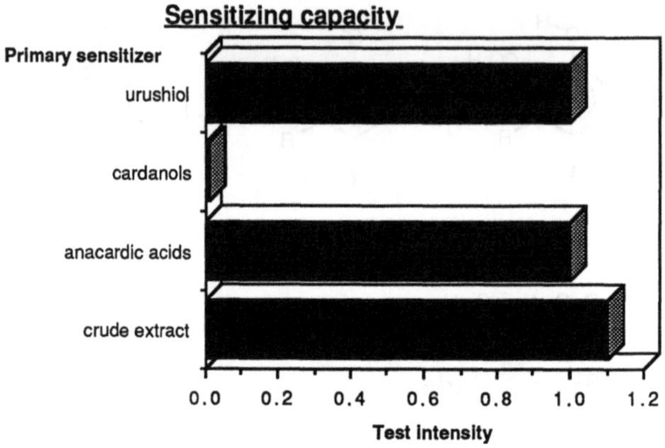

Fig. 3. Elicitation was performed by depositing 25 μL of an acetone solution (crude extract, 3%; anacardic acids, 10%; cardanols, 0.3%; urushiol, 0.05%) on the shaved flank of the animal (on a 2 cm^2 circular area) and tests were read at the 48th h using a 0 (no reaction) to 3 (strong reaction with swelling going beyond the test area). All controls were negatives

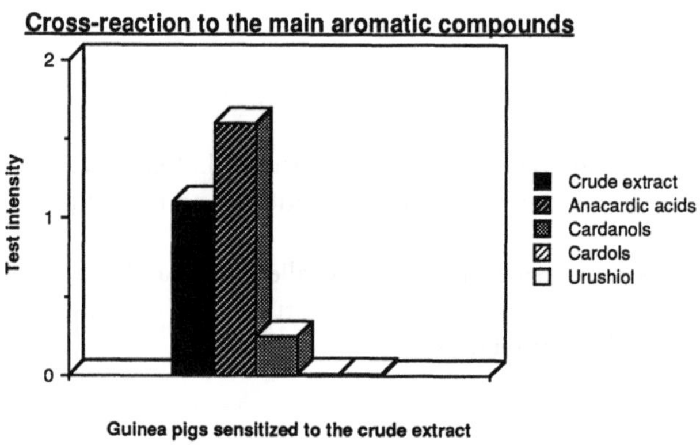

Fig. 4. Elicitation was performed as described in Fig. 3. Concentration: crude extract, 3%; anacardic acids, 10%; cardanols, 0.3%; cardols, 0.1%; urushiol, 0.05%

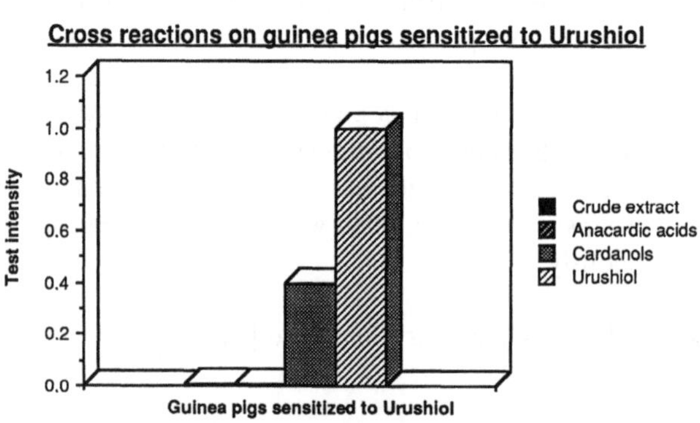

Fig. 5. Elicitation was performed as described in Fig. 3. Concentration: crude extract, 3%; anacardic acids, 10%; cardanols, 0.3%; urushiol, 0.05%

Results

Sensitization Capacity. Figure 3 shows the results of skin testing on different animal groups. Guinea pigs sensitized with the crude extract, ginkgolic acids and urushiol reacted with the primary sensitizer with a significant 1 test intensity. The group treated with cardanols showed no allergic reaction when challenged.

Cross Reactions. Except for the one observed between anacardic acids and crude extract, no clear cross reactions could be observed (Figs. 4, 5).

Discussion

It seems obvious from the above results that ginkgolic acids are the allergens of *Ginkgo biloba* L. and that the hypothesis of a biotransformation of them into catechols is not supported by the experiment.

The more surprising result of this study was the lack of cross reaction between ginkgo and urushiol, cross reactions which are often reported in the literature. Based on these observations, the hypothesis of a biotransformation of anacardic acids into catechols via cardols can no longer be supported. In addition, cardanols, which could have been the precursors of the catechols, were found to be inactive.

The results reported in the literature can be interpreted in the following ways. First, the cross reactions reported are probably true polysensitization, patients being in contact with both urushiol and ginkgo; second, the reactions observed are irritating responses; finally, metabolism in the human skin may be different from that in guinea pig skin.

References

1. Itokawa H, Totsuka N, Nakahara K, Takeya K, Lepoittevin JP, Asakawa Y (1987) Antitumor principles from *Ginkgo biloba* L. Chem Pharm Bull 35: 3016–3020
2. Birch AJ, Donovan FW (1953) Studies in relation to biosynthesis. Some possible routes to derivatives of orcinol and phloroglucinol. Aust J Chem 6: 360–368
3. Kiong LS, Thyman JHP (1981) Long chain phenol. Part 18. Conversion of anacardiac acid into urushiol. J Chem Soc Perkin I, 1942–1952
4. Papageorgiou C, Stampf J-L, Benezra C (1988) Allergic contact dermatitis to tulips: an exemple of enantiospecificity. Arch Dermatol Res 280: 5–7

Addresses

J.-P. Lepoittevin
Laboratoire de Dermatochimie associé au CNRS (UA 31), Université Louis Pasteur, Clinique Dermatologique, CHU F-67091 Strasbourg, France

C. Benezra
Laboratoire de Dermatochimie associé au CNRS (UA 31), Université Louis Pasteur, Clinique Dermatologique, CHU F-67091 Strasbourg, France

Y. Asakawa
Institute of Pharmacognosy, Tokushima Bunri University, Yamashiro-Cho, Tokushima 770, Japan

Contact Dermatitis from *Ficus carica*

G. Angelini, G. A. Vena, and C. L. Meneghini

Summary

It is known that *Ficus carica* (of the Moraceae family), a widely cultivated plant in the Mediterranean area, is able to induce various clinical skin syndromes, whose pathogenetic mechanisms are debatable. It is also well known that in the latex of *Ficus carica* two different compounds, namely ficin and furocoumarins, have been identified. In the last 2 years, we observed eight cases of contact dermatitis from *Ficus carica* with various clinical expressions. In all cases, patch tests and photopatch tests with ethanol extract of cut leaves and pure psoralens (5-methoxypsoralen, 8-methoxypsoralen, 4,5',8-trimethylpsoralen) were carried out. The use of serial dilutions (0.1%–0.0001%) of the psoralens made it possible to differentiate between phototoxic and photoallergic reactions. Three patients showed positive reactions to the extract of cut leaves and 8-methoxypsoralen down to a concentration of 0.0001%. The photopatch tests to the other psoralens were negative. Histopathological examination of the biopsy specimens from positive tests showed changes consistent with photoallergic contact dermatitis.

Key words:

Ficus carica - Phytophotodermatitis - Photoallergy - Furocoumarins

Introduction

Ficus carica, of the Moraceae family, is widely cultivated in the Mediterranean area, the Near and Middle East, and parts of India. Humans come into intimate contact with this plant and its fruits mainly as cultivators, gatherers, packers or consumers. In the latex of *Ficus carica,* two different compounds, namely ficin and furocoumarins, have been identified. Ficin is a proteolytic enzyme with irritant and pruritogenic properties [5, 7, 18, 25]. The furocoumarins present in figs include psoralen [15, 19, 22, 27], 5-methoxypsoralen, 8-methoxypsoralen [3, 6, 18, 19, 22, 27], and 4'-5'-dihydropsoralen [6]. It is known that fig trees are able to induce various clinical skin syndromes, whose pathogenetic mechanisms are debatable. In this study, an investigation by phototesting in eight cases of contact dermatitis from *Ficus carica* is reported.

Material and Methods

Study Population. In the summer and autumn of a 2-year period (1986–1987), we observed eight cases of contact dermatitis from *Ficus carica* with various clinical expressions. In all the patients, cutaneous signs of dermatitis included erythema, edema, vesicles, and bullae in different configurations. The rash usually appeared after a latent period of approx. 10–15 h and reached a maximum within the first 24 h after contact with the plant. Four of eight patients apparently showed an irritant contact dermatitis with scattered erythematovesicular and bullous lesions, mainly localized in a figured way at the limbs or trunk. Another three subjects, all farmers, presented with a severe erythematoedematous and vesicular dermatitis affecting the photoexposed areas, mainly hands, forearms, and face. These three patients had a history of relapsing attacks during the preceding summers. Finally, the eighth case concerned a 17-year-old girl who had used a decoction of fig leaves in order to get tanned. She developed an erythematobullous rash 12 h after a 30-min exposure to the sun (the exposed areas being affected).

By avoiding contact with fig trees and using wet compresses and topical steroids, the cutaneous lesions improved in all the patients in a few days, leaving hyperpigmented sequelae mainly in the last four patients.

Photopatch Tests. Using ethanol extract of cut fig leaves and three pure psoralens, namely 5-methoxypsoralen (bergapten; 5-MOP), 8-methoxypsoralen (xanthotoxin; 8-MOP) and 4,5',8-trimethylpsoralen (trioxalen; TMP) (Sigma Chemical Company, St. Louis, USA) photopatch tests were carried out. The test substances were dissolved in ethanol, and a series of dilutions were prepared. 5-MOP and 8-MOP were tested down to a concentration of 0.0001%; TMP was tested at 0.1% only. The test solutions were applied in duplicate to the backs of the patients under occlusion with the Finn chamber technique [20]. One set of tests was removed after 2 h, and the test sites were immediately irradiated with long-wave ultraviolet light (UVA) from a 150-w xenon arc lamp (Osram XBO) equipped with a Schott BG 38 filter and a window-glass filter. The dose delivered to the test sites was 1.8 J/cm^2 [17]. After irradiation, the test area was covered with opaque aluminized paper. The phototests and the ordinary patch tests were read after 48 and 72 h according to the technique recommended by Fregert et al. [10]. A test was also performed with UVA irradiation only; the test dose was 18 J/cm^2. As controls, 20 healthy volunteers were tested with the same test substances.

Histopathology. Biopsy samples for histological examination were taken in three patients from reactions to 8-MOP at 0.0001% macroscopically considered to be of allergic type.

Results

Photopatch Testing. Three of eight patients reacted to the ethanol extract of leaves and to 8-MOP and UVA down to a concentration of 0.0001%. Photopatch tests with the same substances were negative in the other five patients and in the controls. The positive patch test responses were clinically of the eczematous type, with erythema, edema, and vesicles. The three patients with positive reactions had a history of relapsing photocontact dermatitis with severe itching and erythematoedematous and vesicular lesions on hands, forearms, and face. Tests with 5-MOP and TMP and the responses to all nonirradiated test substances were negative in the patients and the controls, as was the test with UVA only.

Histopathology. The skin biopsies from positive phototest reactions to 8-MOP at 0.0001% revealed changes consistent with an allergic picture: spongiosis and exocytosis in the epidermis and a lymphocytic infiltrate in the dermis, mainly around the vessels.

Discussion

In the literature, various cases of photocontact dermatitis from fig plant have been reported [3, 4, 13, 15, 16]. The condition is not uncommon in Italy, as we observe several cases during the summer months. It is also frequent in Lebanon [27] and more common in Turkey, where about 10% of fig pickers suffer from contact dermatitis to figs [2]. The sap of the shoot or leaf of the fig tree can cause burning sensations of short duration, contact dermatitis, and lasting hyperpigmentation. Dermatitis can also be induced with a decoction of the leaves, as observed in one of our patients. The increased incidence of fig phytophotodermatitis during spring and summer can be attributed to the higher concentrations of the furocoumarins in the plant during these two seasons [22, 27], in addition to other factors that enhance the photoreaction, such as heat, humidity, and increased exposure to sunlight.

The precise pathogenetic mechanisms of the contact dermatitis are still debatable. Phototoxic dermatitis is certainly the more frequent type of reaction due to psoralens. Conflicting statements have been made concerning the direct irritancy and allergy of the sap and the possibility of a photocontact sensitization. In this study, we report eight cases of contact dermatitis from *Ficus carica.* In three subjects, photopatch tests revealed positive reactions to ethanol extract of cut leaves and to 8-MOP down to a concentration of 0.0001%. The histological picture of these reaction sites at 48 h was consistent with contact allergy, with spongiosis and exocytosis in the epidermis and a perivascular lymphomononuclear infiltrate.

In the literature, there are many reported cases of photoallergy to furocoumarins acquired during therapeutic procedures [1, 8, 9, 11, 21, 23, 24, 26]. On the other hand, photoallergic reactions to psoralens from contact with plants are rarely reported. Ljunggren described a patient with photocontact allergy to the psoralens xanthotoxin, bergapten, and imperatorin in parsley *(Petroselium sativum)* [17]. Kavli and Volden exposed themselves repeatedly to psoralen and plant parts from *Heracleum laciniatum*, and after five and six exposures, respectively, photocontact allergy was induced to the psoralens sphondin and isobergapten [14]. Goitre et al. reported two cases of occupational photocontact allergy to leaf, stem, and latex of *Heracleum mantegazzianum* [12].

In conclusion, the plant-induced photoallergy to psoralens is probably overlooked because the dermatitis is considered on all occasions to be phototoxic. Photopatch testing with serial dilutions of furocoumarins seems indicated in suspected cases of phytophotoallergy.

References

1. Angelini G, D'Ovidio R, Vena GA (1987) Allergia da contatto con 8-metossipsoralene. Boll Dermatol Allergol Profession 3: 69–74
2. Behcet H, Ottenstein B, Lion K, Dessauer F (1939) Les dermatitis des figues. Ann Dermatol Syphilig 10: 125–138
3. Benezra C, Ducombs G, Sell Y, Fussereau J (1985) Plant contact dermatitis. Mosby, St Louis
4. Capetanakis JA (1958) Feigendermatitis. Hautarzt 9: 139–140
5. Cohen W (1958) Characterization of ficin. Nature 182: 659–660
6. Dall'Acqua F, Marciani S, Chiaellotto G (1968) Isolation of 4'-5'-di-hydropsoralen from leaves of Ficus carica. Atti Istituto Veneto di Scienze Lettere ed Arti 126: 103–111
7. Englund PT, King PT, Craig LC, Walti A (1968) Studies on ficin. I. Its isolation and characterization. Biochemistry 7: 163–175
8. Fisher T (1985) Topical psoralen ultraviolet radiation. In: Roenigh HH, Maibach HI (eds) Psoriasis. Dekker, New York, pp 493–504
9. Fisher T, Alsins J (1976) Treatment of psoriasis with trioxalen baths and dysprosium lamps. Acta Derm Venereol (Stockh) 56: 383–390
10. Fregert S, Hjorth N, Magnusson B, Bandmann HJ, Calnan CD, Cronin E, Malten K, Meneghini CL, Pirilä V, Wilkinson DS (1969) Epidemiology of contact dermatitis. Trans St. John's Hosp Dermatol Soc 55: 17–34
11. Fulton JE, Willis I (1968) Photoallergy to methoxalen. Arch Dermatol 98: 445–450
12. Goitre M, Roncarolo B, Bedello PG, Romano C, Pira E, Sulotto F, Pavan I, Camerone E (1987) Occupational phytophotodermatitis from Heracleum mantegazzianum: isolation of furocoumarins. Boll Dermatol Allergol Profession 2: 177–184
13. Ippen H (1982) Phototoxische Reaktion auf Feigen. Hautarzt 33: 337–339
14. Kavli G, Volden G (1984) Phytophotodermatitis. Photodermatology 1: 65–75
15. Kitchevatz M (1934) Etiology and pathogenesis of dermatitis due to contact with figs: role of light. Bull Soc Franç Dermatol Syphiligz 41: 1751–1756
16. Lembo G, Lo Presti M, Balato N (1985) Phytophotodermatitis due to Ficus carica. Photodermatology 2: 119–120
17. Ljunggren B (1977) Psoralen photoallergy caused by plant contact. Contact Dermatitis 3: 85–90
18. Mitchell J, Rook A (1979) Botanical dermatology. Greengrass, Vancouver

19. Pathak MA, Daniels F Jr, Fitzpatrik TB (1962) The presently known distribution of furocoumarins (psoralens) in plants. J Invest Dermatol 39: 225–239
20. Pirilä V (1975) Chamber test versus patch test for epicutaneous testing. Contact Dermatitis 1: 48–52
21. Plewig G, Hofmann C, Braun-Falco O (1978) Photoallergic dermatitis from 8-methoxypsoralen. Arch Dermatol Res 261: 201–211
22. Rodighiero G, Antonello C (1959) Ricerche sul contenuto in psoralene e bergaptene delle foglie di Ficus carica. Il Farmaco, Edizione Scientifica 14: 679
23. Sidi E, Bourgeois-Gavardin (1953) Mise au point du traitment du vitiligo par l'Ammi majus. Presse Med 61: 436–440
24. Soihan EM (1979) Contact allergy to methoxalen. Br Med J (2): 20
25. The Merck Index (1976) 9th edn. Merck, Rahway
26. Weissmann J, Wagner G, Plewig G (1980) Contact allergy to 8-methoxypsoralen. Br J Dermatol 102: 113–115
27. Zaynoun ST, Aftimos BG, Abi Ali L, Tenekjian KK, Khalidi U, Kurban K (1984) Ficus carica; isolation and quantification of the photoactive components. Contact Dermatitis 11: 21–25

Addresses

G. Angelini
Department of Dermatology, University of Bari, Bari, Italy

G. A. Vena
Department of Dermatology, University of Bari, Bari, Italy

C. L. Meneghini
Department of Dermatology, University of Bari, Bari, Italy

Metals

Intracutaneous Testing in Doubtful Cases of Contact Allergy to Metals

H. Möller

Summary

In 66 of 1670 consecutively patch-tested patients, an intradermal test with chromium, cobalt, and nickel was additionally performed. Among these 66 patients, there were 49 with one or more doubtful metal reactions: a true allergy was confirmed in 24 cases, but rejected in 54.

Key words:

Intracutaneous test - Chromate - Cobalt - Nickel

Material and Methods

During the 3 years 1985–1987, a standard patch test was performed in 1670 patients. At the time of test application, all patients were questioned on a possible atopic background, which was defined as a personal (previous or present) atopic dermatitis, asthma, and/or hay fever. They were also questioned on a history of metal allergy, which was defined as an eczematous reaction (not only itching) to intimate contact with metals in jewelry or clothing.

The patch tests were supplemented with an intracutaneous test with chromate, cobalt, and nickel in 66 (4%) of the 1670 patients. The reasons for this were (a) a test reaction difficult to read (49 cases), (b) a negative test but a positive history of metal allergy (10 cases), or (c) a previously diagnosed metal allergy, in which case a check-up was wanted (7 cases). There was no case of a positive test with a negative history of metal allergy.

The standard patch test was performed according to International Contact Dermatitis Research Group (ICDRG) recommendations with Finn chambers on Scanpor, test substances being delivered from Chemotechnique Diagnostics, Malmö, Sweden. Thus, the metal salts used were potassium bichromate 0.5%, cobalt chloride 1.0%, and nickel sulfate 5.0%, all in petrolatum. Tests were applied for 48 h and read after a further 24 h. A test was considered positive if erythema *and* papules, vesicles, or infiltration were present. Among cases of doubtful reaction were those consisting of erythema only, of petechiae (usually cobalt), or of follicular papulopustules (porites).

Intracutaneous testing was performed using a 1-ml tuberculin syringe and a needle measuring 0.4 × 19 mm. The test solutions were the same metal salts as above dissolved to 1 m*M* in saline, corresponding for potassium bichromate to 0.029%, for cobalt chloride to 0.013%, and for nickel sulfate to 0.016%. The injection site was the volar aspect of the forearm. Care was taken to raise a wheal of about 4 mm in diameter, which was equivalent to about 0.1 ml fluid. A red and raised dermal infiltration of ≥ 4 mm after 72 h was considered a positive test.

Results

Among the 1670 patients patch-tested, there were 350 (21%) with a contact allergy to one or more metal salts. This is the final result after summation of patch tests clearly positive at the first reading and positive intracutaneous tests performed according to the indications given above.

Doubtful Reactions. The metal incriminated was chromate in 27 cases, cobalt in 19, and nickel in 32 (Table 1); thus, there was more than one metal involved in 22 of the 49 patients. There were 23 patients with atopy and 21 patients with a history of metal allergy, with 12 patients falling into both categories. A positive intracutaneous test to at least one metal was found in 24 instances in the 49 patients, but at the same time contact allergy was rejected in 54 instances (Table 1). Table 1 also shows the outcome of intracutaneous testing with the different metals. It may be seen that chromate and cobalt most often give a negative reaction after a doubtful primary test, but nickel less so.

Test-Negative Patients. In three of the ten patients with a negative patch test in spite of a positive history of metal allergy, a metal allergy was disclosed by intracutaneous testing (nickel in two, cobalt in one); the other seven stayed negative. There were three atopics among these seven test-negative patients.

Table 1. Results of intracutaneous testing in patients with doubtful patch test reactions

Metal	Doubtful patch tests (*n*)	Intracutaneous test (*n*)	
		Positive	Negative
Chromate	27	7	20
Cobalt	19	5	14
Nickel	32	12	20

Check-up Patients. In four of the seven check-up patients, a previously diagnosed contact allergy was still observed on intracutaneous testing; in the remaining three patients, it had disappeared.

Discussion

Patch test reactions to metals are notoriously difficult to interpret. Different methods to overcome this problem have been suggested, such as retesting at a later date [2], testing with a dilution series in water [5], using another vehicle like dimethyl sulfoxide [3], or conducting an open test [1]. In the present study, intradermal testing was found useful to confirm or reject doubtful patch tests.

Doubtful patch test reactions to all three metal salts occurred. In 1987, the incidence of contact allergy in our test laboratory to chromate was 2.5%, to cobalt 5.7%, and to nickel 18.7%. In relation to their actual incidence as contact allergens, therefore, chromate was the metal most difficult to interpret (Table 1), but also the one most commonly showing a negative intracutaneous test. This agrees with retest results [2].

Atopy was observed in 23 of the 49 patients with these doubtful test reactions, a very high frequency (47%). It was recently shown that the combination of a positive history of metal allergy and negative skin tests is an indication of atopy [4].

References

1. Christensen OB, Wall LM (1987) Open, closed and intradermal testing in nickel allergy. Contact Dermatitis 16: 21–26
2. Fischer T, Rystedt I (1985) False-positive, follicular and irritant patch test reactions to metal salts. Contact Dermatitis 12: 93–98
3. van Ketel WG (1978) Patch testing with nickel sulfate in DMSO. Contact Dermatitis 4: 167–168
4. Möller H. Svensson Å (1986) Metal sensitivity: positive history but negative test indicates atopy. Contact Dermatitis 14: 57–60
5. Wahlberg JE, Skog E (1971) Nickel allergy and atopy. Threshold of nickel sensitivity and immunoglobulin E determinations. Br J Dermatol 85: 97–104

Addresses

H. Möller
Department of Dermatology, General Hospital, S-21401 Malmö, Sweden

Is Nickel Vasculitis a Clinical Entity?

N. K. Veien and A. Krogdahl

Summary

Seventeen nickel-sensitive patients (16 women and 1 man) had widespread, symmetrical, pruritic, excoriated, papular lesions. One had purpuric lesions of the lower legs. Histological examination of biopsy samples from 11 of the patients disclosed 2 cases of leukocytoclastic vasculitis, 1 of these in the patient with purpuric lesions. The remaining biopsies showed moderately dense perivascular lymphohistiocytic infiltrates of the superficial plexus with few eosinophils, usually without epidermal involvement. Twelve of the patients were challenged orally with nickel, cobalt, and a placebo in a randomized, double-blind trial. Of these patients, six had flares after oral challenge with nickel, three had no reaction and three had other types of reactions, including placebo reactions.

Key words:

Nickel allergy - Vasculitis - Histology - Oral challenge

Introduction

Hjorth coined the term "nickel vasculitis" to describe an excoriated eruption in a nickel-allergic female patient [1]. We have occasionally encountered nickel-allergic patients with similar clinical lesions, and the following is a description of these patients.

Material and Methods

From 1979 to 1986, we saw 16 female patients and 1 male patient with symmetrical lesions on the extremities who had positive patch tests to 5% nickel sulphate in petrolatum. There were two distinctly different patterns of dermatitis:

1. One patient had pruritic and tender purpuric lesions on the lower legs, as well as painful subcutaneous infiltrates below the knees (Fig. 1).
2. Sixteen patients had symmetrical eruptions comprised of pruritic, excoriated, inflamed papules on the arms and/or legs (Fig. 2). Five patients had similar lesions on the trunk. One patient with typical lesions on the arms and legs also had more confluent lesions on the elbows similar to those previously described by Kaaber et al. [3]. Six patients also had symmetrical hand eczema, usually of the recurrent, vesicular type.

For nine patients, the duration of the eruptions was 1 year or less, while the remainder of the patients had had such eruptions for 1–7 years.

A punch biopsy sample was obtained from 11 patients for routine histological examination. Twelve of the patients were challenged orally with nickel, cobalt and a placebo in a randomized, placebo-controlled fashion [5]. A reproduction or flare of the usual dermatitis within 4 days of the challenge was considered to be a positive

a

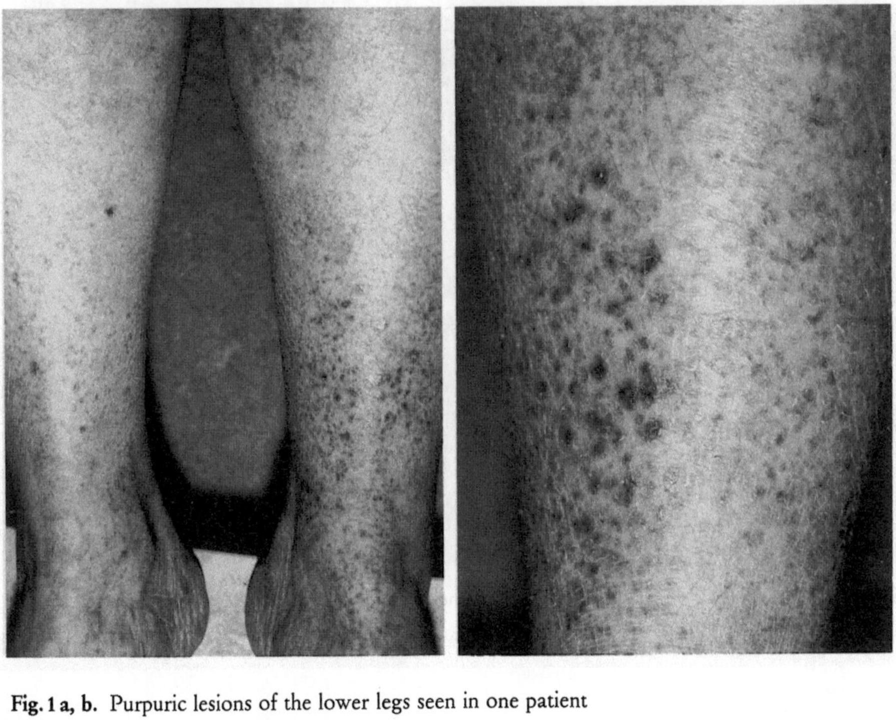

b

Fig. 1 a, b. Purpuric lesions of the lower legs seen in one patient

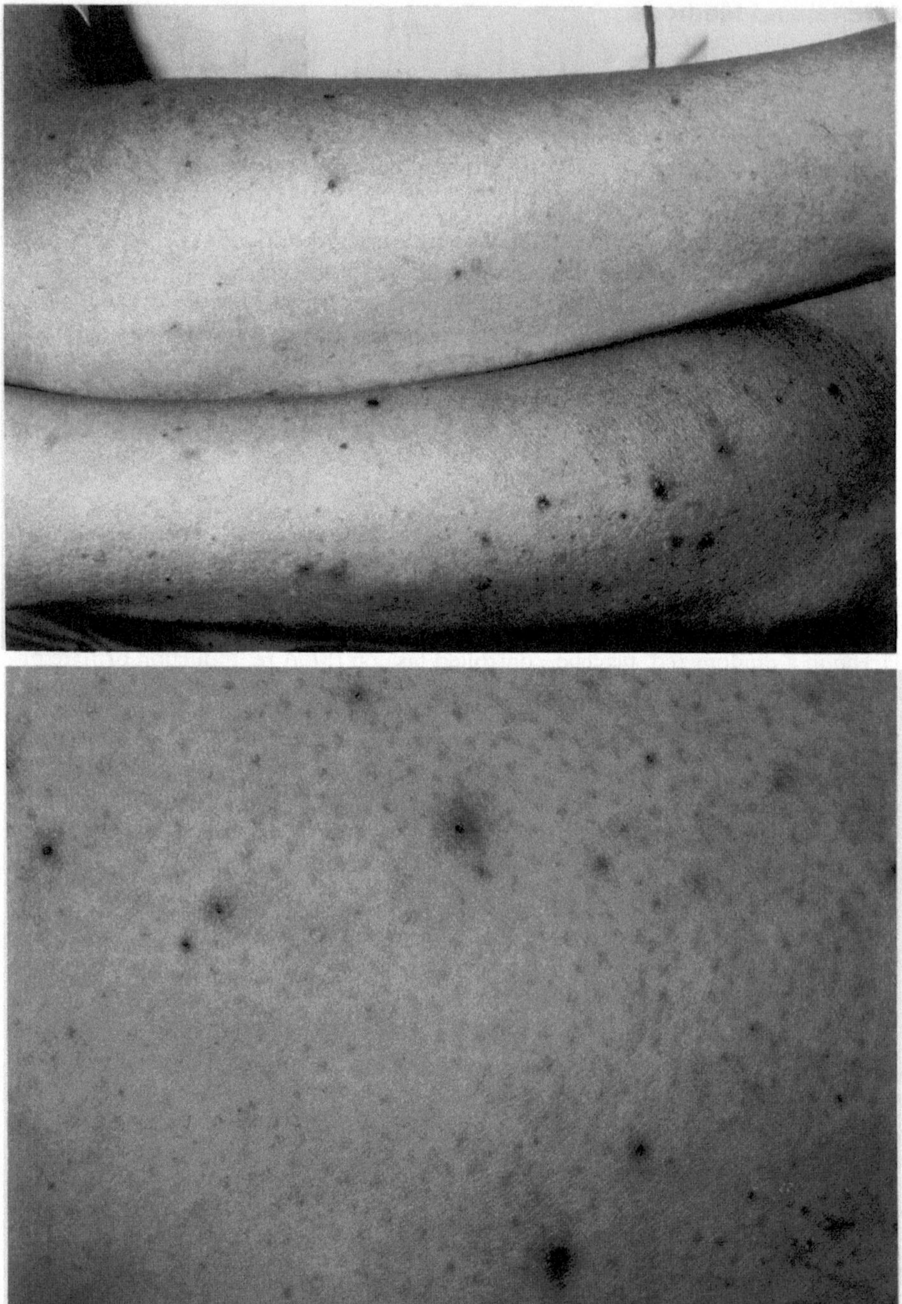

a

b

Fig. 2 a, b. Symmetrical, pruritic, excoriated, inflamed papules, typical in 16 patients reaction. As previously described [4], 14 patients were asked to reduce the intake of nickel in food, and a follow-up examination was carried out when these patients had maintained such a diet for 1–2 months.

Results

Histological examination showed that two patients had classical leukocytoclastic vasculitis. One of these was the patient with purpuric lesions of the lower leg. The other had excoriated papules on the arms and legs. For the remainder of the patients, histological examination showed moderately dense perivascular lymphohistiocytic infiltrates of the superficial plexus with few eosinophils (Fig. 3). In most cases, there was no epidermal involvement, but a punched-out epidermal necrosis was sometimes seen.

Of the 12 patients who were challenged orally, 6 experienced a flare of their usual dermatitis after challenge with nickel, but not after challenge with cobalt or the placebo. One patient reacted to both nickel and the placebo, and three patients had no reaction at all. One patient who did not have a positive patch test to cobalt reacted to cobalt, but not to nickel or the placebo, while one patient reacted to both cobalt and the placebo.

Of the 14 patients who were asked to reduce nickel intake, 3 did not return for the follow-up examination. The eruptions of six other patients (four of whom had

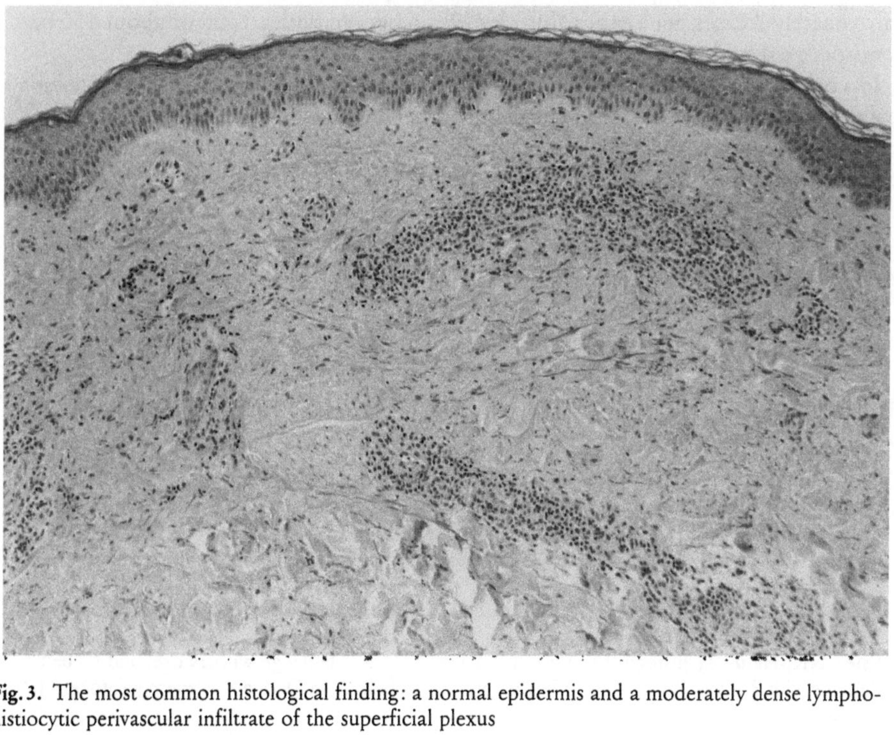

Fig. 3. The most common histological finding: a normal epidermis and a moderately dense lymphohistiocytic perivascular infiltrate of the superficial plexus

had these for more than a year) faded after they had followed the diet for 1–2 months, while in five patients the diet had no effect. Three patients who considered the diet treatment to be effective experienced flares of their usual dermatitis when the diet was not followed.

One patient noticed a flare of a patch of eczema on the abdomen at a site of nickel contact at the same time as the vasculitis-like lesions on the arms and legs flared.

Discussion

Nickel allergy is so common among women that it could be that the clinical lesions seen in the patients described here were unrelated to nickel allergy. However, causal relationship between the nickel allergy and the clinical lesions seen was suggested by the following: (a) a flare of the usual lesions in approximately half of the patients challenged orally with nickel, (b) improvement in approximately half of the patients placed on a nickel-restrictive diet and (c) the occurrence of similar lesions in nickel-allergic patients during disulfiram treatment at a time when serum nickel and the urinary excretion of nickel were very high [2].

If a causal relationship to nickel allergy is proven, the symmetrical appearance and the small papular excoriated lesions indicate systemic rather than topical exposure to the antigen. The mechanism of reaction is uncertain, but it could be caused by immune reactions other than cellular immunity.

The clinical reaction pattern described here is not common: in our clinic, we see aproximately 2 cases per year of this type, as compared with a total of about 150 patients per year with positive patch tests to nickel.

In conclusion, we believe it is possible to distinguish a clinically characteristic reaction pattern in nickel-allergic patients: it can be described as pruritic excoriated papules, which are a few millimetres in diameter, usually on the extremities. Histologically, the most common finding is lymphohistiocytic perivascular infiltrates with few eosinophils in the upper dermis, in most cases with no epidermal involvement. In some patients, a punched-out epidermal necrosis overlying the inflammatory infiltrate was seen.

References

1. Hjorth N (1976) Nickel vasculitis. Contact Dermatitis 2: 356–357
2. Kaaber K, Menné T, Tjell JC, Veien NK (1979) Antabuse treatment of nickel dermatitis. Chelation – a new principle in the treatment of nickel dermatitis. Contact Dermatitis 5: 221–228
3. Kaaber K, Sjølin KE, Menné T (1983) Elbow eruptions in nickel and chromate dermatitis. Contact Dermatitis 9: 213–216
4. Veien NK, Andersen MR (1986) Nickel in Danish food. Acta Dermatol Venereol (Stockh) 66: 502–509
5. Veien NK, Hattel T, Justesen O, Nørholm A (1987) Oral Challenge with Nickel and Cobalt in Patients with Positive Patch Tests to Nickel and/or Cobalt. Acta Dermatol Venereol (Stockh) 67: 321–325

Addresses

N. K. Veien
The Dermatology Clinic, Vesterbro 99, DK-9000 Aalborg, Denmark

A. Krogdahl
The Institute of Pathology, Aalborg Hospital, DK-9000 Aalborg, Denmark

Preliminary Results of a Multicenter Study on the Incidence of Nickel Allergy in Relationship to Previous Oral and Cutaneous Contacts*

I. M. W. van Hoogstraten, K. E. Andersen, B. M. E. von Blomberg, D. Boden, D. P. Bruynzeel, D. Burrows, J. M. G. Camarasa, A. Dooms-Goossens, G. Kraal, A. Lahti, T. Menné, R. J. G. Rycroft, D. Todd, K. J. J. Vreeburg, J. D. Wilkinson, and R. J. Scheper

Summary

Potential relationships between the development of nickel allergy and previous ear piercing or orthodontic treatment with nickel-containing appliances were studied. The preliminary results presented here confirm earlier suggestions that nickel hypersensitivity (as assessed by patch testing) is promoted by ear piercing. It is shown that if orthodontic treatment had preceded the event of ear piercing, the frequency of nickel hypersensitivity was significantly reduced. This supports our view that oral allergenic contacts may induce immunological tolerance.

Key words:

Ear piercing - Nickel sensitivity - Orthodontic treatment - Oral tolerance

Introduction

In industrialized nations the most common allergy among women is nickel allergy [1]. Various population studies indicate that at least 10% of the female and about 1% of the male population is nickel hypersensitive [2–4]. Sensitive subjects may suffer from slight dermatitis at metal contact sites, but others may develop severe hand eczema. It is assumed that various factors promote the development of nickel dermatitis [5]. Atopy represents an important personal factor. External factors include wet work and frequent exposure to irritant and nickel-containing agents. Therefore, a high frequency of nickel dermatitis is observed in occupations such as nursing,

* This work was supported by grant 28-1357 from the Dutch Praeventiefonds

cleaning and hairdressing [6, 7]. Epidemiological studies indicate that both occupational and non-occupational nickel dermatitis are increasing [8, 9].

We recently evaluated the incidence of nickel hypersensitivity in relation to various personal factors in junior hairdressers and nurses [5]. This study revealed that the frequency of nickel sensitivity (as assessed by patch testing) was high in junior hairdressers (26%), compared with junior nurses (12%). Potential relationships between the development of nickel allergy and previous ear piercing or orthodontic treatment with nickel-containing appliances were evaluated in both student groups. Data were obtained suggesting that development of nickel allergy had been promoted by ear piercing. Interestingly, a decreased frequency of nickel hypersensitivity was observed in junior nurses who had received orthodontic treatment during childhood (5.4% vs 18.4%).

In non-sensitized individuals antigenic contacts by the oral route are known to induce tolerance rather than sensitization [10]. In a guinea pig model, we were able to demonstrate the development of tolerance by oral administration of nickel. Attempts to immunize the orally pretreated guinea pigs failed in most animals, whereas non-pretreated guinea pigs became clearly hypersensitive [11]. Recent studies in guinea pigs revealed that oral tolerance to nickel or chromium contact hypersensitivity is dose dependent, allergen specific and long lasting (manuscript in preparation).

At present we are conducting a West European multicenter study to verify whether (a) the sensitizing effect of ear piercing and (b) the tolerogenic effect of orthodontic treatment with metal appliances hold for a large non-selected group of patch-test patients attending dermatological clinics.

Patients and Methods

As of October 1987 in nine West European dermatological clinics all patch-test patients were interviewed by means of a confidential questionnaire. Questions were asked concerning any past or present history of occupational contacts with nickel, problems with (costume) jewellery, wearing of a dental brace for orthodontic treatment (at what age and for how long) and piercing of the ears (at what age). Patch-test results for nickel, cobalt and chromium were recorded.

The questionnaire data were processed on a computer. Statistical calculations were performed with the χ^2 test. At 15 May 1988, 1737 patients had entered the study (1252 females and 485 males). The age of the patients ranged from 2 to 87 years, the mean age being 38.0 years.

Preliminary Results

Of the 1709 patients responding on the question about ear pearcing, 1015 (59.4%) had pierced ears. We evaluated nickel hypersensitivity in relation to age and sex of patients with or without pierced ears. Here we report on patients younger than

Table 1. Effects of ear piercing on the development of nickel hypersensitivity in relation to sex in young patients (age ≤ 31 years)

Piercing	Female patients			Male patients		
	Group size	Nickel-positive		Group size	Nickel-positive	
		Number	Percentage		Number	Percentage
–	48	3	6.3	149	4	2.7
+	568	225	39.6	41	8	19.5

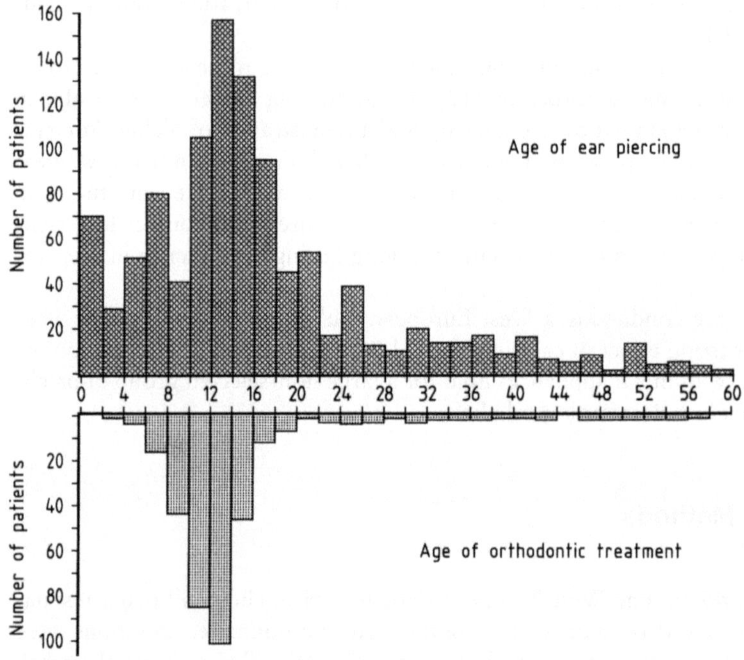

Fig. 1. Age distribution at the time of ear piercing (1103 patients) and at the time of orthodontic treatment (371 patients). The peak of ear piercing coincided with the peak of orthodontic treatment

31 years. In this group 568 females and 41 males had pierced ears (Table 1). The frequency of nickel sensitivity in these groups of patients was 39.6% and 19.5% respectively. In sharp contrast, nickel sensitivity was observed in only 6.3% of 48 unpierced female and in 2.7% of 149 unpierced male patients. The differences between unpierced vs pierced patients were highly significant for both the females ($P<0.001$) and males ($P<0.001$).

Figure 1 shows that many patients had their ear lobes pierced at an early age, with a peak at 12 to 14 years. The age at which this important sensitizing event occurred coincided with the age at which most patients had a dental brace installed. Thus, for evaluating a possible effect of orthodontic treatment on the development of nickel hypersensitivity, each patient had to be studied individually.

Table 2. Effects of orthodontic treatment on the development of nickel hypersensitivity in young patients (age ≤ 31 years)

Orthodontic treatment	Piercing	Group size	Nickel-positive		
			Number	Percentage	
Brace	–	57	2	3.5	
–	–	143	5	3.5	
–	+	431	168	39.0	$P<0.05$
Brace before piercing	+	86	24	27.9	

The results from this study concerning the relationship between orthodontic treatment and nickel sensitization are shown in Table 2. Orthodontic treatment alone did not induce nickel sensitivity (3.5%). Of patients with pierced ear lobes the frequency of nickel hypersensitivity was markedly reduced (from 39.0% to 27.9%; $P<0.05$) when orthodontic treatment had preceded (by more than 1 year) the event of ear piercing.

Discussion

The preliminary results from our study confirm that the incidence of nickel allergic contact sensitivity was highest among young female patients. The high prevalence of nickel dermatitis among young women has been reported earlier in several West and East European studies [12–15]. It has been suggested that this prevalence among younger women may be due to prolonged and heavy exposure to the allergen, for example in costume jewellery. In particular, for a group of Swedish schoolgirls ear piercing has been mentioned as a potentially sensitizing allergenic contact [16]. Our present results confirm a significant correlation between ear piercing and the frequency of nickel sensitivity. Sensitization may be caused by frequent use of inexpensive, nickel-containing ear rings, ear studs, ear clasps and ear clips.

In the present study, we have confirmed that nickel sensitivity is reduced when orthodontic treatment has preceded the event of ear piercing. This supports our view that wearing a dental metal prosthesis can induce tolerance. Thus, sensitization by ear piercing may be prevented by a state of tolerance induced by oro-gastro-intestinal exposure to nickel.

Ear piercing clearly increases the risk of nickel sensitization. Obviously it will be very difficult to curtail this widely spread, charming habit. The use of "safe" alloys with low nickel release might solve part of the problem of nickel sensitization [17]. However, only few alloys have a low nickel release rate. Either these do not have a bright silvery appearance or they are relatively expensive. Results of the present study support our view that oral administration of nickel at an early age may induce a state of cutaneous tolerance and, thus, should be further explored as a possible route to prevent nickel sensitization and related skin disease.

References

1. Cronin E (1980) Contact dermatitis. Churchill Livingstone, Edinburgh
2. Peltonen L (1979) Nickel sensitivity in the general population. Contact Dermatitis 5: 27–32
3. Prytowsky SD, Allen AM, Smith RW, Nonomura JH, Odom RB, Akers WA (1979) Allergic contact hypersensitivity to nickel, neomycin, ethylenediamine and benzocaine. Relationship between age, sex, history of exposure and reactivity to standard patch tests and use tests in a general population. Arch Dermatol 115: 959–962
4. Menné T (1978) The prevalence of nickel allergy among women. An epidemiological study in hospitalized female patients. Derm Beruf Umwelt 26: 123–125
5. Van de Burg CKH, Bruynzeel DP, Vreeburg KJJ, von Blomberg BME, Scheper RJ (1986) Hand eczema in hairdressers and nurses: a prospective study. I. Evaluation of atopy and nickel hypersensitivity at the start of apprenticeship. Contact Dermatitis 14: 275–279
6. Lindemayr H (1984) Das Friseurekzem. Dermatosen 32: 5–13
7. Lammintausta K, Kalimo K, Havu VK (1982) Occurrence of contact allergy and hand eczema in hospital wet work. Contact Dermatitis 8: 84–90
8. Edman B, Möller H (1982) Trends and forecasts for standard allergen in a 12-year patch test material. Contact Dermatitis 8: 95–104
9. Menné T, Borgan Ø, Green A (1982) Nickel allergy and hand dermatitis in a stratified sample of the Danish female population: an epidemiological study including a statistic appendix. Acta Derm Venereol (Stockh) 62: 35–41
10. Tomasi TB (1980) Oral tolerance. Transplantation 29: 353–356
11. Vreeburg KJJ, de Groot K, von Blomberg BME, Scheper RJ (1984) Induction of immunological tolerance by oral administration of nickel and chromium. J Dent Res 63: 124–128
12. Sugai T, Takagi T, Yamamoto S, Takahshi Y (1979) Age distribution of the incidence of contact sensitivity to standard allergens. Contact Dermatitis 5: 383–388
13. Walton S, Nayagam AT, Keckes K (1986) Age and sex incidence of allergic contact dermatitis. Contact Dermatitis 15: 136–139
14. Young E, Houwing RH (1987) Patch test results with standard allergens over a decade. Contact Dermatitis 17: 104–107
15. Schubert H, Berova N, Czernielewski A, Hegyi E, Jirásek L, Kohánka V, Korossy S, Michailov P, Nebenführer L, Prater E, Rothe A, Rudzki E, Stranski L, Süss E, Tarnick M, Temesvári E, Ziegler V, Zschunke E (1987) Epidemiology of nickel allergy. Contact Dermatitis 16: 122–128
16. Larsson-Stymne B, Wildstrom L (1985) Ear piercing – a cause of nickel allergy in schoolgirls? Contact Dermatitis 13: 289–293
17. Menné T, Brandrup F, Thestrup-Pedersen K, Veien NK, Andersen JR, Yding F, Valeur G (1987) Patch test reactivity to nickel alloys. Contact Dermatitis 16: 255–259

Addresses

I. M. W. van Hoogstraten
Department of Pathology, Free University Hospital, P.O. Box 7057, 1007 MB Amsterdam, The Netherlands

B. M. E. von Blomberg
Department of Pathology, Free University Hospital, P.O. Box 7057, 1007 MB Amsterdam, The Netherlands

D. Boden
Department of Pathology, Free University Hospital, P.O. Box 7057, 1007 MB Amsterdam, The Netherlands

R. J. Scheper
Department of Pathology, Free University Hospital, P. O. Box 7057, 1007 MB Amsterdam, The Netherlands

G. Kraal
Department of Cellbiology, Med. Faculty Free University, Amsterdam, The Netherlands

K. E. Andersen
Department of Dermatology, Roskilde, Denmark

D. P. Bruynzeel
Department of Dermatology, Free University Hospital, P. O. Box 7057, 1007 MB Amsterdam, The Netherlands

D. Burrows
Department of Dermatology, Royal Victoria Hospital, Belfast, UK

D. Todd
Department of Dermatology, Royal Victoria Hospital, Belfast, UK

J. M. G. Camarasa
Department of Dermatology, Hospital de N. S. del Mar, Barcelona, Spain

A. Dooms-Goossens
Department of Dermatology, St. Pieter University Hospital, Leuven, Belgium

A. Lahti
Department of Dermatology, University of Oulu, Oulu, Finland

T. Menné
Department of Dermatology, Gentofte Hospital, Hellerup, Denmark

R. J. G. Rycroft
Department of Dermatology, St. John's Hospital, London, UK

K. J. J. Vreeburg
Department of Biomaterials, Free University, Amsterdam, The Netherlands

J. D. Wilkinson
Department of Dermatology, Wycombe General Hospital, Buckinghamshire, UK

Nickel Sensitivity in Schoolchildren in Finland

L. Peltonen and P. Terho

Summary

Schoolchildren, 406 boys and 499 girls aged 7, 11, 14 and 17 years, were tested with nickel sulphate 5% (the 7-year-olds with 2.5%) in petrolatum (pet). The history concerning ear piercing and atopic diseases was taken by a questionnaire. Of the boys 2% and of the girls 16% were found to be allergic to nickel. In 3% of the boys and 75% of the girls the ears were pierced. None of these boys, but 20% of the girls showed a positive reaction to nickel. Nickel allergy was ten fold higher among the girls with pierced ears than in the girls with unpierced ears. It was more frequent (35%) in the girls who had more than one hole per earlobe than in those with only one hole in each earlobe (16%). Seven of the 8 nickel-sensitive boys and 74 of the 78 girls had a positive history of metal sensitivity. Also 20 boys and 30 girls with a negative test reported such a history. Most of them were atopics.

Key words:

Nickel sensitivity - Ear piercing

Introduction

Already in the 1960s in the United States nickel dermatitis was prevalent in adolescent girls following ear piercing [4]. Recently, ear piercing has been shown to involve a considerable risk of nickel sensitization for schoolgirls in Sweden [3, 5]. In Finland, only one of the 90 schoolgirls and one of the 68 schoolboys tested during a population study in 1975 were found to be allergic to nickel [7]. Jeans buttons and wristwatches were the sensitizers in that study. Since then, ear piercing has become very popular among schoolgirls, and to some extent, also among schoolboys in our country. The purpose of this study was therefore to investigate whether an increase in nickel sensitivity has taken place among schoolchildren as a consequence of this fashion.

Material and Methods

The investigation was undertaken between October 1987 and April 1988. It was performed in seven schools in the different areas of the city of Turku in connection of the routine health examination of pupils aged 7, 11, 14 and 17 years. Only a few pupils outright refused to participate in the study, but one-fourth of the 14-year-old boys and nearly one-half of those aged 17 did not come to the readings, mostly because of sports activities.

Patch testing was done with Finn chambers on Scanpor tape. In order to avoid false-positive reactions, nickel sulphate 2.5% in petrolatum (pet.) was used for the youngest age group, while the others were tested with nickel sulphate 5% (Chemotechnic). The test was applied to the upper back for 48 h by one of the authors (P.T.) and read after 72 h by the other (L.P.). Erythema with papules/vesicles and infiltration was required for a positive reaction.

The pupils had together with their parents filled out a questionnaire which they then brought to the reading. They were asked about ear piercing, age at ear piercing, the number of holes and who had made the holes. We further asked whether they had noticed any skin symptoms related to ear piercing, ear rings, metal buttons and other metal objects worn against the skin. Any history of a past or present atopic dermatitis, allergic rhinitis and asthma was also taken by questionnaire.

Results

Of the 406 boys 11 (3%) and 364 of the 499 girls (75%) had had their ears pierced. Among the girls, ear piercing was common already from the youngest age groups (Fig. 1). In 60% of the cases it was done between the ages of 6 and 10 years.

The nickel test was positive in 2% of the boys (Table 1) and in 16% of the girls. None of the boys with pierced ears was allergic to nickel. Nickel sensitivity was present in 2% of the girls with unpierced ears and in 20% of those with pierced ears. The frequencies of nickel allergy in the different age groups are shown in Table 2.

The holes were made by a jeweller in 86% of the cases. Seventy-seven girls had more than one hole per earlobe; 35% of them and 16% of the girls with only one hole in each earlobe were allergic to nickel. Of the 18 girls whose earlobes were pierced when they were 5-years old or younger, 8 developed nickel allergy.

Of the 75 nickel-sensitive girls with pierced ears 63 had noticed itching and dermatitis from cheap earrings. In 35 girls this was the first site of nickel dermatitis; 35 girls experienced skin symptoms from their wristwatch and 19 from jeans buttons (the first site in 8 cases). In all, 67 of the 78 nickel-sensitive girls reported repeatedly having skin symptoms from nickel-plated objects; 7 experienced oozing and suppuration only after ear piercing, and 4 had no history of metal sensitivity. Two nickel-

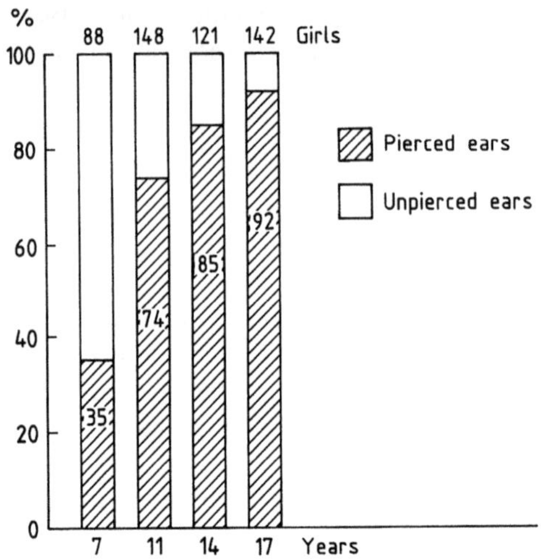

Fig. 1. Frequency of ear piercing in girls in the different age groups

Table 1. Nickel allergy in schoolboys

Age (years)	Nickel-allergic boys/ all tested boys	
	n	%
7	3/108	3
11	3/121	3
14	1/104	1
17	1/73	1
All	8/406	2

Table 2. Nickel allergy in schoolgirls with pierced and unpierced ears

Age (years)	Nickel-allergic girls/all tested girls					
	Pierced ears		Unpierced ears		Total	
	n	%	*n*	%	*n*	%
7	3/31	10	1/57	2	4/88	5
11	11/110	10	2/38	5	13/148	9
14	22/103	21	0/18	0	22/121	18
17	39/132	30	0/10	0	39/142	27
All	75/376	20	3/123	2	78/499	16

sensitive girls had noticed dermatitis from their wrist-watch and metal buttons some years before ear piercing.

Seven of the 8 nickel-sensitive boys had a positive history of dermatitis from buttons in jeans, wristwatch or spectacle frames. In 3 girls and 2 boys nickel dermatitis was present at the time of patch-test reading.

In addition, 30 girls and 20 boys with a negative nickel test reported that they occasionally had had skin symptoms from metal objects; 60% (30/50) of them had a history of present or past atopic dermatitis while 5 had only atopic respiratory symptoms. On examination, they also seemed to have a dry and pruritic skin. Of the total sample, 25% had a history of present or previous atopic dermatitis, asthma or hay fever.

Discussion

The results of the study indicate that a considerable increase in nickel allergy has taken place among schoolgirls in Turku since 1975, but among schoolboys it still remains low. In the girls with pierced ears the frequency of nickel allergy was ten fold higher than that found in the girls with unpierced ears.

Our results confirm the finding of Widström and Larsson-Stymne of a surprisingly high frequency of nickel allergy in schoolgirls [5]. Nickel allergy was even somewhat more frequent among schoolgirls in Finland than in Sweden some years ago. Equally high figures for nickel allergy as in our sample have been reported by Camarasa et al. [2] and Boss and Menné [1]. According to Möller and Svensson, most patients with a history of metal sensitivity and a negative test are atopics [6]. This holds true also in our sample.

References

1. Boss A, Menné T (1982) Nickel sensitization from ear piercing. Contact Dermatitis 8: 211–213
2. Camarasa JMG et al. (1983) Patch tests to metals in childhood. Contact Dermatitis 9: 157–158
3. Fischer T, Fregert S, Gruvberger B, Rystedt I (1984) Nickel release from ear piercing kits and earrings. Contact Dermatitis 10: 39–41
4. Gaul LE (1967) Development of allergic nickel dermatitis from earrings. JAMA 200: 176–178
5. Larsson-Stymne B, Widström L (1985) Ear piercing – a cause of nickel allergy in schoolgirls? Contact Dermatitis 13: 289–293
6. Möller H, Svensson Å (1986) Metal sensitivity: positive history but negative test indicates atopy. Contact Dermatitis 14: 57–60
7. Peltonen L (1979) Nickel sensitivity in the general population. Contact Dermatitis 5: 27–32

Addresses

L. Peltonen
Department of Dermatology, University of Turku, Turku, Finland

P. Terho
Administration of School Health Service, Turku, Finland

Nickel Allergy and Ear Piercing in Young Men

L. Widström and I. Erikssohn

Summary

The aim of this study was to determine the prevalence of nickel allergy and ear piercing in young men. The study was performed on young men enlisted for military service, with 216 18-year-old subjects being examined. Case history was taken by means of a questionnaire. Patch tests with nickel sulphate and cobalt chloride were made. Ear piercing was found to be quite common (22%). In spite of this, the prevalence of nickel allergy in these men was found to be much lower than that known in women. This also applies to the persons with pierced ears.

Key words:

Nickel allergy - Ear piercing - Males - Prevalence

Introduction

An important inducing factor in nickel allergy seems to be ear piercing. From 1982 to 1983, we investigated the incidence of nickel allergy and ear piercing in schoolgirls [1]. We found that 8% of the 8-year-old girls and 12% of the 15-year-old girls were sensitized to nickel. Practically all the nickel-sensitive girls were among those with pierced ears. In 1985, we made a similar study (not published) on women in different professions (hairdressers, cashiers, secretaries). We found a prevalence of nickel allergy of almost 20% in those born in 1960–1969. The correlation to ear piercing was very strong. In recent years, ear piercing has become fashionable among boys and young men. Our aim with this study was to find out if this has caused a correspondingly high frequency of nickel allergy in this group.

Table 1. Results of patch tests

Group	Boys tested (*n*)	Nickel allergy	
		n	%
Total	216	3	1.4
Pierced ears	48	2	4.2
Unpierced ears	168	1	0.6

Material and Methods

Our study population was 244 consecutive young men enlisted for military service, examined on Fridays and Mondays during the autumn of 1987. Of these 244, 28 (11%) were not examined for various reasons, the main ones being organisational difficulties and participation in sports activities. Epicutaneous tests were performed with nickel sulphate (5% petrolatum) and cobalt chloride (0.5% petrolatum). The tests were read after 72 h. The history was taken by means of a questionnaire and personal interview.

Results

The nickel test was positive in 3 (1.4%) of the 216 men investigated and tested. Of these 216, 48 (22%) had had their ears pierced. Of the 48 men with pierced ears, 2 (4.2%) showed a positive reaction. Of the 168 men without pierced ears, 1 (0.6%) showed a positive reaction. The difference between the two groups is not statistically significant (Table 1).

Our conclusion is that ear piercing is quite common among young men, but that the prevalence of nickel allergy is not equal to that among women. The reason for the difference may be hormonal, but probably different clothing and jewellery habits in men and women are important.

Reference

1. Larsson-Stymne, B, Widström L (1985) Ear piercing – a cause of nickel allergy in schoolgirls. Contact Dermatitis 13: 289–293

Addresses

L. Widström
Department of Dermatology, Örebro Medical Center Hospital, Regionsjukhuset, S-70185 Örebro, Sweden

I. Erikssohn
Department of Dermatology, Örebro Medical Center Hospital, Regionsjukhuset, S-70185 Örebro, Sweden

Nickel Dermatitis in Construction Workers

H. J. Schubert, H. Lück, and E. Auermann

Summary

What allergological role does nickel in cement play? Of 1585 consecutive patients at two patch test clinics, 150 were positive to nickel sulphate 5%, 11 of them being construction workers. In 726 workers from two concrete prefabrication plants, we found 12 such cases.

Cement may contain up to 825 ppm nickel. However, this nickel is not water soluble, as we confirmed in 27 brands of cement and several additives examined for nickel by atomic absorption spectrophotometry (detection limit 0.05 ppm). Only out of nickel dross, milled and added by one of the nine cement factories, could 0.28 ppm nickel be extracted by water (30 min). This nickel becomes water insoluble due to alkaline of cement. Our careful examination of all nickel-positive construction workers showed non-occupational nickel sensitisation in every case due to fashion jewellery, jeans buttons and wristwatches, in three cases even before apprenticeship.

Key words:

Nickel dermatitis - Cement - Construction workers

Introduction

Most European cements contain such common contact allergens as chrome, cobalt and nickel [1–4, 6, 7]. Haguenoer et al. (1982) found 16–825 ppm nickel in cements from Northern France and Belgium, its sources being additives such as pyrites (1732 ppm nickel), ashes and dross [4]. Cobalt dermatitis due to cement is well known, and nickel is the twin brother of cobalt not only in mineralogy and metallurgy but also in contact allergy. What allergological role does this nickel play in cement?

Materials and Methods

Patch testing was performed in 1585 consecutive patients with the GDR standard series including nickel sulphate 5% petrolatum. Patch testing was also performed in all willing workers from two concrete prefabrication plants (726 persons). The patches were removed at day 2 and read after removal and again at day 3. Positive reactions were graded according to the International Contact Dermatitis Research Group (ICDRG). All patients with an unambiguous positive nickel reaction were asked for their special history.

The water soluble nickel content of 27 brands of cement and 7 additives was determined by atomic absorption spectrophotometry (AAS): 10 g cement or additive was shaken mechanically with 25 ml deionized water for 30 min and then filtered. The water extract was acidified to pH 1 for stabilisation and sucked into an AAS Perkin-Elmer 300 (232 nm, split 0.2 mm, detection limit 0.05 ppm nickel). Another 10 g cement or additive of the same brands was extracted with 25 ml NH_4OH 2% aqua and analysed in the same way.

Results

Of 1585 consecutive patients at our patch test clinics (with suspected allergic contact dermatitis), 150 (9.5%) were nickel positive (including 11 construction workers). In their history, there was no indication of an occupational cause (Table 1).

The screening of 726 workers in two concrete prefabrication plants in Berlin showed very different results: in plant A, there were 4 nickel-positive reactions among 584 healthy workers (0.7%), and in plant B, 8 positives among 142 workers (11.4%). In plant B, we found many young workers wearing jewellery, etc. and a lot of female apprentices.

The results of AAS are shown in Table 2. All 27 brands of cement were free of traceable water soluble nickel. By NH_4OH extraction, we found nickel (0.05–0.3 ppm) in 8 of 27 cements.

Table 1. Causes of nickel allergy in construction workers

Occupation	Sex	Age at onset (years)	Cause
Concrete construction worker	M	16	Bracelet
Prefabrication plant worker	F	16	Bracelet
Prefabrication plant worker	F	16	Chain, watch
Prefabrication plant worker	F	17	No eczema
Prefabrication plant worker	F	21	Finger rings
Prefabrication plant worker	M	26	Wristwatch
Bricklayer	M	18	Jeans button
Pipe-layer	M	35	Watch bracelet
Underground construction worker	M	22	Watch bracelet
Construction engineer	M	33	Watch bracelet
Construction engineer	M	60	Finger ring

Table 2. Water soluble nickel (expressed in parts per million) in cements and additives

Factory	Material	Extraction	
		Water	NH_4OH 2%
Bernburg			
BT 1	PZ 1/45	ND	0.2
	PZ 5/35	ND	0.05
	PZ 7/35	ND	ND
	PZ 45/F	ND	ND
BT 2	ZZ 1/25	ND	0.18
BT 3	PZ 1/45	ND	ND
	PZ 5/35	ND	ND
	PZ 7/35	ND	0.05
BT 4	PZ 2/30	ND	0.12
Bitterfeld	PZ 1/40	ND	ND
	Gypsum	ND	ND
Deuna	PZ 4/45	ND	ND
	PZ 7/35	ND	0.1
	PZ 45/F	ND	ND
	Blast furnace dross	ND	0.05
Coswig	PZ 1/40	ND	ND
Karsdorf	PZ 4/45	ND	ND
	PZ 7/35	ND	0.05
	PZ 7/35 (BT 3)	ND	0.08
	PZ 45/F	ND	0.3
	Angitporphyrite	ND	ND
	Nickel dross	0.28	1.15
Rüdersdorf	MB 175	ND	ND
	PZ 1/45	ND	ND
	PZ 2/30	ND	ND
	PZ 35/FPZ	ND	0.1
	PZ 45/F	ND	ND
	ZZ 1/25	ND	ND
Rummelsburg	ZZ 1/25	ND	ND
	Cinder	ND	ND
	Clinker	ND	ND
	Gypsum	ND	0.05
Unterwellenborn	ZZ 1/25	ND	ND
Wolfen	PZ 1/40	ND	ND

PZ, Portland cement; MB, ZZ, other cement brands; ND, not detectable by AAS (<0.05 ppm)

Discussion

Cement may contain up to 900 ppm nickel [2, 4, 6, 7]; however, this nickel is not water soluble [2, 3]. This fact was confirmed by us in 27 brands of cement from 9 cement factories and in several additives. Only from nickel dross, milled and added by one of the factories, could 0.28 ppm nickel be extracted by water. The eliciting safety limit of nickel has been put at 0.6 ppm [5]. The amount of milled nickel dross in cement, however, is only 3%, and this nickel becomes insoluble due to alkaline of cement. These insoluble nickel compounds (NiO, $Ni(OH)_2$, NiS, etc.) cannot be dissolved by cysteine and amino acid constituents of body fluids either [3], unlike cobalt. In 2 of 11 cases of nickel dermatitis in construction workers, the doctor suspected cement to be the causing source. By screening another 12 workers were found to be positive too. In all these cases except one, non-occupational nickel contacts could be easily identified as the cause of sensitisation and dermatitis (fashion jewellery, wristwatches, jeans buttons), and no case was caused by cement. In three cases, the first nickel dermatitis had already occurred before apprenticeship.

In conclusion, nickel-caused allergic dermatitis to cement is hardly imaginable, up to now not authentically reported and from a chemical point of view impossible.

References

1. Behrbohm P (1973) Bericht der Konferenz über Arbeitsdermatosen anläßlich des III. Internationalen Symposiums Arbeitshygiene und Arbeitsschutz im Bauwesen, Berlin 1972. Berufsdermatosen 21: 168–182
2. Fregert S, Gruvberger B (1972) Chemical properties of cement. Berufsdermatosen 20: 238–248
3. Fregert S, Gruvberger B (1978) Solubility of cobalt in cement. Contact Dermatitis 4: 14–18
4. Haguenoer JM, Leveque G, Frimat P (1982) Dosage du chrome, du nickel et du cobalt dans les ciments du nord de la France et de Belgique en relation avec les dermatoses professionnelles. Arch Mal Prof Méd Trav Sécur Soc 43: 241–247
5. Malten KE, Spruit D (1969) The relative importance of various environmental exposure to nickel in causing contact hypersensitivity. Acta Derm Venereol (Stockh) 49: 14–19
6. Schaulow I, Zwetanow K (1969) Untersuchungen über den Chrom-, Nickel- und Kobaltgehalt bulgarischer Zemente. II. Internationales Symposium Arbeitshygiene und Arbeitsschutz im Bauwesen, Eisenach 1968. Ergonom Ber 1: 188–189
7. Wahlberg JE, Lindstedt G, Einarsson Ö (1977) Chromium, cobalt and nickel in Swedish cement, detergents, moulds and cutting oils. Berufsdermatosen 25: 220–228

Addresses

H. J. Schubert
Hautklinik der Medizinischen Akademie Erfurt, Erfurt, GDR

H. Lück
Hautabteilung der Zentralen Poliklinik der Bauarbeiter, Berlin, GDR

E. Auermann
Bezirkshygieneinstitut, Karl-Marx-Stadt, GDR

An Investigation of Patients with a History of Nickel Allergy but Negative Epicutaneous Patch Tests

D. J. Todd, D. Burrows, and C. F. Stanford

Patients with a contact allergy to nickel are generally characterised by a good agreement between a history of nickel allergy and the results of epicutaneous patch testing. However, it is reported that 30%–50% of patients who give a positive history of nickel allergy are patch test negative [1–3]. It has been suggested that these patients have a higher than normal incidence of atopy. Moller and Svennson examined 19 such patients for atopic dermatitis, using a constructed score system which they had earlier devised [4], and considered 14 of them to be atopic [5]. Fischer and Rystedt looked at six patients who were nickel history positive but patch test negative and noted that they all had some kind of atopic background, although they did not state their diagnostic criteria for atopy [6]. In contrast, Kieffer found only 4 of 13 such patients to be atopic, using personal and family history as markers [1]. We therefore decided to study the relationship between nickel allergy history with negative patch tests and atopic status more closely.

Age- and sex-matched patients were recruited from the patch test clinic and volunteer student nurses, with 20 patients who were nickel history positive but patch test negative forming the study group. The two control groups were formed from (a) 11 patients who were nickel history positive and patch test positive, and (b) 13 patients who were nickel history negative and patch test negative. The following markers of atopy were assessed in all patients:

1. Personal history
2. Family history
3. Clinical respiratory status
4. Pulmonary function tests
5. Eosinophil counts
6. Serum IgE levels
7. Skin-prick testing

The results are set out in Tables 1, 2. Asthma was diagnosed on clinical history and "atopy" signified allergic rhinitis or history of penicillin allergy. Qualitative data were analysed using Fisher's exact *t* test. Quantitative data were analysed using the independent *t* test and the Mann-Whitney U test.

A simple observation of these results indicates that there is, in general, no difference between the study group and control groups. The only exception is that nine

Table 1. Atopy markers in the study and control groups

Atopy marker	Group		
	+ −	+ +	− −
Current personal history (n)			
Atopic eczema	9*	0*	5
Asthma	1	1	1
Atopy	6	1	5
Family history (n)			
Atopic eczema	4	2	1
Asthma	8	3	3
Atopy	7	4	3
Respiratory status (n)			
3 Chest colds per year	1	1	0
Wheeze with cold	6	5	1
Wheeze with exercise	5	3	1
Taking respiratory drugs	1	1	1
Past history of respiratory drugs	2	1	1
Pulmonary function tests[a]			
FVC (% predicted)	103.8 ± 13.06	102.6 ± 11.46	109.8 ± 10.20
FEV (% predicted)	104.1 ± 12.20	101.2 ± 13.30	112.3 ± 8.74
FEV/FVC (% predicted)	104.3 ± 9.00	100.3 ± 9.70	105.8 ± 5.40
PFR (% predicted)	100.9 ± 25.10	105.3 ± 17.0	119.2 ± 16.89
Eosinophil count (%)			
<4	13	9	6
4–7	5	0	3
>7	1	2	4
Mean	3.0	3.0	4.3
IgE (IU/litre)			
<120	13	8	10
120–400	1	2	2
>400	3	1	1
Mean	179.7	162.0	110.5

+ −, history positive, patch test negative; + +, history positive, patch test positive; − −, history negative, patch test negative; FVC, forced vital capacity; FEV, forced expiratory volume; PFR, peak flow rate

* $P = 0.02$

[a] Values are means ± SD.

patients in the study group gave a personal history of atopic eczema, compared with no patients in one of the control groups. This observation is confirmed by statistical analysis (for this comparison $P = 0.02$). None of the other comparisons between the study group and control groups gave P values less than 0.05. We therefore conclude that patients who have a nickel-positive history but are patch test negative do not have a higher than normal incidence of atopy.

Acknowledgements. We wish to thank Dr. C. Patterson, who performed the statistical analysis; Mrs. Barbara Martin, who performed the respiratory function test; Nurse Liz McCullough, wo performed the skin-prick testing; and Mrs. Jayne Fitz-Gerald for help with the manuscript.

Table 2. Results of skin-prick testing

Skin test diameter	Grass pollens			House dust			House dust mites			Dog			Cat			Aspergillus			Nickel		
	+ −	+ +	− −	+ −	+ +	− −	+ −	+ +	− −	+ −	+ +	− −	+ −	+ +	− −	+ −	+ +	− −	+ −	+ +	− −
Negative (*n*)	11	7	8	11	7	9	10	8	10	12	9	9	11	9	11	19	11	13	19	9	13
1–2 mm (*n*)	1	2	1	2	2	1	3	1	0	2	1	1	2	0	0	1	0	0	0	2	0
>2 mm (*n*)	8	2	4	7	2	3	7	2	3	6	1	3	7	2	2	0	0	0	1	0	0
Mean weal diameter (mm)	2.20	1.36	2.31	1.45	0.82	1.31	2.00	1.55	1.54	1.35	0.45	1.61	1.80	0.73	0.77	0.05	0	0	0.20	0.36	0

+ −, history positive, patch test negative; + +, history positive, patch test positive; − −, history negative, patch test negative

References

1. Kieffer M (1979) Nickel sensitivity: relationship between history and patch test reaction. Contact Dermatitis 6: 398–401
2. Menne T (1981) Nickel allergy – reliability of patch test evaluated in female twins. Dermatosen 29: 156–160
3. Latinga H, Nater JP, Coenraads PJ (1984) Prevalence, incidence and course of eczema on the hands and forearms in a sample of the general population. Contact Dermatitis 10: 135–139
4. Svensson A, Edman B, Moller H (1985) A diagnostic tool for atopic dermatitis based on clinical criteria. Acta Derm Venereol [Suppl] 114: 33–40
5. Moller H, Svensson A (1986) Metal sensitivity: positive history but negative test indicated atopy. Contact Dermatitis 14: 57–60
6. Fischer T, Rystedt I (1985) False-positive, follicular and irritant patch test reactions to metal salts. Contact Dermatitis 12: 93–98

Addresses

D. J. Todd
Departments of Dermatology and Respiratory Medicine, Royal Victoria Hospital, Grosvenor Road, Belfast, Northern Ireland, UK

D. Burrows
Departments of Dermatology and Respiratory Medicine, Royal Victoria Hospital, Grosvenor Road, Belfast, Northern Ireland, UK

C. F. Stanford
Departments of Dermatology and Respiratory Medicine, Royal Victoria Hospital, Grosvenor Road, Belfast, Northern Ireland, UK

Bioimplantation of Metals in Patients with Metal Allergy: The Late Outcome

H. Möller and Å. Carlsson

Summary

In the present follow-up study, it was possible to trace and re-examine 18 patients who had had orthopaedic devices for several years (mean 6.3 years) and who had a contact allergy to the relevant metal before surgery as well as at follow-up. No cutaneous or orthopaedic complications had occurred.

Key words:

Contact allergy - Nickel - Orthopaedic implants

Introduction

In patients with a contact allergy to chromium, cobalt or nickel, orthopaedic implantation of such a metal might elicit an allergic reaction, leading to postoperative or late skin disease as well as prosthetic loosening or other orthopaedic complications. Such an outcome would then be frequent, indeed, since contact allergy to metals – and to nickel in particular – is so common even in healthy populations. As a matter of fact, there is rich anecdotal evidence of eczematous reactions in metal-implanted patients with a previous history of metal sensitivity, but systematic studies are lacking.

In the present study, we wanted to follow patients with a preoperative, test-established metal allergy during the years after bioimplantation, looking for dermatologic and orthopaedic complications. For each individual, it was ascertained that the implant contained a metal agreeing with a positive skin test, and the test was repeated at follow-up including an intradermal confirmation.

Material and Methods

In order to reach patients known to have had a contact allergy to a metal before an orthopaedic bioimplantation, they were traced from two sources:

Group A. Patients found to have a contact allergy to nickel during the 15 years 1962–1976 at the Department of Dermatology ($n = 680$) were looked for in the records at the Department of Orthopaedics. We found 355 patients (52%) with nickel allergy and some medical care at the Department of Orthopaedics. Of these patients, 37 had been operated upon with implantation of a metallic device: 18 were deceased, 19 still living. Of these 19 patients, 15 could be traced and examined.

Group B. In a previously studied series [1], there were nine patients with a positive patch test to nickel before their total hip replacement. Seven of these patients could be evaluated.

A total of 22 patients were thus examined, undergoing dermatologic history-taking and examination, epicutaneous and intracutaneous tests for delayed metal allergy, and clinical and radiographic orthopaedic examination. Patch tests were performed with potassium dichromate 0.5%, cobalt chloride 0.5%, and nickel sulphate 5.0% in petrolatum, using Finn chambers on Scanpor applied for 48 h and read according to the International Contact Dermatitis Research Group (ICDRG) after a further 24 h. Intracutaneous tests were performed on the volar aspect of the right forearm with 1-m*M* saline solutions of the same metal salts and evaluated as a tuberculin reaction after 72 h.

Results

Of the 15 patients in group A, 2 were excluded from the final evaluation, 1 because he had been implanted with a stainless steel (chromium-nickel) prosthesis but at reexamination reacted only to cobalt, and 1 because she had at present no positive metal test. Of the seven patients in group B, two were excluded, one because she had at present no positive metal test, and one because he had been implanted with a vitallium (chromium-cobalt) prosthesis and was allergic to nickel. Thus, there remained 18 patients who had for several years (mean 6.3 years) been exposed to an orthopaedic implant containing a metal to which they were allergic.

From the orthopaedic point of view, no complications were observed that could be attributed to metal allergy. All fractures healed, in one case after revision and a more rigid fixation. One elbow arthroplasty was converted to an arthrodesis because of mechanical loosening of the components, a common complication. The loosening of a knee prosthesis in another case could also be explained by mechanical factors.

In dermatologic history-taking, very little was disclosed. Only 1 of the 18 patients acquired an eczematous dermatitis (leg first, face later) after the operation, while

3 patients saw an eczema disappear. Seven patients had an eczema to about the same degree before and after surgery. Of 15 patients who had a history of metal sensitivity before as well as after the operation, 3 thought that the sensitivity had diminished. Only one patient had had an eczematous reaction at the site and time of the surgical procedure. Of the 15 patients, 8 had had a periodic hand eczema, in most cases before as well as after the operation. In no case had an old eczema deteriorated or a new one appeared.

In group A, 1 of the 18 deceased patients had a skin reaction that could be attributed to a metallic implant. This woman with a previous contact allergy to chromate, cobalt, nickel, and neomycin unknown to the orthopaedic surgeon sustained an ankle fracture at the age of 75 years and was treated with open reduction and internal fixation. Later on, she developed an eczematous dermatitis on the foot and a symmetric papular itching eruption on the trunk. The eczema did not subside until the osteosynthetic material had been removed.

Discussion

This is the first long-term study of patients implanted with metallic devices in which a contact allergy to relevant metals was known before operation and ascertained also at follow-up. Previous studies have shown that preoperative test results are very little changed by orthopaedic bioimplantation, at least by hip arthroplasty [1]. Very few cases of sensitization have been recorded [2, 5], and in some cases metal allergy even disappeared after surgery [3]; this was also observed in our follow-up. Such changes from positive to negative metal tests may be explained by false-positive preliminary tests or by hyposensitization ("hardening") similar to the results of oral administration of a nickel salt [4].

In our 18 patients with persisting metal allergy, several years of wearing metallic implants did not bring about any cutaneous or orthopaedic complications. The procedure apparently is pretty harmless.

References

1. Carlsson ÅS, Magnusson B, Möller H (1980) Metal sensitivity in patients with metal-to-plastic total hip arthroplasties. Acta Orthop Scand 51: 57–62
2. Deutman R, Mulder THJ, Brian R, Nater JP (1977) Metal sensitivity before and after total hip arthroplasty. J Bone Joint Surg 59-A: 862–865
3. Rooker GD, Wilkinson JD (1980) Metal sensitivity in patients undergoing hip replacement. J Bone Joint Surg 62B: 502–505
4. Sjövall P, Christensen OB, Möller H (1987) Oral hyposensitization in nickel allergy. J Am Acad Dermatol 17: 774–778
5. Waterman AH, Schrik JJ (1985) Allergy in hip arthroplasty. Contact Dermatitis 13: 294–301

Addresses

H. Möller
Department of Dermatology, Lund University, S-21401 Malmö, Sweden

Å. Carlsson
Department of Orthopaedics, Lund University, S-21401 Malmö, Sweden

Cobalt, Nickel and PPD Sensitivity in Housewives' Hand Dermatitis

J. Vilaplana, F. Grimalt, and C. Romaguera

Summary

We have been interested in discovering allergens to which housewives with hand dermatitis are sensitive. To avoid coincidence with occupational extradomestic allergens, only housewives with hand dermatitis and with neither previous nor current extradomestic work were selected. The number of women with such characteristics seen during 1986 was 64. The allergens with the highest number of positive reactions were cobalt, nickel and PPD; 37.5%, 36% and 31.25%, respectively. In a previous paper [2, 3], it was demonstrated that Spanish household products contain cobalt and nickel. As we suspected that this high index of PPD sensitization could be due to daily contacts, we analysed 30 household products. We found a spectrophotometric curve pattern compatible with that of PPD in only three shoe creams, in two shoe dyes (household use) and in three household rubber gloves (pink, yellow and black). The possibility of housewives being sensitized to PPD through wearing such gloves is discussed.

Key words:

Rubber gloves - PPD - PPD compounds - Housewives - Household - Shoe creams - Shoe dyes

Introduction

In 1980, on presenting his thesis about sensitization to standard allergens and topical ointments applied to varicose ulcers and varicose complexes in 350 women. Vilaplana [1] referred to the unexplained fact that the allergen with the highest frequency of sensitization in such women (PPD; 12.5% of all sensitivities found in these women). It was followed by benzocaine (11.0%), sulphanilide (10.22%), nickel sulphate (10.0%), neomycin (7.5%), cobalt salts (5.0%) and Novocain (4.0%). As already remarked in a subsequent paper [2, 3], the incidence of cobalt sensitivity increased from 5.0% to 10.0% between 1977 and 1982. We wish to point out that the average age of the varicose women studied was higher than that of the women studied in the subsequent paper.

Despite accepting that, in managing housewives' hand dermatitis, adequate protection of the hand prevents noxious contacts of both irritative and allergic nature, we have been interested in discovering allergens to which housewives with hand dermatitis consulting our Allergy Department are sensitive. To avoid coincidence with occupational extradomestic allergens, only housewives with hand dermatitis and with neither previous nor current extradomestic work were selected. The number of women with such characteristics seen during 1986 was 64.

The results have been surprising. The allergens with the greatest number of positive reactions were cobalt, nickel and PPD (37.5%, 36% and 31.25%, respectively). Of the 17 patients sensitive to PPD, 13 showed positivity to only this substance, 3 patients were sensitive to PPD and Caine mix and 1 case sensitive to PPD and black rubber.

For other allergens sensitivity was as follows: 7.81% were sensitive to rubber (including 6.25% who were allergic to thiram mix); formaldehyde showed 6.25% positivity; 3.12% were allergic to mercury bichloride, and 1.56% to thiomersal; 4.68% were allergic to fragrance mix, and 1.56% to balsam of Peru; and colophony and *p-ter*-butylphenol showed a positivity of 1.56%.

In a previous paper [2, 3] the authors demonstrated that Spanish househould products contain cobalt and nickel. As it is difficult to accept that active sensitization to PPD may occur either from hair dyeing or from textile dye being given off, we suppose that this high index of sensitization may be due to daily household products. Using spectrophotometric methods, we have studied the PPD content in such Spanish products (gloves, shoe creams, cleaners, etc.).

Material and Methods

Determination of chromium, nickel and cobalt in household products by spectrophotometric methods is quite easy. On the other hand, determination of PPD is extraordinarily difficult. Firstly, using pure PPD, chemists establish its spectrophotometric curve pattern, which is later compared with the curve pattern of the studied substances. We studied three popular washing-up liquids, three detergents, three furniture waxes, three floor waxes, six shoe creams, six shoe dyes and six household rubber gloves by atomic absorption spectrophotometric methods, looking for a similar curve pattern to the one obtained using PPD as a standard pattern. The results obtained have been corroborated by manufacturers of the substances studied, which were selected, according to reliable marketing data, as being among the most used products.

Results

The three washing-up liquids studied did not contain any chemical substances compatible with PPD. In a later conversation with the manufacturers, it was discovered that phthalocyanine pigments are used as colourings in such products. We obtained the same results from detergents used for washing by hand. Window-cleaning products showed no presence of chemicals related to PPD, and neither did furniture or floor waxes.

Six shoe creams were studied (black, green, blue, red, yellow and brown). The black, green and blue ones showed negative results, but brown shoe cream showed a spectrophotometric curve pattern almost identical to that of PPD. Yellow and red shoe creams showed curve patterns compatible with that of PPD. In later conversations with manufacturers, we learnt that brown shoe cream contains a fat dye composed of naphthylamine and *m*-phenyldiamine [Color Index (I) no. 11 285]. Yellow shoe cream contains aniline dye (2,4-dichloroaniline). Red shoe cream contains a dye mixture in which 2,5-dichloroaniline (CI no. 12 460) is present.

Manufacturers of shoe and leather dyes state that Spanish consumers use shoe dyes as much as creams, more so than in the rest of Europe. Only two of the six shoe dyes studied showed a spectrophotometric curve pattern compatible with that of PPD. Red shoe dye contains a (phenylazo)aniline (CI no. 26 050), and the yellow one contains yellow aniline (CI no. 11 000).

The housewives' rubber gloves sold under numerous trade marks in this country are manufactured by only three different factories, which use identical chemicals. Of the brands sold, 70% are manufactured in this country, the remaining 30% being imported, chiefly from France and Germany. Of the six different rubber gloves studied, we found curve patterns compatible with PPD in only three: the black, pink and yellow ones.

White rubber gloves contain 2,2-methylene-bis[4-methyl-6-butyl]phenol as antioxidant; zinc diethyldithio carbamate as accelerator; and titanium oxide, zinc oxide and zinc sulphur as pigments. Yellow rubber gloves contain 2,2-methylene-bis[4-methyl-6-butyl]-phenol as antioxidant; zinc diethyldithio carbamate as accelerator; and *arylamide azo dye (dichlorobenzidine + acetoacetanilide).* Green rubber gloves contain 2,2-methylene-bis[4-methyl-6-butyl]-phenol as antioxidant; zinc diethyl dithiocarbamate as accelerator; and chlorinated copper phthalocyanine. Blue rubber gloves contain 2,2-methylene-bis[4-methyl-6-butyl]-phenol as antioxidant; zinc diethyldithio carbamate as accelerator, and non-chlorinated copper phthalocyanine. Pink rubber gloves contain the same antioxidant and accelerator as the blue ones, but the dye is an *azo pigment derived from naphthylamide.* Black rubber gloves contain *phenyl β-naphthylamine* as antioxidant, zinc diethyldithiocarbamate as accelerator and lampblack (of unknown composition; it is not known whether it contains PPD).

We wish to point out that of the three rubber gloves which contain PPD, two (yellow and pink) contain these substances as dyes, but in the black rubber gloves they are used as antioxidants.

Discussion

We have found PPD compounds in three Spanish shoe creams; three shoe dyes; and black, pink and yellow household rubber gloves. As it is difficult to accept that active sensitization to PPD may occur either from hair dyeing or from textile dye being given off, the mechanism of sensitization could be through contacts with PPD contained in the household products mentioned. Some of them contain amine radicals; others can form them by transformation of their chemical structure.

Contact with shoe creams and dyes is usually for a rather short time in normal housewives. We wish to remark that the manufacturers consulted state that shoe dyes are sold in Spain much more than in the rest of Europe. This fact may have practical importance, as generally shoe dye application entails longer hand contact than the application of shoe creams. The higher probability of sensitization could derive from that habit. Unlike shoe creams, contact with rubber gloves can extend to several hours daily. Sensitization to PPD by pink, black and yellow rubber gloves could be an explanation for the rather high percentage of sensitization found in the housewives studied.

Given these results, we have decided to revise the allergy histories of women seen during 1987 with characteristics identical to those reported here. We shall shortly patch-test them with the following substances:

1. Aniline yellow (CI no. 11 000) 1% petrolatum
2. Pigment red 9 (CI no. 12 460) 2% petrolatum
3. Solvent red 19 (CI no. 26 050) 1% petrolatum
4. Solvent brown (CI no. 11 285) 1% petrolatum
5. Phenyl β-naphthylamine 1% petrolatum

Meanwhile, our Allergy Department members will advise women sensitized to PPD not to wear black, pink or yellow rubber gloves, and to use cream, but not dye, for polishing shoes.

References

1. Vilaplana J, Grimalt F, Romaguera C, Mascaró J (1981) Frecuencia de sensibilización a ciertos alergenos en pacientes afectos de tromboflebitis y/o úlceras varicosas. Med Cutan Ibero Lat Am 9: 419–422
2. Vilaplana J, Grimalt F, Romaguera C, Mascaró J (1987) Cobalt content of household cleaning products. Contact Dermatitis 16: 139–141
3. Vilaplana J, Grimalt F, Romaguera C, Mascaró J (1988) Letter to the Editor. Cobalt content of household cleaning products. Contact Dermatitis 18: 254–255

Addresses

J. Vilaplana
Departament de Dermatologia, Hospital Clinic, Casanova 143, 08036 Barcelona, Spain

F. Grimalt
Departament de Dermatologia, Hospital Clinic, Casanova 143, 08036 Barcelona, Spain

C. Romaguera
Departament de Dermatologia, Hospital Clinic, Casanova 143, 08036 Barcelona, Spain

Metalworking Fluids and the Skin

E. M. de Boer, W. G. van Ketel, and D. P. Bruynzeel

Summary

An epidemiological study was performed to estimate the extent of occupational skin problems in metalworkers. In 9 factories, 286 metalworkers were investigated. Skin problems of hands and forearms were common. Exposure to soluble oils caused minor and major skin disease far more often than exposure to neat oils (62% and 25%, respectively). Hypersensitivity was not a major cause of dermatitis (2.8%), in contrast to chronic irritation. A predisposition to occupational dermatitis in atopics was not observed.

Key words:

Metalworking fluids - Occupational dermatitis - Irritant dermatitis - Acrovesicular dermatitis - Biocides - Patch tests - Epidemiology

Introduction

Metalworking fluids (MWF) are used for lubricating and for cooling. For different kinds of metalworking, varying types of fluids are used [1]. Neat oils consist mainly of oils and sometimes contain extreme pressure additives, corrosion inhibitors, antifoams, dyes and fragrances. Water-based fluids, having a far more complex composition, contain oils, emulsifiers, stabilizers, extreme pressure additives, antifoams, corrosion inhibitors, dyes, fragrances and preservatives. Soluble oils contain varying amounts of oil; aqueous solutions contain no oil at all. Water-based fluids are supplied by the producer as a concentrate that has to be diluted with water by the client to about 1%–10% before use.

Exposure to MWF may lead to several dermatoses, such as acne, folliculitis, and hyperpigmentation, and with the old-fashioned fluids, to keratoses and cancer [2]. From the point of view of sick leave due to occupational exposure to MWF, the occurrence of dermatitis is important. In this study, we will confine our attention to dermatitis and dermatitis-like eruptions on hands and forearms.

Materials and Methods

An epidemiological study was performed in nine metalworking plants in the Netherlands. All metalworkers exposed to MWF present at the time of the investigation ($n = 286$) were included in the study. In case of past or present dermatitis of the hands and/or forearms, epicutaneous tests were performed with van der Bend square chambers, fixed with Fixomull tape, removed after 48 h and graded at 72 h as recommended by the International Contact Dermatitis Research Group (ICDRG). The standard series (ICDRG) and a special series of components of MWF, predominantly biocides, were tested. This series was based on data from the literature and information from suppliers of MWF in Holland. Additionally, the workers' own MWF were tested in several dilutions, ranging from undiluted to 10%, and relevant products in each factory.

Results

Of 286 metalworkers, 61 (21%) complained of skin problems of the hands. Dryness and scaling was a common complaint, as was a stinging and burning sensation, sometimes itching, when soluble oil got into small wounds. Mechanical injuries were present among 46% of all operators. Skin changes were divided in to two groups: minor abnormalities (including a dry, rough skin; slight erythema with chapping; and periungual erythema) were present in 31%; major disorders (characterized by more serious erythema, induration and scaling of the skin, and/or chronic paronychia) were present in 27%.

The workers were divided in to three groups according to exposure predominantly to neat oils, to soluble oils or to both types. The occurrence of skin abnormalities was considered in relation to the exposure (Table 1).

Dermatitis of the hands and forearms was present in 14% of all workers. Patch tests were done in all cases and also in two persons with a history of dermatitis. Positive reactions were seen in 8 cases (2.8%). Allergy to one or more biocides was observed in four cases; involving formaldehyde and several releasers, such as Grotan BK, morpholines, isothiazolines and alkanolamineborate complex. The other four workers were sensitized to various allergens: nickel, cobalt and chromate salts; balsam of Peru; and rubber additives. Of 39 persons with dermatitis of the hands, 21 had an acrovesicular eczema. An atopic constitution, diagnosed on history, was present in 21% of all workers. Irritant dermatitis was diagnosed in 15% of atopics and in 10% of non-atopics.

Table 1. The presence and severity of skin abnormalities in relation to the type of metalworking fluid to which workers were exposed

	Metalworking fluid			Total/overall
	Soluble oil	Neat oil	Both types	
No. of workers	181	36	69	286
Skin disease (n)				
Minor	65 (36)	5 (14)	20 (29)	90 (31)
Major	48 (26)	4 (11)	23 (33)	75 (27)

The numbers given in parentheses are percentages.

Discussion

From these data several conclusions may be drawn:

1. Skin problems of the hands and forearms were common in metal workers. Only 42% had no skin disease, the remaining workers having minor or major changes. Data about the incidence of skin problems in metalworkers in the Netherlands are scarce. In the only survey of the incidence of dermatitis, 10.7% of all kinds of metalworkers had dermatitis [3].
2. Contact sensitization was not a major problem. Of the workers with dermatitis, 20% (2.8% of all operators) were allergic. In these cases, the most common cause of sensitization was one or more biocides. This percentage of contact sensitization is difficult to relate to other studies, as most authors consider another group of individuals, and not a "healthy" group of metalworkers. Irritant dermatitis outnumbers allergic dermatitis in almost all observations by far [1, 2, 4–6].
3. Exposure to soluble oils caused minor and major skin disease more often than exposure to neat oils. Both irritant and allergic contact dermatitis have been observed more frequently with soluble oils, but damage to the barrier function of the skin by neat oils has been described [7].
4. Acrovesicular dermatitis as an irritant dermatitis in workers with soluble oils was a common observation. Acrovesicular dermatitis of the hands is often associated with atopy and/or contact sensitization to several allergens, especially to metals [1, 8]. In our study, however, this type of eczema seems to be due to the irritant effect of water-based MWF [9], which confirms the observation of Weidenbach [10].
5. The incidence of atopy was not higher in the group with irritant or allergic dermatitis than in the unaffected group. Figures are small and might be explained by possible selection before or during work.

Limitation of exposure to MWF is important in the prevention of both irritant and allergic contact dermatitis. This might partly be achieved by protective clothing. Furthermore, the concentration of biocides and irritant components in MWF should be kept as low as possible. A higher concentration often means a further rise in the already alkaline character of these fluids, thus adding to the irritating potential. It is therefore very important to use water-based fluids in a correct dilution, which requires regular control. The sensitizing potential of biocides should play a role in their selection.

References

1. Rycroft RJG (1982) Cutting fluids, oil and lubricants. In: Maibach HI, Gellin GA (eds) Occupational and industrial dermatology. Year Book, Chicago, pp 233–236
2. Alomar A (1985) Occupational dermatosis from cutting oils. Contact Dermatitis 12: 129–138
3. Coenraads PJ, Nater JP, van der Lende R (1983) Prevalence of eczema and other dermatoses of the hands and arms in the Netherlands. Association with age and occupation. Clin Exp Dermatol 8: 495–503
4. Rycroft RJG (1985) Soluble oil dermatitis. In: Essentials in industrial dermatology. Griffith and Wilkinson, Oxford, pp 73–85
5. Angelini G, Meneghini CL (1977) Dermatitis in engineers due to synthetic coolants. Contact Dermatitis 3: 219–220
6. Van Ketel WG, Kisch LS (1983) The problem of the sensitizing capacity of some Grotans used as bacteriocides in cooling oils. Dermatosen 31: 118–121
7. Coenraads PJ, Lee J, Pinnagoda J (1986) Changes in water vapor loss from the skin of metal industry workers monitored during exposure to oils. Scand J Work Environ Health 12: 494–498
8. Hornstein OP, Bäurle G (1986) Das chronische Handekzem: Diagnostik und Therapie. In: Braun-Falco O, Schill WB (eds) Fortschritte der praktischen Dermatologie und Venereologie. Springer, Berlin Heidelberg New York, pp 13–25
9. De Boer EM, Bruynzeel DP, Van Ketel WG (1988) Dyshidrotic eczema as an occupational dermatitis in metalworkers. Contact Dermatitis 19: 184–188
10. Weidenbach Th, Rakoski J (1985) Gehäuftes Auftreten von dyshidrosiformen Handekzemen durch eine Öl-in-Wasser-Emulsion bei Metallarbeitern. Dermatosen 33: 121–124

Addresses

E. M. de Boer

Department of Occupational Dermatology, Academic Hospital Free University, de Boelelaan 117, 1081 HV Amsterdam, The Netherlands

W. G. van Ketel

Department of Occupational Dermatology, Academic Hospital Free University, de Boelelaan 117, 1081 HV Amsterdam, The Netherlands

D. P. Bruynzeel

Department of Occupational Dermatology, Academic Hospital Free University, de Boelelaan 117, 1081 HV Amsterdam, The Netherlands

Cutting Oil Dermatitis: A Review of 115 Patients

J. S. C. English and R. J. G. Rycroft

Summary

We have investigated 115 patients presenting with dermatoses, who worked with cutting oils. The study period was from 1986 to 1987. There were 111 men and 4 women, with ages ranging from 16 to 66 years (mean 42 ± 14.3 years). The final diagnoses were as follows: 28 patients had endogenous hand eczema and irritant contact dermatitis (ICD); 22 allergic contact dermatitis (ACD) and ICD; 21 ICD alone; 19 ACD alone; 12 endogenous hand eczema; 6 other (non-eczematous) conditions; 4 ACD, ICD and endogenous hand eczema; and 3 ACD and endogenous hand eczema. Formaldehyde-releasing biocides were the commonest cause of allergic reactions in the cutting oil series. Reactions were also seen to colophony, formaldehyde, nickel, rubber, dichromate and epoxy resin in the International Contact Dermatitis Research Group (ICDRG) standard series. As 42% of the patients had relevant positive patch tests, patch testing remains an essential investigation in the management of cutting oil dermatitis.

Key words:

Cutting oil dermatitis - Irritant - Allergic - Formaldehyde-releasing biocides - Colophony - Occupational

Introduction

Most physicians probably think of cutting oil dermatitis as an irritant contact dermatitis, yet its aetiology can involve both irritant and allergic contact dermatitis, an endogenous factor, or combinations of all three. We have reviewed our patients with suspected cutting oil dermatitis over the past 2 years to see to what extent allergic factors were contributing to their dermatitis, and to determine the usefulness of a cutting oil series.

Materials and Methods

All patients with suspected work-related dermatitis from cutting oils who presented to the St John's Hospital Contact Clinic in the years 1986 and 1987 were included in the study. The patients were usually referred by their occupational physician. After having dermatological and occupational histories taken, with a clinical examination and review of contact factors, each patient was patch-tested with the ICDRG standard series, a cutting oil series (Table 1) and a face series, which included phosphorus sesquisulphide, if the dermatitis had spread to the face. The patch tests were applied with Finn Chambers and Scanpore tape and read at 2 and 4 days.

Work-related dermatitis was defined as that which was caused or made worse by the patient's work, that is worse during the working week and better or cleared

Table 1. Cutting oil series adapted from Chemotechnique Diagnostics AB

Allergen	Dilution (%)
Abietic acid	10
PCMC	1
PCMX	0.5
Dichlorophen	0.5
O-Phenylphenol	1
Propylene glycol	5 aqua
Triethanolamine	2
p-tert-Butylbenzoic acid	1
1,2-benzisothiazolin-3-one	0.1 aqua
Grotan BK	1 aqua
Bioban P1487	1
Chloroacetamide	0.2
n-Methylol-chloroacetamide	0.1
Benzotriazole	1
Irgasan DP300	2
Bioban CS1246	1
Bioban CS1135	1
Tris Nitro	1
Merthiolate	0.1
Hydrazine sulphate	1
Trichlorocarbanilide	1
Amerchol L101	As is
Dipentene	1
Sodium omadine	0.1 aqua
Coconut diethanolamide	0.5
Kathon 886 MW	0.02
Tektamer 38	0.1
Araldite CY 184	1

The vehicle is petrolatum unless otherwise stated.

away from work. Endogenous eczema was diagnosed by a combination of the clinical pattern of the eczema and the fact that it was not caused by work, housework or hobbies. ICD was diagnosed if the dermatitis was work related, the patient was in contact with known irritants and relevant patch tests were negative. ACD was diagnosed if positive patch tests to allergens which the patient was in contact with were obtained.

Results

We investigated 111 men and 4 women, with ages ranging from 16 to 66 years (mean 42 ± 14.3 years). The length of history of dermatitis prior to presentation ranged from 1 month to 50 years (mean length 4.8 years $\pm$ 8.7 SD). The final diagnoses were as follows: 28 (24%) of the patients had endogenous hand eczema and ICD; 22 (19%) ACD and ICD; 21 (18%) ICD alone; 19 (17%) ACD alone; 12 (10%) endogenous hand eczema; 6 (5%) other (non-eczematous) conditions; 4 (4%) ACD, ICD and endogenous hand eczema; and 3 (3%) ACD and endogenous hand eczema.

Patch Tests. The number of positive patch tests to particular allergens is shown in Table 2. Colophony followed by formaldehyde were the commonest.

Discussion

From our results, there is no doubt about the value of patch testing in patients with suspected cutting oil dermatitis. Other studies [1, 2] have shown as high a percentage of patients working with cutting oils with ACD. However, it is not only the al-

Table 2. The most frequent positive allergens

Allergen	Positive tests (*n*)
Colophony	12
Formaldehyde	10
Nickel	10
Dowicil 200	7 (4)
Bioban CS1135[a]	7 (6)
Neomycin	7
Fragrance	6
Thiram	6
Araldite CY 184[a]	5
Chromate	4
Epoxy resin	4
Phosphorus sesquisulphide	4
Grotan BK[a]	4 (3)
Bronopol	3

The number of HCHO positive tests is given in parentheses.
[a] In cutting oil series.

lergenic additives in the oils that are the source of the dermatitis but also other allergens with which the patients come into contact, such as rubber gloves, and preservatives in barrier creams, liquid soaps and after-work creams; for example, the source of the Dowicil 200 in three of the seven Dowicil-positive patients, was a hand cleanser.

The incidence of the various causes of ACD will depend upon exposure to allergens, and this will vary from factory to factory and country to country. Alomar et al. [1] in Spain found 21% of their patients positive to benzisothiazolone, whereas we did not have any. However, 10% of our patients were allergic to colophony, compared with only 3% in Alomar's series.

Regarding the usefulness of a cutting oil series, in our patients 11% of relevant positive allergic reactions would have been missed if the series had not been applied. A cutting oil series, therefore, is a useful diagnostic tool when investigating cutting oil dermatitis, though not a complete substitute for patch testing with non-irritant dilutions of potentially allergenic products to which the patient is exposed.

Patch testing in patients with suspected cutting oil dermatitis is essential, even though ICD remains the major cause. ACD plays a powerful supporting role in the often multifactorial aetiology of cutting oil dermatitis.

References

1. Alomar A, Conde-Salazar L, Romaguera C (1985) Occupational dermatoses from cutting oils. Contact Dermatitis 12: 129–138
2. Angelini G, Meneghini CL (1977) Dermatitis in engineers due to synthetic coolants. Contact Dermatitis 3: 219–220

Addresses

J. S. C. English
Department of Occupational Dermatoses, St John's Hospital for Diseases of the Skin, 5 Lisle Street, London WC2H 7BJ, UK

R. J. G. Rycroft
Department of Occupational Dermatoses, St John's Hospital for Diseases of the Skin, 5 Lisle Street, London WC2H 7BJ, UK

Medicaments

Contact Hypersensitivity in Patients with Chronic Otitis Externa

P. K. Buxton, D. G. Keay, and I. M. Smith

Summary

Positive reactions were found in 22 (58%) of 37 patients with chronic otitis externa who were investigated for delayed hypersensitivity using standardised patch testing. This incidence is higher than the 40% found in the only similar previous study [1] and is within the range of 32% [2]–72% [3] found in patients with contact dermatitis. The average age of subjects showing a positive reaction was 56.7 years, and for those with negative tests it was 34.9 years. This age difference suggests that in the younger patient, contact hypersensitivity is a less significant aetiological factor. Neomycin was the commonest sensitising agent, tests being positive in 12 (32%) of the patients.

Key words:

Otitis externa - Allergy - Contac dermatitis

Introduction

Patients treated in hospital clinics represent the more severe cases of otitis externa and can be slow to respond. Previous studies [1, 4, 5] have suggested that the development of allergy to topical medication may be an aetiological factor in these patients. This study adopted the standard method for patch testing and limited inclusion to those patients suffering solely from otitis externa for a minimum of 3 months.

Materials and Methods

Between January 1986 and February 1988, 37 patients suffering from otitis externa for a minimum of 3 months, who were referred to the otolaryngology outpatient department of the Royal Infirmary, Edinburgh, were studied. Those with generalised skin pathology, viral or malignant otitis externa, or a coexistent otitis media were excluded. A clinical history established the presence of previous atopy, contact sensitivity and drug allergy. The condition of the pinna and both external auditory canals was recorded, and patch testing was carried out using the standard European battery, supplemented by specific eardrop constituents.

Results

Throughout this study, Student's *t* test was used for statistical analysis. There was no significant sex difference between those with negative and those with positive responses. The age distribution for those with and without topical hypersensitivity is shown in Fig. 1. The mean ages of the groups were 56.7 years and 34.9 years, respectively, a statistically significant difference ($P<0.001$). Patients reacted to 24 of the 49 agents tested. The substances more frequently responsible are recorded in Table 1.

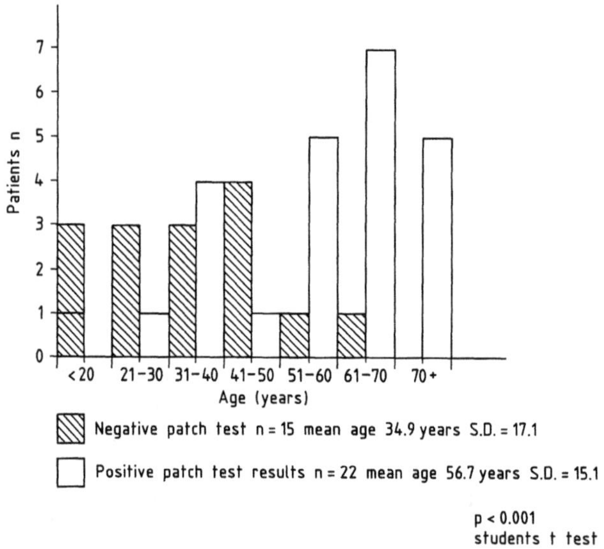

Fig. 1. Age distribution for patients with positive and negative patch tests

Table 1. Positive patch tests in patients with otitis externa and contact dermatitis

Test substance	Positive tests		
	Otitis externa		Contact dermatitis[a]
	n	% of total[b]	
Neomycin 20%	12	55	14
Framycetin	10	45	–
Fragrance mix	5	23	18
Benzalkonium chloride 0.1%	4	18	–
Graneodin ointment	3	14	–
Quinolone mix 6%	3	14	–
Audicort drops	2	9	–
Nickel sulphate 5%	2	9	39
Chloramphenicol	2	9	–
Thiuram mix 1%	2	9	8
Balsam of Peru 25%	2	9	7
Gentamycin sulphate 1%	2	9	–

[a] Percentage of total positives (from [6]).
[b] A total of 22 patients showed positive tests.

Agents relevant to the treatment of otitis externa which did not produce hypersensitivity are as follows:

1. Clioquinol 5%
2. Polymyxin B sulphate 5%
3. Terracotril ointment
4. Canesten cream
5. Fucidin ointment
6. Clycerine and ichthammol 10%
7. Nystaform ointment

Of the 22 patients with hypersensitivity, 14 (63%) gave responses to two or more agents. Neomycin hypersensitivity was associated with a cross-reaction to framycetin in 10 of 12 patients and to gentamycin in 2 of 12 patients.

Discussion

The incidence of positive patch tests in this group was 58%, which is higher than the 40% reported in a previous Scandinavian study [1]. Among patients with suspected allergic contact dermatitis in the Lothian Region, 68% showed positive patch tests [6] (Table 1). The problem of allergic contact dermatitis has also been found in patients with leg ulcers, who show an incidence of 55% [7]–85% [8]. It would appear, therefore, that hypersensitivity is as common in chronic otitis externa as in these other conditions.

Allergy to these agents in otitis externa appears to be particularly relevant in the older age group, in contrast to the age distribution of hypersensitivity in contact dermatitis, with incidence peaks at 20–30 years and 50–70 years [9]. This difference in age distribution has not been previously observed. The increased hypersensitivity seen with ageing has been attributed to the loss of suppressor-cell regulation of the immune system, as found in experimental animals [10].

Neomycin was the most common allergen, giving a positive patch test result in 32% (12) of the patients tested. This is much higher than the incidence found in either leg ulcers (0%–25% [8, 11]) or contact dermatitis (3.7%–6% [3, 12]), and it is far in excess of that found in the normal population (0.55%–1.8% [13]). Our 83% cross-over sensitivity between neomycin and framycetin is in agreement with values found elsewhere [14], but the 17% cross-over with gentamycin is rather less than the 40% level we would have expected from previous work [15]. Although the avoidance of neomycin in otitis externa has been previously advocated [16], exposure to neomycin must have occurred in 32% (12) of our patients for hypersensitivity to have developed. We would, therefore, stress that neomycin-containing preparations should not be used in the treatment of otitis externa.

References

1. Fraki Jorma E, Kirsti Kalimo, Pekka Tuohimaa, Eero Aantaa (1985) Contact allergy to various components of topical preparations for the treatment of external otitis. Acta Otolaryngol (Stock) 100: 414–418
2. Hammershoy Ole (1980) Standard patch test results in 3225 consecutive Danish patients. Contact Dermatitis 6: 263–268
3. Ruoner EJ et al. (1973) North American contact dermatitis group – The epidemiology of contact dermatitis in North America: 1972. Arch Dermatology 108: 537–540
4. Holmes RC, Johns AN, Wilkinson JD, Black MM, Rycroft JG (1972) Medicament contact dermatitis in patients with chronic inflammatory ear disease. JRS Med 75: 27–30
5. Rasmussen PA (1974) Otitis externa and allergic contact dermatitis. Acta Otolaryngol
6. Vestey JP, Gawkrodger OJ, Wong WK, Buxton PK (1986) The analysis of 501 consecutive contact clinic consultations. Contact Dermatitis 15: 119–125
7. Parasmothy Y, Collins M, Smith AG (1988) Contact dermatitis in patients with leg ulcers. Contact Dermatitis 18: 30–36
8. Blondell A, Oleffe J, Achten G (1978) Contact allergy in 330 dermatological patients. Contact Dermatitis 4: 270–276
9. Tetsuro Sugai, Takashi Takagi, Sachiyo Yashimoto, Yohko Takahashi (1979) The age distribution of the incidence of contact sensitivity to standard allergens. Contact Dermatitis 5: 383–388
10. Polak L (1978) Recent trends in the immunology of contact sensitivity I and II. Contact Dermatitis 4: 249–263
11. Brian RG, Nater JP (1973) Ulcus crurisen contacticzeem. Naederlandse Tijdschrisft of Geneeskunde 117: 561–565
12. Fregert S, Hjorth V, Magnusson B, Bandmann H-J, Calnan CD, Cronin E, Malten K, Meneshini CL, Perilia V, Wilkison DS (1969) Epidemiology of contact dermatitis. In: Transactions StJohn's Hospital Dermatological Society 55: 17–35
13. Prystovsky A (1979) Allergic contact hypersensitivity. Archives Dermatology 115: 960–962
14. Carruthers JA, Cronin E (1976) Incidence of neomycin and framycetin sensitivity. Contact Dermatitis 2: 269–270
15. Parila V, Hirvonen ML, Rouhunkoskis (1968) The pattern of cross sensitivity to neomycin secondary sensitisation to gentamycin. Dermatologica 136: 321–324
16. Jensen CO, Allen HJ, Mordecai CR (1966) Neomycin contact dermatitis superimposed on otitis externa. JAMA 195: 175

Addresses

P. K. Buxton
Department of Dermatology, The Royal Infirmary, Edinburgh, Scotland, UK

D. G. Keay
Department of Otolaryngology, The Royal Infirmary, Edinburgh, Scotland, UK

I. M. Smith
Department of Otolaryngology, The Royal Infirmary, Edinburgh, Scotland, UK

Mafenide - Still an Allergen of Importance?

R. Breit and P. Seifert

Summary

Mafenide contact allergy was found in 149 (3.5%) of 4270 patients tested in Munich (FRG) between 1976 and 1987. In spite of the fact that the main mafenide-containing product, Marfanil-Prontalbin-Puder, was removed from the market in 1974, 40 patients reported an onset of dermatitis less than 1 year ago; in addition, 28 patients were under the age of 40. It was demonstrated that mafenide-containing products are still on the market, mainly in veterinary medicine. Therefore, mafenide should remain incorporated in standard test series, at least in Germany.

Key words:

Mafenide - Veterinary medicine - Contact dermatitis - Test results

Introduction

Mafenide [4-(aminomethyl)benzenesulfonamide] was used as a topically applied chemotherapeutic agent in Germany from 1941 up to 1974, when the marketing of the main mafenide-containing product, Marfanil-Prontalbin-Puder, ceased for human purposes. According to Jelenko et al. [6], "During the years that Mafenide has been known, it has been involved in an amazing mosaic of history, including war, politics, murder, and espionage." In addition, mafenide used to be a notorious sensitizer, with 1.5%–5.5% positive reactions in several investigations [1–4, 7]. Because the incidence of sensitization will directly reflect the use of the allergenic chemical, one would expect the rate of sensitization in the German population to decline gradually after 1974. If this assumption is correct, today mafenide should only be an allergen of historical importance.

Materials and Methods

To test this hypothesis, we continued to investigate mafenide sensitivity in the allergy unit of the Department of Dermatology and Allergology of the City-Hospital, Munich-Schwabing. Between 1976 and 1987, 4270 patients were tested with 10% mafenide hydrochloride in petrolatum, following the International Contact Dermatitis Research Group (ICDRG) rules.

Results

We found 149 positive patients, which is an overall percentage of 3.5. There was a small but only insignificant decline over the investigation period. The mean age of the mafenide-positive patients was high (58.7 years). Of the 149 patients 18.8% (28) were under the age of 40 years. The two largest clinical diagnostic categories were stasis dermatitis and allergic dermatitis (40.9% and 38.3%, respectively; Table 1). First localization of dermatitis was the lower leg in 41.6% of all cases, but in 20.1% it was the hand. In 46.3%, the history ranged backwards more than 5 years, but 26.8% reported an onset of dermatitis less than 1 year previously. Nearly half the mafenide-positive patients were not sensitized to a chemically related substance of the so-called para group (Table 2) and 28 (18.8%) of the patients showed a mono-

Table 1. Clinical diagnosis in 149 mafenide-positive patients

Diagnosis	Patients	
	n	%
Dermatitis		
Stasis	61	40.9
Allergic	57	38.3
Unclassified	13	8.7
Atopic	11	7.4
Other types	8	5.4
Other	3	2.0

Table 2. Concomitant allergies in 149 mafenide-positive patients

Allergens	Patients	
	n	%
Para group −, other −	28	18.8
Para group +, other −	19	12.8
Para group +, other +	62	41.6
Para group −, other +	40	26.8

Table 3. First localization(s) of dermatitis of less than 1 year's duration in nine monovalent mafenide-positive patients

Localization	No. of cases
Hand	2
Foot	2
Flexures	1
Lower leg	1
Face	0
Trunk	0
Generalized	1
Other	2

valent allergy against mafenide. Of these 28 patients, 10 (35.7%) were under the age of 40 years, and 9 (32.1%) reported dermatitis of less than 1 year's duration (Table 3).

Discussion

As expected, the "typical" mafenide-positive patient is in the second half of his or her life, so he or she had the opportunity to come into contact with mafenide decades ago. Marfanil-Prontalbin-Puder was used especially for treating infected wounds, for instance, leg ulcers in stasis dermatitis. This diagnosis is always correlated to history of long duration. Sensitization to medicaments is very frequent in stasis dermatitis [5]. In this group of patients, mafenide is only of historical importance.

However, there is still another type of mafenide-positive patient, those under the age of 40 years: the clinical diagnosis is contact allergy, the history can be traced back only less than a year, and the site of the first involvement is not infrequently the hand. The mafenide allergy cannot be explained as a concomitant allergy in patients originally sensitized to chemicals of the so-called para group. To our surprise, not only was mafenide used to treat burns up to 1984, but it is still on the German market in eyedrops and two preparations for wound dressing. Even more important is its continuing use in veterinary medicine. Also, the famous Marfanil-Prontalbin-Puder is still marketed here in unknown but probably large amounts [8]. Careful examinations revealed that several of our patients could very well be exposed to mafenide via these routes. In addition, the old Marfanil-Prontalbin-Puder is probably still dangerously present in many old-fashioned first-aid kits in home and business locations. Even the possibility of veterinary medicaments being used for human purposes cannot be ruled out in rural regions. Therefore, still being an allergen of importance, mafenide should remain incorporated in standard test series, at least in Germany.

References

1. Bandmann HJ (1966) Die Kontaktallergie durch Arzneimittel. Pharm Zeit 111: 1470–1479
2. Bandmann HJ, Breit R (1973) The Mafenide story. Br J Dermatol 89: 219–221
3. Barthel C (1979) Zur Kontaktallergie gegen Neomycin, Lanolin und p-Hydroxybenzoesäure. Thesis, Munich
4. Braun W (1970) Iatrogene Sensibilisierung und Beinleiden. Med Klin 65: 506–509
5. Breit R (1977) Allergen change in stasis dermatitis. Contact Dermatitis 3: 309–311
6. Jelenko C, Jelenko JM, Mendelson JA, Buxton RW (1966) The Marfanil mystery. Surg Gyn Obst 122: 121–127
7. Lämmer D (1979) Testergebnisse von 1008 Patienten mit Kontaktallergie. Z Hautkr 54: 571–579
8. Seifert P (1988) Mafenid – immer noch ein Allergen von Bedeutung? Untersuchung zur Häufigkeit von Mafenidkontaktallergien im Raum München (1975–1987). Thesis, Munich

Addresses

R. Breit

Dermatologische und Allergologische Abteilung des Städt. Krankenhauses München-Schwabing, Kölner Platz 1, 8000 München 40, FRG

P. Seifert

Dermatologische und Allergologische Abteilung des Städt. Krankenhauses München-Schwabing, Kölner Platz 1, 8000 München 40, FRG

Systemic Drugs and Palmar Eczema

B. Edman

Summary

A statistical study of the relationship between vesicular palmar eczema and various clinical variables was carried out. Vesicular palmar eczema was found in 153 patients (38%), whom 113 (74%) were women. Of all the cases found, 92% could be regarded as pompholyx. Three new pathogenetic factors were suggested in vesicular palmar eczema: use of acetylsalicylic acid (Aspirin), contraceptives and smoking. Furthermore, the relationship between pompholyx and contact allergy to nickel was confirmed. No correlation to atopy was found; however, both atopy and sex were found to constitute certain risk groups. The study was based on information from 425 consecutively patch-tested patients (74% women) from our local database DA-LUK.

Key words:

Hand eczema - Pompholyx - Systemic drugs - Contact dermatitis - Atopy - Acetylsalicylic acid - Contraceptive drugs - Smoking

Introduction

Pompholyx (vesiculosis, dyshidrosis) is a common type of hand dermatitis. In one study, pompholyx was found in about 20% of all cases of hand eczema [1]. The pathogenesis of pompholyx is still obscure, although a hereditary predisposition may exist [2]. The view that the sweat glands play a role has been virtually abandoned today [3].

At our clinic, many of the patch-tested patients with vesicular palmar eczema (VPE) stated that the only systemic or topical drug used at the time of their latest eczematous eruption was acetylsalicylic acid. Furthermore, B. Björkner (Section for Occupational Dermatology, Malmö) had seen a suspected case of correlation between the use of contraceptives and pompholyx. In addition, it has been reported that the pathogenesis of another chronic palmoplantar disease, *viz.* pustulosis, is correlated to smoking. Thus, a study was designed to investigate further the association between these causes and VPE (pompholyx in particular). In addition, evaluation of correlations between VPE and contact allergy to nickel, cobalt, chromate, neomycin and balsam of Peru was included since they have all been described before.

Material and Methods

During a 9-month period (1986–1987), the following information about 425 consecutively patch-tested patients was recorded at the time of application of the patch tests:

1. Age and sex.
2. Atopy.
3. Smoking habits.
4. VPE (eczema elsewhere in addition was permitted).
5. Pompholyx (eczema elsewhere in addition was *not* permitted).
6. Systemic drugs. The reported drugs were classified in groups, e.g. diuretics, contraceptives, etc., except for analgesics, which were divided into acetylsalicylic acid, paracetamol and other analgesics.
7. Patch test results.

VPE as solitary or associated manifestation of eczema was found in 153 cases (38%), consisting of 113 women (74%) and 40 men (26%). Of these 153 patients, 15 had eczema elsewhere: 3 on the soles (included in the pompholyx cases), 2 on the legs, 3 on the arms, 4 on the wrists and 3 elsewhere; thus, pompholyx was found in 141 cases (33%), i.e. in 92% of all cases of VPE.

Results

It was found that a statistical relationship exists between VPE and smoking ($P<0.05$). The correlation was observed mainly in men, and a special risk group is non-atopic men. Furthermore, smoking was correlated to low age ($P<0.05$), but not to sex.

Thirty-one different groups of systemic drugs were registered. The most frequent drugs/groups were found to be acetylsalicylic acid (ASA) (15%), paracetamol (13%), contraceptives (12%) and diuretics (11%). It was confirmed that VPE is correlated to the use of ASA and contraceptives. The positive correlation between the use of contraceptives and VPE has not been reported before. Atopic women predominate in this group.

Discussion

The correlation between VPE or pompholyx and the use of ASA, also not reported before, is of great interest due to the high frequency of use of ASA. ASA is known to provoke a variety of skin reactions, including urticaria, angioneurotic oedema, purpura and pustular psoriasis [5]. ASA is known also to provoke a non-specific-type reaction of urticaria [6] and the same might be considered for VPE and pompholyx. This correlation was dominated by men and atopic women. The correlation between VPE and smoking, which has never been reported before, was also confirmed. It was found that men constituted a certain risk group.

Finally, contact allergy to nickel was found in 81 (19%; including 73 women) of the 425 patch-tested patients, to neomycin in 13 patients (3.0%) and to balsam of Peru in 13 patients (3.0%). VPE was found to be positively correlated only to contact allergy to nickel in women, as shown earlier [4]. No correlations were found between VPE and balsam of Peru, neomycin, cobalt or chromate, although such correlations have been shown by others, as described by [1]. This may be due to the small numbers of patients allergic to these substances. Nor could a relationship between VPE and atopy be demonstrated, as has been suggested by other authors concerning pompholyx [2]. A possible explanation for this could be that different definitions of atopy and/or various selection criteria have been used. Furthermore, VPE was found to be correlated to low age, i.e. to occur, predominantly in the age group 20–40 years, which is at variance with an earlier study [2].

References

1. Burton JL, Rook A, Wilkinson DS (1986) Eczema, lichen simplex, erythroderma and prurigo. In: Rook A et al. (eds) Textbook of dermatology. Blackwell, Oxford, p394
2. Lorincz AL, Grauer FH (1958) Arch Dermatol 74: 245
3. Wolff HH, Kutzner H (1986) How do I treat dyshidrosiform eruptions? Z Haut Kr 61 (11): 815–818
4. Christensen O, Möller H (1975) Nickel allergy and hand eczema. Contact Dermatitis 1: 129–135
5. Andersson RH (1984) Autoimmune progesterone dermatitis. Cutis 33: 490–491
6. Michaelsson G, Juhlin L (1973) Urticaria induced by preservatives and dye additives in food and drugs. Br J Dermatol 88: 525

Addresses

B. Edman
Department of Dermatology, S-21401 Malmö, Sweden

Cutaneous Reactions to Estraderm

R. M. Adams

Summary

Transdermal delivery systems have been devised and marketed for clonidine, nitroglycerine, scopolamine, and estrogen. The estrogen system is especially valuable because the route of administration bypasses the liver, where normal estrogen detoxification takes place. For maximum effectiveness, the patch must remain on the skin for 3 or 4 days. Many patients have experienced dermatitis at the site of application of the estrogen patches. Some possible causes of these reactions will be discussed.

Key words:

Transdelivery system - Estrogen - Estradiol - Ethyl alcohol - Hydroxypropyl cellulose - Irritant and allergic contact dermatitis

Estraderm is a transdermal therapeutic system for delivering estradiol-17β through intact skin to raise serum levels of estradiol to physiologic premenopausal levels. The system was developed in the early 1980s by the Alza Corporation (Palo Alto, Calif) [1] and Ciba Geigy (Summit, NJ). Since then, it has been widely promoted and used, especially in the United States. The purpose of this route of administration is to avoid the effects of hepatic metabolism, which include enzyme induction, leading in some cases to hypertension, cholelithiasis, and intravascular clotting. At the same time, it is proposed that this method of therapy will relieve postmenopausal vasomotor symptoms, minimize atrophic changes in the vagina, and prevent osteoporosis, all of which have been the aims of oral estrogen therapy for decades. The two most commonly used oral estrogens are conjugated equine estrogens (Premarin, Ayerst, NY) and micronized estradiol-17 (Estrace, Mead Johnson, Evansville, Ind).

Estraderm was developed to provide a uniform, steady release of estradiol through the skin. The system has four layers. The backing consists of a transparent polyester film impermeable to the drug. Next is the drug reservoir, consisting of estradiol (United States Pharmacopeia) and ethyl alcohol gelled with hydroxypropyl cellulose. A rate-controlling membrane follows, composed of ethylene vinyl acetate copolymer, which allows diffusion of the estradiol at a controlled rate into the skin. An adhesive layer consisting of light mineral oil and polyisobutylene is next, and over this a plastic film, which is removed prior to use.

The patches are applied to the abdomen most commonly and left in place for 3 or 4 days. Because the patches adhere to the skin for several days with complete occlusion, cutaneous reactions could be expected. The most frequent is irritation resulting from occlusion, in which the ethyl alcohol probably acts as the chief irritant. Allergic sensitization to several of the ingredients has been suspected. Schwartz and Clendenning recently reported allergic contact dermatitis to the hydroxypropyl cellulose (HPC) present in the reservoir layer. Positive results were seen at 72 and 96 h to HPC in 70% ethyl alcohol and in mineral oil, but negative results in water [2]. In recent studies, McBurney et al. [3] described nine patients with dermatitis from use of the system. Four patients showed reactions to a component of the drug reservoir, four reacted to the adhesive, and two patients had reactions suggesting sensitivity to estradiol.

During the past 4 months, I have observed two patients with reactions to this novel method of estrogen administration:

1. A 51-year-old housewife began to experience dermatitis under the Estraderm patches several weeks after beginning use (Fig. 1). Itching appeared about 12 h after each application and increased until the patches were removed 3–4 days

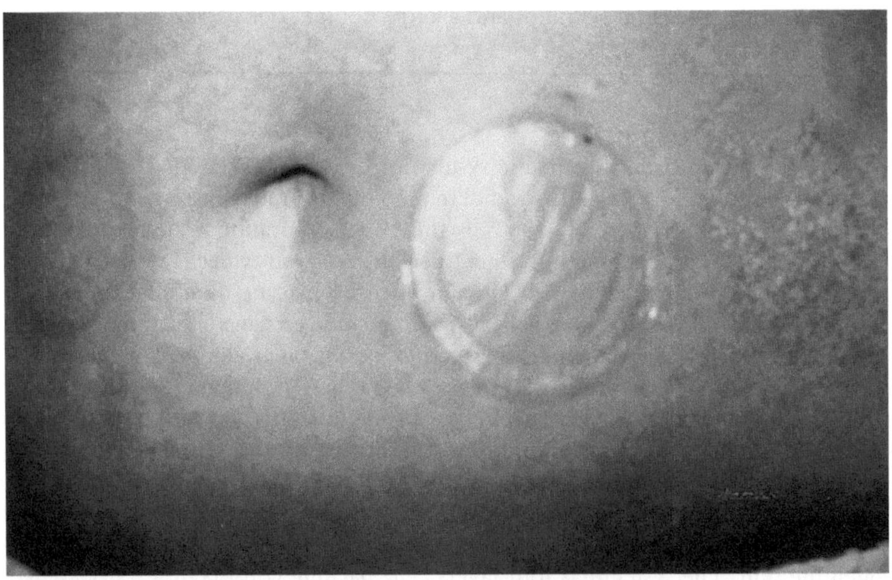

Fig. 1. Reaction, presumably irritant, to Estraderm patch. On patch testing, this patient (case 1) showed an irritant reaction to ethyl alcohol

later. There was no history of atopy. Patch testing to the Estraderm patch and the following ingredients was performed: (a) estradiol, 2% petrolatum; (b) petrolatum control; (c) estradiol, ethyl alcohol, and hydroxypropyl cellulose; (d) polyisobutylene/mineral oil and ethyl alcohol; (e) glyceryl monooleate, estradiol and ethylene vinyl acetate; and (f) same as (e) without estradiol. Positive reactions were seen from the patch and at (c) and (d) above, in which ethyl alcohol was the only common ingredient. Further patch testing to ethyl alcohol, 30% aqua was positive when applied immediately after application to the test patch, but negative if the alcohol was allowed to evaporate for 3–4 min.

2. A 63-year-old nonatopic woman had used the Estraderm patches for 3 months. She is receiving hemodialysis for polycystic kidneys, diagnosed 4 years ago. She has been quite satisfied with the patches, in spite of experiencing a burning sensation and redness beginning within 6–8 h after each application. Patch testing with the transdermal system with and without the drug, and to various concentrations of ethyl alcohol, revealed positive irritant reactions at all test sites. By waiting 10–15 min before application of Estraderm, she has been able to avoid reactions.

It is apparent from studies thus far that the etiology of reactions to Estraderm is not always clear. When the manufacturer provides the ingredients individually for testing, and when appropriate dilutional testing is done, using a sufficient number of controls, we will have a better understanding of the nature of these reactions, which appear to be fairly common in the United States. At present, it appears most likely that irritancy will explain most of these reactions (Hurkmans et al. 1985), but contact allergic sensitization to estradiol and perhaps to other ingredients, even to ethyl alcohol (Fregert et al. 1969), remains a challenging possibility.

Acknowledgements. My thanks to Alfred Amkraut, PhD, of Alza Corporation (Palo Alto, Calif.) for his most helpful cooperation and advice, and to my colleague David South, MD, of Freedom, California, for referring patient 2.

References

1. Place VA, Powers M, Darley PE et al. (1985) A double-blind comparative study of Estraderm and Premarin in the amelioration of postmenopausal symptoms. Am J Obstet Gynecol 152: 1092–1099
2. Schwartz BK, Clendenning WE (1988) Allergic contact dermatitis from hydroxypropyl cellulose in a transdermal estradiol patch. Contact Dermatitis 18: 106–107
3. McBurney EI, Noel SB, Collins J (1988) Allergic contact dermatitis to transdermal estradiol system. Submitted for publication
4. Hurkmans JFGM, Bodde HE, van Driel LMJ et al. (1985) Skin irritation caused by transdermal drug delivery systems during long-term (5 days) application. Br J Dermatol 112: 461–467
5. Fregert S, Groth O, Hjorth N et al. (1969) Alcohol dermatitis. Acta Derm Venereol 49: 493–497

Addresses

R. M. Adams
Department of Dermatology, Stanford University, Stanford, California, USA

Corticosteroid Contact Allergy: A Reality

A. Dooms-Goossens, H. Degreef, and S. Coopman

Summary

Contact allergy to corticosteroids seems to be quite common but often goes undetected. The case histories of 19 patients with a corticosteroid contact allergy are presented. Sixteen of these patients reacted to tixocortol pivalate (1% petrolatum), a corticosteroid that is known in France to be a sensitizer. However, this substance was not available at the time on the Belgian market so it is highly unlikely to have been used by our patients. The patients who reacted to tixocortol pivalate also reacted to other corticosteroid molecules and particularly to hydrocortisone, which could explain exacerbations of the eczema in most of these cases. Therefore, tixocortol pivalate may be a useful, though certainly not infallible, marker for screening patients for contact sensitivity to a good number of corticosteroids.

Moreover, we found that associations of positive patch tests for corticosteroids occur approximately six to seven times more frequently in well-defined groups of structurally related substances than between corticosteroids belonging to different groups.

Indeed, an analogous substitution pattern on the steroid D-ring or the carbon side chain (C-20, C-21) seems to have a significant influence on the occurrence of associations of positive patch test results, while this is not the case for other structural variables, such as the presence of a double bond in the steroid A-ring or fluor substitutions on the B-ring.

Key words:

Contact dermatitis - Cross reactions - Hydrocortisone - Tixocortol pivalate - Topical corticosteroids

Introduction

In 1986 [5], we reported a case of a patient sensitive to pure hydrocortisone who also reacted to tixocortol pivalate, a topical corticosteroid not available on the Belgian market but present in our corticosteroid test series for research purposes. Thioesters such as tixocortol pivalate are capable of hydrolyzing rapidly and freeing the tixocortol, which only differs by a thiol group instead of a hydroxyl group at C-21. Therefore, we considered a cross-reaction to be likely. Allergic reactions to tixocortol pivalate have been reported in France [2, 10], where it has been marketed for nondermatological applications, such as the treatment of rhinitis. It was introduced on the Belgian market only in march 1988. The development of eczematous reactions as early as 1–3 days after the first exposure led us to wonder if these patients were already sensitive to corticosteroids. Indeed, further studies showed that some of these tixocortol pivalate sensitive patients reacted to other corticosteroids such as hydrocortisone [8, 9].

To clarify the situation, we gathered additional data on contact allergies to topical corticosteroids, including tixocortol pivalate (see also [4]).

Material, Methods, and Results

Between January 1984 and December 1986, we tested all patients in whom we suspected a corticosteroid allergy also with tixocortol pivalate (1% pet.). We verified six cases of corticosteroid sensitivity, five of which also reacted to tixocortol pivalate.

In January 1987, we added tixocortol pivalate to our standard series, with which 692 patients have been tested as of February 1988. In this group, we discovered 13 new cases of corticosteroid contact allergy of which 11 (1.6% of the patients tested) involved sensitivity to tixocortol pivalate. Moreover, within the EECDRG, we even obtained a frequency of 1.9% (data to be published), which is comparable to the frequencies of parabens, formaldehyde, and ethylene diamine, classic allergens in our routine standard series. The reactions to tixocortol pivalate we observed ranged from erythematopapular and edematous to papulovesicular and even vesiculobullous. One patient, who showed an extremely positive result, reacted positively down to 1 ppm, which was confirmed a year later when this test concentration was tested by itself.

All 19 patients were later tested with other corticosteroids, and most of them with an extensive corticosteroid series, the details of which will be published in a separate article.

All 16 patients who reacted to tixocortol pivalate also reacted to other corticosteroids. However, in some cases we had to alter the test concentrations and vehicles in order to avoid some of the pitfalls in the detection of steroid sensitivity: for example, hydrocortisone never produced a reaction when tested 25% in petrolatum, but we obtained reactions with 2% in ethanol. In some cases, only a dilution with a mixture of DMSO and ethanol gave a positive result.

Hydrocortisone gave positive results in 12 of the 16 tixocortol pivalate positive

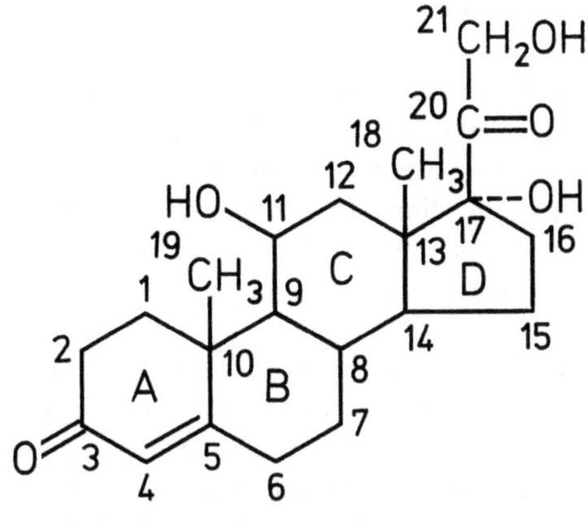

Fig 1. The structure and nomenclature of adrenocorticosteroids. The prototype is cortisol (hydrocortisone)

patients; two of the others reacted to prednisolone/prednisone, and the other two to hydrocortisone-17-butyrate, among other corticosteroids.

We also noted that multiple positive reactions to corticosteroids occurred almost constantly and in certain associations. In order to investigate this further, we systematically analyzed our corticosteroid patch test results and those reported in the literature.

We analyzed the principal variants in the A-, B-, C-, and D-rings of the corticosteroid structure (see Fig. 1):

A-ring: double bonding C-1–C-2
B-ring: substitutions at C-6, C-9, C-7 (fluorine, chlorine, and methyl groups)
D-ring: -16,17-*cis*-diol with *cis*-ketal formation
-16-methyl substitute
Side chain: esterification C-17 and/or C-21

We considered whether the parameters than can preferentially explain associated positive patch-test results between corticosteroids are structural variations in the A- and B-rings of the molecule (hypothesis 1) or in the D-ring or C-20, C-21 side chain (hypothesis 2).

In contrast to the randomly distributed pattern of associated positive patch-test reactions produced by Hypothesis 1, the pattern produced by Hypothesis 2 is situated within well-defined structural groups. Moreover, they occur approximately six to seven times more frequently within groups of structurally related substances than between corticosteroids belonging to different groups (data submitted for publication).

Discussion

In agreement with the literature [1,6,7,11],we noted that corticosteroid hypersensitivity is particularly common among patients with chronic eczema and coexistent hypersensitivity to numerous ingredients of topical medications. In 12 of our patients sensitive to corticosteroids, intolerance to topical medications, including corticosteroid preparations, had been suspected by the referring dermatologist. In the seven other cases, contact allergy to such preparations was not suspected but was detected only by means of a reaction to tixocortol pivalate in our standard series.

Only two tixocortol pivalate positive patients reacted to hydrocortisone-17-butyrate (1% ethanol), which Reitamo and coworkers proposed as a marker [11]. However, three patients who did not react to tixocortol pivalate (1% petrolatum) showed positive reactions to other corticosteroids, including hydrocortisone-17-butyrate (1% ethanol). Of course, contact allergy to corticosteroids could even be more frequent than we found, since, in this period, we routinely tested only tixocortol pivalate.

With regard to the associations of positive reactions to corticosteroids, we could demonstrate that an analogous substitution pattern on the steroid D-ring or the carbon side chain (C-20, C-21) seems to be important, while this is not the case for other structural variables, such as the presence of a double bond in the steroid A-ring or fluor substitutions on the B-ring. These results suggest a classification into four classes [3], which, however, does not match with their potency scale:

Class A: Hydrocortisone type: corticosteroids without substitution on the corticosteroid D-ring or C-20, C-21 carbon chain, but including C-17 and/or C-21 short chain (acetate) esters *and* the C-21 thioester, tixocortol pivalate.

Class B: Triamcinolone acetonide type: corticosteroids with a C-16, C-17 *cis*-ketal or -diol structure.

Class C: Betamethasone type: corticosteroids with a C-16 methyl substitution.

Class D: Hydrocortisone- and clobetasone-17-butyrate type: corticosteroids with a long-chain ester at C-17 and/or C-21, and with or without a C-16 methyl substitution.

The detection of corticosteroid contact allergy is complex. Moreover, tixocortol pivalate seems at present to be a good marker for group A, and hydrocortisone-17-butyrate and clobetasone-17-butyrate good markers for group D.

We are currently attempting to optimize the choice of appropriate allergy markers and test conditions for groups B, C, and D, since we think that the most reliable strategy for the detection of corticosteroid allergy consists in patch testing certain representatives of the four groups indicated by our analysis. We have indeed demonstrated that our patients' allergic conditions improved when they were treated with a corticosteroid of a group to which no reactions were obtained.

References

1. Alani SD, Alani MD (1976) Allergic contact dermatitis and conjunctivitis to corticosteroids. Contact Dermatitis 2: 301–304
2. Boujnah-Khouadja A, Brändle I, Reuter G, Foussereau J (1984) Allergy to 2 new corticoid molecules. Contact Dermatitis 11: 83–87
3. Coopman S, Dooms-Goossens A (1988) Cross-reactions in allergic contact dermatitis caused by topical corticosteroids. Contact Dermatitis 19: 145–146

4. Dooms-Goossens A (1988) Identification of undetected corticosteroid allergy. Contact Dermatitis 18: 124–125
5. Dooms-Goossens A, Verschaeve H, Degreef H, Van Berendoncks J (1986) Contact allergy to hydrocortisone and thixocortol pivalate: problems in the detection of corticosteroid sensitivity. Contact Dermatitis 14: 94–102
6. Förström L, Lassus A, Salde L, Niemi K-M (1982) Allergic contact eczema from topical corticosteroids. Contact Dermatitis 8: 128–133
7. Guin JD (1984) Contact sensitivity to topical corticosteroids J Am Acad Dermatol 10: 773–782
8. Jelen G (1986) Un nouveau cas d'allergie au pivalate de tixocortol. Allergie croisée avec l'hydrocortisone. La lettre du Gerda 3: 27–29
9. Jelen G, Dooms-Goossens A (1986) A propos de l'allergie à l'hydrocortisone. La lettre du Gerda 3: 76
10. Jelen G, Grosshans E, Foussereau J (1985) Une autre forme d'allergie au pivalate de tixocortol. La lettre du Gerda 5: 16
11. Reitamo S, Lauerma AI, Stubb S, et al. (1986) Delayed hypersensitivity to topical corticosteroids. J Am Acad Dermatol 15: 582–589

Addresses

A. Dooms-Goossens
Department of Medical Research (Dermatology), Katholieke Universiteit Leuven, University Hospital, 3000 Leuven, Belgium

H. Degreef
Department of Medical Research (Dermatology), Katholieke Universiteit Leuven, University Hospital, 3000 Leuven, Belgium

S. Coopman
Department of Medical Research (Dermatology), Katholieke Universiteit Leuven, University Hospital, 3000 Leuven, Belgium

Drug-Induced Dermatitis with Acetonides of Corticoids

O. M. Maucher, H. Knipper, and M. Faber

Summary

A 58-year-old female patient with recurrent ulcus cruris in connection with chronic venous insufficiency, as well as a known allergy to neomycin sulfate, benzocaine (Anesthesin), formalin, and (possibly) penicillin, developed severe eczema through treatment with triamcinolone acetonide (Volon A) shaking mix. Tests indicated an extensive eczematous cross-sensitivity to acetonide-substituted corticoids, such as triamcinolone acetonide, fluocinonide, fluocinolone acetonide, flurandrenolone, desonide, and halcinonide; in addition, allergies to adjuvants such as benzyl alcohol and sodium disulfite were diagnosed. Such cases of ulcus cruris often result in epidermal sensitization, which can also include topically applied corticoids. It is suspected that the lability of the acetonide group allows for the development of a common antigen determinant.

Key words:

Acetonide-substituted corticoids - Cross-sensitivity - Allergic contact dermatitis - Adjuvants

Introduction

Compared with other allergies, corticoid allergies are certainly not common, but they occur by no means as infrequently as is often believed to be the case. These allergies are just not recognized very often, due to the fact that they are rarely taken into consideration, and potential hypersensitivity reactions to medication are usually attributed to other substances. Since allergic contact dermatitis is the most common allergic reaction to corticoids [6], this possibility must be taken into account, particularly in the treatment of allergy sufferers such as patients with ulcus cruris.

Case Report

Medical History. The familiy medical history of the 58-year-old female patient was not contributory. The childhood diseases were measles, mumps, scarlet fever, chickenpox, German measles (?), and whooping cough, and at the age of 2 years paratyphoid. Since 1954, she had had ulcus cruris with chronic venous insufficiency. From 1960 to 1969, there were four or five instances of phlebothrombosis and, in addition, erysipelas. In 1960, allergy to penicillin was suspected after using penicillin to treat sinusitis. In 1961, she had hepatitis. In 1963, an umbilical hernia operation was performed. In 1967, there was radiological exclusion of gallstones due to gallstone colic; in addition, pulmonary embolism occurred, and phenprocoumon (Marcumar) therapy (for 7 years) was begun. In 1968, appendectomy was performed. Since 1970, recurrent allergic reactions had occurred to topical treatment of ulcus cruris. In 1971, allergies to neomycin sulfate, benzocaine (Anesthesin), and formalin were diagnosed.

Present Illness. In 1983, eczema surrounding an ulcus cruris was topically treated with i.a. Volon A shaking mix. During treatment, the eczema became worse. Patch screen tests with Volon A shaking mix and parallel tests with Volon A soluble

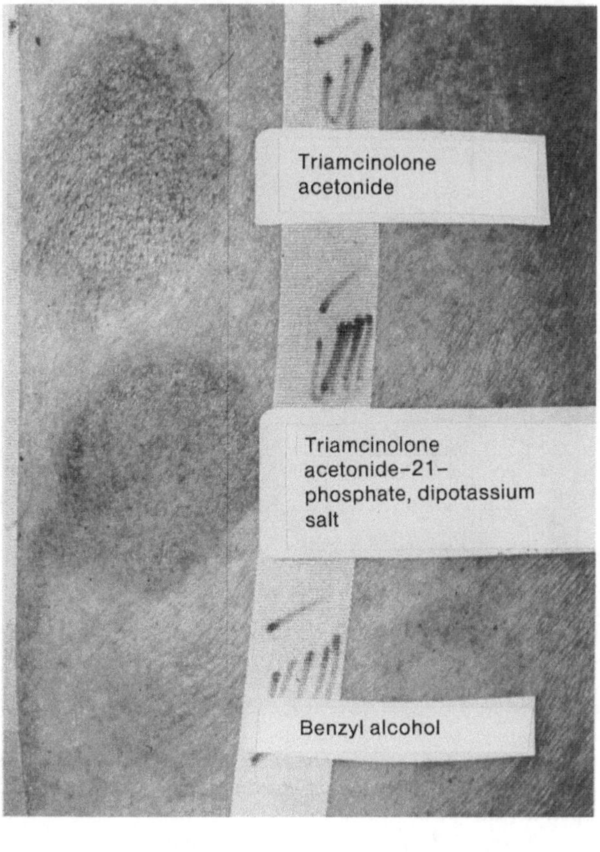

Fig. 1. Positive patch tests showing both a papuloerythematous reaction (initially vesicular) to triamcinolone acetonide and triamcinolone acetonide-21-phosphate, dipotassium salt, and a papuloerythematous reaction to benzyl alcohol after 24 h

yielded eczematous reactions, which led us to suspect an allergy to triamcinolone acetonide. Furthermore, the spectrum of ulcus allergens was found to include gentamicin sulfate, framycetin sulfate, paromomycin, and balsam of Peru.

Results of Glucocorticoid Tests. Our suspicion of a triamcinolone acetonide allergy was confirmed in the patch test by contact dermatitis reactions to the pure substances triamcinolone acetonide (0.1% petrolatum) and triamcinolone acetonide-21-phosphate, dipotassium salt (0.1% aqueous) (Fig. 1). Patch tests with added substances found in the above-mentioned commercial corticoid preparations yielded positive allergic reactions to benzyl alcohol (in Volon A shaking mix) and sodium disulfite (in Volon A soluble). Extensive testing with pure substances in acetonide-substituted corticoids resulted in positive eczematous reactions (Fig. 2) to fluocinonide (0.05% petrolatum), fluocinolone acetonide (0.03% petrolatum), flurandrenolone (0.05% petrolatum), desonide (0.05% petrolatum), and halcinonide (0.1% petrolatum).

In further patch tests, it was shown that the following pure corticoid substances were tolerated without eliciting any reaction: betamethasone NF micr.; betametha-

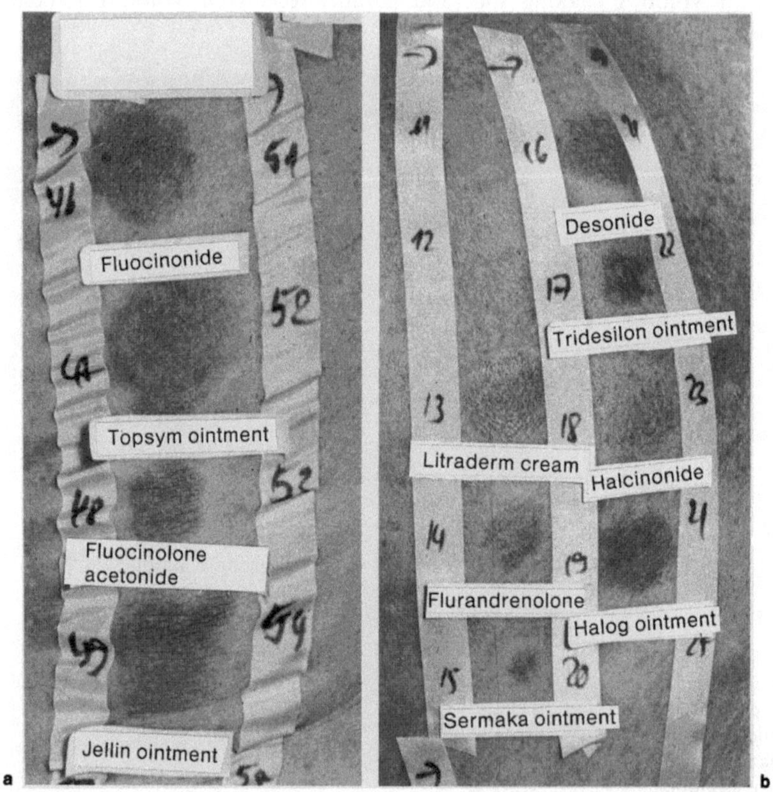

Fig. 2 a, b. Positive patch tests showing erythematous and papuloerythematous reactions to fluocinonide, fluocinolone acetonide, flurandrenolone, desonide, and halcinonide, as well as the respective specifics, after 48 h sone-17-benzoate; betamethasone-21-dihydrogen phosphate, disodium salt; betamethasone-17,21-dipropionate; betamethasone-17-valerate; clobetasol-17-propionate; clobetasone butyrate; clocortolone-21-hexanoate; clocortolone-21-pivalate; desoxymethasone; dexamethasone; dexamethasone-21-dihydrogen phosphate, disodium salt; diflorasone-17,21-diacetate; diflucortolone-21-valerate; flumethasone-21-pivalate; fluocortolone butyl; fluocortolone; fluocortolone monohydrate; fluocortolone-21-hexanoate; fluocortolone-21-pivalate; fluprednilidene-21-acetate; hydrocortisone acetate; hydrocortisone-17-butyrate; methylprednisolone; methylprednisolone-21-hydrogen succinate, sodium salt; prednisolone; prednisolone acetate, and triamcinolone.

It still had to be clarified which corticoids can be orally or parenterally administered in the case of emergency allergy therapy. Due to the extensive testing already performed (as well as the patient's diagnosed stomach sensitivity), we only tested three specifics (by exposure) which had been negative in the screening test (patch/scratch test). Results showed that the patient tolerated 100 mg fluocortolone (Ultralan oral); 80 mg methylprednisolone (Urbason tablet); and 80 mg methylprednisolone-21-hydrogen succinate, sodium salt (Urbason soluble).

Discussion

Of a group of 1835 contact dermatitis patients (Alani et al.) [1], 23 were found to have an epidermal corticoid allergy, 17 of whom suffered from ulcus cruris. From this it follows that patients suffering from allergies (long-term application of various topical preparations on morphologically and functionally damaged skin, i.e., ideal conditions for epidermal sensitization) are susceptible to the development of not only a wide range of iatrogenic allergies but also an occult corticoid hypersensitivity. While allergic contact eczema to glucocorticoids is not that rare, urticaria, Quincke's edema, exanthema, anaphylactoid purpura, contact urticaria, and anaphylactic shock, by contrast, are described as being less common allergy syndromes [6]. Unlike most other cases in which patients have been found to have allergies to a wide variety of corticoid substances (mostly single observations), our investigation has demonstrated extensive sensitization to acetonide-substituted corticoids, in addition to several known ulcus allergens and adjuvants. Contact allergies to benzyl alcohol and sodium disulfite are important in so far as these substances are found, e.g., in injectable drugs.

An allergy to triamcinolone in connection with urticaria was first reported by Robinson et al. [8]; an eczematous triamcinolone allergy (also in connection with ulcus cruris) was first reported by Bandmann et al. [2]. It is interesting to note that Bandmann's patient only exhibited an allergic reaction to triamcinolone acetonide, while tests with triamcinolone turned out negative, and at the same time other acetonides such as fludroxycortide produced no reaction. Wulf [12] and Wiegel [11] have reported other allergies to triamcinolone acetonide (Wulf also reported a simultaneously occurring allergy to triamcinolone). However, Wiegel's tests cannot be regarded as sufficient since he carried them out exclusively with specifics, and not with pure substances.

One case similar to ours, which is the basis of research by Coskey [4], involves an allergy to four corticoids with an acetonide substituent in positions 16 and 17. It is difficult to explain why the fluocinolone acetonide belonging to this group did not yield a positive result in his investigation. On the one hand, it is known that cross-sensitivities can be partial. On the other hand, special cases involving corticoids might be explicable by the possibility that pharmacologically potent corticoids which just elicit weak allergies treat their own contact dermatitis reaction. In terms of desonide [1, 9], there are single reports of allergies to single-entity drugs having this configuration without a broader clarification of acetonide-substituted corticoids. Boujnah-Khouadja et al. [3] have reported the cross-sensitivity of amcinonide, a substance very similar in structure, with two drugs belonging to the acetonide group (desonide, triamcinolone acetonide). Hausen et al. [5] have reported an allergy to fludroxycortide. Unfortunately, the pure substances amcinonide [3] and budesonide [7, 10], which are of interest in terms of the allergy spectrum of our patient, were unavailable. Critical observation of the allergen corticoids involved has led us to suspect that the responsiveness of the acetonide group allows for the development of a common antigen determinant.

Due to the unpredictable range of corticoid allergies, it is recommended to perform extensive tests with the most important corticoids used in topical, oral, and parenteral applications, especially with those corticoids which are structurally related to the allergologically relevant corticoid, e.g., the various salts of a corticoid, stereoisomeric corticoids [6], and corticoids with similar substituents. Tests should also be performed with all other ingredients of a preparation. More importantly, tolerable glucocorticoids should be found for cases of emergency treatment.

Acknowledgments. We would like to express our gratitude to the following companies, which supported us by providing us with information, as well as the specifics and their ingredients: Asche AG, 2000 Hamburg 50; Basotherm GmbH, 7950 Biberach an der Riss 1; Beiersdorf AG, 2000 Hamburg 20; Cassella-Riedel Pharma GmbH, 6000 Frankfurt/M.; Ciba-Geigy GmbH, 7867 Wehr; Desitin-Werk Carl Klinge GmbH, 2000 Hamburg 63; Essex Pharma GmbH, 8000 München 33; Glaxo Pharmazeutika GmbH, 2060 Bad Oldesloe; Goedecke AG, 1000 Berlin; Grünenthal GmbH, 5190 Stolberg; Von Heyden GmbH, 8000 München 19; Hoechst AG, 6230 Frankfurt/M. 80; Klinge Pharma GmbH, 8000 München 80; Eli Lilly GmbH, 6380 Bad Homburg; Merck, 6100 Darmstadt 1; Schering AG, 1000 Berlin 65; Dr. Karl Thomae GmbH, 7950 Biberach an der Riss 1; Upjohn GmbH, 6148 Heppenheim. We would also like to thank Mrs U. Fissun, MTA, for her technical assistance, and Mrs L. Goerke and Mr F. Kaut for the photographic reproductions.

References

1. Alani MD, Alani SD (1972) Allergic contact dermatitis to corticosteroids. Ann Allergy 30: 181–185
2. Bandmann HJ, Huber-Riffeser G, Woyton A (1966) Kontaktallergie gegen Triamcinolanacetonid. Hautarzt 17: 183–185
3. Boujnah-Khouadja A, Brändle I, Reuter G, Foussereau J (1984) Allergy to 2 new corticoid molecules. Contact Dermatitis 11: 83–87
4. Coskey RJ (1978) Contact dermatitis due to multiple corticosteroid creams. Arch Dermatol 114: 115–117
5. Hausen BM, Kulenkamp D (1985) Kontaktallergie auf Fludroxycortid und Cetylalkohol. Dermatosen 33: 27–28
6. Maucher OM, Faber M, Knipper H, Kirchner S, Schöpf E (1987) Corticoidallergie. Hautarzt 38: 577–582
7. Meding B, Dahlberg E (1986) Contact allergy to budesonide in a nasal spray. Contact Dermatitis 14: 253–254
8. Robinson HM jr, Robinson RCV, Raskin J (1959) Triamcinolone in dermatologic therapy. Southern Medical Journal 52: 330–341
9. Sturtz RP, Rau RC (1983) Contact dermatitis to desonide. Arch Dermatol 119: 1023
10. Van Hecke E, Temmerman E (1980) Contact allergy to the corticosteroid budesonide. Contact Dermatitis 6: 509
11. Wiegel O (1968) Kontaktallergie durch Kortikosteroid-haltige Externa (Triamcinolon-acetonid und Dexamethason). Med Welt 13: 828–829
12. Wulf K (1967) Beitrag zur Triamcinolon-Kontaktallergie. Z Haut-Geschl Kr 42: 765–768

Addresses

O. M. Maucher
Universitäts-Hautklinik, Hauptstr. 7, D-7800 Freiburg im Breisgau, FRG

H. Knipper
Universitäts-Hautklinik, Hauptstr. 7, D-7800 Freiburg im Breisgau, FRG

M. Faber
Universitäts-Hautklinik, Hauptstr. 7, D-7800 Freiburg im Breisgau, FRG

Optimal Testing for Contact Allergy to Topical Corticosteroids*

S. Reitamo, A. I. Lauerma, and L. Förström

Summary

Patch testing with hydrocortisone-17-butyrate (H-17-B) is a reliable screening method for the detection of topical glucocorticosteroid allergy. Patch testing is usually performed with corticosteroid preparations in a petrolatum base, which in our hands frequently show false-negative test results. The purpose of the present study was to further define the vehicle effect on H-17-B patch and use test reactions. Patch testing was performed with H-17-B in ethanol and in white petrolatum in nine patients with previously known contact hypersensitivity to topical corticosteroids. H-17-B was used at 1.0%, 0.1% and 0.01% concentrations. Additionally, a commercial H-17-B ointment preparation was tested. Positive patch test reactions were seen most consistently with 1.0% and 0.1% H-17-B in ethanol; 0.01% H-17-B in ethanol gave positive test reactions at a rate and intensity similar to those seen with both 1.0% and 0.1% H-17-B in petrolatum, and with the commercial Locoid ointment. Use tests were positive in four of nine patients; the ethanol preparation was superior to the commercial ointment. The present results suggest that patch testing with 1.0% or 0.1% H-17-B is the optimal method for screening of topical corticosteroid allergy.

Key words:

Glucocorticosteroids - Topical allergens - Patch test reactions

* These studies were supported by the Paulo Foundation and the Sigrid Jusélius Foundation.

Introduction

Patch testing with corticosteroid derivatives for topical use has shown that positive test reactions are most often seen with hydrocortisone-17-butyrate (H-17-B) in ethanol [1, 3]. However, epicutaneous testing for corticosteroid allergy is usually performed with corticosteroid preparations in a petrolatum base, which in our hands frequently show false-negative test results. The purpose of the present study was to further define the vehicle effect on H-17-B patch and use test reactions.

Material and Methods

Patients. Nine patients with previously known contact hypersensitivity to topical corticosteroids were tested. All nine patients had shown positive test reactions to H-17-B when tested approx. 2 months earlier.

H-17-B Preparations. We obtained H-17-B preparations in lyophilized form, dissolved in 94% ethanol or mixed into white petrolatum. The lyophilized preparations were gifts from the manufacturer (Gist-Brocades, supplied through Algol Oy, Helsinki). H-17-B was tested at 1.0%, 0.1% and 0.01% in ethanol; at 1.0% and 0.1% in white petrolatum; as commercial 0.1% Locoid ointment; and as 0.01% mixture containing one-tenth 0.1% Locoid ointment and nine-tenths white petrolatum. Ethanol and petrolatum withouth H-17-B were included as controls.

Epicutaneous Testing. Using the aluminium Finn Chamber (Epitest Ltd., Helsinki, Finland) technique [2], epicutaneous testing was performed on the patient's backs. A filter paper disk was used, with ethanol as vehicle. The chambers were fixed with Scanpor surgical tape on intact skin and removed after 24 h of exposure (day 1). The results were read at days 1, 2, 4 or 5, and 7 or 8. The test reactions were defined according to the terminology of the International Contact Dermatitis Research Group [5]: – (negative), ?+ (doubtful reaction), +[weak (non-vesicular) reaction], ++ [strong (oedematous or vesicular) reaction], +++ [extreme (bullous or ulcerative) reaction] and IR (irritant reaction).

Use Testing. Use tests were performed with three applications a day on clinically normal skin of the flexor side of the arms. The applications were continued until a positive reaction occurred or up to 10–12 days. The preparations used for testing were 1.0% or 0.1% H-17-B in ethanol and 0.1% Locoid ointment. The test reactions were defined as negative or positive (acute eczema at the site of testing).

Results

The combined results of epicutaneous tests with H-17-B are shown in Fig. 1. The most intense test reactions were seen with 1.0% and 0.1% H-17-B in ethanol. Posi-

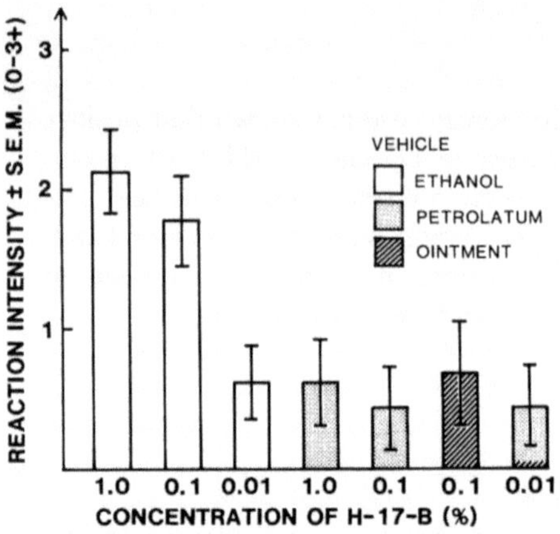

Fig. 1. Combined results ($n = 9$) of epicutaneous tests with hydrocortisone-17-butyrate *(H-17-B)* in various vehicles (reaction intensities: *0*, −; *1*, ?+; *2*, +; *3*, ++)

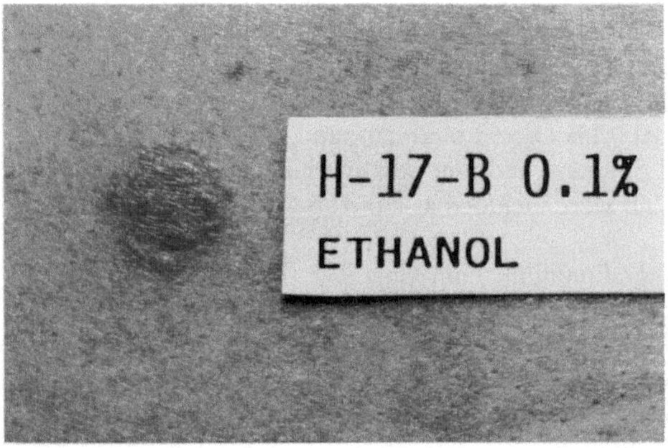

Fig. 2. A positive patch test reaction to 0.1% hydrocortisone-17-butyrate *(H-17-B)* in ethanol

tive test reactions with 1.0% or 0.1% H-17-B in ethanol were seen in six patients (Fig. 2), and with 0.1% Locoid ointment in three patients. Use testing was positive in four patients. There were positive results with 1.0% or 0.1% H-17-B in ethanol in four patients, and with 0.1% Locoid ointment in two patients.

Discussion

In the present study, H-17-B gave positive test results most consistently in both patch and use tests when tested in an ethanol vehicle. The results with H-17-B in petrolatum were less intense than those with H-17-B in ethanol. The present results suggest that patch testing with 1.0% or 0.1% H-17-B in ethanol is the optimal method for screening of topical corticosteroid allergy. As we have seen more patients with positive test reactions to 1.0% than to 0.1% H-17-B in ethanol, we recommend 1.0% H-17-B in ethanol for routine screening of corticosteroid allergy. With this method we have detected approx. 50 new patients with topical corticosteroid allergy since 1985 [4].

Acknowledgements. The technical help of Ms Liisa Kannas is gratefully acknowledged.

References

1. Lauerma AI, Visa K, Pekonen M, Förström L, Reitamo S (1987) Cellular kinetics of delayed hypersensitivity test reactions to topical glucocorticosteroids. Arch Dermatol Res 279: 379–384
2. Pirilä V (1972) Chamber test versus patch test for epicutaneous testing. Contact Dermatitis 1: 48–52
3. Reitamo S, Lauerma AI, Stubb S, Käyhkö K, Visa K, Förström L (1986) Delayed hypersensitivity to topical corticosteroids. J Am Acad Dermatol 14: 582–589
4. Reitamo S, Lauerma AI, Förström L (1989) Detection of contact hypersensitivity to topical glucocorticosteroids with hydrocortisone-17-butyrate. (submitted for publication)
5. Wilkinson DS, Freger S, Magnusson B, Bandmann HJ, Calnan CD, Cronin E, Hjorth N, Maibach HJ, Malten KE, Meneghini CL, Pirilä V (1970) Terminology of contact dermatitis. Acta Derm Venereol (Stockh) 50: 287–292

Addresses

S. Reitamo
Department of Dermatology, Helsinki University Central Hospital, Snellmaninkatu 14, SF-00170 Helsinki, Finland

A. I. Lauerma
Department of Dermatology, Helsinki University Central Hospital, Snellmaninkatu 14, SF-00170 Helsinki, Finland

L. Förström
Department of Dermatology, Helsinki University Central Hospital, Snellmaninkatu 14, SF-00170 Helsinki, Finland

Cross-Allergy to Non-steroidal Antiphlogistic Drugs

U. Beller

Key words:

Contact dermatitis - Cross-allergy - Topical anti-inflammatory agents

Along with the frequent use of non-steroidal antiphlogistic drugs on the skin, the number of cases of contact dermatitis is increasing. Contact dermatitis has been reported to pyrazolone derivates [1], bufexamac [2], etofenamat [3], diclofenac [4], indomethacin [5], etc. Since cross-sensitivity between pyrazolone derivates is well known [6], we investigated whether such cross-reactivity exists between bufexamac, etofenamat, diclofenac and indomethacin.

In the last 2 years we had observed nine patients with contact dermatitis to bufexamac (5 cases), etofenamat (3 cases) and indomethacin (1 case) (Table 1). These patients were re-evaluated by patch tests, using 0.5%, 1%, 2% and 5% of bufexamac, etofenamat, diclofenac and indomethacin in petrolatum (Vaseline). We found no cases of cross-sensitivity in the nine patients tested (Table 1). It is remarkable that

Table 1. Patch test results in patients with contact dermatitis to non-steroidal antiphlogistic drugs

Case no.	Sex	Age (years)	Reaction							
			Diclofenac		Indomethacin		Bufexamac		Etofenamat	
			48 h	72 h	48 h	72 h	48 h	72 h	48 h	72 h
1	F	39	0	0	0	0	0	0	+++	+++
2	F	49	0	0	0	0	0	0	++	+++
3	F	47	0	0	0	0	0	0	+++	+++++
4	F	77	0	0	0	0	0	+	0	0
5	M	24	0	0	+++	++	0	0	0	0
6	M	44	0	0	0	0	0	++	0	0
7	F	18	0	0	0	0	+	++	0	0
8	M	39	0	0	0	0	+	++	0	0
9	F	62	0	0	0	0	0	+	0	0

between bufexamac and diclofenac (both derivates of phenylcarbon acid) no cross-sensitivity occurred. This implies that the phenylcarbon acid group seems not to be the sensitizing structure. We conclude also that bufexamac, etofenamat, diclofenac and indomethacin could replace each other in case of sensitization to one of them.

References

1. Meneghini CL et al. (1979) Contact dermatitis 5: 197–198
2. Frosch PJ et al. (1987) Hautarzt 38: 331–334
3. Lang E et al. (1985) Akt Dermatol 99–100
4. Przybilla B et al. (1986) Allergologie 9: 8–15
5. Beller U et al. (1987) Contact dermatitis 17: 121
6. Ebner H (1986) Akt Dermatol 12: 197–199

Addresses

U. Beller
Department of Dermatology, University of Ulm, Oberer Eselsberg 40, D-7900 Ulm, FRG

Acute Generalized Dermatitis to Orally Administered Disulfiram

E. van Hecke

Summary

A severe reaction with an urticarial as well as an eczematous aspect is described after intake of 400 mg disulfiram on 2 consecutive days. The patient had a disulfiram implant 4 years ago.

Key words:

Disulfiram - Antabuse - Systemic eczematous contact dermatitis

Case Report

A 36-year-old man was brought to the emergency unit of the University Hospital, Gent, with the tentative diagnosis of angioedema or cutaneous infection of the face. He showed gross edema of the face, making vision and speech almost impossible. The eyelids and cheeks were swollen and erythematous, with patches of vesicles, exudation, and yellowish crusts (Fig. 1). At various sites on the body, shoulders, arms, back, and legs, erythematous, edematous, and vesicular patches occurred. A patch with an urticarial aspect was present around an operation scar on the lower right abdominal skin (Fig. 2). The dermatological diagnosis was contact dermatitis.

The history of the patient revealed that he had a disulfiram implant 4 years ago to try to control his alcoholism. However, the implant had to be removed because it "inflamed". Since alcohol has continued to be a problem – the patient drinks more than ten pints of beer a day – he decided on his own initiative to take one tablet of 400 mg disulfiram (Antabuse) 2 days before admission. The next day, he experienced the first symptoms of itch and redness in the face, but he took a second tablet of 400 mg Antabuse.

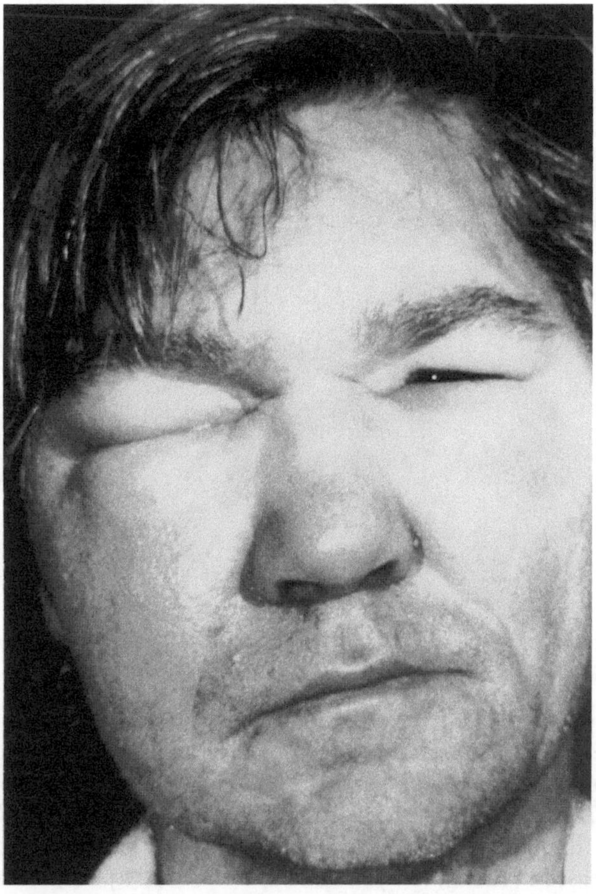

Fig. 1. Acute dermatitis of the face

After clearing of the dermatitis, he was tested. Patch tests with the European standard series revealed sensitivity to thiuram mix and epoxy resin. Patch tests with the Trolab rubber series, consisting of 20 rubber chemicals, revealed sensitivity to all thiurams tested: tetramethylthiuram disulfide, tetramethylthiuram monosulfide, tetraethylthiuram disulfide and dipentaethylenethiuram disulfide.

The patient has worked for 11 years in a factory where mentally disabled people are employed. He has been assigned to various jobs, like assembly of electronic devices and metal machinery; now, he is a storekeeper.

Discussion

Disulfiram is tetraethylthiuram disulfide. It has been advocated as a therapeutic drug in psychiatry and in dermatology. In dermatology, orally administered disulfiram is used as a chelating agent in nickel-sensitive people with chronic hand dermatitis [2]. The aim of the treatment is a reduction of the nickel deposits in the skin with conse-

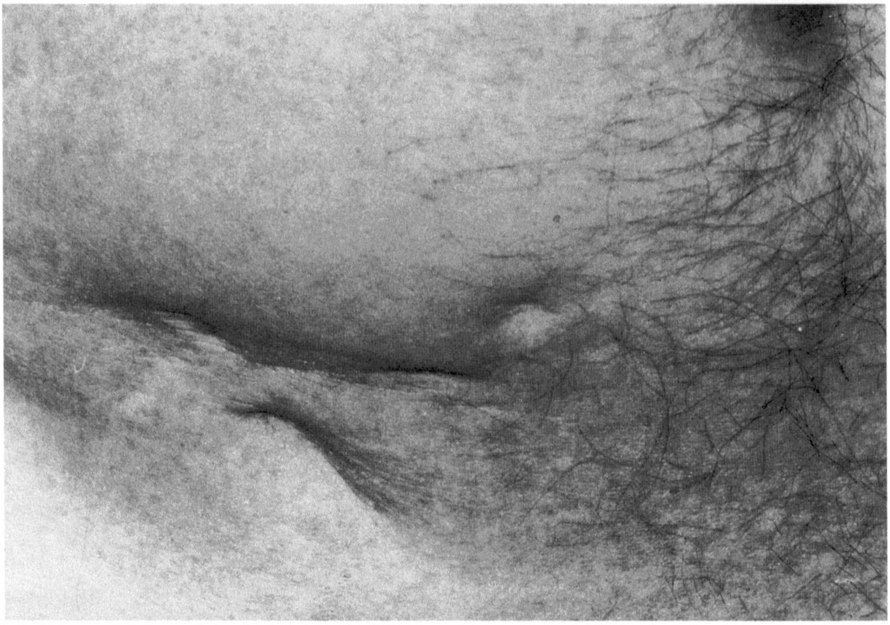

Fig. 2. Urticarial eruption around operation scar

quent healing of the dermatitis. It has remained an exceptional approach in the treatment of nickel dermatitis. No disulfiram sensitivity has been reported from this source, as could be expected.

Disulfiram was introduced into psychiatry in 1948 [1]. When alcohol is drunk after disulfiram intake, a series of unpleasant sensations occur, such as flushing, increased sweating, tachycardia, hypotension, dyspnea, nausea, vomiting, vertigo, and a sense of fear. Even life-threatening complications such as myocardial infarction and hemiplegia have occurred. Urticaria and dermatitis are not included in this type of reaction, but flares of dermatitis after ingestion of alcohol without intake of disulfiram have been described in disulfiram-sensitive patients [7]. The pharmacological action of disulfiram – accumulation of the alcohol metabolite acetaldehyde by enzymatic blocking – only partly explains the symptoms [6]. It has been suggested that the disulfiram effect is at least partly due to the patient's expectation of becoming sick. This is particularly true for disulfiram implants. The dose of the implantation is very low, considering the oral dose necessary to induce alcohol intolerance: 1 g for at least 6 months v 1 g a day. Moreover, disulfiram blood levels after implantation only rise in the 1st week and do not come near the values of the oral intake. No disulfiram metabolite is found in the expired air after implantation [4]. It is thus understandable that the disulfiram implant practice has been abandoned in many countries. However, it remained very popular in Belgium, where alcoholics eventually receive multiple implants. This might explain why sensitivity to disulfiram implants was reported from this country [3].

In our patient, sensitivity could have been acquired by a former disulfiram implant, but more common ways of sensitization could have occurred, such as occupational contact or simple everyday contact with utensils and garments. Generalized dermatitis due to disulfiram intake was first mentioned at the 11th International Congress of Dermatology and has been described occasionally since then [5]. Our patient had a particularly severe reaction, which started the morning after the first intake of 400 mg Antabuse. Since the cause of the reaction was not recognized, a second 400 mg tablet was taken. The dose he took was in fact too low to induce alcohol intolerance. The allergic reaction was nevertheless severe. It is advisable that patients should be patch-tested with the thiuram mixture of the standard series before they start disulfiram treatment, particularly if there is a history of problems with a former implant. The dermatological implications of disulfiram sensitization by implantation should be considered by psychiatrists in the discussion on the pros and cons of disulfiram implants.

References

1. Hald J, Jacobsen E (1948) A drug sensitizing the organism to ethylalcohol. Lancet 255: 1001–1004
2. Kaaber K, Menne T, Tjell JC, Veien N (1979) Antabuse treatment of nickel dermatitis. Contact Dermatitis 5: 221–228
3. Lachapelle JM (1975) Allergic "contact" dermatitis from disulfiram implants. Contact Dermatitis 1: 218–220
4. Malcolm MT, Madden JS, Williams AE (1974) Disulfiram implantation critically evaluated. Br J Psychiatry 124: 485–490
5. Pirilä V (1957) Dermatitis due to rubber. In: Proceedings 11th International Congress of Dermatology, vol 2, pp 252–255
6. Raby K (1954) Relation of blood acetaldehyde levels to clinical symptoms in the disulfiram-alcohol reaction. J Stud Alcohol 15: 21–32
7. Van Ketel WG (1968) Rubber, alcohol and eczema. Dermatologica 136: 442–444

Addresses

E. van Hecke
Department of Dermatology, University Hospital, B-9000 Gent, Belgium

Relevant Allergens in Perianal Contact Dermatitis

K.-P. Peters, A. Heese, and H. Hahn

Summary

Hemorrhoids may cause pruritus ani and microbial dermatitis in the perianal region and on the buttocks. The first therapy is usually performed by the physician or by patients themselves with ointments containing sensitizers such as peruvian balsam, lanolin, or neomycin. Our results of patch tests in patients suffering from contact dermatitis of the perianal region are presented.

The most common allergens in topical medicaments were balsam of Peru and its cross-reacting substances, like benzoic acid. Another important group of sensitizers were mercury compounds, especially phenylmercuric salts and mercury bichloride (sublimate). In addition, lanolin and neomycin, various conservatives, and other contents of the ointments compose the extensive list of these allergens.

Key words:

Contact dermatitis - Hemorrhoids - Peruvian balsam - Mercurials

Introduction

Hemorrhoids and sometimes fissures or perianal fistulas may cause pruritus ani or a microbial dermatitis, which can be superinfected by *Candida albicans.* First therapy is usually done by patients themselves or by the physician, using ointments and suppositories, which partly contain sensitizers such as balsam of Peru, antiseptics, and antibiotics. The purpose of our study is to assess the incidence of allergens in patients suffering from perianal contact dermatitis.

Materials and Methods

The positive patch test results of 60 patients (19 women, 41 men) with perianal contact dermatitis treated in our university hospital between 1974 and 1987 were studied. The mean age was 51 years (range 21–79 years). The patch test series consisted of the European standard, vehicles and emulsifiers, preservatives, antibiotics, antimycotics, and substances for inflammatory anal diseases.

Results

All allergens are listed below except those without any pathogenetic significance for perianal contact dermatitis (e.g., nickel sulfate). In the 60 patients tested, the most frequent allergens were as follows:

	No. of patients
Balsam of Peru	14
Benzoic acid	11
Mercury bichloride	16
Phenylmercuric borate	9
Resorcin	6
Lanolin	5
Mafenide (Marfanil)	5
Neomycin	5

Less frequent allergens, partly cross-reacting with those listed above, were as follows:

1. Allergens partly cross-reacting with balsam of Peru	
	No. of patients
Tincture of benzoin	3
Colophony	1
Tars of wood	2
Fragrance mix (Trolab)	2
Carvacrol	4
Vanilla	1
Turpentine	2
2. Preservatives and antimicrobials	
Phenylmercuric acetate	3
Merthiolate	1
Formalin	3
Benzalkonium chloride	2
Chlorhexidine digluconate	2
Chloramine-T	2
Hexachlorophene	2
Kathon CG	2

Bronopol	1
Paraben mixture	1
Phenol	3
Sorbic acid	3
Clioquinol	1
3. Antibiotics	
Chloramphenicol	2
Gentamycin	1
Bacitracin	1
Erythromycin	1
4. Miscellaneous allergens	
Benzocaine	4
p-Aminobenzoic acid	1
Eucerin	1
Cetylstearyl alcohol	1
Bufexamac	1
Hexylresorcinol	4
Quinine	2
Arnica	1
Menthol	1
Thymol	1

Discussion

Allergens. The following conclusions may be drawn concerning allergens:

1. The high rate of sensitization to *balsam of Peru* is caused by the general presence of this mixture of substances and its components (fragrances, spices, benzoic acid, tincture of benzoin, and tars of wood). Proctological and phlebological patients are exposed to this allergen by the local application of peruvian-balsam-containing remedies. Possible cross-reactions occur with other components such as spices and artificial flavors; for instance, these ingredients in chocolate and cola drinks may induce hematogenic allergic contact dermatitis.
2. The frequent use of *inorganic and organic mercurials* as antiseptics used to be more widespread. Frequent sensitizations restricted their application to a few substances (phenylmercuric acetate, merbromin, and merthiolate). Due to their reduced importance, the rate of positive patch test reactions to mercury bichloride as a marker substance for inorganic mercurials decreased. Mercurials as antimicrobials in proctological lubricants should be treated with caution.
3. *Resorcin* is still common in dermatology for its antiseptic and keratolytic effect (for example, Castellani's paint and some commercial drugs).
4. As an emulsifier used especially in local therapeutics, *lanolin* has lost importance because of the allergenic risk.

5. In the past, *mafenide* (a sulfonamide) was locally applied and created frequent cross-reactions to other sulfonamides and the derivates of *p*-aminobenzoic acid (benzocaine and procaine).
6. *Neomycin* is an aminoglycoside antibiotic with local and enteral application. Attention should be paid to possible cross-reactions with other aminoglycoside antibiotics (for example, bacitracin and framycetin).
7. Concerning the huge variety of different *preservatives,* there is a low risk of allergic contact dermatitis.

Test Series. In conclusion, we propose the following patch test series for patients with perianal contact dermatitis:

1. European standard
2. Vehicles and emulsifiers
3. Preservatives
4. Antibiotics
5. Additional allergens
   a) Benzoic acid
   b) Mercury bichloride (sublimate)
   c) Resorcin
   d) Hexylresorcinol
   e) Phenol
   f) Hexachlorophene

References

1. Cronin E (1980) Contact dermatitis. Churchill Livingstone, Edinburgh
2. Fisher AA (1986) Contact dermatitis, 3rd edn. Lea and Febiger, Philadelphia
3. Nater JP, de Groot AC (1985) Unwanted effects of cosmetics and drugs used in dermatology, 2nd edn. Elsevier, Amsterdam

Addresses

K.-P. Peters
Department of Dermatology, University of Erlangen-Nürnberg, 8520 Erlangen, FRG

A. Heese
Department of Dermatology, University of Erlangen-Nürnberg, 8520 Erlangen, FRG

H. Hahn
Department of Dermatology, University of Erlangen-Nürnberg, 8520 Erlangen, FRG

Bacitracin and Polymyxin B: Important Contact Allergens in Patients with Leg Ulcers

D. Kleinhans

Summary

Bacitracin and polymyxin B are frequent and therefore important contact allergens in patients with leg ulcers. Of 317 patients with leg ulcers tested between 1984 and 1987 (patients with and without eczema), 25 (7.9%) were sensitized towards bacitracin (5% in petrolatum) and 32 patients (10.1%) were sensitized towards polymyxin B (5% in petrolatum). Bacitracin and polymyxin B should routinely be tested in patients with leg ulcers.

Key words:

Bacitracin - Polymyxin B - Leg ulcer patients

Some practical aspects of contact dermatitis in leg-ulcer patients are considered in this report. From 1984 to 1987, we patch-tested 317 leg-ulcer patients with and without dermatitis. The overall rate of positive reactions was 76.3%, with 78.8% for males and 75.2% for females (Table 1).

Bacitracin

Contact allergy to bacitracin has been reported for more than 20 years. The published rate of occurrence has varied even in the Scandinavian countries, with 7.8% in Finland [6] and 0.3% in Sweden [1]. Contact allergy towards bacitracin has been said to be rare [2], and it is this controversial situation that probably led Katz and Fisher to publish a review on bacitracin in 1987 [3].

At the Allergy Unit of the Department of Dermatology in Stuttgart we have been patch-testing bacitracin in leg-ulcer patients for about 15 years. During the past

Table 1. Patch test results in leg-ulcer patients 1984–1987

Total	Positive (*n*/%)
99 Males	78/78.8
218 Females	164/75.2
317 Males + females	242/76.3

Table 2. Bacitracin[a] contact allergy in leg-ulcer patients 1984–1987

Total	Positive (*n*/%)
99 Males	9/9.1
218 Females	16/7.3
317 Males + females	25/7.9

[a] Patch tested 5% pet., applied 48 h, read up to day 7

Table 3. Polymyxin B[a] contact allergy in leg-ulcer patients 1984–1987

Total	Positive (*n*/%)
99 Males	13/13.1
218 Females	19/ 8.7
317 Males + females	32/10.1

[a] Patch tested polymyxin B sulphate 5% pet., applied 48 h, read till day 7

4 years, 317 leg ulcer patients were patch-tested with bacitracin 5% petrolatum (pet.; Table 2). Twenty-five patients, i.e. 7.9%, gave a positive patch-test result (only clear-cut reactions were taken into account). This percentage is slightly lower than the sensitization rate in leg-ulcer patients seen, for example, by Lindemayr and Drobil [4]. In many cases, our patients had used the bacitracin-containing Nebacetin ointment. Bacitracin seems to be a rather frequent contact allergen in leg-ulcer patients. In addition to dermatologic ointments, there are many ophthalmic and some otologic preparations containing bacitracin. Bacitracin, as an antibiotic produced by a strain of *Bacillus subtilis,* may also cause an immediate-type allergic reaction (for details see Katz and Fisher [3]).

Polymyxin B

The peptide antibiotic polymyxin B is obtained from *Bacillus subtilis* as is bacitracin, so that a cross sensitization might exist. Our own data do not favour this hypothesis: only 5 out of 35 polymyxin-B allergic patients, i.e. 14.3%, were also allergic to bacitracin, and all 5 bacitracin-positive patients also had a positive patch test with neomycin, probably being sensitized by Nebacetin ointment (our own earlier data, unpublished).

Polymyxin B is thought to be a rare sensitizer [2]. There are very few publications demonstrating that polymyxin B might be more important [4, 5]. We have been patch testing polymyxin B in all our leg-ulcer patients for 7 years now, using polymyxin B sulphate 5% pet. We chose this concentration, because we had been using the same with bacitracin, being aware of the 3% concentration used by Möller [5]. This 5% concentration of polymyxin B obviously does not liberate histamine, as our

20 controls gave a negative scratch test. Our own results for the past 4 years were the following (Table 3): 32 out of 317 patients were sensitized, i.e. 10.1%. Most of these patients had applied Terramycin ointment, containing polymyxin B and oxytetracycline in a wool alcohol-free base. In conclusion, polymyxin B is a frequent, and therefore important, contact allergen – at least in our own leg-ulcer patients. Again, it is used in ophthalmic and otologic preparations, as is bacitracin. Polymyxin B should be offered as a patch substance commercially.

References

1. Björkner B, Möller H (1973) Bacitracin: a cutaneous allergen and histamine liberator. Acta Derm Venereol (Stockh) 53: 487–491
2. Cronin E (1980) Contact dermatitis. Churchill Livingstone, Edinburgh
3. Katz BE, Fisher AA (1987) Bacitracin: a unique topical antibiotic sensitizer. J Am Acad Dermatol 17: 1016–1024
4. Lindemayr H, Drobil M (1985) Unterschenkelekzem und Kontaktallergie. Hautarzt 36: 227–231
5. Möller H (1976) Eczematous contact allergy to oxytetracycline and polymyxin B. Contact Dermatitis 2: 289–290
6. Pirilä V, Förström L, Rouhunkoski S (1967) Twelve years of sensitization to neomycin in Finland. Arch Derm Venereol (Stockh) 47: 419–425

Addresses

D. Kleinhans
Department of Dermatology, Allergy Unit, 7000 Stuttgart-Bad Cannstatt, FRG

Contact Dermatitis to Minoxidil

J. G. Camarasa, E. Serra-Baldrich, B. García-Bravo, and J. F. Vozmediano

Key words:

Contact dermatitis - Minoxidil

Different adverse skin reactions secondary to the use of topical solutions of minoxidil have been documented, namely, irritative contact dermatitis [1], allergic contact dermatitis to minoxidil or to propylene glycol used as a vehicle [2, 3], paraphenylenediamine (PPDA)-crossed allergic contact dermatitis [4], and photoallergic dermatitis [5]. With regard to the incidence of contact dermatitis to minoxidil, Van der Willingen et al. [3] reported three cases among 95 patients, Tosti et al. [5] found three cases in a series of 465 patients, and Roenigk et al. [1] described one case in a group of 777 patients who had been topically treated with minoxidil.

We report ten patients with contact dermatitis on the scalp out of a total of 1050 individuals with androgenic alopecia who had been using topical solutions of minoxidil. All patients 1 ml of a solution of minoxidil from different commercial manufacturers had been applied onto the alopecic area, twice a day, for 1 to 2 years uninterruptedly. The incidence of contact dermatitis to minoxidial was 0.5%.

Six of the ten patients were men and four were women, ranging in age from 25 to 57 years (mean, 36 years). Contact dermatitis developed between 3 and 9 months (mean, 5.4 months) after treatment with minoxidil was begun. Four patients presented with an acute pruriginous vesicular dermatitis, whereas the remaining six experienced localized erythema, edema and pruritus. Only one patient used a proprietary product; the other nine employed magistral formulas according to their physicians's prescriptions which contained unverifiable concentrations of minoxidil. In six cases, the formula possibly contained minoxidil at 3%, and in the remaining four, including the case of the proprietary product, the drug concentration would be 2%.

In the entire group of 1050 patients, only 60 employed proprietary minoxidil preparations (2% in ethanol, prolylene glycol and aqueous solution). The other pa-

Table 1. Results of patch tests (read at 96 h)

Substance tested	Case no. 1	2	3	4	5	6	7	8	9	10
Minoxidil										
0.5% Ethanol solution	NT	NT	++	−	++	−	−	−	−	−
1% Ethanol solution	+	+	NT	NT	NT	NT	−	−	−	+
2% Ethanol solution	++	++	++	++	++	−	−	−	−	++
2% Petrolatum	NT	NT	++	−	−	−	−	−	−	NT
Propylene glycol 20%	−	−	++	−	−	−	−	−	−	−
Propylene glycol 10%	−	−	++	−	−	−	−	−	−	−
Placebo	−	−	−	−	−	−	−	−	−	−

NT, not tested; ++, positive result; −, negative result

tients used equal or similar formulas of undetermined sources for which the percentage of minoxidil was unknown.

The ten patients were patch-tested with a series provided by the commercial manufacturer who had the drug registered (Table 1). Results were read at 48 and 96 h. Six patients were reactive (++) to an epicutaneous test of minoxidil 2% in ethanol solution; three patients were reactive to minoxidil 1% and 2% in ethanol solution; two were positive to minoxidil 2% and 0.5% in ethanol solution, and one of these last two patients was also positive to minoxidil 2% petrolatum. Only one patient was reactive (++) to minoxidil and propylene glycol. None of the epicutaneous tests showed an irritative reaction. The results were interpreted as true allergic reactions.

The four patients with negative patch-testing results had clinical manifestions of erythema and pruritus solely. Therapy with minoxidil was successfully reinitiated after a period of withdrawal. Four of the six patients with minoxidil sensitivity suffered from vesicular contact dermatitis, and the remaining two had intense pruritus, erythema and marked oedema.

Topical solutions of 2% and 3% minoxidil may cause contact dermatitis in a small number of patients; either irritative- and/or allergic-type dermatitis can be observed. Propylene glycol may also be responsible for intolerance to such agents.

References

1. Roenigk HH, Pepper E, Kuruvilla S (1987) Topical minoxidil therapy for hereditary male pattern alopecia. Cutis 37: 337–342
2. Valsecchi R, Cainelli T (1987) Allergic contact dermatitis to minoxidil. Contact Dermatitis 17: 58–59
3. Van der Willingen AH, Dutree-Meulemberg ROGM, Stolz E et al. (1987) Topical minoxidil sensitization in androgenic alopecia. Contact Dermatitis 17: 44–45
4. Degreef M, Hendrickx I, Dooms-Goossens A et al. (1985) Allergic contact dermatitis to minoxidil. Contact Dermatitis 13: 194–195
5. Tosti A, Bardazzi F, De Padora MP et al. (1985) Contact dermatitis to minoxidil. Contact Dermatitis 13: 275–276

Addresses

J. G. Camarasa
Department of Dermatology, Hospital del Mar, Autonomous University of Barcelona, Barcelona, Spain

E. Serra-Baldrich
Department of Dermatology, Hospital del Mar, Autonomous University of Barcelona, Barcelona, Spain

B. García-Bravo
Cátedra de Dermatología M. Q. y Venereología, Hospital Universitario, Seville, Spain

J. F. Vozmediano
Cátedra de Dermatología, Hospital Universitario, Cádiz, Spain

Contact Lens Intolerance, Astigmatism, and Atopy

P. Guerra, A. Aguilar, and A. Garcia-Perez

Summary

The results of a study of 34 patients suffering from contact lens intolerance were compared with the data obtained from a survey in a normal population (1113 individuals). Only 9 of the 34 patients showed some significant positive reactions to the patch tests. On the other hand, contact lens intolerance, refraction defects, and especially astigmatism were more frequent among the atopic individuals of the survey ($P < 0.02$).

Key words:

Contact lens intolerance – Astigmatism – Atopy – Atopic dermatitis – Contact dermatitis

Introduction

Intolerance to contact lenses is frequent due to several different causes, including mechanisms comparable to both allergic and irritant contact dermatitis [2, 8]. In this study, 34 cases of contact lens intolerance are reviewed, and the data from a survey on the same subject done in a normal population are also shown.

Material and Methods

The 34 patients with contact lens intolerance who were studied were referred by the Department of Ophthalmology (Hospital Clinico, Madrid). Personal and family data in relation to an atopic background were obtained. Patch tests were performed

Table 1. Composition of survey population

Profession	Sex (*n*)		Total
	Male	Female	
Doctor	77	172	249
Medical student	112	301	413
Nurse	0	134	134
Beautician	0	252	252
Other	3	62	65
Total	192	921	1113

with the following substances (including a battery of solutions for cleaning or preserving the lenses and some of the substances contained in the solutions or used to manufacture the lenses):

1. Spanish standard series
2. Benzalkonium chloride (0.1% petrolatum)
3. Boric acid (as is)
4. Chlorhexidine gluconate (1% alcohol)
5. EDTA sodium (1% water)
6. Lauryl ether sulfate sodium (1% and 0.2% water)
7. Phenyl mercury nitrate (0.05% petrolatum)
8. Thiomersal (0.1% petrolatum)
9. Methyl methacrylate (1% olive oil)
10. Hydroxypropyl methacrylate (10% olive oil)

Also, some of the results of a survey of 1113 healthy individuals were evaluated. This survey included, among other data, questions about the existence or nonexistence of a personal or family history of atopy, about the existence or not of refraction defects (myopia, hypermetropia, or astigmatism), and about the use of contact lenses and intolerance to them. The composition of our sample population is shown in Table 1.

In order to study the possible relation between atopy and some other parameters, the sample was divided into two arbitrary groups: group A, made up of those individuals who had or had had asthma, hay fever, any kind of eczema, or urticaria ($n = 496$) and group B, those who had not had any of these processes ($n = 617$). We considered that in group A most of the atopic subjects would probably be found, and in group B the nonatopic individuals.

The data were processed in a PC 640 X INVES computer, and the statistical data were calculated with the chi-square test, using the EPISTAT calculation program.

Results

Patients with Contact Lens Intolerance. The patch test results are given in Table 2. Of the 34 patients, 13 (38.2%) presented one or more positive reactions to the Spanish standard series. In 25 (73.4%), some positive reactions to the solutions for cleaning or preserving the lenses or to some of their components were found. A personal history of atopy was found in 20 (58.8%) of the 34 patients, but only 14 (41.2%) had a family history of it.

Normal Population. The overall results of the survey are given in Table 3. The results obtained in group A ("atopics") as compared with group B ("nonatopics") are shown in Table 4.

Table 2. Results of patch tests in patients with contact lens intolerance

Test substance	Positive reactions (n)
Nickel sulfate (2.5% petrolatum)	5[a]
Benzalkonium chloride (0.1% petrolatum)	3
Formaldehyde (2% water)	2
Mercury metal (0.5% petrolatum)	2
Caine mix (amethocaine, 1% petrolatum)	1
Phenyl mercury nitrate (0.05% petrolatum)	2
Chlorhexidine gluconate (1% alcohol)	1
Lauryl ether sulfate (1% water)	12[b]
Solutions[b]	
Lentiflex	9
Solensa	4
Lenticon	1

[a] Only women.
[b] Nonspecific irritant response.

Table 3. General findings of the survey ($n = 1113$)

Finding	No. of cases
Asthma	52 (4.6)
Hay fever	129 (11.6)
Urticaria	210 (18.2)
Hand eczema	167 (15.0)
Other eczemas	201 (18.0)
Family history of atopy	534 (47.9)
No refraction defects	507 (45.6)
1 or more refraction defects[a]	606 (54.4)
Myopia	407 (36.5)
Hypermetropia	82 (7.3)
Astigmatism	248 (22.2)
Using contact lens	223/606 (36.7)
Contact lens intolerance	73/223 (32.7)

The numbers given in parentheses are percentages.
[a] Presbyopia was not included in the study.

Table 4. Results obtained in group A ("atopics"; $n=496$), as compared with group B ("nonatopics"; $n=617$)

Parameter	No. of cases		Significance
	Group A	Group B	
1 or more refraction defects	289 (58.2)	317 (51.3)	$P<0.05$
Myopia	189 (38.1)	218 (35.3)	NS
Hypermetropia	42 (8.4)	40 (6.5)	NS
Astigmatism	128 (25.8)	120 (19.4)	$P<0.02$
Using contact lenses	110 (38.0)	113 (35.6)	NS
Contact lens intolerance	40 (8.1)	33 (5.3)	$P<0.02$

The numbers given in parentheses are percentages.

Discussion

Contact lens intolerance can be caused by keratitis, corneal ulcers, infections due to different germs, and/or unspecific conjunctivitis. Only the latter, which does not represent more than 10% of the total cases of intolerance [7], can be compared to both irritant and allergic contact dermatitis.

Of our 34 patients, 13 showed positive reactions to some of the standard patch test series. Of these substances, nickel (5 of 25 women) was not considered to be related to the clinical findings. Two patients having a positive patch test reaction to formaldehyde had contact dermatitis on the eyelids from a nail hardener. Two patients were positive to mercury metal and also to phenyl mercury nitrate, but none of them were positive to thiomersal. Three patients were positive to benzalkonium chloride, and one to amethocaine found in an anesthetic eyewash.

Of the patients tested with the battery of solutions for cleaning or preserving the lenses and their components, one was positive to chlorhexidine. We interpreted the rest of the positivities (lauryl ether sulfate, some of the solutions) as irritant responses, not only because of the characteristics of the response but also because frequent positivities were found in a control group. However, the possible role of this factor in producing irritative conjunctivitis should be taken into consideration.

Regarding the data of our survey, the incidence of intolerance to lenses found in the atopic group (group A) was 8%, somewhat more than that in the rest of the population (group B 5.3%; $P<0.02$). We also found significant differences in the incidence of refraction defects between the atopic group (58.2%) and the nonatopic group (51.3%; $P<0.05$). This difference was especially significant for astigmatism (group A 25.8% as against group B 19.4%; $P<0.02$).

We have found no references to this datum in the classical [1] or modern [5, 6] dermatology literature. We have only found two mentions of this factor in the ophthalmology literature: Kornerup and Lodin in 1959 [3] mentioned a high incidence of irregular corneal astigmatism among atopic dermatitis patients, and more recently, Muir et al. in 1987 [4] reported significant differences in corneal thickness and corneal curvature, with a high incidence of against-the-rule astigmatism in 40 atopic patients compared with normal control individuals.

Astigmatism, which has several clinical types, is a common phenomenon to a higher or lower degree. Our data suggest that some cases of astigmatism could be related to atopy. We believe that the frequency of this finding could be considered high enough for it to affect the data of our survey in a significant way. On the other hand, it is a different matter from keratoconus, whose relation to atopy is well known, but whose frequency is very low.

We consider that our observations could have some important biases, although the high number of subjects in the survey population and the large quantity of doctors, medical students, or nurses participating in it might partially compensate for some of the deviation. Furthermore, it is not possible to establish an exact criterion to classify what atopy is or is not; thus, our groups A and B are unavoidably imperfect. It is necessary to compare these preliminary findings with ophthalmologic studies on series of atopic patients and conversely, with evaluations of atopic features in series of ophthalmologic patients.

References

1. Baer RL (1955) Atopic dermatitis. New University Press, Philadelphia
2. Fisher AA (1985) Allergic reactions to contact lens solutions. Cutis 36: 209–211
3. Kornerup T, Lodin A (1959) Ocular changes in 100 cases of Besnier's prurigo (atopic dermatitis). Acta Ophthalmol 37: 508–521
4. Muir MGK, Woodward EG, Leonard TJK (1987) Corneal thickness, astigmatism and atopy. Br J Ophthalmol 71: 207–211
5. Rajka G (1975) Atopic dermatitis. Saunders, London
6. Rich LF, Hanifin JM (1985) Ocular complications of atopic dermatitis and other eczemas. Int Ophthalmol Clin 25: 61–76
7. Ruben M (1966) Acute eye disease secondary to contact-lens wear. JAMA 195: 901
8. Van Ketel WG, Melzer-van Riemsdijk FA (1980) Conjunctivitis due to soft lens solutions. Contact Dermatitis 6: 321–324

Addresses

P. Guerra
Department of Dermatology, Hospital Clínico de San Carlos, Universidad Complutense, Madrid, Spain

A. Aguilar
Department of Dermatology, Hospital Clínico de San Carlos, Universidad Complutense, Madrid, Spain

A. Garcia-Perez
Department of Dermatology, Hospital Clínico de San Carlos, Universidad Complutense, Madrid, Spain

Allergic Contact Conjunctivitis Due to Ophthalmic Solutions

A. Tosti and G. Tosti

Summary

In 136 patients affected by allergic contact conjunctivitis (ACC) due to eyedrops, patch tests were performed with the standard International Contact Dermatitis Research Group (ICDRG) series, the personal eyedrops, and, when available, the individual constituents thereof. The results show that preservatives (and particularly thimerosal) are the most common sensitizers in eyedrops. Preservative-induced ACC is generally not accompanied with eyelid CD and is frequently associated with a negative patch test to the causative eyedrops. ACC due to the active ingredients of eyedrops is rare, usually associated with eyelid CD, and frequently accompanied with a positive patch test to the causative eyedrops.

Key words:

Allergic contact conjunctivitis - Eyedrops - Thimerosal - Benzalkonium chloride - Dexamethasone

Introduction

Although contact lens solutions are a well-known cause of sensitization in contact lens wearers [1–3, 5], the real incidence of allergic contact conjunctivitis (ACC) due to eyedrop constituents in eyedrop users is actually unknown. Moreover, the clinical diagnosis of ACC is rarely made when the conjunctivitis is not associated with contact dermatitis (CD) of the eyelids. Our study, which has been carried out on 136 patients affected by contact conjunctivitis (CC), identifies some important sensitizers in ophthalmic preparations and evidences the need for patch testing in ophthalmology.

Material and Methods

Sensitization to ophthalmic preparations was suspected by the ophthalmologist in 136 patients (35 men and 101 women; age 14–84 years, average 36 years), who had consulted him for long-standing conjunctivitis, which in 60 cases was associated with eyelid CD. All these patients were subjected to patch tests according to the International Contact Dermatitis Research Group (ICDRG) directions, using the standard series, the patients' personal ophthalmic solutions, and the individual constituents thereof (when available). An ocular provocation test was routinely made to confirm the patch test results.

Results

The causative agent of the ACC was detected in 75 of our patients, with the clinical relevance of the patch test results being confirmed by the prompt resolution of the clinical manifestations after eyedrop instillation was stopped.

As shown in Table 1, preservatives were responsible for ACC in 61 patients, and thimerosal was by far the most common cause of conjunctivitis in our series. Thimerosal CC is generally not associated with eyelid CD: in fact, 36 of the 52 patients with thimerosal-induced CC were only affected by long-standing follicular conjunctivitis, which, in most of the cases, had been previously diagnosed as viral conjunctivitis. The patch tests with the thimerosal-containing eyedrops were negative in all but 2 of the 52 patients, probably because of the low concentration of this preservative in eyedrops (0.01%–0.0001%).

ACC due to active ingredients of ophthalmic preparations was diagnosed in only 14 patients who had presented a positive patch test reaction to the causative eyedrops: aminoglycosides were the responsible allergens in 6 patients, 3 of them also

Table 1. Causative agents of allergic contact conjunctivitis in 75 patients

Substances	Patients affected (*n*)			Positive patch test to causative eyedrops (*n*)
	Total	ACC	ACC+ECD	
Preservatives	61	39	22	
Thimerosal	52	36	16	2
Benzalkonium chloride	7	3	4	1
Parabens	2	0	2	2
Active ingredients	14	4	10	14
Aminoglycoside antibiotics	6	2	4	
Phenylephrine	2	0	2	
Dexamethasone	2	2	0	
Tropicamide	1	0	1	
Idoxuridine	1	0	1	
Chloramphenicol	1	0	1	
Nitrofurazone	1	0	1	

ACC, allergic contact conjunctivitis; ECD, eyelid contact dermatitis being affected by eyelid eczema; phenylephrine caused ACC in 2 patients, both presenting acute dermatitis of the face; and corticosteroids were the cause of ACC in 2 patients who were sensitized to dexamethasone. A 66-year-old woman reacted to her eyedrops Visumidriatic 0.5%, which according to the manufacturer (MSD) only contain tropicamide; unfortunately, the manufacturer refused to furnish us with this parasympatholytic agent for patch testing. Chloramphenicol, idoxuridine, and nitrofurazone were the agents responsible for three further cases of ACC associated with eyelid CD.

Discussion

Preservatives are certainly the most important sensitizers in eyedrops, and since each preservative is contained in a large number of ophthalmic preparations, not only does ACC due to these compounds frequently go undetected but it is actually prolonged by the very eyedrops that are prescribed to relieve the patient's ocular discomfort. Thimerosal sensitization is probably the main allergological problem in eyedrop users, as well as in contact lens wearers, and this compound should not, in our opinion, be used in ophthalmic formulations [4].

Since preservative sensitization is the main cause of ACC, monodose eyedrops are probably the best strategy in the prevention and management of this condition. Unfortunately, this approach is not always possible. In fact, benzalkonium chloride sensitization, although rare, is a real problem in glaucomatous patients since the most effective antiglaucomatous agents, β-blockers, are, in our country, only available as multidose benzalkonium-preserved eyedrops.

Although corticosteroid sensitization has never been previously described in ophthalmology, the presence in our series of two patients sensitized to dexamethasone suggests that CC due to corticosteroids may not actually be rare.

Since patients sensitized to preservatives generally present a negative patch test reaction to the causative eyedrops, these compounds must be routinely tested in patients with ACC; sensitization to active eyedrop constituents, on the other hand, is almost always associated with a positive patch test reaction to the eyedrops as is, and therefore testing all the eyedrop constituents is not strictly necessary for a presumptive diagnosis. Ophthalmic preservatives and patients' eyedrops are, in our opinion, a simple and reliable patch test approach for patients with ACC.

References

1. Fisher AA (1985) Allergic reactions to contact lens solutions. Cutis 9: 209–211
2. Pedersen NB (1978) Allergic contact conjunctivitis from merthiolate in soft contact lenses. Contact Dermatitis 4: 165
3. Rietschel RL, Wilson LA (1982) Ocular inflammation in patients using soft contact lenses. Arch Dermatol 118: 147–149

4. Tosti A, Tosti G (1988) Thimerosal: a hidden allergen in ophthalmology. Contact Dermatitis 18: 268–273
5. Van Ketel WG, Melzer-van Riemsdijk PA (1980) Conjunctivitis due to soft lens solutions. Contact Dermatitis 6: 321–324

Addresses

A. Tosti
Department of Dermatology, University of Bologna, via Massarenti 1, 40138 Bologna, Italy

G. Tosti
Department of Ophthalmology, University of Bologna, via Massarenti 9, 40138 Bologna, Italy

Various Allergens

Formaldehyde and Glyceryl Monothioglycolate: Results of the German Contact Dermatitis Research Group

P. J. Frosch, D. Kleinhans, T. Fuchs, A. Schnuch, H. Ippen, J. Ring, B. Przybilla, J. Rakoski, A. Stary, H. Merk, G. Lischka, J. Brasch, F. Bahmer, and G. Goerz

Summary

Today, for the detection of formaldehyde sensitivity most authors recommend a 1% aqueous solution. Even at this concentration irritant reactions may occur. Furthermore, an aqueous solution is impractical for new ready-to-use systems such as the Epiquick or True Test. Therefore, the German Contact Dermatitis Research Group studied two vehicles as an alternative to water: Softisan 649 (a lanolin substitute containing vegetable fatty acids) and a carboxymethyl cellulose gel. Based on preliminary studies the concentrations of formaldehyde (F) were 1.5% in Softisan (S) and 1% in the gel (G), compared to 1% F in water (W).

A total of 1428 patients was tested in 10 hospitals. The number of positive reactions with formaldehyde in different vehicles was as follows: 35 (S), 32 (W), 31 (G) at 48 h, and 41 (S), 46 (W), 38 (G) at 72 h. Doubtful or irritant reactions at 72 h were also in a similar range (16, 18 and 17 respectively). These differences were not significant (χ^2 test). Control testing with the vehicles showed slightly more irritant reactions with the gel. We therefore conclude that 1.5% formaldehyde in Softisan 649 is a suitable alternative to the 1% aqueous solution.

In the second study the sensitization to glyceryl monothioglycolate (GMT) was assessed based on the report of Storrs (1984) that this ingredient of "acid" permanent waves is a much more relevant sensitizer than ammonium thioglycolate (AMT). A total of 196 patients was tested in 9 clinics. 43 (21.9%) reacted to 1% GMT in petrolatum whereas only 4 (2%) showed a reaction to 1% AMT in petrolatum. Of 87 hairdressers 33 (37.9%) were positive to 1% GMT; in 70% these reactions were considered to be of clinical relevance. Thus, GMT is also in Germany a very important allergen for hairdressers and should be added to the supplementary tray for this profession.

Key words:

Formaldehyde - Softisan 649 - Vehicle - Glyceryl monothioglycolate - Ammonium thioglycolate - Hairdressers

In March 1987 the German Contact Dermatitis Research Group was formed as a subgroup of the German Dermatological Society (Deutsche Kontaktallergie-Gruppe in der Deutschen Dermatologischen Gesellschaft). At present, 16 Departments of Dermatology are represented by 21 members[1].

Our main goals are multicenter trials in regard to standardization and updating of patch testing as well as collection of computerized data under the aspects of epidemiology of contact dermatitis in the general population and in various professions [1].

In order to standardize the patch testing with formaldehyde we have tested three different vehicles. Most authors now recommend a 1% aqueous solution of formaldehyde. However, even at this concentration irritant reactions may occur and an aqueous solution is impractical for new ready-to-use devices such as the Epiquick or True test. We therefore studied alternatives to water such as Softisan 649 and a carboxymethyl cellulose gel.

Based on a report of Storrs [3] from the United States glyceryl monothioglycolate (GMT) as the active ingredient of "acid" permanent waves is a much more relevant sensitizer than ammonium thioglycolate (AMT). Preliminary results in Heidelberg and Stuttgart confirmed this conclusion for Germany. We therefore tested GMT nationwide in order to establish its relevance for hairdressers at the present time in this country.

Materials and Methods

1. Formaldehyde Study

Formaldehyde (F), stabilized with 10% methanol (Formaldehydlösung min. 37%; Merck, Darmstadt) was diluted for patch testing in three different vehicles: 1% (F) in water, 1.5% (F) in Softisan 649 (Dynamit-Nobel, Troisdorf), 1% (F) in carboxy methylcellulose gel (Thylose CB 4000; Hoechst). The formaldehyde free vehicles served as controls. All materials were simultaneously supplied by Hermal (Reinbek).

Most centers used Finn-chambers on Scanpor tape applied for 48 h with readings taken at 48 and 72 h (in doubtful cases at 96 h) according to the scale of the ICDRG.

2. Glyceryl Monothioglycolate Study

Glyceryl monothioglycolate (GMT) (Merck, Darmstadt) was diluted to 0.5% and 1.0% respectively in vaselinum album (DAB 9). Ammonium thioglycolate (AMT) (Merck, Darmstadt) was prepared at 1% and 2.5% in the same vehicle.

The materials were primarily tested on hairdressers but in some centers also included into the standard series for a short period of time.

[1] *German Contact Dermatitis Research Group:* P.J. Frosch (Chairman – Heidelberg), F. Bahmer (Homburg), J. Brasch (Kiel), T. Fuchs (Göttingen), M. Gloor (Karlsruhe), G. Goerz (Düsseldorf), J. Görtz (Essen), B. Hausen (Hamburg), H. Ippen (Göttingen), F. Klaschka (Berlin), D. Kleinhans (Stuttgart), J. Knop (Münster), G. Lischka (Tübingen), H. Merk (Köln), K.P. Peters (Erlangen), B. Przybilla (München), J. Rakoski (München), J. Ring (München), A. Schnuch (Göttingen), K.H. Schulz (Hamburg), A. Stary (Dortmund)

Results

1. Formaldehyde Study

A total of 1428 patients was tested in 10 centers. 67 patients were positive to at least one of the three formaldehyde formulations at 72 h (Table 1). The positivity rate ranged from 1.8% to 8.7% with a mean of 4.7%. Table 2 lists the number of positive cases at 48 and 72 h in regard to the three different vehicles used. The differences were only slight and not significant (Chi-Square test, $p > 0.3$). The intensity of test reactions was also in the same range (Table 3); this applied also to doubtful (+/−) reactions.

Table 1. Formaldehyde study. Results of patients tested with formaldehyde in 3 different vehicles – number of total positive cases at 72 h to at least one formaldehyde formulation

Center	Patients tested	Positive 72 h	Percent
TU-München	218	19	8,7%
LMU-München	271	13	4,8%
Göttingen	277	5	1,8%
Heidelberg	166	12	7,2%
Köln	135	3	2,2%
Tübingen	130	6	4,6%
Stuttgart	107	3	2,8%
Kiel	56	4	7,1%
Homburg	47	1	2,1%

Table 2. Formaldehyde study. Positive cases at 48 h and 72 h in regard to 3 different formaldehyde formulations.

	1,5% F (Softisan)	1,0% F (Water)	1,0% F (Gel)
48 h reading	35	32	31
72 h reading	41	46	38

Chi-Square test: not significant ($p > 0{,}3$)

Table 3. Formaldehyde study. Intensity of test reactions at 72 h.

	1,5% F (Softisan)	1,0% F (Water)	1,0% F (Gel)
±	16	18	17
+	17	25	18
++	17	15	13
+++	7	6	7
≥+	41	46	38

Table 4. Formaldehyde study. Reactions to the formaldehyde free vehicles in 1428 patients.

	Softisan		Water		Gel	
	48 h	72 h	48 h	72 h	48 h	72
±	2	2	1	1	1	4
+	0	1	0	0	2	1
++ and +++	0	0	0	0	0	0

24 of 67 formaldehyde positive patients showed a positive reaction to formaldehyde simultaneously in all three vehicles (35.8%). 12/67 (17.9%) were only positive to formaldehyde in Softisan, 10/67 (14.9%) only positive to formaldehyde in water, and 3/67 (4.5%) were only positive in formaldehyde dissolved in the carboxy methylcellulose gel. Various combinations (positive reaction to one formulation and negative to the others) were observed in 18 cases (26.9%).

Only few reactions were noticed with the formaldehyde free vehicles in 1428 patients (Table 4). The gel formulation produced the highest incidence with 4+/− reactions at 72 h and 1+/− reaction at 48 h. However, the differences to the other vehicles were not significant (Chi-Square test, $p > 0,05$).

2. Glyceryl Monothioglycolate Study

A total of 196 patients was tested in 9 hospitals. 43 patients were positive to 1% glyceryl monothioglycolate in vaseline (21.9%) as opposed to only 4 to 1% AMT (2.0%) (Table 5). Of 196 patients 87 were hairdressers. The number of positive results to both concentrations of GMT and AMT are shown in Table 6. Over 30%

Table 5. Glyceryl monothioglycolate study. Positive cases in a total of 196 patients

196 Patients tested in 9 hospitals (Dortmund, Tübingen, Heidelberg, Stuttgart, TU-München, LMU-München, Homburg, Düsseldorf, Köln)	
43 Positive to 1% GMT (V)	21,9%
4 Positive to 1% AMT (V)	2,0%

Table 6. Glyceryl monothioglycolate study. Positive reactions in 87 hairdressers at 72 h.

GMT		AMT	
0,5%	1,0%	1,0%	2,5%
30	33	4	5
34,5%	37,9%	4,6%	5,7%
clinical relevance: 23/33 (69,7%)		clinical relevance: 4/5 (80,0%)	

reacted to GMT with a minimal difference between 0.5% and 1% GMT (34.5% and 37.9% respectively). Clinical relevance of these reactions has been ascertained in 23 of 33 cases (69,7%). In contrast, only 4 hairdressers reacted to 1% AMT and 5 to 2.5%. Clinical relevance was given in 4 cases.

Discussion

The results of the formaldehyde study show that this allergen is still of great importance and must be maintained in the standard series. Regional deviations may be explained by differences in usage of formaldehyde containing products. However, the nearly twofold difference in one large city (München) rather reflects differences in methodology, particularly the reading of "positive" cases at 72 h. Further standardization in technique and interpretation of test results seem to be important.

The number of positive cases was highest with 1.5% formaldehyde in Softisan at 48 h and with 1% formaldehyde in water at 72 h. However, this difference was not significant. The number of doubtful allergic or irritant reactions was also in the same range with all three formaldehyde formulations. The intensity of positive reactions showed a similar pattern as well. Positive reactions of slight to moderate degree were observed with all three vehicles. Although statistically not significant, there was the tendency that the gel is more irritating than the others.

On the basis of these results we conclude that 1.5% formaldehyde in Softisan 649 and 1% formaldehyde in carboxymethylcellulose gel produce comparable patch test results to 1% formaldehyde in water. 1.5% formaldehyde in Softisan may be preferable to the gel because the vehicle produced less irritant reactions and the concordance with 1% formaldehyde in water was slightly better.

In order to solidify these conclusions it would have been desirable to obtain data on clinical relevance of formaldehyde reactions and to perform a repeated open application test (ROAT) in all doubtful cases. These data have been provided only in a minority of patients so far, in others these are still to be evaluated.

Softisan 649 is a new lanolin substitute based on vegetable fatty acids. It is stable to oxydation and there is no change in appearance and consistency on storage. It is miscible with fats and oils and its capacity for water uptake is more than 200%. It is non-sensitizing and well tolerated by the skin [2]. Väänänen and Hannuksela [4] have successfuly used Softisan 649 as a patch test vehicle for nickel sulphate.

Our results with glyceryl monothioglycolate confirm the conclusion of Storrs [3] that this is a much more relevant contact allergen in hairdressers than ammonium thioglycolate. Nearly 40% of 87 hairdressers were sensitized; clinical relevance was given in the majority of cases. We have tested GMT at 0.5% and 1.0% in vaseline. Based on the results of Storrs and on our own experience in Heidelberg, 2.5% GMT in vaseline is irritating. It might be possible that even at 1.0% GMT some irritant reactions may occur.

This study is continued in the German Contact Dermatitis Research Group with 0.5% and 1% GMT in vaseline, 1% GMT in an aqueous buffer (Chemotechnique) and 2.5% in water (Trolab-Hermal).

The histories taken from sensitized hairdressers suggest that these frequently do not apply the "acid perms" as recommended by the manufacturer. They do not wear gloves, splash the material over the fingers of the left hand when applying it to the curled hairs or touch the GMT contaminated hair when they test the waves for appropriate stability. According to the patch test results with various gloves most thin vinyl gloves do not provide protection against the penetration of glyceryl monothioglycolate [3]. As heavy duty gloves are impractical in this profession extreme care must be taken to avoid direct skin contact in order to reduce the sensitization rate to glyceryl monothioglycolate. Contact dermatitis caused by glyceryl monothioglycolate in clients receiving a hair treatment has been reported [3] and was also observed in our group. However, this seems to be much more infrequent than in the daily exposed hairdressing personal.

References

1. Frosch PJ, Bäurle G, Bahmer FA, Kietzmann H, Stary A (1988) Einheitliche Berücksichtigung von Allergenen bei berufsdermatologischen Testungen. In: Aktuelle Beiträge zu Umwelt- und Berufskrankheiten der Haut (Hornstein O, Klaschka F, Hrsg) Grosse Berlin 1: 147–161
2. Hermsdorf H (1982) Eigenschaften und Einsatzmöglichkeiten eines neuen Wollwachssubstitutes. Fette, Seifen, Anstrichmittel 3: 126–129
3. Storrs FJ (1984) Permanent wave contact dermatitis: Contact allergy to glyceryl monothioglycolate. J Am Acad Dermatol 11: 74–85
4. Väänänen A, Hannuksela M (1986) Softisan – a new vehicle for patch testing. Contact Dermatitis 14: 215–216

Addresses

P. J. Frosch
Universitäts-Hautklinik, Voßstr. 2, 6900 Heidelberg

D. Kleinhans
Hautklinik Stuttgart-Bad Cannstatt, Prießnitzweg 24, 7000 Stuttgart 50

T. Fuchs
Universitäts-Hautklinik, von-Siebold-Str. 3, 3400 Göttingen

A. Schnuch
Universitäts-Hautklinik, von-Siebold-Str. 3, 3400 Göttingen

H. Ippen
Universitäts-Hautklinik, von Siebold-Str. 3, 3400 Göttingen

J. Ring
Dermatologische Universitäts-Klinik, Frauenlobstr. 9, 8000 München 2

B. Przybilla
Dermatologische Universitäts-Klinik, Frauenlobstr. 9, 8000 München 2

J. Rakoski
Dermatologische Klinik und Poliklinik der Technischen Universität, Biedersteinerstr. 29, 8000 München 40

A. Stary
Hautklinik der Städtischen Kliniken, Beurhausstr. 40, 4600 Dortmund 1

H. Merk
Universitäts-Hautklinik, Joseph-Stelzmann-Str. 9, 5000 Köln-Lindenthal

G. Lischka
Universitäts-Hautklinik, Liebermeisterstr. 25, 7400 Tübingen

J. Brasch
Universitäts-Hautklinik, Schittenhelmstr. 7, 2300 Kiel

F. Bahmer
Universitäts-Hautklinik, 6650 Homburg/Saar

G. Goerz
Universitäts-Hautklinik, Moorenstr. 5, 4000 Düsseldorf

Comparative Patch Testing with PPD-Base and PPD-Dihydrochloride: Human and Animal Data Compiled by the European Environmental Contact Dermatitis Research Group

A. Dooms-Goossens, R. J. Scheper, K. E. Andersen, D. Burrows, J. G. Camarasa, P. J. Frosch, A. Lahti, and J. Wilkinson

Summary

The replacement of PPD-base 1% petrolatum (pet.) by PPD-dihydrochloride 0.5% pet. in the ICDRG standard series in 1984 seems to have reduced considerably the number of positive reactions to PPD. Therefore, the EECDRG decided to perform comparative patch tests with PPD-base and PPD-dihydrochloride. The results in human testing showed that most of the PPD sensitivities were missed by the PPD-dihydrochloride. Guinea pig experiments confirmed that PPD-dihydrochloride was less able to elicit hypersensitivity reactions than PPD-base. Similar results were obtained with groups of guinea pigs sensitized by intradermal injection to either allergen preparation. The difference in molecular weights, different liabilities in oxidative degradation to the sensitizing intermediate, or different skin penetration capabilities may account for this phenomenon.

Key words:

Contact dermatitis - PPD-base - PPD-dihydrochloride - Paraphenylenediamine - False-negative reactions

Introduction

Before 1984, PPD-base 1% petrolatum (pet.) was routinely tested in the ICDRG standard series to detect contact allergic reactions to PPD and para-amino-benzene derivatives in general.

Since its replacement by PPD-dihydrochloride 0.5% pet., the number of contact dermatitis reactions to PPD seems to have dropped considerably. Indeed, in a comparable number of patients tested in Leuven, Belgium, (A.D.G.) between 1981 and

1983, we found a frequency of PPD sensitivity of 6.6%. Between 1985 and 1987, this frequency dropped to 1.3%. Other centers reported an even lower rate: 0.7% (K.A., Denmark), 0.4% (A.L., Finland), and 0% (J.W., England).

Several factors might contribute to this phenomenon.

1. By changing the PPD-base 1% pet. to 0.5% PPD-dihydrochloride, the concentration of PPD is reduced by more than threefold. Indeed, considering the respective molecular weights (PPD-base, 108.14; PPD-dihydrochloride, 181.07) 1% of the base is equivalent to 1.7% of the dihydrochloride.
2. From a chemical point of view, the pure base will undergo oxidative degradation much more easily than will the dihydrochloride. This is why the PPD-base darkens more rapidly upon exposure to air than does PPD-dihydrochloride. The same thing applies to the patch-test sites. Of course, we do not know the exact identity of the PPD-allergen, for it has been said that one or more of its intermediate oxidation products are the probable allergens. Individual differences in skin metabolism may well be why some patients do react to PPD-dihydrochloride (cf. [1]).
3. As regards the PPD-derived hair dyes, as with many other chemicals, "changes in structure that increase lipophilicity also increase percutaneous absorption" [2]. PPD-base is more lipophilic than PPD-dihydrochloride, so it could well be that PPD-base penetrates the horny layer more easily.

To investigate further the differential capacity of PPD-base and PPD-dihydrochloride to elicit PPD-specific skin hypersensitivity reactions, comparative testing with PPD-base and PPD-dihydrochloride was performed in humans and experiments were performed in guinea pigs.

Materials and Methods

Human Study

Members of the EECDRG tested 2070 consecutive patients with PPD-base and PPD-dihydrochloride (following the ICDRG patch-testing guidelines) at concentrations of 0.5% and 1% in petrolatum.

Guinea Pig Study

Outbred albino female guinea pigs of the Himalayan strain (TNO, The Netherlands) weighing 250–350 g were used. Groups of guinea pigs were sensitized by one intradermal injection of 0.1 ml PPD-base (0.1% in propylene glycol), 0.1 ml PPD-dihydrochloride (0.1% in propylene glycol), or 0.1 ml solvent only.

On the 10th day after sensitization, all the animals were given patch tests on shaved and depilated flanks: PPD-base and PPD-dihydrochloride, 0.5% and 1.0% in petrolatum. The patches were removed 20 h later, and the reactions were evaluated by two observers at 24, 48, 72, and 96 h by grading the intensity of erythema as follows: equivocal or no reaction, 0; pink spots, 0.5; red, confluent, 1; intense red, 2.

Results

Human Study

Although the figures from the different centers of the respective members varied considerably (Table 1), most of the PPD sensitivities were missed when testing with PPD-dihydrochloride, irrespective of the concentration. Out of a total of 2070 patients tested with PPD-base and PPD-dihydrochloride, 47 reactions occurred to PPD-base, most of which were considered relevant. Only six of them also clearly reacted to PPD-dihydrochloride.

Guinea Pig Study

All the guinea pigs that received one intradermal injection of either PPD-base or PPD-dihydrochloride developed PPD hypersensitivity (Fig. 1). Interestingly, no dif-

Table 1. PPD-base versus PPD-dihydrochloride (number of positive reactions)

	n	PPD-dihydrochloride	PPD-base
DB (Ireland)	650	1	3
JC (Spain)	62	4	6
ADG (Belgium)	331	1	17
PF (F.R.G.)	111	1 (?)	3
AL (Finland)	302	0	3
JW (England)	614	0	15

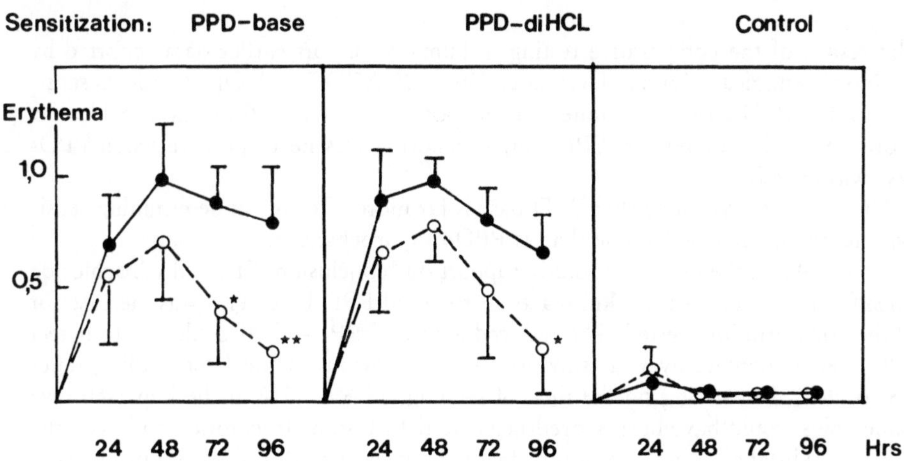

Fig. 1. Skin-test reactivity in guinea pigs sensitized to PPD-base (*left*; $n = 11$), PPD-dihydrochloride (*middle*; $n = 10$), or injected with solvent only (*right*; $n = 7$). Skin tests were performed on day 10 by epicutaneous application of 0.5% PPD-base (●—●) or 1.0% PPD-dihydrochloride (○—○). The means + SD are shown at 24, 48, 72, and 96 h after skin testing. $^{*}P<0.05$, $^{**}P<0.01$ (Wilcoxon) compared with PPD-base skin tests

Table 2. Frequency of positive skin test reactions to PPD-base and PPD-dihydrochloride in guinea pigs sensitized to either substance

Sensitization	Skin test	48 h	72 h	96 h
PPD-base	Base/dihydrochloride[a]	11/9[b]	11/8	11/4
PPD-dihydrochloride	Base/dihydrochloride	10/8	10/8	10/5
% Responders[c]		100/81	100/76	100/43

[a] 0.5% PPD-base/pet., respectively 1.0% PPD-dihydrochloride/pet.

[b] Numbers of animals manifesting positive reactions (erythema > 0.3) to PPD-base and PPD-dihydrochloride, respectively

[c] Percentages of animals in both groups manifesting positive reactions to PPD-base and PPD-dihydrochloride, respectively

ferences emerged between the groups as to their reactivity to either test substance. In both groups, PPD-base consistently elicited stronger skin reactions than did PPD-dihydrochloride. This was especially obvious at the later reading times (72 and 96 h). Note that these results were obtained with the lower dose of the PPD-base. Testing with 1.0% PPD-base resulted in slightly stronger reactions (average increase of 0.2), but no significant difference in skin test reactivity was detected for 0.5% or 1.0% PPD-dihydrochloride (data on file).

In Table 2, the skin-test data show the percentages of positively reacting animals (erythema at least 0.3) in each group for all reading times. With PPD-dihydrochloride, the number of animals scoring negatively increased from 48 on (19% to 57%).

Discussion and Conclusion

The results of the comparative testing in humans support earlier data reported by the North American Contact Dermatitis Group (NACDG) [3]. Of 22 patients sensitive to 1% PPD-base, only nine reacted positively to 1% PPD-dihydrochloride. Moreover, as in our results, PPD-dihydrochloride was never positive when PPD-base was negative.

Therefore, we conclude that PPD-base is far more effective in determining sensitivity to paraphenylenediamine than is PPD-dihydrochloride.

The results of the guinea pig study support our conclusion. PPD-dihydrochloride consistently elicited weaker skin reactions than did PPD-base. This was the case for all the concentrations tested. The reduced ability of PPD-dihydrochloride to detect PPD-specific contact hypersensitivity was most obvious at the later reading times (48 to 96 h). Depending on the time of reading, 19% to 57% of the hypersensitive guinea pigs would have been scored negative if PPD-dihydrochloride had been the only test substance. These data, too, favor the view that PPD-base should be preferred in clinical skin testing.

Although it may be too early to decide on the exact test concentration of PPD-base – 0.5% or 1% – we conclude that we all are now definitely testing the wrong substance.

Acknowledgements. We would like to thank Mr. J. de Groot for his skillful assistance in the guinea pig sensitization study.

References

1. Schmidt RJ, Fernandez de Corres L (1987) Allergic contact dermatitis from proprietary topical analgesic sprays containing 32-(aminomethyl)-pyridyl salicylate. Dermatologica 174: 272–279
2. Bronaugh RL, Congdon ER (1984) Percutaneous absorption of hair dyes: correlation with partition coefficients. J Invest Dermatol 83: 124–127
3. Storrs FJ, Taylor J, Jordan WP, Maibach HI (1979) Paraphenylenediamine hydrochloride. Contact Dermatitis 5: 126

Addresses

A. Dooms-Goossens
Department of Medical Research (Dermatology), University Hospital, Leuven, Belgium

R. J. Scheper
Department of Pathology, Free University Hospital, Amsterdam, The Netherlands

K. E. Andersen
Hudklinikken, Roskilde, Denmark

D. Burrows
Department of Dermatology, Royal Victoria Hospital, Belfast, Ireland

J. G. Camarasa
Department of Dermatology, Universitat Autònoma de Barcelona, Spain

P. J. Frosch
Universitäts-Hautklinik, Heidelberg, Germany

A. Lahti
Department of Dermatology, University of Oulo, Oulo, Finland

J. Wilkinson
Department of Dermatology, Wycombe General Hospital, High Wycombe, England

Colour Developing Agents: High-Performance Liquid Chromatography Analysis of Test Preparations Used in Guinea Pig Maximization Testing

C. Lidén, A. Boman, and J. Sollenberg

Summary

Colour developing agents which are derivatives of *p*-phenylenediamine (PPDA), e.g. CD-2, CD-3 and CD-4, are known to cause allergic contact dermatitis and lichenoid reactions in workers at film laboratories and in photographers. Some of these patients show positive patch test reactions to more than one colour developer, and also to developers that they have not been occupationally exposed to. The aims of the study were to determine the sensitizing potential of CD-2, CD-3 and CD-4, and to study cross-sensitization between the colour developing agents and PPDA. In three separate series of guinea pig maximization tests (GPMT), animals were exposed to CD-2, CD-3 and CD-4, respectively. Challenge testing was done with CD-2, CD-3, CD-4 and PPDA in all series. CD-2, CD-3 and CD-4 were analysed with respect to purity, common contaminants and reaction products, using high-performance liquid chromatography (HPLC). Test substances used in the GPMT were analysed before and after testing, and remaining substances on the patches and on the skin were analysed, as well as bulk chemicals and tank solutions. CD-2, CD-3 and CD-4 were shown to be extremely potent sensitizers – 100% of the animals were sensitized. Simultaneous reactions to the other tested colour developing agents were found in 75%–100%, while reactions to PPDA were not seen. No contaminants or reaction products in common were detected by the HPLC analysis. The simultaneous test reactions were interpreted as cross-sensitization. Metabolization of these chemicals within the skin was, however, beyond the scope of this study.

Key words:

Colour developing agents – p-Phenylenediamine – Contact allergy – Cross-sensitization

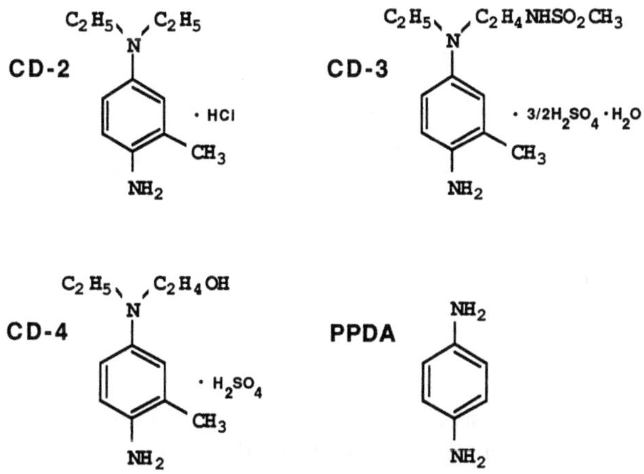

Fig. 1. Structural formulas of CD-2, CD-3, CD-4 and *p*-phenylenediamine (PPDA)

Introduction

The process of developing colour film has been established for 50 years. CD-2, CD-3 and CD-4, which are derivatives of *p*-phenylenediamine (PPDA), are the most frequently used colour developing agents (Fig. 1). For 30 years, it has been known that they can cause contact allergy [9] and lichenoid reactions [2]. Occupational skin disease from colour developing agents is still a problem [3, 5, 6] It has been claimed that CD-2 is a more potent sensitizer than CD-3 [1]. The question of cross-sensitivity between the colour developing agents and PPDA has been discussed in connection with patients with multiple patch test reactions [4]. The aims of this study were to determine the sensitizing potential in the guinea pig of CD-2, CD-3 and CD-4, and to study cross-sensitization between the colour developing agents and PPDA. Parallel to the animal experiments, the test substances, as well as bulk chemicals and tank solutions, were analysed with respect to purity, common contaminants and reaction products, using high-performance liquid chromatography (HPLC).

Materials and Methods

Chemicals. CD-2, CD-3 and CD-4 were from Merck, of technical quality (Fig. 1). *p*-phenylenediaminedihydrochloride (PPDA) was from Fluka AG, of purest quality.

Guinea Pig Maximization Tests. Using the method of Magnusson and Kligman [8], guinea pig maximization tests (GPMT) were carried out in three separate series (for details see [7]). Induction was done with CD-2, CD-3 and CD-4, respectively (0.2% intradermally on day 0 and 25% in petrolatum topically on day 7). Challenge was performed with CD-2, CD-3, CD-4 and PPDA in all series (0.5 and 0.1 mol/kg in petrolatum for CD-2, CD-3 and CD-4, and 0.06 mol/kg in petrolatum for PPDA).

Table 1. Analytical system used for separation of CD-2, CD-3, CD-4 and *p*-phenylenediaminedihydrochloride with high-performance liquid chromatography

Parameter	Value
Column	Hypersil ODS (5 μm), 200 × 5 mm
Mobile phase	Methanol: KH_2PO_4 (50 mmol/litre), heptanesulphonic acid sodium salt (3 mmol/litre) + triethylamine to pH 6.1 (40:60)
Flow	2 ml/min
Temperature	45 °C
Injection	20 μl
Detector	UV, 246 nm

Each series consisted of approx. 20 exposed animals and 20 sham-treated controls. Challenge reactions were read blindly 48 and 72 h after application.

HPLC Analysis. PPDA and different samples of CD-2, CD-3 and CD-4 were separated and analysed for purity and stability [10] using a Hewlett-Packard 1084 B HPLC instrument. The analytical parameters are shown in Table 1. Samples for HPLC analysis were drawn from the GPMT with CD-2, CD-3 and CD-4 at different stages as follows:

1. Intradermal induction	0 h
2. Topical induction	0 h
3. Topical induction (filter paper)	48 h
4. Challenge	0 h
5. Challenge (test patch, skin surface)	24 h

The remaining substances on filter paper pads, on Finn chambers and on the skin surface at test sites were analysed. Other samples of CD-2, CD-3 and CD-4 for analysis were bulk chemicals (12 batches), tank solutions from 6 machines, patch test preparations for clinical use and aqueous solutions of the colour developing agents. The petrolatum preparations were dissolved in ligroin and extracted with water before analysis.

Statistics. For statistical analysis the χ^2test or Fisher's exact test were used.

Results

The results from the GPMT are shown in Table 2. All animals induced with CD-2, CD-3 and CD-4, respectively, were sensitized to the corresponding substance. The cross-sensitization challenge tests showed that the animals were also positive to the other colour developing agents applied ($P < 0.001$). A few reactions to PPDA were seen, but they were not significantly more frequent among exposed animals than among controls, nor were they more frequent than reactions to the petrolatum vehicle control (NS).

Table 2. Results from three separate guinea pig maximization tests: positive reactions in exposed (e) and control (c) animals

Induction substance	No. of animals (e/c)	No. of positive reactions to challenge (e/c)				
		CD-2[a]	CD-3[a]	CD-4[a]	PPDA[b]	Petrolatum
CD-2	20/19	20/1	15/0	18/0	3/1	1/2
CD-3	20/20	20/2	20/1	20/1	1/1	1/0
CD-4	21/20	20/0	17/1	21/0	3/0	1/0

[a] Concentration 0.5 mol/kg.
[b] Concentration 0.06 mol/kg.

The retention times for CD-2, CD-3, CD-4 and PPDA in HPLC analyses were 3.3, 2.7, 2.2 and 1.2 min, respectively. No contaminants or reaction products in common were shown in the test preparations of CD-2, CD-3 and CD-4 from the GPMT procedure, or in the bulk chemicals. The colour developing agents were stable in petrolatum preparations but unstable in water solutions.

Discussion

The colour developing agents CD-2, CD-3 and CD-4 were shown to be extremely potent sensitizers (Table 2). It is suggested that the lower grading in the study cited [1] was an underestimation due to the use of a less sensitive test method (a modified Landsteiner test). Simultaneous reactions to the other tested colour developing agents were shown to a great extent (Table 2), which was interpreted as cross-reactivity. This was based on the results from the HPLC analyses. No contaminants or reaction products in common were detected in the different samples of the colour developing agents.

Petrolatum was regarded as the most suitable vehicle for testing the colour developing agents in guinea pigs and patients. Pre-tests had shown that aqueous solutions, but not petrolatum preparations, caused irritation and staining of the skin. HPLC analysis showed that aqueous solutions were unstable while petrolatum preparations were stable. Patch testing with petrolatum preparations has been shown to be adequate in clinical practice [5, 6].

The results do not exclude the possibility that other potent allergens might develop from these substances in e.g. aqueous solutions or tank solutions. In this study, however, the stable petrolatum preparations were shown to be potent sensitizers with cross-reactivity, in accordance with clinical experience. An investigation of the metabolization of the substances within the skin was beyond the scope of this work.

References

1. Bent RL, Dessloch JC, Duennebier FC et al. (1951) Chemical constitution, electrochemical, photographic and allergenic properties of *p*-amino-*N*-dialkylanilines. J Am Chem Soc 73: 3100–3125
2. Buckley WR (1958) Lichenoid eruptions following contact dermatitis. Arch Dermatol 78: 454–457
3. Cronin E (1980) Contact dermatitis. Churchill Livingstone, Edinburgh, pp 861–865
4. Goh CL, Kwok SF, Rajan VS (1984) Cross sensitivity in colour developers. Contact Dermatitis 10: 280–285
5. Lidén C (1984) Occupational dermatoses at a film laboratory. Contact Dermatitis 10: 77–87
6. Lidén C (in press) Occupational dermatoses at a film laboratory. Follow-up after modernization. Contact Dermatitis
7. Lidén C, Boman A (1988) Contact allergy to colour developing agents in the guinea pig. Contact Dermatitis 19: 290–295
8. Magnusson B, Kligman A (1969) The identification of contact allergens by animal assay. The guinea pig maximization test. J Invest Dermatol 52: 268–276
9. Massmann W, Zschunke E (1954) Allergische Hautreaktion nach Einwirkung von *p*-Amino-*N*-diäthylanilin, einen Farbfilmentwickler. Arch Derm Syph 197: 496–504
10. Sollenberg J, Lidén C, Hansén L, Arvidson A (in press) Contact allergy to colour developing agents. Analysis of test preparations by high-performance liquid chromatography. Dermatosen

Addresses

C. Lidén

Division of Occupational Dermatology, National Institute of Occupational Health, and Department of Occupational Dermatology, Karolinska Hospital, S-10401 Stockholm, Sweden

A. Boman

Division of Occupational Dermatology, National Institute of Occupational Health, S-17184 Solna, Sweden

J. Sollenberg

Division of Analytical Chemistry, National Institute of Occupational Health, S-17184 Solna, Sweden

Contact Dermatitis and Vitiligo Due to Colour Developers

F. M. Brandão, A. Dinis, and R. Silva

Summary

A 54-year-old man working in a photographic laboratory developed eczema on both hands and on his face and, 2 years later, vitiligo-like macules on the same areas. Patch tests were positive to several colour developers, but not to *p*-phenylene-diamine or to hydroquinone. Two months later, lichenoid reactions were observed at the site of positive patch tests, but no achromia. Progressive repigmentation occurred over the following months.

Key words:

Contact dermatitis - Contact vitiligo - Colour developers - Hydroquinone

Introduction

Contact dermatitis due to photographic chemicals is nowadays an uncommon finding due to the automatization of this industry. However, sporadic cases still occur, mainly among amateur photographers, who develop their own films manually [1]. Contact vitiligo may be produced by developers containing hydroquinone, but only a few cases have been reported in the literature [1–4].

Case Report

A 54-year-old man had worked in a photographic laboratory for the past 8 years. After 2 years, eczematous lesions appeared, first on the dorsa of both hands and fingers, and later on his face, mainly on the right side. Some months afterwards, depigmented macules were seen on roughly the same areas and on the anterior aspect of his right wrist. He was patch-tested with the standard and photography series. Tests were strongly positive (+++) to several colour developers (CD1, CD2, CD3, CD4, CD32, TSS; all 1% petrolatum), but negative to *p*-phenylenediamine (PPD) and hydroquinone. Two months later, the patient was reviewed. Having taken great care and having had no further contact with the developers, he had no eczema, and repigmentation had begun on his face. On the back, looking for achromia at the hydroquinone patch test site, only lichenoid reactions were observed at the site of previous positive tests. Unfortunately, biopsy was refused by the patient. Over the following months, there was an almost complete repigmentation on the face and a moderate improvement of the leucoderma on the dorsa of the hands.

Discussion

The allergy to several colour developers was probably due to cross-reactions; as far as we could tell, the patient was in contact with a CD4-containing developer and had previously worked with another one containing CD3. All these chemicals are PPD derivatives with a similar structure, which explains the possible cross-reactions. However, in accordance with most cases reported, there was no allergy to PPD. Clinically, contact allergy to colour developers may assume either an eczematous picture or a lichenoid pattern. In our patient, clinical lesions were of eczema, but the patch test sites developed a lichenoid aspect after 2 months.

Hydroquinone is used widely in industry as a reducing agent, as a photographic developer and as a stabiliser for certain materials that polymerise, like acrylic and polyester systems [5]. It is known to induce depigmentation by inhibiting the conversion of tyrosine to melanin [6], but it can also have a cytotoxic effect on the melanocyte [7]. Occupational leucoderma due to hydroquinone in photography workers has seldom been reported [1–4]. This is probably due to the low concentration used in film developers, although it has been reported to reach 7% in black-and-white developers [2]. Unlike its monobenzyl ether, it usually does not induce permanent depigmentation and therefore has been largely used in bleaching creams in concentrations of 2%–5%. In this case, the responsibility of hydroquinone may be questioned. However, the localisation of leucoderma on exposed areas and the partial regression observed after diminution of contact with the developer are strongly suggestive of its playing a role in the pathogenesis of the vitiligo. The simultaneous occurrence of dermatitis and vitiligo is quite rare and, as far as we know, has been reported only once before [4].

References

1. Fisher AA (1986) Contact Dermatitis, 3rd edn. Lea and Febiger, Philadelphia, pp 495–496
2. Duffield JA (1952) Depigmentation of skin by quinol and its mono-benzyl-ether. Lancet I: 1164
3. Frenk E, Loi-Zedda P (1980) Occupational depigmentation due to a hydroquinone-containing photographic developer. Contact Dermatitis 6: 238–239
4. Kersey P, Stevenson CJ (1981) Vitiligo and occupational exposure to hydroquinone from servicing self-photographing machines. Contact Dermatitis 7: 285–287
5. Fisher AA (1986) Contact Dermatitis, 3rd edn. Lea and Febiger, Philadelphia, pp 681–684
6. Denton CR,Lerner AB, Fitzpatrick TB (1952) Inhibition of melanin formation by chemical agents. J Invest Dermatol 18: 119–135
7. Jimbow K, Obata H, Pathak MA, Fitzpatrick TB (1974) Mechanism of depigmentation by hydroquinone. J Invest Dermatol 62: 436–449

Addresses

F. M. Brandão
Department of Dermatology, Santa Maria Hospital, P-1699 Lisbon Codex, Portugal

A. Dinis
Department of Dermatology, Santa Maria Hospital, P-1699 Lisbon Codex, Portugal

R. Silva
Department of Dermatology, Santa Maria Hospital, P-1699 Lisbon Codex, Portugal

Thiourea Contact Sensitivity in Portugal

A. Azenha, F. M. Brandão, M. S. J. Marques, M. Pecegueiro, A. Pinto Soares, G. Saudade, A. Sousa Basto, and T. Vale

Summary

In 1986, with the objective of assessing contact sensitivity to thioureas in Portugal, the Portuguese Contact Dermatitis Group carried out an overall study, which included four thioureas from Trolab. The total number of patients tested was 2025, of whom only 3 reacted positively to thioureas. The cause of the affection in every case was their footwear.

Key words:

Thioureas - Allergic contact dermatitis - Dibutylthiourea - Diethylthiourea - Diphenylthiourea - Ethylene thiourea

Introduction

Thiourea compounds are at present used widely in several industrial sectors, either as intermediated in the manufacture of various general-purpose products or as basic components of many others [1–9]. Despite their multiple uses (namely, as antioxidants, anticorrosive agents, fixing agents, and rubber vulcanization accelerators), the contact sensitivity capacity of thioureas seems to be weak.

Material and Methods

A total of 2025 patients were tested in seven contact allergy centers during 1986 with the Portuguese standard series and other special series, including four thioureas from Trolab: dibutylthiourea, diphenylthiourea, diethylthiourea, and ethylene thiourea. Of these patients, 1137 presented positive reactions to several types of allergens, and only 3 reacted positively to thioureas (0.15%). In one case (a 43-year-old man), only ethylene thiourea affected the patient. In the remaining two cases, positive reactions were observed to diphenylthiourea and ethylene thiourea (a 39-year-old woman) and to diphenylthiourea, dibutylthiourea, and ethylene thiourea (a 45-year-old woman).

Case Reports

Case 1. A 43-year-old metalworker presented an itchy erythematosquamous eruption on both insteps. The lesions had appeared after use of Ritex Sport athletic shoes for 2 months. Standard patch tests were negative except for nickel sulfate (+ +) and quinoline mix (+ +). Special patch tests (including rubber allergen series, dyes and colorants, plastics, and resins) were negative except for ethylene thiourea (48 h+ +; 96 h+ +). Positive patch test reactions were observed to the foam in the tongue of the shoe (+ +) and to the lining (+ +). The dermatitis disappeared completely after a few days of local corticosteroid therapy and no further use of the athletic shoes.

Case 2. A 39-year-old housewife developed recurrent erythematous scaling skin lesions on the soles, sides, and dorsa of the feet. The dermatitis had appeared 3 years before and recurred in the summer. The patient usually wore rubber shoes. Standard patch tests were negative except for colophony (+ + +). Results from special patch tests (including rubber series, dyes and colorants, plastics, and resins) were negative except for diphenylthiourea (48 h+ +; 96 h+ + +) and ethylene thiourea (48 h+ + +; 96 h+ + +). Patch tests were also positive to the lining (+ + +) and insole (+ + +).

Case 3. A 45-year-old woman developed an erythematosquamous dermatitis on the distal soles after wearing Tiger athletic shoes for 4 months. She referred to identical episodes occurring in recent summers. She also had a history of contact eczema to stockings and brassieres. Standard patch tests were negative for mercapto mix (+ + +). Special patch tests with rubber series, dyes and colorants, plastics, and resins were read at 48 and 96 h and gave the following positive results: CBS (+ + +) MBT (+ + +), MBTS (+ + +), MOR (+ + +), dibutylthiourea (+ + +), diphenylthiourea (+ + +), and ethylene thiourea (+ + +). Patch tests were also positive to the foam (+ + +) and insole (+ + +). The patient was probably already sensitized to the mercapto mix (history of eczema episodes on the feet and after local contact with elastics). The recent increase of the dermatitis after use of athletic shoes may be related to the presence of the two allergens – mercapto in the sole and thiourea in the foam. It was impossible to confirm this because we could not contact the manufacturer (Taiwan).

Discussion

All of the cases presented the same topographic location and were caused by footwear. From the patch test results we can admit the presence of thiourea compounds in the footwear, and particularly ethylene thiourea, used as an accelerator in the vulcanization of various elastomers [4] and present in rubber materials [4]. Allergic contact dermatitis to ethylene thiourea is rare because its allergenicity is very low [4]; however, we could find three cases which had in common positivity to ethylene thiourea in rubber material. From the results obtained it can be concluded that in Portugal, thiourea contact allergy is not frequent, and its contact sensitivity capacity is confirmed to be weak. Nevertheless, thioureas must be included in the shoes contact series.

References

1. Adams RM (1982) Contact allergic dermatitis due to diethylthiourea in a wetsuit. Contact Dermatitis 8: 277
2. Aloamar A, Vilaltella I (1985) Contact dermatitis to dibutylthiourea in swimming goggles. Contact Dermatitis 12: 348–349
3. Andersen KE (1983) Diethylthiourea contact dermatitis from an acidic detergent. Contact Dermatitis 9: 146
4. Bruze M, Fregert S (1983) Allergic contact dermatitis from ethylenethiourea. Contact Dermatitis 9: 208–212
5. Camarasa JG, Romaguera C, et al. (1985) Thiourea reactivity in Spain. Contact Dermatitis 12: 220
6. Dooms Goossens A, Boyden B, et al. (1979) Dimethylthiourea: an unexpected hazard for textile workers. Contact Dermatitis 5: 367–370
7. Dooms Goosens A, Chrispeels MT, et al. (1987) Contact and photocontact sensivity problems associated with thiourea and its derivatives: a review of the literature and case reports. Br J Dermatol 116: 573–579
8. Fregert S, Trullsson L, Zimerson C (1982) Contact allergic reactions to diphenylthiourea and phenylisothiocyanate in PVC adhesive tape. Contact Dermatitis 8: 38–42
9. Kanerva L, Jolanki R, et al. (1984) Contact dermatitis from dibutylthiourea. Report of a case with fine structural observations of epicutaneous testing with dibutylthiourea. Contact Dermatitis 10: 158–162
10. Kellet JK, Beck MH, Auckland G (1984) Contact sensitivity to thiourea in photocopy paper. Contact Dermatitis 11: 124
11. Lidén C (1984) Contact allergy to the photographic chemical PBA-1. Contact Dermatitis 11: 256
12. Masmoudi ML, Lachapelle JM (1987) Occupational contact dermatitis to dihidroxydiphenyl and diphenylthiourea in neoprene gloves. Contact Dermatitis 16: 290–291
13. Nurse D (1980) Sensitivity to thiourea in plant printing paper. Contact Dermatitis 6: 153–154
14. Roberts JL, Hanifin JM (1979) Athletic shoe dermatitis. Contact allergy to ethylbutylthiourea. JAMA 241: 275–276
15. Roberts JL, Hanifin JM (1980) Contact allergy and cross reactivity to substituted thiourea compounds. Contact Dermatitis 6: 138–139
16. Romaguera C, et al. (1988) Contact dermatitis to thioureas. Contact Dermatitis 18: 175–176

17. Taylor J (1984) Contact dermatitis from goggles. Patch test symposium of the American Academy of Dermatology Meeting, Washington DC
18. White WC, Wickers HR (1970) Diethylthiourea as a cause of dermatitis in a car factory. Br J Ind Med 27: 167–169

Addresses

A. Azenha
Hospital de São Marcos, Serviço de Dermatologia, 4700 Braga, Portugal

F. M. Brandão
Hospital de São Marcos, Serviço de Dermatologia, 4700 Braga, Portugal

M. S. J. Marques
Hospital de São Marcos, Serviço de Dermatologia, 4700 Braga, Portugal

M. Pecegueiro
Hospital de São Marcos, Serviço de Dermatologia, 4700 Braga, Portugal

A. Pinto Soares
Hospital de São Marcos, Serviço de Dermatologia, 4700 Braga, Portugal

G. Saudade
Hospital de São Marcos, Serviço de Dermatologia, 4700 Braga, Portugal

A. Sousa Basto
Hospital de São Marcos, Serviço de Dermatologia, 4700 Braga, Portugal

T. Vale
Hospital de São Marcos, Serviço de Dermatologia, 4700 Braga, Portugal

Allergic Contact Dermatitis from the Insecticide Dichlorvos

J. de la Cuadra and G. Serrano

Summary

Despite the widespread domestic use of commercial insecticide sprays, toxic or allergic adverse reactions to them are unusual. A 60-year-old woman developed an acute contact dermatitis on exposed areas (neck, arms, and legs) 25 days after applying a marketed insecticide spray onto her skin. Patch tests showed strong positive reactions to dichlorvos, one of the active ingredients of the spray (0.1% and 0.01%), and to the fragrance. The patient also reacted to one of the spray solvents, *n*-C_{14} (tetradecane; 1% in petrolatum). In this case, sensitization was favored by abnormal usage conditions.

Key words

Allergic contact dermatitis - Insecticide - Dichlorvos - Fragrance - Tetradecane - Domestic sprays

Introduction

Dichlorvos (2,2-dichlorovinyl dimethyl phosphate; DDVP; Fig. 1) is an aliphatic organophosphate compound with high vapor pressure, which gives it strong fumigant properties. It acts as an insecticide either by direct contact or by indirect contact with vapors. It is used in fumigation operations and in sprays for domestic use. It has been incorporated into plastic pet collars and pest strips; vapor action from impregnated plastics may last several months, and for this reason the insecticide is very effective in controlling fleas. Dichlorvos is marketed under a variety of names: Derriban and Maton (Spain), Apavap (Italy, Sweden), Nogos and Nuvan (Switzerland), Vapona, Atgard, and Task (USA), etc.

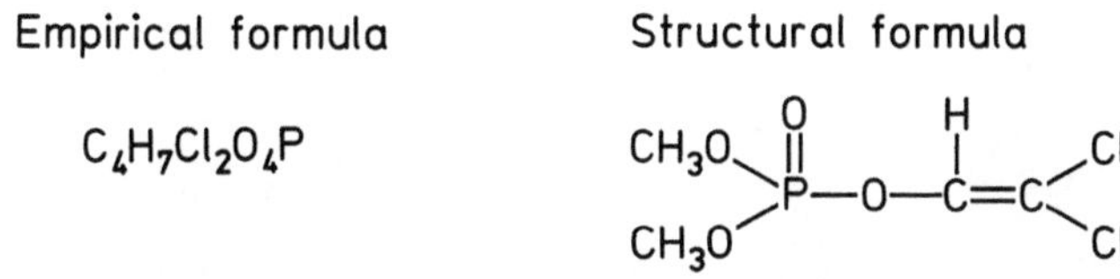

Fig. 1. Empirical and structural formulas of dichlorvos

This insecticide is capable of producing primary skin irritation in dogs, with hair loss from the neck and even chemical burns, reported as fleao-collar dermatitis [2]. An unusual feature of flea-collar dermatitis is its persistence several months after the flea collar is removed. Muller [3] cites occasional widespread reactions as evidence of sensitization. In humans, skin reactions are rare, but primarily irritation may occur, resulting from accidental skin contamination [4] or from handling a flea collar, handling a dog wearing it, or both [1].

This case report describes a vegetable seller who developed an acute dermatitis of the exposed areas several days after applying a marketed insecticide spray (Maton) containing dichlorvos onto the skin. The clinical picture, as well as the patch test results, suggests that the dermatitis was allergic in nature.

Case Report

A 60-year-old white female vegetable seller with no previous history of dermatitis was seen in our clinic on 3 July 1986 with a pruritic, acute dermatitis on exposed areas of the neck, arms, and legs. Upon questioning, she recognized the misuse of a marketed insecticide spray (Maton). The cutaneous eruption began 25 days after she started sporadically applying such spray onto the skin. As she worked outdoors, in a market, she thought the insecticide would have no effect when sprayed into the air. She claimed that fleas were causing her such discomfort that she decided to spray it directly onto the skin.

On examination, there were erythematous, oozing vesicular and bullous lesions over the lateral aspects of the neck, the arms, and the anterior aspect of the legs (Figs. 2, 3). The patient did not complain of other symptoms. Determination of cholinesterase blood levels was not done.

Material and Methods

The patient was tested a month after clearing of the eruption, using Finn chamber patches. Patch tests were done in duplicate with the different chemicals contained in the insecticide spray used by the patient. All substances were initially diluted in ethanol. The composition of the insecticide spray is shown in Table 1. A row of chemicals was occluded for 24 h and then irradiated by means of a PUVA 500 unit with a dose of 7 J/cm^2. We also performed further patch tests with the Spanish Contact

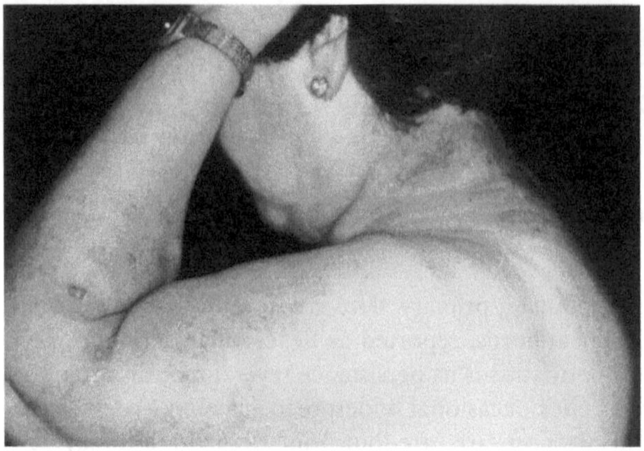

Fig. 2. Erythematous and oozing lesions on the side of the neck. Over the arms, there were isolated vesiculobullous lesions within an erythematous base

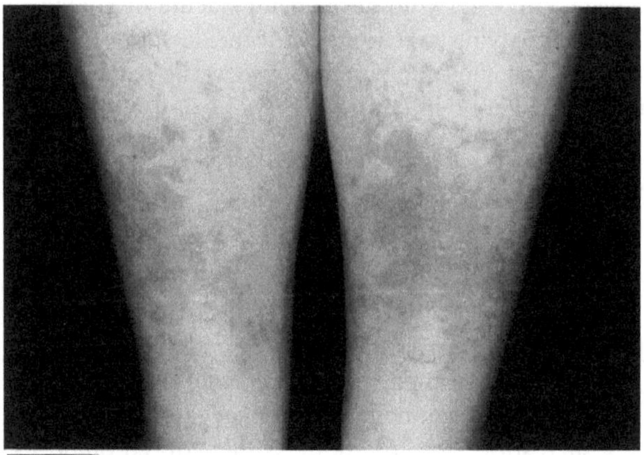

Fig. 3. Eczematous lesions over the anterior aspect of the legs

Table 1. Composition of the insecticide spray

Substance	Content (%)
Active ingredients	
Dichlorvos	1
Neopynamin (tetramethrin)	0.05
Synergistic agents	
Epichlorohydrin	0.15
Piperonyl butoxide	0.21
Solvents	
Methylene chloride	36
n-C_{14} (tetradecane)	7.18
Fragrance	
Fragrance 817 (lemon oil)	0.87
Propellent	
Deodorized butane	54.54

Dermatitis Research Group (GEIDC) standard series and the pesticide and fragrance Trolab series.

Due to the initial patch test findings, and in order to rule out an angry-back skin syndrome, the patient was tested again 1 year later with the chemicals to which she had shown positive reactions. At this time, we used water and petrolatum as vehicles.

Results

The results of first patch testing with the components of the insecticide spray, and with the GEIDC standard, fragrance, and pesticide series, are shown in Table 2. No differences were seen when the dark and the irradiated patches were compared. Patch tests were positive to the spray fragrance 1% and 0.1%; to dichlorvos 1%, 0.5%, and 0.1%; to tetradecane 10%; and to piperonyl butoxide 10% (all in ethanol). In 20 controls tested with these substances at the same concentration, the results were all negative. Patch testing with the standard series showed positive cross-reactions to malathion 0.5%, and to geraniol and lemon oil 2% (all in petrolatum).

Results of the patch tests performed 1 year later are shown in Table 3. Patch tests were positive to dichlorvos 0.1% and 0.01%, both in water and in petrolatum, and to tetradecane 1% in petrolatum.

Table 2. Results of the first patch tests with components of the spray, and with the standard, pesticide, and fragrance series

Chemical	Concentration (%)	Reaction 48 h	Reaction 96 h
Spray components[a]			
Fragrance 817	0.1	++	++
Fragrance 817	1	+++	+++
Dichlorvos	0.1	+++	+++
Dichlorvos	0.5	+++	+++
Dichlorvos	1	+++	+++
Methylene chloride	10	–	–
Tetradecane	10	++	++
Neopynamin	0.1	–	–
Neopynamin	1	–	–
Epichlorohydrin	0.1	–	–
Epichlorohydrin	1	–	–
Piperonyl butoxide	1	+?	+?
Piperonyl butoxide	10	+	+
GEIDC standard series		–	–
Malathion	0.5	++	++
Geraniol	1	++	++
Lemon oil	2	++	++
Lemon grass oil	2	–	–

[a] Ethanol vehicle.

Table 3. Results of the second patch tests with components of the spray

Chemical	Concentration (%)	Reaction	
		48 h	96 h
Dichlorvos	0.1	+++	+++
Dichlorvos	0.01	+++	+++
Piperonyl butoxide	1	−	−
Tetradecane	1	−	++

Water and petrolatum vehicles were used.

Discussion

Toxic and allergic skin reactions to dichlorvos in humans are very unusual. In our case, the appearance of the dermatitis was clearly due to the misuse of a marketed insecticide spray, despite a warning note on the bottle to prevent its direct application to the skin.

The distribution of the lesions, mainly in the exposed areas, initially suggested photodermatitis, an assumption also suported by the patient's profession: she used to sell a variety of vegetables, some of them (celery) related to phototoxic reactions. This assumption was soon discarded on obtaining the results of the patch and photopatch tests. We presumed the patient had been sensitized to the spray fragrance. It was, however, very difficult to decide whether the results of patch tests initially performed with dichlorvos and other spray components were irritative or allergic in nature (angry back). Our first impression, favoring an allergic basis, was merely speculative since dichlorvos is a well-known chemical irritant in dogs and in humans, and (to our knowledge) no case of allergic contact dermatitis to this substance has been previously reported. The positive patch test performed 1 year later with concentrations of dichlorvos as weak as 0.01% and the cross-reactivity with the related chemical malathion led us to label the reaction suffered by our patient as allergic in nature.

It is not the purpose of this contribution to advise against the use of dichlorvos in domestic insecticide sprays. Like antiflea pet collars, they have been proven to be an effective aid in controlling fleas and other insects, and despite their widespread use, toxic or allergic reactions to them are unusual. In our case, sensitization was favored by abnormal usage conditions.

References

1. Cronce PC, Alden HS (1968) Flea-collar dermatitis. JAMA 206: 1563–1564
2. Muller GH, Kirk RW (1969) Flea collar dermatitis. In: Small animal dermatology. Saunders, Philadelphia
3. Muller GH (1970) Flea collar dermatitis in animals. JAVMA 157: 1616–1626
4. Toby Mathias CG (1983) Persistent contact dermatitis from the insecticide dichlorvos. Contact Dermatitis 9: 217–218

Addresses

J. de la Cuadra
Servicio de Dermatologia, Hospital General, 46014 Valencia, Spain

G. Serrano
Servicio de Dermatologia, Hospital General, 46014 Valencia, Spain

Contact Dermatitis
Due to Naphazoline Intermediates

A. Rothe

Key words:

Contact dermatitis - Naphazoline intermediates - α-Chloromethyl naphthalene - α-Naphthyl acetonitrile - Pharmaceutical industry

Introduction

In the synthesis of imidazoline derivatives used in medicaments, only 2-chloromethyl imidazoline was described as a strongly sensitizing intermediate [12]. However, the synthesis of the sympathomimetic naphazoline proceeds in a different way (Fig. 1), producing in step 1 α-chloromethyl naphthalene (CMN; α-naphthylmethylchloride, α-menaphthalene chloride) and α-naphthyl acetonitrile (NAN; naphthylcyanide, nitrilomethyl naphthalene) in step 2. Only CMN has been mentioned as being harmful to the skin, although no details are available [1]. Our report concerns contact dermatitis caused by both intermediates.

Case Reports

Case 1. Initially, on 5 February 1986, we saw a 24-year-old female chemist. Her sister suffers from atopic dermatitis and asthma, and 3 years ago she herself suffered from an outbreak of hand eczema lasting 3 months. The cause was unknown. She was working on a new method of naphazoline synthesis, but she only came into contact with CMN and NAN a few times of a 2-month period. After working with CMN for the first time, she noticed a burning sensation in her eyes. First, she developed dermatitis in a skin area directly contaminated with CMN. This was followed 2 days later by widespread eczema, affecting both the hands and skin areas covered by clothes. The eczema cleared up completely, and 4 months later we ordered a supervised reexposure. Within 2 days, the patient had developed hand eczema again.

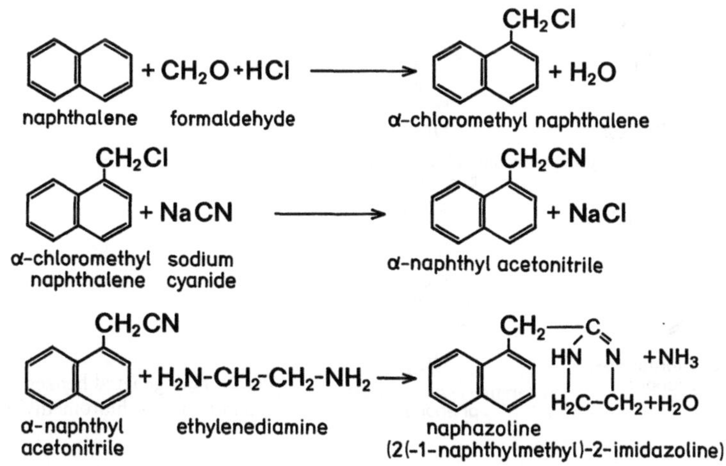

Fig. 1. Naphazoline synthesis

Table 1. Positive patch test results

Substance	Concentration (%)	Results	
		Case 1	Case 2
α-Chloromethyl naphthalene	0.01	+/++/++	+/++/++
α-Naphthyl acetonitrile	0.1	+/+/++	+/++/+++

Case 2. In November 1986, we saw a 35-year-old chemical worker, who was employed in the same plant in the production of naphazoline. After a period of 1 month, he contracted widespread eczema too, which involved the skin covered by clothes in particular. He had no personal or family history of dermatitis, but he had had seasonal asthma for the previous 3 years. His dermatitis cleared up rapidly within 4 weeks.

Methods and Results

Path tests were performed with the GDR standard series, and with naphthalene, CMN 0.01%, and NAN 0.1% in water. Positive allergic reactions were obtained only with the two above-mentioned intermediates (Table 1). Controls with NAN 0.1% were negative in 10 unexposed subjects. Controls with CMN were applied only to the investigator's own skin. CMN 0.1% caused an irritation. Both patients remained free of eczema after cessation of exposure.

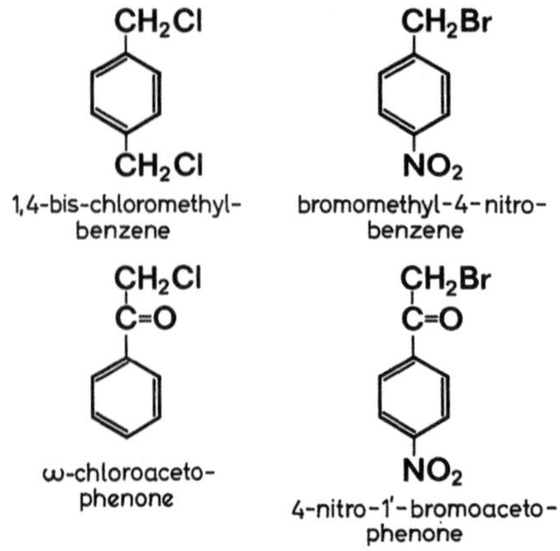

Fig. 2. Halogenated benzene derivatives corresponding to α-chloromethyl naphthalene

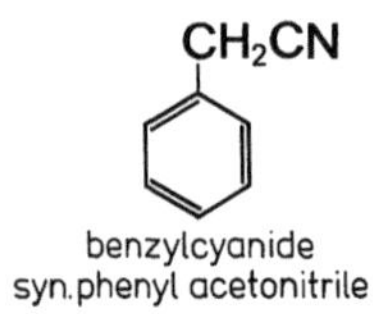

Fig. 3.

Discussion

The clinical data mentioned above should furnish sufficient evidence that the naphazoline intermediates were acting as allergens. The result of the supervised reexposure in case 1 in particular should serve to underline that. In addition, both substances are strong irritants. It is not quite clear why, in both patients, skin areas covered by clothes were affected. Possible explanations would be either systemic eczema or the effect after the chemicals penetrated the clothes.

It is noticeable that some of the halogenated benzene derivatives corresponding to CMN (Fig. 2) are both well-known strong allergens and irritants too [2–7, 9–11], possibly because of the halogenated methyl radical in terminal position. As regards irritant properties, the same can be said of NAN and phenylacetonitrile [9] (Fig. 3). Highly reactive halogenated substances such as CMN have to be regarded as powerful sensitizers; therefore, we intentionally refrained from further control testing with CMN, thus avoiding sensitization by patch testing.

References

1. Berg V, Weichard H (1953/1954) Berufsdermatosen in der chemischen Industrie und ihre Verhütung. Berufsdermatosen 2: 92–97
2. Chung CW, Giles AL (1972) Sensitization of guinea pigs to alpha-chloroacetophenone (CN) and ortho-chlorobenzylidenemalononitrile (CS), tear gas chemicals. J Immunol 109: 284–293
3. Fuchs T, Ippen H (1986) Kontaktallergie auf CN- und CS-Tränengas. Derm Beruf Umwelt 34: 12–14
4. Holland P, White RG (1972) The cutaneous reactions produced by o-chlorobenzylidenemalononitrile and ω-chloroacetophenone when applied directly to the skin of human subjects. Br J Dermatol 86: 150–154
5. Horn T, Mulders A (1986) Kontaktdermatitis auf 2-Chloracetophenon nach Tränengasexposition. Hautarzt 37: 287–290
6. Ippen H, Liebeskind H (1978) Kontaktekzem durch 1,4-Bis-chlormethylbenzol. Derm Beruf Umwelt 26: 97
7. Kleine-Natrop HE, Pinzer B, Horn K (1975) Hautschäden durch Tränengas. Dermatol Monatsschr 161: 678–680
8. Lob M (1983) Toluene and derivatives. In: Parmaggiani L (ed) Encyclopaedia of occupational health and safety, vol 2, 3rd edn. International Labour Organization, Geneva, p 2185
9. Maucher O, Stengel R, Schöpf E (1986) Chloracetophenonallergie. Hautarzt 37: 397–401
10. Pickering FC, Ive FA (1983) Allergic contact dermatitis due to highly reactive halogenated compounds. Contact Dermatitis 9: 500–503
11. Saynisch F (1959) Hautschäden bei der Chloromycetinherstellung. Berufsdermatosen 7: 198–204
12. Schulz KH, Schöpf E (1967) Klinische und experimentelle Untersuchungen zur Kontaktallergie durch Chlormethylimidazolin. Hautarzt 18: 547–550

Addresses

A. Rothe

Department of Dermatology, Central Institute of Occupational Medicine of the GDR, DDR-1134 Berlin, Noeldnerstr. 40–42, GDR

The Significance of Positive Patch Test Reactions to 4,4′-Diaminodiphenylmethane

G. Gailhofer, J. Smolle, and M. Ludvan

Summary

4,4′-Diaminodiphenlymethane (DDM), an isocyclic diamine, is commonly used in the production of rubber, plastics, dyes and adhesives. Exposure via germicides, insecticides, surfactants and corrosion inhibitors may also occur. From 1979 to 1987, we observed positive patch test reactions to DDM in 3.57% of all patients tested. To determine the significance of these reactions, data concerning age, sex and profession; type, localisation and duration of skin lesions; and combined positive allergens were evaluated for 202 DDM-positive patients. The results obtained were compared by chi-square test with those of 3397 consecutive, unselected contact dermatitis patients with negative test reactions to DDM.

We can state the following:

1. In many patients, the positive patch test reaction to DDM is a "marker" for allergy to *p*-amino compounds usually contained in externals.
2. In 39 of 202 patients with isolated positive test reactions to DDM, the source of the allergen remained undetected.
3. Workers at chemical laboratories seem to have an increased risk of being sensitised to DDM.
4. In accordance with the literature, clinical relevance could be proven in only a few patients.

Key words:

4,4′-Diaminodiphenylmethane - Methylenedianiline - Aniline compounds - *para*-amino compounds - Patch test - Contact dermatitis

$H_2N\text{-}C_6H_4\text{-}CH_2\text{-}C_6H_4\text{-}NH_2$

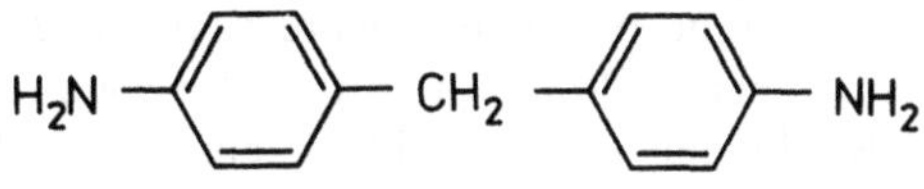

Fig. 1. Chemical formula of 4,4′-diaminodiphenylmethane

Introduction

4,4′-Diaminodiphenylmethane (DDM) is an isocyclic diamine with the chemical formula $C_{13}H_{14}N_2$ (Fig. 1). Synonyms are methylenedianiline and bis-[4-aminophenyl]-methane. The pure substance occurs as a powder or blocks, and the molecular weight is 198.26. The melting point is 92 °C, the boiling point about 398 °C–399 °C. DDM is odourless and hardly soluble in water but easily soluble in alcohols, acetone, esters and ethers [1, 2].

DDM is used as a curing agent for epoxy resins and as a vulcaniser, antioxidant or retarding agent in the manufacture of rubber and in the production of adhesives and dyes. It is also an intermediate in the production of germicides, phosphate insecticides, detergents, isocyanates, polyamides and corrosion inhibitors and also in the pharmaceutical industry.

The frequency of positive patch test reactions to DDM varies in earlier reports, as do the interpretations of the results obtained. Argup and Fregert [3] observed positive patch test reactions to DDM in 3.8% of their patients, Cronin [4] in 2.76% and the Spanish Contact Dermatitis Research Group even in 8.5% of the patients tested [17]. Simultaneous positive reactions to *p*-amino compounds were frequently seen. Clinical relevance could be proven in only a few patients, and the significance of the positive DDM patch test reactions remained unclear [4, 5, 17]. Rubber, plastics and epoxy resins were assumed as the source of the allergen [7, 9–11, 13]. Proven clinical relevance of DDM was reported by Levine [8] (photoallergic contact dermatitis caused by DDM contained in isolation material of electric wires) and by Alomar [12] (contact dermatitis due to a fashion watchband containing DDM). Direct exposure to DDM may cause yellow staining of the skin, hair and nails, and this may even be a “marker” for DDM exposure [6].

In our department, DDM has been included in the routine patch test series since 1979, and we could see a nearly constant frequency of positive patch tests to DDM in 3.57% of all patients tested. The present study aimed to elucidate the clinical significance of positive DDM patch test reactions.

Patients and Methods

Data concerning sex, age and profession; type, duration and localisation of skin lesions; atopy; and combined positive allergens were obtained from a sample of 202 patients (120 women, 82 men) with positive test reactions to DDM. These data were compared by chi-square test with those of 3397 consecutive, unselected contact dermatitis patients negative to DDM. Data management and evaluation was done on a personal computer [15].

The routine patch tests were performed by the classical method according to Bandmann and Dohn [14] with test substances provided by Trolab (Reinbek, FRG), Dr. Brinkmann (Greven, FRG) and HAL (Haarlem, Netherlands). In particular, DDM was tested at a concentration of 0.5% in petrolatum (Trolab; as commonly recommended [16]).

Results

Age and Sex Distribution. In male patients, positive reactions to DDM are more frequent, as expected due to the reference group ($P<0.01$). The mean age of DDM-positive patients (53.3 ± 17.2 years) is significantly higher than that of the controls (40.2 ± 18.7 years; *t* test $P \leqslant 0.05$).

Type and Location of Eczema. In DDM-positive women, there is a noticeably increased frequency of subacute-type eczema ($P<0.05$). The main locations are lower leg (35.9%), hands (21.2%), and face and neck (18.2%). In DDM-positive male patients, the incidence of acute-type eczema is markedly higher than in the controls ($P<0.01$), and the skin lesions are mainly located on the face and neck (35.3%) and the lower leg (26.7%).

In DDM-allergic women, the incidence of eczema of the hands is significantly lower ($P<0.01$), and skin lesions of the lower leg and the perianal region are markedly more frequent ($P<0.01$) than in the controls. In DDM-positive men, the incidence of eczema of the lower leg is as much increased ($P<0.01$) as in women. Disseminated eczematous reactions are significantly less frequent ($P<0.01$).

Atopy. There is no case of atopy in male DDM-positive patients ($P<0.01$). Atopic women are of similar frequency in both groups ($P>0.05$).

Occupations. All professions evaluated were similarly distributed in both groups except female chemical laboratory workers, who were predominantly found in the DDM-positive group ($P<0.01$). These patients had eczematous lesions on the hands (2 patients), with *p*-phenylenediamine and nickel sulphate, and benzocaine, respectively, as combined positive allergens. One further patient was "prophetically" tested and showed a single positive reaction to DDM. The incidence of retirement was increased in female and male DDM-positive patients ($P<0.01$) with skin lesions located on the lower leg (64%), hand and forearms (15%) and face and neck (10%).

Relationship to Other Allergens. Frequently combined positive allergens ($P<0.05$) in patients with DDM allergy are *p*-amino compounds and substances related to local therapy (*p*-amino compounds as cross-reactants and substances chemically not related to DDM) (Table 1).

Table 1. Relative frequency of positive allergens in patients with 4,4'-diaminodiphenylmethane (DDM) allergy and in controls

Substance	Relative frequency (%)		Significance[a]
	DDM-positive patients	Controls	
Amino-azobenzene	1.98	0.29	$P<0.01$
Aniline	0.99	0.03	$P<0.01$
Balsam of Peru	25.25	7.54	$P<0.01$
Benzocaine	30.19	1.53	$P<0.01$
Epoxy resin	1.98	0.38	$P<0.01$
Formaldehyde	3.46	0.85	$P<0.01$
Fragrance mix	12.37	6.97	$P<0.01$
Gentamycin	4.45	0.91	$P<0.01$
Neomycin	14.35	3.62	$P<0.01$
Parabens	10.39	2.44	$P<0.01$
p-Phenylenediamine	21.28	0.58	$P<0.01$
Phenylmercuric nitrate	3.96	1.41	$P<0.01$
Triethanolamine	2.47	0.91	$P<0.05$
Wood tars	5.94	1.44	$P<0.01$
Wood alcohols	5.45	2.62	$P<0.01$

[a] Chi-square test.

Isolated Sensitization to DDM. In 39 patients (21 women, 18 men), isolated positive test reactions to DDM were seen.The mean age of the patients was 47.7 years (SD 17.9). In 13 of 39 patients, the skin lesions were located on the hands, in 5 on the forearms and in 9 in the face/neck region. Eczematous lesions of the lower leg could be seen in only four of the patients, while eight suffered from generalised contact dermatitis. There were no further characteristic data in these patients.

Discussion

Case histories indicate that in 50.5% of all cases, positive test reactions to DDM take place in patients sensitised to externals mainly used in the treatment of leg ulcers of different origin, perianal dermatoses and face dermatoses. In 64% of these patients, positive reactions to other drug-related *p*-amino compounds occur.

In our leg ulcer patients, we do not think that DDM allergy was caused by elastic leg-support bandages and support hose. The material these therapeutics are made of did not give any positive reactions in any patients. The manufacturers of the support bandages (Lohmann GmbH & Co. KG, Neuwied, FRG and Sigvaris GmbH, Vienna, Austria), frequently used in our patients, informed us that DDM is not contained in their products.

The insignificant low number of workers in the rubber and plastic industries among our patients is to be pointed out. Due to the reports at issue, we expected more of these workers to be sensitised to DDM. A significant connection between DDM allergy and profession could only be seen in female chemical laboratory workers, but in two of three patients clinical relevance could not be definitively proven (positive test reactions to other commonly used *p*-amino compounds). In the third patient, the isolated positive reaction to DDM, without any history of contact dermatitis, seems to be – at the time of testing – irrelevant.

The clinical significance of isolated positive reactions to DDM is difficult to determine. None of the evaluated parameters indicated possible sources of the allergen. However, the localisation of the lesions indicates that allergen exposure by manual work seems to be possible (13 of 39 patients showed eczematous lesions on the hands). Additionally, contact in the face and neck area may also play an important role (9 of 39 patients had eczema in the face/neck region). The occurrence of generalised eczematous reactions in 8 of 39 DDM-allergic patients remains to be explained. There was no anamnestic information in any of these patients which could clarify the source of the allergen.

Photodynamic eczematous reactions due to DDM were evident in 2 of 202 patients (a 23-year-old male student and a 49-year-old farmer). They showed single positive reactions to DDM (classical patch test), but the allergen source remained undetected.

Summing up our results, we can state the following:

1. A positive patch test reaction to DDM often represents a marker of allergy to *p*-amino compounds usually contained in externals.
2. There seems to be an increased risk of sensitisation to DDM in chemical laboratory workers.
3. In 39 patients with an isolated positive reaction to DDM, the source of the allergen is still unknown.
4. In accordance with the literature, clinical relevance of the positive patch test reactions to DDM could be proven in only a few patients.

References

1. Neumüller OA (1981) Römpps Chemie-Lexikon. Franckh'sche Verlagsbuchhandlung, Stuttgart
2. Beilsteins Handbuch der Organischen Chemie, 4th edn. (1985) Volume 13. Springer, Berlin Heidelberg New York
3. Argup G, Fregert S (1969) Contact Allergy to 4,4'-Diaminodiphenylmethane. Contact Dermatitis Newsletter: 92
4. Cronin E (1980) Contact dermatitis. Churchill Livingstone, Edinburgh
5. Goldmann P (1963) Betriebsbedingte Hauterkrankungen in der chemischen Industrie. Z Haut Geschl Kr 35: 14–29
6. Cohen SR (1985) Yellow staining caused by 4,4'-methylenedianiline exposure. Arch Dermatol 121: 1022–1027
7. Romaguera C, Grimalt F, Vilaplana J (1985) Paratertiary butylphenol formaldehyde resin in prostheses. Contact Dermatitis 12: 174
8. Levine MJ (1983) Occupational photosensitivity to diaminodiphenylmethane. Contact Dermatitis 9: 488–490
9. Malten KE, Kuiper JP, von der Staak WBJM (1973) Contact allergic investigations in 100 patients with ulcus cruris. Dermatologica 147: 241–254
10. Malten KE (1973) Occupational dermatoses in the processing of plastics. Trans St. John's Hosp Dermatol Soc 59: 78–113

11. van Joost T, Heule F, de Boer J (1987) Sensitisation to methylenedianiline and para-structures. Contact Dermatitis 16: 246–248
12. Alomar A (1986) Contact dermatitis from a fashion watch. Contact Dermatitis 15: 44–45
13. Malten KE, Nater JP, van Ketel WG (1976) Patch testing guidelines. Dekker and van de Vegt, Nijmegen
14. Bandmann HJ, Dohn W (1967) Die Epikutantestung. Bergmann, Munich
15. Gailhofer G (1988) Computerunterstützte Erfassung und Auswertung von Epikutantestdaten – Ein Modell. Dermatosen 36: 10–12
16. Fisher AA (1986) Contact dermatitis. Lea and Febiger, Philadelphia
17. Romaguera C, Garcia-Perez A, Martin-Pascual A, Miranda A (1981) Diaminodiphenylmethane in standard patch tests. Contact Dermatitis 7: 347–348

Addresses

G. Gailhofer
Department of Dermatology, University of Graz, Auenbruggerplatz 8, A-8036 Graz, Austria

J. Smolle
Department of Dermatology, University of Graz, Auenbruggerplatz 8, A-8036 Graz, Austria

M. Ludvan
Department of Dermatology, University of Graz, Auenbruggerplatz 8, A-8036 Graz, Austria

Contact Dermatitis of the Face

A. Tosti, M. Melino, and S. Veronesi

Summary

The authors report the patch test results in 377 patients affected by contact dermatitis of the face. In 163 cases, the cause of dermatitis was definitively determined. In our series, positive patch test reactions to preservatives were as frequent as positive patch test reactions to fragrances. Kathon CG was the preservative responsible for the majority of positive reactions, while among the fragrances, balsam of Peru, isoeugenol, and oak moss were the most common causes of positive reactions. Hair dyes, colophony, topical drugs, and colorants were less frequently responsible for the clinical manifestations. Occupational airborne dermatitis was diagnosed in four patients: two were sensitized to epoxy resin, and two to primin. We point out that the large number of positive patch test reactions to Kathon CG in our country is presumably related to the high concentration of this preservative in cosmetics here, as permitted by EEC regulations.

Key words:

Contact dermatitis - Face - Fragrances - Preservatives

Introduction

This study was carried out on a group of 377 patients with contact dermatitis involving the face. In all these patients, patch tests with standard series were performed according to the International Contact Dermatitis Research Group (ICDRG) recommendations. Following an allergological investigation, one or more of the following substances were patch-tested in some of our patients: fragrances, preservatives, hair dyes, colorants, toluenesulfonamide formaldehyde resin, cosmetic products and topical drugs used by the patients, and (whenever possible) several or all of the products' individual ingredients. Photopatch tests were done when photoallergy was suspected. The use test was performed when cosmetic patch tests were negative or doubtful.

Results

We were able to determine the cause of dermatitis definitively in 163 of the 377 tested patients affected by contact dermatitis of the face. Of these 163, 138 were women (84.7%) and 25 were men (15.3%); the age ranged from 2 to 81 years (mean 40 years). The positive patch test reactions in these 163 patients are shown in Table 1. In our series, positive patch test reactions to preservatives were as frequent as patch test reactions to fragrances, followed by topical drugs and their active ingredients. Hair dyes, colophony, colorants, and nail polish were less frequently responsible for the clinical manifestations.

Table 1. Positive patch test reactions in 163 patients

Substance	No. of reactions
Fragrances[a]	
Fragrance mix	42
Balsam of Peru	26
Isoeugenol	10
Oak moss	8
Propolis	6
Eugenol	2
Cinnamic aldehyde	2
Hydroxycitronellal	2
Musk ambrette	2
Clove oil	2
Others[b]	8
Preservatives[c]	
Kathon CG	38
Parabens	7
Formaldehyde	7
Thimerosal	7
Captan	4
Imidazolidinyl urea	3
Triclosan	2
Chloracetamide	2
Others[b]	8
Topical drugs	20
Colophony	10
Hair dyes	9
Colorants	5
Toluenesulfonamide formaldehyde resin	4
Others[b]	9

[a] Positive reactions were seen in 62 patients.
[b] Substances causing one reaction each.
[c] Positive reactions were seen in 63 patients.

An occupational airborne contact dermatitis was diagnosed in four patients: two were sensitized to epoxy resin, and two to primin.

As regards fragrances, in 21 cases the individual fragrance component responsible could not be determined, but when it could, the most common causes of positive reactions were balsam of Peru, propolis, isoeugenol, and oak moss (Table 1). Among preservatives, the most frequent cause of reactions was Kathon CG, followed by parabens, thimerosal, and formaldehyde. The other preservatives causing positive patch test reactions are listed in Table 1. In 17 patients, positive reactions to both preservatives and fragrances were seen.

In all the 163 patients, we endeavored to find a relationship between patch test positivity and personal use of end products containing these ingredients. Clinical relevance was easy to assess in all the patients with a positive reaction to topical drugs, colophony, hair dyes, and nail polish. In 19 of the 108 patients with suspected cosmetic-related contact dermatitis, we observed a positive patch test reaction or a positive use test to the cosmetic alone, but we were not able to find the ingredient responsible for the positive reaction.

Discussion

Since the face is one of the body sites most frequently affected by contact dermatitis, we investigated causes closely related to facial dermatitis. We therefore collected much-needed information about the use of products containing the ingredients responsible for the majority of the positive patch test reactions. In our series, the cosmetic components that gave the highest incidence of positive reactions, as has been previously reported [1–4], are preservatives and fragrances. The other most frequent causes were topical drugs, which caused positive reactions due to their active ingredients or to preservatives.

We observed four cases of occupational airborne contact dermatitis localized to the face due to epoxy resin and primin. In these cases, the clinical manifestations caused by volatile or evaporated compounds were typical and symmetrically involved the upper eyelids and the perioral area.

On the basis of the results of our study, we can confirm, in agreement with previous data, that cosmetic ingredients are the main cause of contact dermatitis of the face. Finally, it should be pointed out that the large number of positive patch test reactions to Kathon CG in our country is presumably related to the high concentration of this preservative in cosmetics here, as permitted by EEC regulations.

References

1. Adams RM, Maibach HI (1982) A five-years study of cosmetic reactions. J Am Acad Dermatol 13: 1062–1069
2. Emmons WW, Marks JG (1985) Immediate and delayed reactions to cosmetic ingredients. Contact Dermatitis 13: 258–265
3. De Groot AC, et al. (1986) Contact allergy to preservatives (I). Contact Dermatitis 15: 120–122
4. De Groot AC, et al. (1986) Contact allergy to preservatives (II). Contact Dermatitis 15: 218–222

Addresses

A. Tosti
Clinica Dermatologica, Università di Bologna, via Massarenti, 1, 40138 Bologna, Italy

M. Melino
Clinica Dermatologica, Università di Bologna, via Massarenti, 1, 40138 Bologna, Italy

S. Veronesi
Clinica Dermatologica, Università di Bologna, via Massarenti, 1, 40138 Bologna, Italy

The Allergens in Cosmetics*

A. C. de Groot and J. W. Weyland

Systematic investigation of the allergens in cosmetics has rarely been performed. In this study by the Dutch Contact Dermatitis Group, the allergens responsible for cosmetic allergy were identified in 119 patients (102 women, 17 men; age 12–78 years; average age 36 years). More than half of all reactions were caused by skin care products ($n = 67$, 56%). Next came nail cosmetics ($n = 16$, 13%), followed by perfumes ($n = 10$, 8%), hair cosmetics ($n = 7$, 6%), deodorants ($n = 6$, 5%), and lip cosmetics ($n = 5$, 4%). Of the 119 patients, 81 (68%) were tested with all the ingredients of the suspected cosmetic products, and 38 (32%) were tested with 1 or more allergens known to be present in cosmetics used. A total of 53 cosmetic allergens were found (Table 1). The most frequent contact allergen was Kathon CG, causing reactions in 33 patients (28%). Second most frequent was toluene sulfonamide/formaldehyde resin, causing reactions in 15 patients (13%), followed by unspecified fragrances ($n = 15$, 13%) and oleamidopropyl dimethylamine ($n = 13$, 11%). The classes of cosmetic allergens are shown in Table 1. Due to the large number of patients reacting to Kathon CG, preservatives were the most important category implicated, with 47 reactions (32%), followed by fragrances with 39 reactions (27%) and emulsifiers (mostly oleamidopropyl dimethylamine) with 21 reactions (14%).

Key words:

Cosmetic allergy - Ingredient patch testing

* The full details of this study will be published in [1].

Table 1. Classes of causative ingredients in 119 patients with cosmetic allergy

Allergens	No. of patients
Preservatives	47 (32)
Kathon CG (100 ppm a.i. aqua)	33
Diazolidinyl urea (2% pet)	3
Quaternium-15 (1% pet)	3
Imidazolidinyl urea (2% aqua)	2
Propylparaben (5% pet)	2
Others[a]	4
Fragrances	39 (27)
Unspecified (10% pet)	15
Specified	24
Eugenol (5% pet)	4
Hydroxycitronellal (2% pet)	4
Cinnamic alcohol (5% pet)	2
Citronellol (2% pet)	2
Geraniol (5% pet)	2
Isoeugenol (3% pet)	2
Others[a]	8
Emulsifiers	21 (14)
Oleamidopropyl dimethylamine (0.4% aqua)	13
Cocamidopropyl betaine (0.1% and 1% aqua)	3
Cocamide DEA (0.5% aqua)	2
Others[a]	3
Toluenesulfonamide/formaldehyde resin (10% pet)	15 (10)
Lanolin (derivatives)	4 (3)
Miscellaneous	21 (14)
4-Isopropyl-dibenzoylmethane (5% pet)	2
3-(4-Methylbenzylidene)-camphor (2% pet)	2
Myristyl alcohol (5% pet)	2
Others[a]	15

The numbers in parentheses are percentages of the total number of *reactions* ($n = 147$).
pet, petrolatum
[a] Substances causing one reaction each.

Reference

1. De Groot AC, Bruynzeel DP, Bos JD, van der Meeren HLM, van Joost T, Jagtman BA, Weyland JW (1988) The allergens in cosmetics. Arch Dermatol 124: 1525–1529

Addresses

A. C. de Groot
Department of Dermatology, Carolus & Willem-Alexander Hospital, P.O. Box 90152, 5200 MD 's Hertogenbosch, The Netherlands

J. W. Weyland
Food Inspection Service, Department of Cosmetics, P.O. Box 777, 7500 AT Enschede, The Netherlands

Adverse Reactions to Artificial Nails

B. Felix, G. Ducombs, and M. Geniaux

Summary

We have seen ten women presenting intolerance to artificial nails (involving onychomycosis, irritation, or sensitization). The clinical aspect was onycholysis, perionyxis, nail discoloration (chloronychia, xanthonychia), and eczema of the fingertips. The products used are similar to products used in dentistry or industry: triethylene glycol dimethacrylate, ethylene glycol dimethacrylate, and benzoyl peroxide. Patch testing was performed with manicure products and Hermal-Chemie allergens.

Key words:

Articifial nails - Diamalust - Ethylene glycol dimethacrylate - Triethylene glycol dimethacrylate

Introduction

Recently, numerous shops have opened all over France, offering a new method for making artificial nails to onychophagists or subjects with too short, dystrophic, or even normal nails. The manicurist moulds a nail closely against the natural nail with products (Diamalust) imported from the United States. Diamalust compounds are (a) polymer powder composed of methacrylate polymer, ethylene methacrylate copolymer, and benzoyl peroxide and (b) monomer liquid composed of triethylene glycol dimethacrylate and ethylene methacrylate. These products are similar to industrial products (glue, paints, printed ink, and jointings), and to dentistry and medical products (cements, surgical prostheses, and soft lenses).

Method for Making Artificial Nails

Artificial nails are made in several stages:

1. Natural nail is brushed with a sandpaper roll to increase the adhesion of the resin to the nail and provoke thinning of the nail plate.
2. Application of a disinfectant called Sterilizer.
3. Application with a brush of a liquid called Primer to promote resin adhesion on the nail.
4. Application of an adhesive support all around the natural nail to protect the skin.
5. The manicurist dips the brush in polymer liquid, and then in polymer powder, and applies the mixture rapidly to the natural nail to mould the artificial nail.
6. Finally, the new nail can be varnished, with the natural nail still growing under the artificial nail. It is necessary to touch the artificial nail up every 2 or 3 weeks.

Adverse Reactions to Artificial Nails

We observed ten patients with adverse reactions to artificial nails. These complications are not too numerous in proportion to the number of users. Most of these reactions disappear in a few months (4 or 6 months) after removal of artificial nails.

Monomer liquid, and less often polymer powder, provokes irritation and sensitization. Preexistent onychopathy (psoriasis, pelade, or lichen) may increase, and Koebner's phenomenon may even appear, with localization on the nail of a preexistent dermatosis. Monthly manicures promote irritation of the nail plate. Artificial nails also promote onychomycosis by occlusion and maceration of the nail bed. *Candida albicans* is the fungus most often isolated. As usual, the clinical aspect is chloronychia or xanthonychia (yellowish, greenish, or brownish dyschromia of the nail plate) with subungual hyperkeratosis and partial or total onycholysis. The

Table 1. Clinical aspects in ten patients with adverse reactions

Case no.	Irritation	Allergic reactions	Mycologic infestations
1	+	−	*Cephalosporium*
2	+	−	*Candida albicans*
3	−	+	−
4	+	−	−
5	−	−	*Candida albicans*
6	−	+	−
7	−	−	*Candida albicans*
8	−	+	*Candida albicans*
9	+	−	*Candida albicans*
10	−	+	−
Total	4	4	6

symptoms of irritant or allergic reactions can have different aspects: hyperkeratosis of the nail bed; thinning of the nail plate, which becomes chapped and unstuck; partial or total onycholysis; and desquamation and fissures of the fingertips. Paronychia, onychia, paresthesia, and persistent pain can handicap patients in their ordinary daily activities. Dyschromia is not always due to mycologic contamination and could be due to the irritant effect of acrylates on natural nail. Perionyxis and allergic eczema spread over the skin around the nail. Table 1 sums up the different clinical aspects of our ten cases.

Patch Testing and Mycologic Examination

Patch testing was performed with the following Diamalust products (10% in petrolatum) and Hermal-Chemie allergens:

1. Diamalust products
   a) Primer
   b) Polymer powder
   c) Monomer liquid
   d) Glue
   e) Adhesive protective frame
2. Hermal-Chemie battery
   a) Methyl methacrylate 2%
   b) Bisphenol A
   c) Triethylene glycol dimethacrylate
   d) Ethylene glycol dimethacrylate
   e) Phenol formaldehyde resin acid catalyzed
   f) Benzoyl peroxide
   g) Butyl acrylate

Ten patients presented adverse reactions; of the six patients with mycologic infestation (five *Candida albicans*, one *Cephalosporium*), one was also allergic to acrylates (methyl methacrylate, ethylene glycol diamethacrylate, and monomer liquid) (Table 1). Four patients presented allergic reactions: three of them were allergic to

Table 2. Results of patch testing with Diamalust products

Product	Reaction				
	Controls[a]	Allergic patients			
		1	2	3	4
Primer	–				
Powder	–				
Liquid	–	+	++	++	
Glue	–		++		
Adhesive	–		++		

[a] $n = 22$.

Table 3. Results of patch testing with the Hermal-Chemie battery

Product	Reaction				
	Controls[a]	Allergic patients			
		1	2	3	4
Methyl methacrylate 2%	–		++	++	++
Bisphenol A	–				
Triethylene glycol dimethacrylate	–		++		
Ethylene glycol dimethacrylate	–	+	++	++	++
Phenol formaldehyde resin acid catalyzed	–				
Benzoyl peroxide	–				
Butyl acrylate	–				

[a] $n = 22$.

Diamalust products (monomer liquid); the fourth one reacted only to Hermal-Chemie allergens (Tables 2, 3). One patient reacted to Diamalust glue and adhesive. The 22 controls tested were all negative to Diamalust products.

Discussion

Monomer liquid is a potential sensitizer. Polymerization at room temperature is much less perfect than at high temperature. After the hardening of the nail, persistent monomer residues can perforate the table of the natural nail or the skin around it and provoke irritation or contact allergy. In the United Stated, methyl methacrylate was forbidden and replaced by butyl methacrylate and ethyl methacrylate. Irritation and sensitization due to artificial nails are reported in Great Britain [4, 5], Spain [3], and the United States [6–10]. Sensitization to ethyl methacrylate of artificial nail is also described. Marks et al. [11] proposed patch testing with methyl methacrylate and *n*-butyl methacrylate at 1% in ethanol because cross-sensitization is possible between the two molecules. Several clinical aspects have been reported [1, 3, 4, 6, 9, 11, 13, 14]:

1. Yellowish or greenish dyschromia of nail table without mycologic infestation. Dyschromia could be due to irritant effects of acrylates on natural nail.
2. Hyperkeratosis of nail bed with thinning, chapping, and unsticking of the nail table.
3. Partial or total onycholysis.
4. Paronychia and onychia with paresthesia and persistent, handicapping pain.
5. Perionyxis and eczema around the nail.
6. Cracked eczema of the fingertips.
7. Contact eczema of eyelids and lateral areas of the neck by contact with the nails.

Persistent anonychia after 7 years has been described [8].

References

1. Baran R (1985) Conséquences de l'utilisation des cosmétiques sur l'appareil unguéal. Nouv Dermatol 4: 22–24
2. Chung CW, Giles AL (1977) Sensitization potentials of methyl, ethyl and *n*-butyl methacrylates and mutual cross sensitivity in guinea pigs. J Invest Dermatol 68: 187–190
3. Conde-Salasar L, Guinaraens D, Romero L, Gonzalez M (1986) Allergic contact dermatitis from sculptural artificial nails. In: 8th international symposium on contact dermatitis, Cambridge, 20–22 March 1986
4. Cronin E (1976) Onycholysis due to acrylic nails. Clin Exp Dermatol 1: 191–192
5. Cronin E (1980) Contact dermatology. Churchill Livingson, Edinburgh, pp 583–584
6. Fisher AA, Francks A, Glick H (1959) Allergic sensitization of the skin and nails to acrylic plastic nails. J Allergic 23: 84–89
7. Fisher AA (1973) Contact dermatitis, 2nd edn. Lea and Febiger, Philadelphia, p 185, 233, 82, 83
8. Fisher AA (1980) Permanent loss of finger nails from sensitization and reaction to acrylic in a preparation designed to make artificial nails. J Dermatol Surg Oncol 6: 70–71
9. Goodwin (1976) Onycholysis due to acrylic nail application. Clin Exp Dermatol 1: 191–192
10. Maibach H, et al. (1978) Butyl methacrylate monomer and ethyl methacrylate monomer frequency of reaction. Contact Dermatitis 4: 60
11. Marks JE, Bishop ME, Willis WF (1979) Allergic contact dermatitis to sculptural nails. Arch Dermatol 115: 100
12. Pillet J, Guyaux MC, Le Gall CA (1987) Prothèses unguéales. Ann Dermatol Venereol 114: 425–428
13. Scher RK (1982) Cosmetics and ancillary preparation for the care of nails. J Am Acad Dermatol 6: 523–528
14. Scott EA, Scher RK (1985) Exogeneous factors affecting the nails. Dermatol Clin 3: 409–413

Addresses

B. Felix
Clinique Dermatologique, Hôpital Pellegrin, F-33076 Bordeaux Cedex, France

G. Ducombs
Clinique Dermatologique, Hôpital Pellegrin, F-33076 Bordeaux Cedex, France

M. Geniaux
Clinique Dermatologique, Hôpital Pellegrin, F-33076 Bordeaux Cedex, France

Contact Dermatitis in the Textile and Garment Industry

M. Gasperini, M. Farli, P. Lombardi, and A. Sertoli

Reports in the literature [1] indicate that dermatological risk is low in the textile and garment industry. To date, there have been reports of only individual cases of contact dermatitis, and the major risk has been shown to be for the workers who do the dyeing operations [2, 3, 6–8]. The causes of sensitization often remain unknown, but the substances most often cited as responsible are potassium bichromate [4], antiwrinkling resins with formaldehyde base [3], antispotting agents [2], antiinflammatory agents [2], optical whiteners [9], and biocidal agents [3, 5].

As part of an investigation sponsored by the Dipartimento Sicurezza Sociale della Regione Toscana (Social Security Department of Tuscany, Italy) during 1986 and 1987, we examined 161 subjects with occupational contact dermatitis; 104 (11 men and 93 women) were garment industry workers. We found a higher incidence of ir-

Table 1. Number of cases of irritant contact dermatitis in high-risk jobs for contact dermatitis in textile ($n = 57$) and garment industry workers ($n = 104$)

Job	No. of cases
Textile industry	
Dyeing	9
Spinning	8
Finishing	4
Carding	2
Spooling	2
Weaving	1
Printing	1
Sorting	1
Total	28
Garment industry	
Sewing	30
Cutting	13
Ironing	9
Generic	9
Finishing	7
Patterns	2
Mechanic	1
Total	71

Table 2. Incidence of allergic contact dermatitis in high-risk jobs for contact dermatitis in textile ($n = 57$) and garment industry workers ($n = 104$)

Job	No. of cases
Textile industry	
Finishing	9
Dyeing	7
Spinning	4
Weaving	4
Spooling	3
Scouring	1
Carbonizing	1
Total	29
Garment industry	
Sewing	14
Ironing	6
Finishing	5
Cutting	4
Generic	4
Total	33

ritant contact dermatitis (ICD; 68.3%) than allergic contact dermatitis (ACD; 31.7%) in the garment workers, while in the textile workers the incidence of the two types of dermatitis was approximately the same (49.2% ACD and 50.8% ICD). The different jobs presenting the highest risk of ICD and ACD in the garment and textile groups in our study are listed in Tables 1, 2.

Our allergological study of the 161 subjects (53 men and 108 women) with suspected occupational contact dermatitis was done using a battery of haptens prepared according to the recommendations in the literature [2, 3] and our experience using the Rapid Patch Test (RPT) technique [10].

Table 3 shows the results of the patch tests for the textile and garment workers separately. We note that among the textile workers there were 12 positive reactions to chromium compounds, 9 each to dyes and para-group (paraphenylenediamine, diaminodiphenylmethane, *p*-aminoazobenzene) haptens, and 4 to 2 different resins (2 each to phenol formaldehyde resin and *p-tert*-butylphenol formaldehyde resin).

Table 3. Results of patch tests in 62 textile and garment industry workers with allergic contact dermatitis

Test substance	Concentration (%)	Positive reactions (*n*)	
		Textile industry	Garment industry
Nickel sulfate	5	5	18
Cobalt chloride	1	5	8
Potassium dichromate	0.5	9	0
Chromium trichchloride	2	3	0
Disperse Blue 124	1	2	6
Disperse Yellow 3	1	2	2
Disperse Black 1	1	1	1
Disperse Orange 76	1	0	2
Disperse Yellow 54	1	1	0
Disperse Red 17	1	1	0
Disperse Blue 35	1	1	0
Disperse Orange 3	1	1	0
Acid Black 48	1	0	1
Paraphenylenediamine	0.5	2	0
Diaminodiphenylmethane	0.5	4	8
p-Aminophenol	1	1	0
p-Aminoazobenzene	0.25	1	0
p-Dimethylaminoazobenzene	1	1	0
Phenol formaldehyde resin	5	2	3
p-tert-Butylphenol formaldehyde resin	1	2	0
Triethanolamine	5	1	0
Thiuram mix		2	0
Mercapto mix		2	0
Carba mix		2	0
Thimerosal	1	1	0
Ammoniated mercury	1	3	0
Rosin	20	1	0
Wool alcohols	30	2	0
Fragrance mix		3	2

The vehicle used was petrolatum.

Among the garment workers with ACD, there were no cases of reaction to chromium compounds, but there were 26 positive reactions to other metals (18 to nickel sulfate and 8 to cobalt chloride), as well as 12 to dyes (half of them to Disperse Blue 124), 8 to diaminodiphenylmethane, and 3 to phenol formaldehyde resin.

Sensitization to nickel and cobalt was more frequent in the garment industry because of the use of metal instruments and accessories in making the clothing; the majority of the workers involved in these particular phases of manufacture are women. ACD from chromium compounds was found only in the textile workers because of the substances used in the dyeing operations (e.g., mordants and premetallized dyes). On the other hand, we found the same frequency among textile and garment industry workers for ACD due to dyes and para-group haptens (paraphenylenediamine, diaminodiphenylmethane, *p*-aminophenol, *p*-aminoazobenzene, *p*-dimethylaminoazobenzene, and chemical intermediaries used in the synthesis of dyeing agents). In our experience, the results of tests with paraphenylenediamine and diaminodiphenylmethane are not trustworthy indications of sensitization to dyes in general, and to azoic dyes in particular. The resins responsible for ACD were phenol formaldehyde resin and *p-tert*-butylphenol formaldehyde resin, which are used in waterproofing the materials. Furthermore, in the textile workers we found cases of sensitization to the haptens in substances used in washing materials, i.e., softeners (triethanolamine), deodorants (perfume mixes), and preservatives (mercury compounds), as well as to rosin and the lanolin alcohols sometimes used in the operations to finish the materials. Sensitization to rubber haptens (MBT and thiuram and carbamate mixtures) is understandable in the textile workers because they often use rubber gloves or aprons, for example, to prevent contact with noxious substances, unlike the garment industry workers.

References

1. Adams RM (1983) Occupational skin disease. Grune and Stratton, New York
2. Cronin E (1980) Contact dermatitis, 2nd edn. Churchill Livingston, Edinburgh
3. Fisher AA (1986) Conctact dermatitis, 3rd edn. Lea and Febiger, Philadelphia
4. Fregert S, Gruvberg B, Goransson K, Normak S (1978) Allergic contact dermatitis from chromate in military textiles. Contact Dermatitis 4: 223–224
5. Hatch KL, Maibach MI (1980) Textile chemical finish dermatitis. Contact Dermatitis 14: 1–13
6. Kiec-Swierczynska M (1982) Occupational contact dermatitis in the workers employed in production of Texas textiles. Berufsdermatol 30: 41–43
7. Mathur NK, Mathur A, Banerje E (1985) Contact dermatitis in tie and dye industry workers. Contact Dermatitis 12: 38–41
8. Newhouse ML (1974) Dermatitis in a clothing factory. Contact Dermatitis Newsletter 16: 478–480
9. Osmundsen PE (1969) Contact dermatitis due to an optical whitener in washing powders. Br J Dermatol 81: 779–801
10. Sertoli A, Farli M, Francalanci S, Gola M, Lombardi P (1987) Vantaggi di un nuovo metodo (Rapido) per l'esecuzione di patch test. 8a Riunione G.I.R.D.C.A. Riassunto 57

Addresses

M. Gasperini
Clinica Dermosifilopatica, Universitá di Firenze, Via Alfani 37, Firenze, Italy

M. Farli
Clinica Dermosifilopatica, Universitá di Firenze, Via Alfani 37, Firenze, Italy

P. Lombardi
Clinica Dermosifilopatica, Universitá di Firenze, Via Alfani 37, Firenze, Italy

A. Sertoli
Clinica Dermosifilopatica, Universitá di Firenze, Via Alfani 37, Firenze, Italy

Contact Dermatitis in a Shamrock Painter

P. Podmore

Key words:

Fat oil - Pottery worker - Turpentine - Cobalt - Pigments

Case History

A 30-year-old pottery worker presented with a localised patch of vesicular eczema on the palmar aspect of her right hand. Treatment with topical steroids resulted in clearance, but it subsequently recurred. She had recently returned to work after maternity leave, and prior to this she had had no problems with her hands. In her past history, she had suffered from psoriasis on her legs and chronic blepharitis with lower eyelid eczema. She also had a 4- to 5-year history of nickel intolerance, in that she was unable to tolerate cheap earrings.

Her first job was as a nylon-tights examiner from the age of 16 to 17 years. She then joined the pottery, where she trained as a shamrock painter and continued in this job for 13 years. This is a highly skilled job, in which the painter has to mix four different pigments into a paste of the required shade, using turpentine or a more viscous substance known as fat oil. The paste is mixed on a slab, using a wooden-handled carbon steel knife. The paste is then painted onto the pottery, using a brush made out of camel hair, a goose quill, brass wire and wood. The rash on the patient's right hand corresponded to the area in contact with the brush. The pigment-turpentine or pigment-fat oil paste tended to run down the brush.

Patch Tests

The patient was initially tested to the standard battery and found positive to nickel sulphate 5% petrolatum (pet.), cobalt chloride 1% pet., colophony 20% pet. and fragrance 8% pet. As we thought her cobalt sensitivity (despite its rarity) was the answer [4], she was then tested to the pigments waterleaf green, holly leaf green, light green and meadow green mixed in petrolatum. The first three of these pigments contain cobalt. However, she had no positive reactions. As the eczema on her hands had cleared completely with a break from work but recurred on returning to work, her contactants were reassessed, and she was then patch-tested to the brush hair, the turpentine she used to mix the pigments (10% in olive oil), the fat oil she used for the same purpose and some related allergens we owned, namely, turpentine peroxide 0.3% pet., Venice turpentine 20% pet., α-pinene 15% pet., abitol 10% pet., abietic acid 5% pet., geraniol 1% pet., lemon oil 2% pet., and hydroxycitronella 1% pet. She reacted to the fat oil, her own turpentine 10% in olive oil and Venice turpentine 20% pet.

The fat oil is a distillate of turpentine, pine oil and wood resin. Having obtained the constituents from the makers, we tested her with the wood resin 10% pet., turpentine 10% in olive oil, the pine oil 5% pet., and the fat oil itself 1% and 10% in olive oil. She reacted to all of these except the pine oil 5% in pet.

Discussion

The turpentine used to mix with the pigments is genuine gum turpentine from Portugal. Turpentine, like pine oil, rosin (colophony), rosin oils and wood tars, is extracted from pine trees. It is an oleoresin which contains terpenes such as α-pinene, β-pinene, limonene and Δ^3-carene. Δ^3-Carene is recognised as the most potent sensitiser [3], whereas the pinenes are less allergenic. Turpentine is obtained in two different ways: in hot climates such as Portugal, the turpentine exudes from the trees to give gum turpentine, whereas in cold climates such as Sweden, the turpentine is extracted from the trees by a process known as sulphation to yield sulphate turpentine, which is high in Δ^3-carene. This lady was definitely using Portuguese gum turpentine to mix her pigments. However, the type of turpentine used in fat oil distillation is unknown. It is also recognised that exposure of turpentine to air increases its allergenicity and irritancy, as hydroperoxides are formed [2].

This lady's total positive were: nickel sulphate 5% pet., cobalt chloride 1% pet., fragrance mix 8% pet., colophony 20% pet., Portuguese turpentine 10% in olive oil, fat oil 1% and 10% in olive oil, wood resin 10% pet. and fat oil turpentine 10% in olive oil. Her nickel sensitivity is probably irrelevant, in that both her knife and the wire on the paintbrush were negative using the dimethylglyoxime spot test for nickel. Her cobalt sensitivity may be relevant, in that cobalt is contained in three of the pigments. Turpentine cross-reacts with fragrance mix. The remaining positives (colophony, Portuguese turpentine, fat oil turpentine, fat oil and wood resin) are all extracts of pine trees, with common allergens in the terpenes such as Δ^3-carene. Foussereau and Benezra (1970) [1] have previously reported turpentine allergy in porcelain painters.

References

1. Foussereau J, Benezra C (1970) Les eczémas allergiques professionnels. Mason et Cie, Paris, p 377
2. Kirton V (1972) Reactions to ageing turpentine. Contact Dermatitis 11: 302
3. Pirila V, Kilpio O, Okkonen A, Pirila L, Siltanen E (1969) Chemical nature of eczematogens in oils of turpentine. Patterns of sensitivity to different terpenes. Dermatologica 139: 183
4. Rystedt I (1979) Evaluation and relevance of isolated test reactions to cobalt. Contact Dermatitis 5: 233–238

Addresses

P. Podmore
Altnagelvin Area Hospital, Londonderry, Northern Ireland, UK

Occupational Contact Dermatitis to Arsenic Trioxide

S. Gonçalo, M. S. Silva, M. Gonçalo, and A. P. Baptista

Summary

Occupational contact dermatitis to arsenic trioxide was observed in three men working at an atelier of composition in the glass industry. Cutaneous lesions (pruritic maculopapules, pustules, and folliculitis) were localized mainly in exposed and moist areas. Rhinitis and pharyngitis were mentioned by two patients. All had concomitant signs of peripheric polyneuropathy. Dosage of arsenic in the hair and nails varied between 17 and 35 mg/100 g and in the urine between 11.6 and 46.6 µg/100 ml. Patch tests with the manipulated products as is gave a pustular and follicular reaction to arsenic trioxide in two patients. Negative reactions were observed at concentrations of 5%, 2%, and 1% in petrolatum, and also in 25 controls. The irritative nature of the lesions is discussed, and the authors point out the importance of cutaneous lesions in calling attention to other signs of chronic intoxication by arsenic, e.g., neurological signs.

Key words:

Arsenic trioxide - Folliculitis - Occupational dermatitis

Arsenic trioxide (AT) is a thin, easily diffusible white powder, used mainly in the glass industry, ceramics, metallurgy, insecticides, weed killers, and feeds. Cutaneous lesions (either irritative or allergic) due to contact with AT were observed by several authors [1, 3, 5] in patients at copper- and gold-smelting factories and in the glass industry. Lesions were mainly eczematous and pustulous, with folliculitis and cutaneomucous ulcerations, localized in exposed and moist areas. Occasionally, neurological symptoms (sensorial neuropathy of the limbs) were described after cutaneomucous absorption [2]. The process begins slowly, is often subclinical, and is due to wallerian degeneration, mainly on long axons [4].

Patients and Methods

We studied three male patients, aged 23–50 years, with occupational dermatitis to AT. They had been working in the atelier of glass composition in two different factories for periods varying between 6 months and 20 years. In a polluted environment, with deficient protection, they weighed and mixed different powders for glass composition, including AT.

The observation was complemented by general clinical examination; neurological study; electromyography; laboratory study of hematic, hepatic, and renal functions; and thorax X-ray. At regular intervals, the concentration of arsenic in urine, hair, and nails was determined by spectrophotometry with Gutzeit apparatus. Hair and nails were carefully cleaned to avoid external contamination. Patch tests were done with the standard test series of the International Contact Dermatitis Research Group (ICDRG), all the powders the patients worked with (as is), and AT at 1%, 2% and 5% in petrolatum. Biopsies of a cutaneous lesion and of the patch test at 48 h were done.

Results and Discussion

Cutaneous manifestations of a multiform aspect, always pruriginous, began within the first months of exposure. We observed erythematous or scaling lesions, vesicles, pustules, ulceration, and folliculitis, localized mainly to exposed areas and the more sweating ones – antecubital and axillary folds. In one patient, lesions were also present in the bald area of the scalp. Rhinitis, pharyngitis, and conjunctivitis were mentioned by two patients. Evolution was similar in all three cases: worsening in summer, improvement in winter, and regression during holidays. All patients also mentioned distal numbness. Neurological examination revealed peripheral neuropathy with a decrease in pain sensation in a symmetrical "stocking-glove" distribution, mainly in the lower limbs. No other systemic manifestation was found (Table 1).

Table 1. Details of dermatitis to arsenic trioxide in three patients

Case no.	Age (years)	Exposure period	Cutaneous lesions	Localization	Neurological symptoms	Other symptoms
1	33	5 Years	Erythemato-squamous, vesicular and pustular	Face, neck, presternal area, axillary folds, thighs, and scrotum	Sensorial neuropathy	Rhinitis and conjunctivitis, pharyngitis
2	23	6 Months	Ulcerations, erythemato-papules, and vesicles	Dorsal aspect of the hands, face, neck, axillary folds	Sensorial neuropathy	Rhinitis and conjunctivitis
3	50	20 Years	Erythemato-squamous and papulopustular folliculitis	Folds of the face, neck, bald scalp	Sensorial neuropathy	

Table 2. Arsenic concentrations in exposed and unexposed individuals (normal values)

	Arsenic concentration	
	Hair and nails (mg/100 g)	Urine (µg/100 ml)
Unexposed individuals	0.001–0.008	1–2
Case 1	17–35	11.6–12[a]
Case 2	23.8	25–35
Case 3	32	46.6–10

[a] No arsenic was found in the urine 3 months after suspension of work.

Arsenic concentrations varied between 17 and 35 mg/100 g in hair and nails, and between 11.6 and 46.6 µg/100 ml in urine (Table 2), values that highly exceed those of unexposed individuals. Histopathological study of two of the cutaneous lesions showed vesiculopustule with sharp limits, necrosis of epidermis, and no inflammatory reaction (case 1), and typical folliculitis of the whole depth of the follicule, with a discrete inflammatory lymphomonocytic infiltrate (case 3), which may suggest an irritative reaction. Patch tests were positive only to AT as is and fairly reproduced the clinical and histopathological pattern of pustular folliculitis. At 5%, we observed only a weak positive reaction, histopathologically showing a discrete vascular congestion with slight perivascular lymphoplasmocytic infiltrate. No reaction was found at 1% and 2%. Of 25 controls, 23 were negative to the 3 concentrations; 2 showed a discrete irritative reaction.

In our patients, the cutaneous lesions and their localization are similar to the ones mentioned by Birmingham et al. [1]. The high diffusibility and lightness of the powder of AT contribute to its localization in moist areas and in those rich in sebum, mainly the follicular infundibulum, where it induces an inflammatory reaction. The early development of lesions, which affected all the workers of the atelier; their clinical and histopathological aspect; the negativity of patch tests at 1%–5%; and the reproduction of the morphology of cutaneous lesions with AT as is suggest that this is an irritative reaction.

This dermatitis is well tolerated, but it is important in calling attention to possible systemic lesions, particularly neurological ones. According to most authors, cutaneous exposure seldom is the cause of systemic compromise. However, as systemic absorption is confirmed, a long period of exposure may, eventually, induce systemic intoxication or even predispose to neoplasia [6].

After a change of activity, total regression of cutaneous symptoms, slight improvement of neurological signs, and disappearance of arsenic from urine within 3 months were observed in one patient. In the other patients, with improvement of working conditions, cutaneous symptoms decreased, as well as urinary arsenic. The other workers of the department in the two factories were observed (a total of five), and all occasionally mentioned similar symptoms.

References

1. Birmingham DJ, Key MM, Holaday DA, Perone VB (1965) An outbreak of arsenical dermatosis in a mining community. Arch Dermatol 91: 457–466
2. Heyman A, Pfeiffer JB Jr, Willet RW, Taylor HM (1956) Peripheral neuropathy caused by arsenical intoxication. A study of 41 cases with observations on the effects of BAL. N Engl J Med 5: 1–6
3. Holmquist I (1951) Occupational arsenical dermatitis. A study among employees at a copper ore smelting work including investigations of skin reactions to contact with arsenic compounds. Acta Derm Venereol (Suppl 26): 1–214
4. Ohta M (1976) Ultrastructure of sural nerve in a case of arsenical neuropathy. Acta Neuropathol (Berl) 16: 233–242
5. Paschoud JM (1964) Notes cliniques au sujet des eczémas de contact professionnels par l'arsenic et l'antimoine. Dermatologica 129: 410–415
6. Thiers H, Colomb D, Moulin G, Collin L (1967) Le cancer cutané arsenical des viticulteurs du Beaujolais. Am Dermatol Syphyligr 94: 133–158

Addresses

S. Gonçalo
Clínica de Dermatologia, Hospitais da Universidade, 3000 Coimbra, Portugal

M. S. Silva
Clínica de Dermatologia, Hospitais da Universidade, 3000 Coimbra, Portugal

M. Gonçalo
Clínica de Dermatologia, Hospitais da Universidade, 3000 Coimbra, Portugal

A. P. Baptista
Clínica de Dermatologia, Hospitais da Universidade, 3000 Coimbra, Portugal

Reduction of the Allergenicity of Colophony (Rosin) by Hydrogenation

A.-T. Karlberg, A. Boman, J. L. G. Nilsson, and J. E. Wahlberg

Summary

Colophony (rosin) and its derivatives are common causes of contact dermatitis. The aim of the present study was to diminish the allergenicity of gum rosin. Since the allergenicity is due mainly to oxidation products, it will be decreased by chemical reduction of these products. Further, hydrogenation of the conjugated double bonds in abietic-type acids will decrease oxidation of the resin. Gum rosin was hydrogenated over palladium catalyst on charcoal. The allergenic activity of the modified rosin was determined both in animal experiments and in patch testing. The allergenicity was found to be considerably reduced.

Key words:

Abietic acid - Colophony - Contact allergy - Hydrogenation - Rosin

Introduction

Colophony (rosin) and its derivatives are common causes of allergic contact dermatitis. An increasing incidence of allergic reactions to rosin has been reported [9]. The exact origin of a patient's contact allergy may be difficult to determine since modified or unmodified rosin is present in many different products [5]. The global production of rosin is about one million tons a year. The main areas of use are paper size, adhesives, emulgators, and soldering fluxes. It is also used in products in close contact with the skin, e.g., cosmetics and plasters [3, 16]. Three types of rosin (gum rosin, wood rosin, and tall oil rosin) are distinguished depending on the method of recovery. In our research on colophony allergy, we have studied both gum rosin and tall oil rosin [5, 7]. However, in the search for the allergens we have concentrated

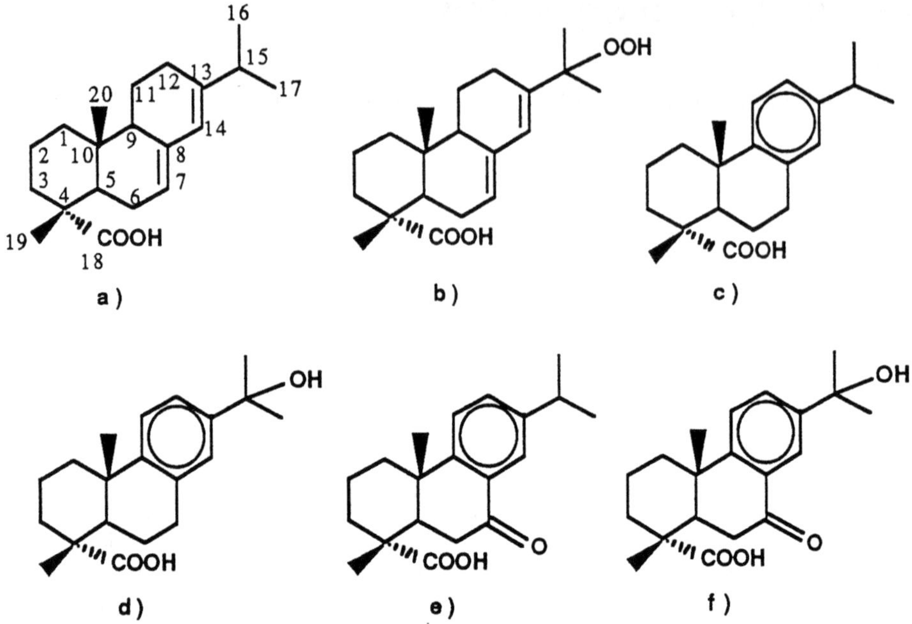

Fig. 1. **a** Abietic acid. **b** 15-Hydroperoxyabietic acid. **c** Dehydroabietic acid. **d** 15-Hydroxydehydroabietic acid. **e** 7-Oxodehydroabietic acid. **f** 15-Hydroxy-7-oxodehydroabietic acid

on gum rosin since this is the common screening material when patch-testing dermatitis patients [9, 16].

Rosin has a complex chemical composition, consisting of 90% resin acids and 10% neutral matter. The main component is abietic acid (Fig. 1 a), which is not allergenic in itself but rather acts as a prohapten [6]. Abietic acid is readily oxidized in air, and one oxidation product, 15-hydroperoxyabietic acid (Fig. 1 b), has been demonstrated to be a main allergen in Portuguese gum rosin [8]. Further, oxidation products of dehydroabietic acid (Fig. 1 c–f) have been shown to be allergenic [10].

The aim of the present study was to diminish the allergenicity of gum rosin. Since the allergenicity is due mainly to oxidation products, it will be decreased by chemical reduction of these products. Further, hydrogenation of the conjugated double bonds in abietic-type acids will decrease oxidation of the resin.

Methods and Results

Hydrogenation of Gum Rosin. Portuguese gum rosin was hydrogenated over palladium catalyst on charcoal. To estimate the degree of unsaturated nonaromatic material still left after hydrogenation, the ^{1}HNMR spectrum of the hydrogenated rosin was compared with that of unmodified rosin. No signals of vinylic protons appeared in the spectrum of the hydrogenated rosin, indicating the presence of $<1\%$ of compounds with nonaromatic double bonds.

Sensitization Experiments in Guinea Pigs. The eliciting activity of the hydrogenated rosin was determined in animals induced with unmodified gum rosin according to the guinea pig maximization test (GPMT) method [1, 15]. When challenge-tested, a response was obtained to unmodified rosin. However, no significant response was found to hydrogenated rosin (Fig. 2).

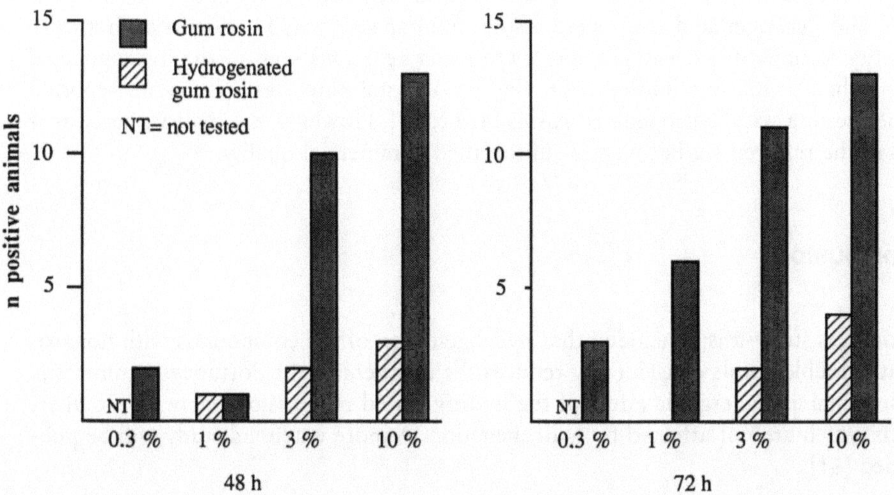

Fig. 2. Eliciting activity of hydrogenated rosin when tested according to the guinea pig maximization test (GPMT) ($n = 15$). Induction material: Unmodified gum rosin 5% intradermally and 25% epidermally. Challenge material: Unmodified gum rosin 10%–0.3% and hydrogenated gum rosin 10%–1% (w/w) in petrolatum. The number of positive animals at 48 h *(left)* and 72 h *(right)* after application is given

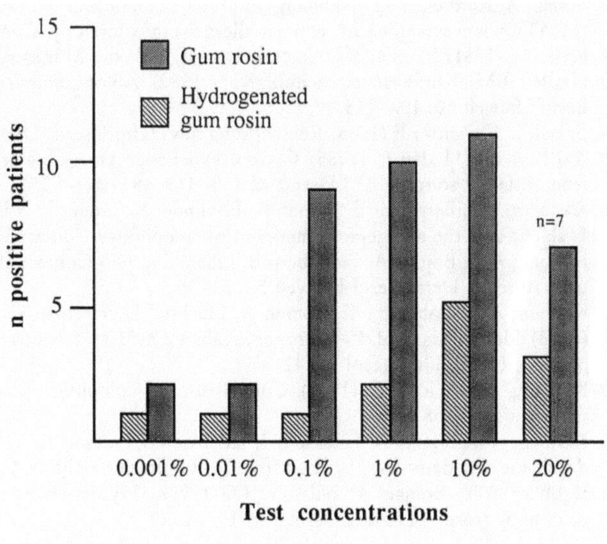

Fig. 3. Positive patch test reactions to hydrogenated and unmodified gum rosin in 11 patients with known allergy to unmodified gum rosin

The sensitizing capacity of the hydrogenated rosin was determined according to both the GPMT method and the Freund's complete adjuvant test (FCAT) method [1, 14]. There was a significant response to the highest test concentration (10% in petrolatum) in the GPMT study, while no significant reactions were found in the FCAT experiment.

Patch Testing in Patients. Patch testing was carried out according to the internationally accepted method for diagnosis of contact allergy [2]. Serial dilutions of unmodified and hydrogenated rosin were tested simultaneously in 11 patients with known allergy to unmodified rosin. There were fewer reactions seen to the hydrogenated rosin than to the unmodified rosin (Fig. 3). Varying patch test results are reported when testing with hydrogenated rosins [4, 12, 13]. However, the hydrogenated rosins in the referred studies were of unspecified commercial quality.

Conclusion

From this study it is concluded that hydrogenation of the compounds with nonaromatic double bonds considerably reduces the allergenicity of Portuguese gum rosin. The remaining allergenic effect of the hydrogenated rosins is probably due to allergens which are not affected by hydrogenation. A more extended study will be published [11].

References

1. Boman A, Karlberg A-T, Wahlberg JE (1988) Experiences with Freund's complete adjuvant test (FCAT), when screening for contact allergens in colophony. Contact Dermatitis 18: 25–29
2. Fregert S (1981) Manual of contact dermatitis, 2nd edn. Munksgaard, Copenhagen, pp 71–81
3. Hausen BM, Kuhlwein A, Schulz KH (1982) Kolophonium-Allergie (1. Mitteilung). Derm Beruf Umwelt 30: 107–115
4. Jirasek L, Kvicalova E (1965) Reizwirkung des Heftpflasters. Derm Wochenschr 151: 384–394
5. Karlberg A-T, Lidén C (1985) Clinical experience and patch testing using colophony (rosin) from different sources. Br J Dermatol 113: 475–481
6. Karlberg A-T, Bergstedt E, Boman A, Bohlinder K, Lidén C, Nilsson JLG, Wahlberg JE (1985) Is abietic acid the allergenic component of colophony? Contact Dermatitis 13: 209–215
7. Karlberg A-T, Boman A, Holmbom B, Lidén C (1986) Contact allergy to acid and neutral fractions of rosin. Derm Beruf Umwelt 34: 31–36
8. Karlberg A-T, Bohlinder K, Boman A, Hacksell U, Hermansson J, Jacobsson S, Nilsson JLG (1988) Identification of 15-hydroperoxyabietic acid as a contact allergen in Portuguese colophony. J Pharm Pharmacol 40: 42–47
9. Karlberg A-T, Lidén C (1988) Comparison of colophony patch test preparations. Contact Dermatitis 18: 158–165
10. Karlberg A-T, Boman A, Hacksell U, Jacobsson S, Nilsson JLG (1988) Contact allergy to dehydroabietic acid derivatives isolated from Portuguese colophony. Contact Dermatitis 19: 166–174
11. Karlberg A-T, Boman A, Nilsson JLG (1988) Hydrogenation reduces the allergenicity of colophony (rosin). Contact Dermatitis 19: 22–29

12. Keil H (1943) Hypersensitivity to adhesive tape. J Ind Hyg Toxicol 25: 238–242
13. Keil H (1943) Dermatitis due to resin-finished shorts and fabrics. J Allergy 14: 477–491
14. Klecak G (1985) The Freund's complete adjuvant test and the open epicutaneous test. A complementary test procedure for realistic assessment of allergenic potential. Curr Probl Derm 14: 152–171
15. Magnusson B, Kligman AM (1970) Allergic contact dermatitis in the guinea pig. Identification of contact allergens. Thomas, Springfield Illinois
16. Taylor JS (1986) Adhesives, Gums, and Resins. In: Fisher AA (ed) Contact dermatitis, 3rd edn. Lea and Febiger, Philadelphia, pp 666–674

Addresses

A.-T. Karlberg
Division of Occupational Dermatology, National Institute of Occupational Health, S-171 84 Solna, Sweden

A. Boman
Division of Occupational Dermatology, National Institute of Occupational Health, S-171 84 Solna, Sweden

J. L. G. Nilsson
Apoteksbolaget AB, Central Laboratory, S-105 14 Stockholm, Sweden

J. E. Wahlberg
Division of Occupational Dermatology, National Institute of Occupational Health, S-171 84 Solna, Sweden

Contact Allergy Towards Ninhydrin in a Marking Pen for Patch Testing

J. Roesler and D. Kleinhans

Summary

A 73-year-old male patient when patch tested because of long-standing leg ulcers, showed an eczematous contact dermatitis in exactly those skin areas where the patch tests had been marked by a special marking pen. The pen contained ninhydrin, gentian violet and disulphine blue. Ninhydrin 5% mek (open test) led to a positive patch-test reaction, whereas gentian violet and disulphine blue gave negative results.

Key words:

Ninhydrin - Patch testing - Marking pen dermatitis

We present a case where we first observed an eczematous contact dermatitis in those skin areas marked by a special marking pen during patch testing. This marking pen had been used by our Allergy Department in approximately 3000 patch-test patients without similar reactions.

Case History

In October 1987, a 73-year-old male patient was patch tested because of long-standing leg ulcers. He proved to be sensitized towards benzocaine, parabenes and probably wool alcohols due to the topical therapy of the ulcers. To our surprise, he showed an eczematous contact dermatitis in exactly those skin areas where the patch test had been marked by a special marking pen.

Table 1. Results of patch tests

	Day 1	Day 2	Day 3	Day 4
Ninhydrin 5% mek, open[a]	+	++	++	++
Gentian violet 1% aq.[b]	–	–	–	–
Disulphine blue 1% aq.[b]	–	–	–	–
Butanol 1% aq.[b]	–	–	–	–

[a] Ninhydrin (Merck, Darmstadt, FRG): MW 178.15 g/mol, minimum purity grade 99%
[b] Closed tests, Finn chamber on Scanpore

Marking Pen

The marking pen used was supplied by Hermal Chemie (Reinbek, FRG) under the name "Epikutan-Markierungsstift", being produced by Ethicon (Norderstedt, FRG). It is identical with the "Codman surgical marking pen violet-43-1030 CD". The marking pens contain 5% ninhydrin (2,2-dihydroxy-1,3-indandione), 0.0075% gentian violet (C.I. 42535), 0.0032% disulphine blue (C.I.42045), dissolved in butandiol, propanediol and distilled water.

Patch Test Results

The results of the patch tests are shown in Table 1.

Ninhydrin

Ninhydrin forms colourless crystals. In aqueous solution ninhydrin together with amino acids, peptides and proteins produces a blue colour. It has therefore been used since 1911 for chemical analysis. During this ninhydrin reaction NH_3 is released; the reduced ninhydrin with the help of NH_3 combines with a further molecule of non-reduced ninhydrin to produce the blue dye. Ninhydrin is therefore used in chemical analysis, in criminology to reveal fingerprints and in skin marking pens.

Comment

The source of the patient's sensitization towards ninhydrin remains obscure. In the review of the literature going back to 1966, only one relevant Soviet publication from 1974 was found [1]. It concerned a 29-year-old chemist who had contact with 2%–50% ninhydrin solutions during analysis. Three months after starting this work he developed contact dermatitis on fingers and dorsa of the hands. The patch test (0.25% ninhydrin aqueous, closed test) was positive. In the meantime we have been informed of two analogous cases of marking pen dermatitis seen in the Göttingen Dermatology Department and obviously also caused by ninhydrin.

Reference

1. Kystaubalewa KS, Shaparjenko MW (1974) Case of occupational eczema caused by ninhydrin. Gig Tr Prof Zabol 18: 46–47

Addresses

J. Roesler
Department of Dermatology, Allergy Unit, 7000 Stuttgart-Bad Cannstatt, FRG

D. Kleinhans
Department of Dermatology, Allergy Unit, 7000 Stuttgart-Bad Cannstatt, FRG

Plastics

Acrylic Reactions - Ten-Years' Experience

J. S. Taylor

Summary

Sixteen cases of adverse reactions to acrylics seen over a 10-year period reflect the increasing use of these chemicals for industrial and consumer application. Fourteen patients had contact dermatitis typically of the hands and/or face (11 allergic, 1 irritant, and 2 undetermined) and two had nail dystrophy. Sources of the acrylics were nail chemicals (5 cases), adhesives (3 cases), research laboratories (3 cases), dental acrylics (3 cases), histology embedding medium (1 case), and printing plates (1 case). Eleven cases were occupational. Highest patch-test reactivity rates were for THFMA, HPMA, EGDMA, HDDA, and TMPTM. In screening for acrylic allergy MMA, n-AA and PEGDMA are suggested as a minimum.

Key words:

Acrylics - Acrylates - Methacrylates - Contact dermatitis- Nail dystrophy

Reports of adverse reactions from acrylics have been increasing in recent years [2, 3, 10] and parallel the vastly increased commercial use of these chemicals [17]. This paper reviews our patch-test clinic experience with acrylic reactions over the past 10 years.

Methods

A list of 16 patients with skin and nail reactions to acrylics from 1978 to 1987 was retrieved by computer. Most were patch-tested according to standard methodology with Finn chambers on Scanpore. Patch testing was usually performed with the standard screening series of the North American Contact Dermatitis Group (NACDG) and one or more acrylic chemicals [13]. Other plastics and glues and work and environmental contactants were tested in several patients. Acrylics tested (in petrolatum (pet.) unless otherwise specified) include: hydroxyethyl methacrylate (HEMA) 5%; polyethyleneglycol dimethacrylate (PEGDMA) 5%; hydroxypropyl methacrylate (HPMA) 5%; tetraethyleneglycol diacrylate (TEGDA) 0.1%; hexanediol diacrylate (HDDA) 0.1%; trimethylolpropane trimethacrylate (TMPTMA) 0.2%; n-amyl (pentyl) acrylate (n-AA) 1%; butyl acrylate (BA) 0.1%; ethylhexyl acrylate (EHA) 5%; methacrylic acid (M acid) 5%; methyl methacrylate (MMA) 5%; 10% olive oil and rarely 1%; ethyl methacrylate (EMA) 5%; n-butyl methacrylate (n-BMA) 5%; isobutyl methacrylate (iBMA) 5%; trimethylolpropane trimethacrylate (TMPTMA) 5%; tetrahydrofurfuryl methacrylate (THFMA) 5%; diethyleneglycol dimethacrylate (DEGDMA) 5%; ethyleneglycol dimethacrylate (EGDMA) 5%; and isobornyl methacrylate (i-Bornyl MA) 1%.

Summary of Cases

There were 16 cases, 13 in females and three in males ranging in age from 22–62 years. More than one-half of the cases were seen since 1985. Five were atopic.

The sources of acrylic exposure were acrylic nails and newer variants in five cases, industrial adhesives in three cases (Loctite in two and an acrylic-propyleneimine vinyl adhesive in one), chemicals in research laboratories in three cases, dental chemicals (two in dental assistants and one patient with stomatitis) in three cases, histology laboratory embedding medium in one case, and printing-plate photopolymers in one case.

Eleven were occupational. The five cases which were not occupationally caused included four of the five nail cases and the patient with the denture reaction. An acrylic was considered to be the sole or major cause of the dermatitis or nail reaction in most cases.

Thirteen had contact dermatitis, two had nail dystrophy, and one had both contact dermatitis and nail dystrophy. Of the 14 cases of contact dermatitis, 11 were allergic, one was irritant and two were not determined. Sites of dermatitis in the 14 cases were: hands or fingers, 7; hands and face, 3; face and eyelids, 3; and mouth, 1. Mucosal irritation from acrylic vapors was reported by two patients and urticaria (localized and later generalized) accompanied contact dermatitis in one.

Acrylic exposure prior to onset of reaction ranged from 1 day to 18 years with the usual being several months to 3 years.

Details of the nail cases will be reported elsewhere (J.S.Taylor, in preparation) and one of the Loctite adhesive cases has previously been described in detail [15].

Results of patch testing with acrylics are presented in Tables 1 and 2. The highest reactivity rates were seen from THFMA, HPMA, EGDMA and derivatives, n-AA, and TMPTMA. Negative reactions occurred from MMA, BMA, iBMA, and i-Bornyl MA. Some positive responses represent cross reactions rather than reactions

Table 1. Positive patch tests

Chemical	No. positive/ no. tested	Acrylic source[a]
Methacrylates 5%		
Hydroxyethyl	6/9	N A Path
Hydroxypropyl	3/6	N A
Tetrahydrofurfuryl	5/6	N A D
Ethyl	2/11	N
Dimethacrylates 5%		
Ethyleneglycol	7/9	N A P D
Diethyleneglycol	6/8	N A P D
Polyethyleneglycol	4/5	N A P
Acrylates		
N-amyl 1%	3/5	N A
Butyl 0.1%, 1%	2/4	N C
Hydroxyethyl 1%	1/1	C
Diacrylates 0.1%		
Hexanediol	4/6	N A P
Tetraethylene glycol	2/5	N P
Triacrylate 0.2%		
Trimethylolpropane	3/5	N P

[a] Acrylic source in patients with positive patch tests. Some are cross reactions and not reactions from primary sources of the chemicals

%, Patch-test concentration; N, nails; A, adhesive; P, printing; D, dental; Path, pathology laboratory; C, chemical laboratory

Table 2. Negative patch tests

Chemical	No. negative/ no. tested
Methacrylates 5%	
Methyl	9/10[a]
Butyl	11/11
Isobutyl	10/10
Isobornyl 1%	2/2
Trimethacrylate	
Trimethylolpropane 5%	5/9[a]
Acrylate	
Ethylhexyl 5%	4/5
Other	
Other plastic and glue chemicals	7/7

[a] Other reactions were doubtful

from primary sources of the chemicals. We documented the following acrylics with their primary sources: THFMA and DEGDMA, sculptured nails; PEGDMA, Loctite adhesive and a Japanese printing plate; HEMA, pathology embedding medium and a chemical research laboratory; EGDMA, cross linker in dental acrylics; and HDDA, an American printing plate.

Discussion

Acrylic compounds are thermoplastic chemicals formed by polyaddition chain propagation reactions and have in common a basic similarity in chemical structure to acrylic acid ($CH_2 = CH-COOH$) [10, 17]. Acrylic monomers can be made to combine with themselves or with other monomers to form more complex polymers and copolymers known as acrylic resins [17]. Malten has summarized the many products and processes employing acrylics. These include cosmetics, medical prostheses, adhesives, textiles, utensils, and the construction and printing industries. This widespread use of acrylics has resulted in the exposure of many people in industrial and household environments.

Our limited experience with patients exposed to acrylics over the past 10 years reflects the evolving and expanding use of these chemicals. After seeing a few patients between 1978–1980, we adopted the acrylic nail chemicals identified by Fisher [5] as our "acrylic" patch-test tray. However, instead of identifying patients with allergy to acrylic nails, we found a number with acrylic reactions from other causes. In 1986–1987, we saw our first cases of acrylic nail allergy.

The use of acrylic nails is expanding rapidly in the United States, especially in California. Most are applied in salons, but recently they have been sold directly to consumers. Manicurists may be exposed to a number of occupational hazards, including vapors from acrylic monomers and solvents, fiberglass, and particulates from sanding of nails. Local exhaust ventilation may help as well as use of 1-component gels which emit less vapor. The latter are replacing the older 3-component sculptured nail chemicals. Recently MMA (banned for use in acrylic nails in the USA in 1975) has been measured in the workroom air of nail salons but it was found to be below the threshold limit value of 100 ppm [6, 7].

Loctite and other anaerobic acrylic industrial adhesives continue to be used worldwide. In the USA, they are now sold for consumer use under the Permatex label. Most anaerobic adhesives are applied from small containers, but some applications are automated [15].

Acrylics are used in a number of other adhesive formulations which have previously been reviewed [18]. In particular, there are extensive numbers of acrylic monomers used in pressure-sensitive adhesives. Recently, allergic contact dermatitis has been reported from cyanoacrylate adhesives [1]. Patch tests with cyanoacrylates were negative in the three patients we tested who had dermatitis and/or nail dystrophy associated with using nail acrylics.

Cases of adverse acrylic reactions similar to ours have been reported and Malten's recent review lists clinical reports by individual acrylic compound [10]. Malten has also reviewed acrylics used in printing-plate manufacturing processes [11].

Local and systemic reactions from acrylic exposure have occurred [8, 9, 12, 14]. Two of our patients reported mucosal irritation. One of the manicurists developed eye and nasal irritation when applying 3-component sculptured nails. One of the dental technicians also reported mild mucosal irritation when handling acrylic monomers. Urticaria in one of the laboratory research workers was temporally related to acrylic exposure.

Although penetration of rubber and polyvinyl gloves by acrylics is well known [4, 8], several of our patients reported temporary benefit from careful donning and removal of gloves, and wearing them for short periods of time. Nitrile gloves have been recommended recently [16].

The search for one more monomer to screen for acrylic allergy remains elusive. Rietschel [16], following a review of the literature, suggests the combination of MMA and pentyl (amyl) or neopentyl acrylate as a good but imperfect screening tool. Based on our experience, I would also include PEGDMA in screening for acrylic allergy.

One manufacturer suggested to me that i-Bornyl MA was "less sensitizing"; it *was* negative in two of our nail patients who were positive to a number of other acrylics. This information is obviously anecdotal.

Kanerva [8] has recently demonstrated active patch-test sensitization to acrylates and recommends testing EA, 2HEA, and HPA at 0.167% in petrolatum. False-negative reactions have not been excluded.

In conclusion, when patch-testing with a battery of acrylics, many strong positive reactions may occur in highly sensitive patients. In these cases, the excited skin syndrome may require exclusion by retesting the positive acrylics individually and possibly at lower concentrations. It is also important to remember that delayed irritant reactions resembling allergic reactions have been reported from 1,6-HDDA and 1,4-butanediol diacrylate [16].

References

1. Belsito DV (1987) Contact dermatitis to ethyl-cyanoacrylate-containing glue. Contact Dermatitis 17: 234–236
2. Bjorkner B (1984) Sensitizing capacity of ultraviolet cured acrylic compounds. Thesis, Department of Occupational Dermatology, University of Lund, Sweden
3. Fisher AA (1986) Contact dermatitis, 3rd edn. Lea and Febiger, Philadelphia, pp 555–560 and 652–653
4. Fisher AA (1986) Reactions to acrylic bone cement in orthopedic surgeons. Cutis 37: 425–426
5. Fisher AA (1980) Cross reactions between methyl methacrylate monomer and acrylic monomers presently used in acrylic nail preparations. Contact Dermatitis 6: 345–368
6. Froines JR, Garabrant DH (1986) Quantitative evaluation of manicurists' exposure to methyl, ethyl and isobutyl methacrylate during production of synthetic fingernails. Appl Ind Hyg 1: 70–74
7. Hiipakka D, Samimi B (1987) Exposure of acrylic fingernail sculptors to organic vapors and methacrylate dusts. Am Ind Hyg Assoc J 48: 230–237
8. Kanerva L, Verkkala E (1986) Electron microscopy and immunohistochemistry of toxic and allergic effects of methylmethacrylate on the skin. Arch Toxicol [Suppl] 9: 456–459

9. Lozewicz S, et al. (1985) Occupational asthma due to methyl methacrylate and cyanoacrylates. Thorax 40: 836–839
10. Malten KE (1987) Old and new, mainly occupational dermatological problems in the production and processing of plastics. In: Maibach HI (ed) Occupational and industrial dermatology, 2nd edn, chapt 31. Yearbook, Chicago, pp 290–340
11. Malten KE (1987) Printing plate manufacturing processes. In: Maibach HI (ed) Occupational and industrial dermatology, 2nd edn, chapt 34. Yearbook, Chicago, pp 351–366
12. Mathias CGT, et al. (1979) Contact dermatitis and gastrointestinal symptoms from hydroxyethylmethacrylate. Br J Dermatol 100: 447–449
13. Patch Testing in Dermatology (1984) American Academy of Dermatology, Evanston, Illinois
14. Rajaniemi R (1986) Clinical evaluation of occupational toxicity of methyl methacrylate monomer to dental technicians. J Soc Occup Med 36: 56–59
15. Ranchoff R, Taylor JS (1985) Contact dermatitis to anaerobic sealants. J Am Acad Dermatol 13: 1015–1020
16. Rietschel RL (1986) Contact allergens in ultraviolet-cured acrylic resin systems. Occup Med: State of the Art Reviews 1: 301–306
17. Rycroft RR (1977) Contact dermatitis from acrylic compounds. Br J Dermatol 96: 685–687
18. Taylor JS (1986) Adhesives, gums and resins. In: Fisher AA (ed) Contact dermatitis, chapt 37. Lea and Febiger, Philadelphia, pp 644–674

Addresses

J. S. Taylor
Department of Dermatology, Section of Industrial Dermatology, A-61, The Cleveland Clinic Foundation, 9500 Euclid Avenue, Euclid, OH 44106, U.S.A.

Occupational Allergic Contact Dermatitis from Acrylates: Observations Concerning Anaerobic Acrylic Sealants and Dental Composite Resins

L. Kanerva, T. Estlander, and R. Jolanki

Summary

Three cases of allergic contact dermatitis from anaerobic acrylic sealants (all from Loctite products) and seven cases of allergic acrylate contact dermatitis from dental composite resins have been detected. The different types of acrylate patch test reactions are described.

Key words:

Epoxy acrylates - Epoxy resin - Methacrylate - Dental personnel - Loctite - Plastics

Introduction

Currently, the most prominently increasing group of allergens causing occupational dermatoses are the plastics [1]. Here, we present occupational allergic dermatoses caused by two types of acrylic plastics: anaerobic acrylic sealants (AAS) [2–10] and dental composite resin products (DCR). Two of the three patients allergic to AAS and five of the seven allergic to DCR have been tested with an extensive (meth)acrylate series, giving new information on cross-allergy and concomitant sensitization to acrylates. A more detailed report of DCR allergy is published elsewhere [11].

Patients and Methods

Patients. Patch testing at our clinic has been performed since 1946 (see [1]). Here, all the patients who have been diagnosed as having allergic contact dermatitis from AAS ($n=3$) or DCR ($n=7$) are reported. Patch testing (and prick testing to detect atopy) was performed as described earlier [1, 11, 12].

Patch Testing with Acrylates. Before 1982, only methyl methacrylate and substances brought in by the patient were patch-tested when contact allergy to acrylates was suspected. In 1982–1985, seven acrylates were used (see [12]); since 1985, the commercial (meth)acrylate series of Chemotechnique Diagnostics AB (Malmö, Sweden) containing 28 substances has been used (see [12] and Table 2).

Patch Tests with AAS and Active Ingredient in Loctite Products. Allergic contact dermatitis (from AAS) has been detected only from Loctite products. These have been tested in petrolatum at 0.5%–5% (w/w) or undiluted (see Table 1). Our last patient was also tested with a dilution series of polyethylene glycol dimethacrylate (kindly supplied by the manufacturer of Loctite products; see Table 2) in petrolatum.

Patch Testing with DCR. Resins brought in by the patients were tested at 1% (w/w) petrolatum except in case 3, for which the patch test concentrations have been reported in detail earlier [13].

Results

Patients Allergic to Anaerobic Acrylic Sealants. Three patients have been detected who have occupationally become sensitized to Loctite AAS. The characteristics and patch test results of the patients are shown in Tables 1, 2.

Case 1 had had a mild hand dermatitis for 13 years and been exposed to many chemicals, including Loctite 221 and 573. He did not suspect allergy towards his Loctite products, which was patch-tested amongst many other chemicals he had been exposed to. Patch testing with the Loctite products he used gave an allergic reaction (Table 1). He was not patch-tested with other (meth)acrylates. He has changed his job and is no longer exposed to Loctite sealants, but he has been exposed to solvents, mineral oils, and metal dust, and he has suffered from mild to moderate hand eczema, which has been considered irritant occupational eczema from solvents.

Case 2 had had atopic eczema as a child. Prick tests with common allergens gave positive results for cat epithelium, and this allergy was confirmed by a positive RAST test (score 3). She had had hand eczema in the 1970s, which became accentuated in 1985, when she had been working as a car furnisher for 3 years. At the same time, she also developed eczema on her lower arms, body, and the folds of the knees and elbows, partly due to allergic contact dermatitis from black rubber chemicals.

Table 1. Characteristics of the patients sensitized to Loctite anaerobic acrylic sealants (AAS)

	Case		
	1	2	3
Occupation	Filer	Car furnisher	Pipe fitter
Sex	Male	Female	Female
Year of diagnosis	1978	1986	1987
Exposure to AAS before sensitization (years)	5	3	12
Personal/family atopy	–/–	+/+	–/–
No. of patch test sessions	2	3	3
Protective gloves used	None	None	None
Associated causes of hand eczema	Solvents (irritant)	Rubber (allergic); atopy	Solvents (irritant)
Epicutaneous tests			
Loctite sealants	Loctite 221 2% 2+ 1% 2+ 0.5% 2+	Loctite 572 100% 4+ 5% 2+ Loctite 242 100% 4+ 5% 2+	Loctite 242 5% 3+ 2% 3+ Loctite 542 1% 3+ 1% 3+ Polyethylene glycol dimethacrylate 2% 3+ 0.67% 3+ 0.2% 3+ 0.067% 3+ 0.02% 2+ 0.0067% (+)
(Meth)acrylate series	Not done	See Table 2	See Table 2
Other work contactants	Negative	Negative (except rubber chemicals)	Negative

Case 3 had been working in the same place since 1973. Loctite products came into use in 1975. The patient had had hand eczema since 1975, probably due to the solvents to which he was exposed. His hand eczema was clearly accentuated in 1987, and this was probably due to sensitization to Loctite products.

Patients Allergic to Dental Composite Resins. Seven patients have been detected who have become sensitized to DCR through their work. Some of the characteristics of the sensitized patients and patch test results are summarized in Tables 2, 3. Cases 1–6 were dental nurses, and case 7 a dentist. Three were atopics and two others had a history of atopy in their family. All patients had hand eczema, especially on their fingers; in addition, three occasionally had dermatitis on the face. All patients had concomitant allergies to their protective gloves or disinfectants (see [11]; not shown in Table 3). All patients showed a positive patch test reaction to at least one of the DCR they had been exposed to (Table 3). The names of the DCR are shown in Table 3. Cases 3–7 were patch-tested with an extensive (meth)acrylate series, and all the dental nurses (cases 3–6), but not the dentist, were patch test positive to 2,2-bis[4-(2-hydroxy-3-methacryloxypropoxy)phenyl]propane (BIS-GMA)

Table 2. Patch test results in two patients allergic to Loctite products and five patients allergic to dental composite resin products (adapted from [11])

Compound	Concentration (w/w) (%)	Results						
		Loctite case		Dental composite resin case				
		2	3	3	4	5	6	7
Ethyl acrylate	0.167–0.5	–	–	–	1+	–	–	3+
Butyl acrylate	0.5	–	–	–	2+	–	–	3+
2-Ethylhexyl acrylate	0.5	–	–	–	–	–	–	–
2-Hydroxyethyl acrylate	0.167–0.5	–	–	–	2+	–	–	3+
2-Hydroxypropyl acrylate	0.167–0.5	–	–	–	2+	–	–	3+
Methyl methacrylate	2	–	2+	3+	–	–	–	2+
Ethyl methacrylate	2	–	2+	–	–	–	–	3+
n-Butyl methacrylate	2	–	–	–	–	–	–	2+
2-Hydroxyethyl methacrylate	2	2+	2+	–	1+	–	2+	3+
2-Hydroxypropyl methacrylate	2	2+	2+	–	2+	–	2+	3+
Ethylene glycol dimethacrylate	2		3+	–	–	–	3+	2+
Triethylene glycol dimethacrylate	2	3+	3+	–	3+	–	4+	2+
1,4-Butanediol dimethacrylate	2	–	3+	–	–	–	–	1+
Urethane dimethacrylate	2	–	–	–	–	–	–	–
2,2-bis[4-(2-methacryloxyethoxy) phenyl]propane	1	–	–	–	3+	–	–	–
2,2-bis[4-(methacryloxy)phenyl] propane	2	–	–	–	–	–	–	–
2,2-bis[4-(2-hydroxy-3-meth-acryloxypropoxy)phenyl]propane	2	–	–	4+	3+	2+	2+	–
1,4-Butanediol diacrylate	0.1	–	–	–	2+	–	–	2+
1,6-Hexanediol diacrylate	0.1	–	–	–	2+	–	–	–
Diethylene glycol diacrylate	0.1	–	–	–	3+	–	–	2+
Tripropylene glycol diacrylate	0.1	–	–	–	–	–	–	–
Trimethylolpropane triacrylate	0.1	–	–	–	–	–	–	–
Pentaerythritol triacrylate	0.1	–	–	–	–	–	–	–
Oligotriacrylate 480	0.1	–	–	–	–	–	–	–
Epoxy diacrylate	0.5	–	–	4+	2+	2+	2+	–
Urethane diacrylate (aliphatic)	0.1	–	–	–	–	–	–	–
Urethane diacrylate (aromatic)	0.1	–	–	–	–	–	–	–
Triethylene glycol diacrylate	0.1	2+	2+	–	3+	–	2+	3+
Epoxy resin	1	–	–	3+	3+	3+	3+	–

The case numbers are the same as in Table 1 for Loctite-allergic patients and Table 3 for dental composite resin-allergic patients.

and epoxy diacrylate (BIS-GA). Three of the patients (4, 6, and 7) reacted to a large number of aliphatic acrylates, including triethylene glycol dimethacrylate (TREGDMA) and triethylene glycol diacrylate (TREGDA); case 5 reacted only to epoxy acrylates (BIS-GMA and BIS-GA). Case 3 was patch test positive to methyl methacrylate (MMA) and epoxy acrylates. The dentist's patch test results closely resembled those of the patients allergic to AAS (especially case 3); she was allergic to a large number of acrylates, including MMA, but not to epoxy acrylates. Nor was she allergic to epoxy resin, whereas cases 3–6 were. Urethane acrylates caused no positive patch test reactions.

Table 3. Characteristics of the seven patients sensitized to dental composite resins (DCR) (adapted from [11])

	Case						
	1	2	3	4	5	6	7
Occupation	Dental nurse	Dental nurse	Dental nurse	Dental nurse	Dental nurse	Dental nurse	Dentist
Sex	Female	Female	Female	Female	Female	Female	Female
Year of diagnosis	1979	1982	1985	1986	1986	1987	1986
Hand eczema onset	1970	1982	1984	1984	1979	1974	1985
Age at diagnosis (years)	60	22	20	34	28	41	41
Probable duration of exposure to DCR before sensitization (years)	1	1	3[a]	9	1	5	14
Personal/family atopy	–/–	+/–	–/–	+/+	–/+	+/+	–/+
Positive patch tests to personal DCR	Concise Resin A and B 3+	Concise Resin A and B 2+	Miradapt Universal Paste 2+	Silar Paste A and B 3+	Silar Paste A and B 2+	Silar Paste A and B 3+	Silar Paste A and B 2+
	Concise Paste A and B 3+/2+	Silar Paste A and B 2+	Miradapt Catalyst Paste 2+	Silux Universal Opaque Paste 3+	Silux Universal Opaque Paste 2+	Delton Pit & Fissure Sealant Universal and Catalyst 3+	Aurafill 2+
			Bonding Agent Universal Resin and Catalyst Resin 2+	Aurafill 3+			Delton Pit & Fissure Sealant Curing 3+

[a] Months.

Discussion

Allergic contact dermatitis to AAS and DCR can reliably be diagnosed with products brought in by the patients, as was the case with all our patients. A clear positive reaction was obtained with AAS tested at 0.5% in petrolatum (in case 1), but with this concentration some cases may remain undetected. The concentration of 1% (w/w) in petrolatum gave reliable test results for DCR. MMA is not a good screening product for AAS or DCR. Of our 2 AAS patients tested, 1 was positive to MMA, but only 4 of the 65 earlier reported cases have shown a positive patch test (not all patients have been tested) to MMA (Table 4). If possible, the active ingredient of Loctite products, i. e., polyethylene glycol dimethacrylate, should be used as a test substance. In our case, it gave a positive reaction even at 0.02%, while Ranchoff and Taylor's [9] case was positive with 1% and 5%, but negative with 0.1% in petrolatum.

Except for the large number of people sensitized in a car factory in Germany (34 patients) [5], the number of allergic contact dermatitis cases from Loctite products is relatively small (Table 4). Soubrier et al. [8] reported that their patients had been sensitized to cyanoacrylates, but apparently the sensitization was due to Loctite AAS. Our patients had been exposed to AAS for 3–12 years before they became sensitized. It was apparent that our patients had had hand eczema before they had become sensitized to AAS. They had not used protective gloves. The sensitizing capacity of Loctite products is apparently not very high, but workers should still be informed that Loctite products are sensitizers.

AAS cases 2 and 3 were tested with an extensive (meth)acrylate series, and showed reactions very similar to the patient of Ranchoff and Taylor [9]; these three patients reacted positively, e. g., to 2-hydroxyethyl methacrylate and 2-hydroxypropyl methacrylate. Case 3 was positive to ethylene glycol dimethacrylate, as was that of Ranchoff and Taylor's [9], whereas case 2 was negative. Both of our patients reacted strongly to TREGDMA, but this was probably not tested by Ranchoff and Taylor [9]. According to the manufacturer, Loctite products 242 and 572 are based

Table 4. Published cases of allergic contact dermatitis due to anaerobic acrylic sealants

Reference	Year	No. of sensitized patients	No. of patients allergic to methyl methacrylate
[3]	1967	7	
[4]	1972	7	2
[5]	1975	34	
[2]	1980	4	1
[6]	1982	2	1
[7]	1984	3	0
[8]	1984	6	
[9]	1985	1	0
[10]	1987	1	ND
This paper		3	1[a]

ND, not determined

[a] Of 2 patients tested.

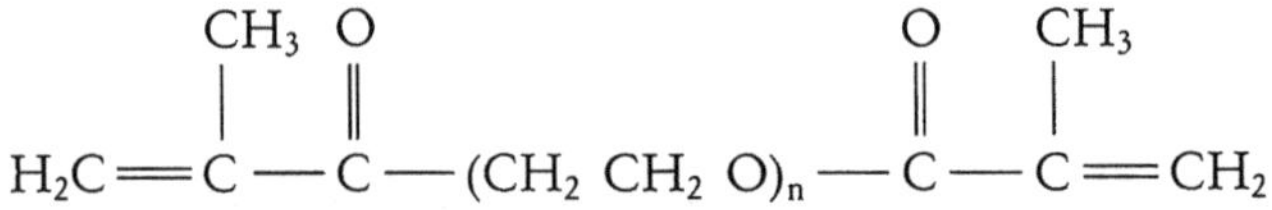

Fig. 1. The structural formula of polyethylene glycol dimethacrylate. In anaerobic acrylic sealants, $n=3$

on polyethylene glycol dimethacrylate (PEGDMA), and they contain no other methacrylates or acrylates. Accordingly, the other (meth)acrylate reactions would represent signs of cross-sensitivity, which is known to occur with (meth)acrylates [11]. The structural formula of PEGDMA is seen in Fig. 1. Ranchoff and Taylor [9] stated that *n* in this formula is usually 4, while the manufacturer informed us that PEGDMA contains a significant quantity (about 40%) of TREGDMA, i.e., where *n* equals 3, and both of our patients reacted strongly to this compound.

Most DCR are based on aromatic dimethacrylate monomers (see [11]). DCR contains at least the following allergens: (a) aromatic epoxy acrylate; (b) other aliphatic monofunctional and difunctional acrylates; (c) additives, such as initiators (e.g., benzoyl peroxide), activators (e.g., tertiary aromatic amines), and inhibitors (e.g., hydroquinone); and (d) impurities, possibly, e.g., epoxy resin (ER) molecular weight (MW) 340. Two types of independent allergies to DCR were observed: from aromatic epoxy and/or from low-viscosity aliphatic acrylates. ER MW 340 allergy may have been due to impurities since it is believed that epoxy acrylates and ER MW 340 do not cross-react. More data about allergic contact dermatitis from DCR have been reported elsewhere [11].

References

1. Kanerva L, Estlander T, Jolanki R (1988) Occupational skin disease in Finland. An analysis of 10 years of statistics from an occupational dermatology clinic. Int Arch Occup Environ Health 60: 89–94
2. Cronin E (1980) Plastics. In: Contact dermatitis. Churchill Livingstone, Edinburgh, pp 585–587
3. Allardice JT (1967) Dermatitis due to an acrylic resin sealer. Trans St Johns Hosp Dermatol Soc 53: 86–89
4. Magnusson B, Mobacken H (1972) Contact allergy to a self-hardening acrylic sealer for assembling metal parts. Berufsdermatosen 20: 199–200
5. Jansen K (1975) Zur Häufigkeit und Prophylaxie allergischer Kontaktekzeme durch Acrylat-Klebstoffe. Arb Med Soc Med Prav 9: 206–207
6. Dempsey KJ (1982) Hypersensitivity to Sta-Lok and Loctite anaerobic sealants. J Am Acad Dermatol 7: 779–784
7. Mathias CG, Maibach HI (1984) Allergic contact dermatitis from anaerobic acrylic sealants. Arch Dermatol 120: 1202–1205
8. Soubrier R, Bresson JR, Chabeau G (1984) Manifestations d'intolérance aux cyanoacrylates. Arch Mal Prof 45: 6, 460–464
9. Ranchoff RE, Taylor JS (1985) Contact dermatitis to anaerobic sealants. J Am Acad Dermatol 13: 1015–1020

10. Kokelj F, Patussi V, Basei R, Marcolina M (1987) Contact dermatitis to Loctite 221 and 270. Contact Dermatitis 17: 51
11. Kanerva L, Estlander T, Jolanki R (1989) Allergic contact dermatitis from dental composite resins due to aromatic epoxy acrylates and aliphatic acrylates. Contact Dermatitis (in press)
12. Kanerva L, Estlander T, Jolanki R (1988) Sensitization to patch test acrylates. Contact Dermatitis 18: 10–15
13. Kanerva L, Jolanki R, Estlander T (1986) Occupational dermatitis due to an epoxy acrylate. Contact Dermatitis 14: 80–84

Addresses

L. Kanerva
Section of Dermatology, Institute of Occupational Health, Topeliuksenkatu 41 a A, SF-00250 Helsinki, Finland

T. Estlander
Section of Dermatology, Institute of Occupational Health, Topeliuksenkatu 41 a A, SF-00250 Helsinki, Finland

R. Jolanki
Section of Dermatology, Institute of Occupational Health, Topeliuksenkatu 41 a A, SF-00250 Helsinki, Finland

Contact Allergy to Cycloaliphatic Epoxy Resins

R. Jolanki, M.-L. Sysilampi, L. Kanerva, and T. Estlander

Summary

We have patch-tested 18 patients with skin symptoms who were exposed to cycloaliphatic epoxy resins (CA-ERs) in a factory where CA-ERs have been used to manufacture outdoor electrical insulators. The CA-ERs were Araldit CY 184 and Lekutherm X 100. Based on mass spectrometry and nuclear magnetic resonance (NMR) investigations, the CA-ERs were found to contain diglycidyl ester of hexahydrophthalic acid. Most of the patients were also exposed to diglycidyl ether of bisphenol A (DGEBA)-based epoxy resin modified by diglycidyl aniline (Lekutherm X 287). Insulators made of DGEBA-based epoxy resin are used for indoor mountings. The amount of DGEBA molecular weight (MW) 340 was 43% in Lekutherm X 287, and its highest concentration was 0.5% in CA-ERs. The highest total amount of nine reactive diluents [*n*-butyl glycidyl ether (GE), allyl GE, phenyl GE, cresyl GE, butanediol diglycidyl ether (DGE), hexanediol DGE, neopentyl glycol DGE, glycidyl ester of synthetic fatty acids (Cardura E 10), and glycidyl ether of aliphatic alcohols (Epoxide 8)] in the three epoxy resins was 0.4%. Diglycidyl ester of hexahydrophthalic acid was the main component of Araldit CY 184 and Lekutherm X 100, and the amounts were 50% (w/w) and 70% (w/w), respectively.

Patch tests were performed with the following epoxy compounds: DGEBA epoxy resin of standard series [1% petrolatum (pet.)]; the reactive diluents except butanediol DGE (0.25% pet.); and Araldit CY 184, Lekutherm X 100, and Lekutherm X 287 (each 1%, 0.3%, and 0.1% pet.). Of 18 patients, 12 showed allergic patch test reactions to CA-ERs (12 to Araldit CY 184 and 11 to Lekutherm X 100) and 7 patients to Lekutherm X 287, but only 1 patient to DGEBA epoxy resin. Of the 12 patients, 5 had patch test reactions to 1–4 of the diluents tested, possibly indicating cross-reactivity between CA-ERs and reactive diluents. Six patients had no allergic reactions to the epoxy compounds. None of the patients were allergic to the anhydride hardeners of the resins. The tests showed considerable irritation in 3 of 32 control patients with Araldit CY 184 and Lekutherm X 100 at the concentration of 1% pet., but lower concentrations provoked no reactions in the patients.

The present study indicates that CA-ERs are strong sensitizers in humans, and that CA-ER allergy is not revealed by testing with DGEBA epoxy resin. The most suitable test concentration for CA-ERs may be 0.5% pet. In most cases, minimization of exposure and certain industrial hygienic improvements will make it possible to continue work despite sensitization. The highest risk of exposure to CA-ERs occurs in the electrical industry, e.g., the manufacture of insulators.

Key words:

Cycloaliphatic epoxy resins - Diglycidyl ester of hexahydrophthalic acid - Occupational contact allergy - Electrical industry - Epoxy compounds

Introduction

Aromatic diglycidyl ether bisphenol A (DGEBA) epoxy resin, oligomer molecular weight (MW) 340, is a strong sensitizer. Epoxy-reactive diluents, both aliphatic and aromatic compounds, are moderate to strong sensitizers [10]. Based on their chemical structure, cycloaliphatic epoxy resins (CA-ERs) can be considered potential sensitizers, but little is known about their sensitizing capacity [3]. Epoxy resins of cycloaliphatic structure were initially investigated by Shell and Bayer in Europe [4]. These products have low viscosities and are highly reactive. A typical commercial product is based on hexahydrophthalic acid. In Finland, some 95% of outdoor electrical insulators are now made of cycloaliphatic epoxy resins. Here, we present 12 cases of contact allergy to cycloaliphatic epoxy resins containing the monomer diglycidyl ester of hexahydrophthalic acid (Fig. 1), MW 284. To our knowledge, only one report of contact allergy to diglycidyl ester of hexahydrophthalic acid has been published [1].

Materials and Methods

Patients. Of a total of 80 people working in a department manufacturing insulators from epoxy resins, 18 workers with present or previous skin eruptions participated in a dermatological investigation. We found 12 cases of contact allergy to CA-ERs.

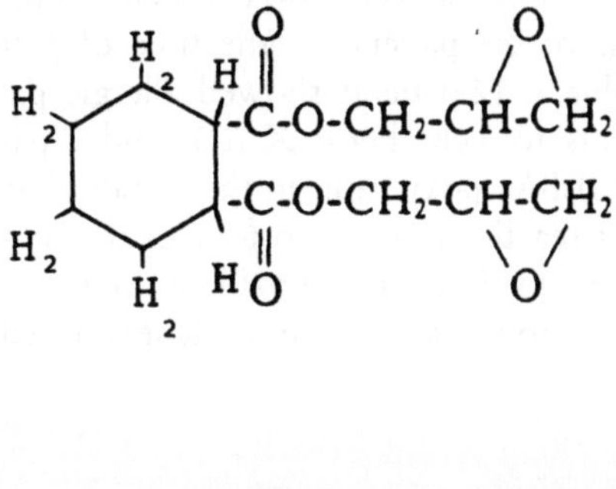

Fig. 1. *o*-Diglycidyl ester of hexahydrophthalic acid

Prick Tests. Using common environmental allergens [9], prick tests were performed only when the anamnesis gave reason to suspect atopy. The results were negative in 4 of the 12 patients tested.

Patch Tests. All of the patients were patch-tested, using Finn chambers, on the upper back; the occlusion time was 24 h. The tests were read at least 24 h and 72 h after removal of the chambers. In addition to the European standard series, containing epoxy resin (1% pet.), the patients were tested with five substances from the plastics and glue series (Epikon Oy, Finland): bisphenol A (1% pet.), epichlorohydrin (1% pet.), diaminodiphenyl methane (1% pet.), ethylene diamine (1% pet.), and triethylene tetramine (0.5% pet.). Epoxy-reactive diluents (see below), except butanediol diglycidyl ether (DGE), were patch-tested at 0.25% in pet. The three epoxy resins and four organic anhydride hardeners used in the factory were tested in dilution series (1%, 0.3%, and 0.1% pet.). The intensity of patch test reactions was scored as previously described [8]. Patch tests with the same epoxy resins were also performed for 32 unexposed control patients.

Epoxy Resins. According to the material safety sheets, Araldit CY 184 (Ciba-Geigy, Switzerland) is diglycidyl ester of hexahydrophthalic acid, Lekutherm X 100 (Bayer AG, FRG) a CA-ER with an average MW of less than 700, and Lekutherm X 287 (Bayer AG) an epoxy resin with an average MW of less than 700 and containing a plasticizer. Warnings about the risk of allergy were given in every case. Lekutherm X 100 and Araldit CY 184 were analyzed by mass spectrometry and nuclear magnetic resonance (NMR) investigations. The method will be published in detail elsewhere (M.L.Henriks-Eckerman, unpublished). The amounts of the monomer, bisphenol A-type epoxy resin oligomers, and nine reactive diluents [*n*-butyl glycidyl ether (GE), allyl GE, phenyl GE, cresyl GE, butanediol DGE, hexanediol DGE, neopentyl glycol DGE, glycidyl ester of synthetic fatty acids (Cardura E 10), and glycidyl ether of aliphatic alcohols (Epoxide 8)] in the three insulator resins were analyzed by gas chromatography (GC) and high-performance liquid chromatographic determination (HPLC), as described earlier [5–6].

Results

The results of the GC and HPLC studies on epoxy resins are summarized in Table 1. The main monomer was found to be diglycidyl ester of hexahydrophthalic acid. All of the 12 patients had hand dermatitis, 7 also having dermatitis on the face or neck. Nine were also exposed to diglycidyl aniline before the patch testing. Analysis of the patients at the time of patch testing is given in Table 2. As shown in Table 3, 12 patients showed allergic patch test reactions to Araldit CY 184, 11 patients to Lekutherm X 100, and 7 patients to Lekutherm X 287, but only 1 to DGEBA epoxy resin in the standard series. Five of the patients had positive patch test reactions to one to four of the diluents tested (Table 4). *n*-Butyl GE, allyl GE, Cardura E 10, and Epoxide 8 provoked no reactions. None of the patients were allergic to the anhydride hardeners tested.

Table 1. Amounts of diglycidyl ester of hexahydrophthalic acid, bisphenol A-type epoxy resin oligomers, and nine reactive diluents [6] in insulator resins

Substances	Amount (%)		
	Araldit CY 184	Lekutherm X 100	Lekutherm X 287
Diglycidyl ester of hexahydrophthalic acid MW 284[a]	About 50	About 70	–
Epoxy resin oligomers[b]			
MW 340	Below 0.002	0.5	43
MW 624	–	0.05	2.5
Reactive diluents[a]			
1,4-Butanediol diglycidyl ether	0.4	–	–
Glycidyl ethers of aliphatic alcohols	–	0.02	0.06

[a] Gas chromatography study.
[b] High-performance liquid chromatography study.

Of the 12 patients, 1 continued working despite persistent skin symptoms (case 8), and another (case 10) was able to work without symptoms until retirement. The symptoms of cases 2 and 4 disappeared after these patients changed jobs, becoming coil winders in the same department. Of the 12 patients, 5 were able to continue working with CA-ERs, and 3 others (cases 1, 3, and 11) were able to continue the working with indoor resins without symptoms, even though 2 of these 3 have contact allergy to Lekutherm X 287, the indoor resin (Table 3).

Control patch tests were performed for 32 patients. The testing showed considerable irritation in three cases with Araldit CY 184 and Lekutherm X 100 at the concentration of 1% pet., but 0.3% and 0.1% provoked no reactions.

Discussion

Contact allergy to CA-ERs was found in 12 cases. The actual allergen molecule was not purified, but it is obviously diglycidyl ester of hexahydrophthalic acid. The previously reported cases of allergic contact sensitization to diglycidyl ester of hexahydrophthalic acid were in fact due not to epoxy resins, but to a cutting oil containing the compound as an additive [1]. However, in our previous material, 3 of 71 epoxy-sensitized patients had an allergic reaction only to their own epoxy products, possibly because the reaction was due to a CA-ER compound [7]. The present study indicates that CA-ERs are strong sensitizers in humans. CA-ER allergy was not revealed by testing with DGEBA epoxy resins. Because of the irritation caused by CA-ERs in 1% pet., we prefer testing with 0.5% pet.

The test reactions to epoxy-reactive diluents possibly indicate cross-reactivity between CA-ERs and the diluents. Butanediol DGE was not included in the series of epoxy-reactive diluents when the 12 patients were patch-tested. Case 6 reacted only to Araldit CY 184, containing 0.4% of butanediol DGE (Tables 1, 3), but unlike our

Table 2. Details of the 12 patients at the time of patch testing

Case no.	Sex	Age (years)	Work at onset of first symptoms	Total duration of exposure at work site (years)	Exposure to CA-ERs		Exposure to aniline ER	
					Before symptoms	After symptoms	Before symptoms	After symptoms
1	Female	19	Casting	1	1 Month	2 Months	–	10 Months
2	Female	49	Casting	7	6 Months	6 Months	6 Months	6 Months
3	Female	45	Casting	11	1 Month	–	–	7 Years
4	Female	46	Casting	5	6 Months	–	4 Months	–
5	Male	46	Repair	10	4 Years	6 Years	4 Years	6 Years
6	Female	41	Casting	2	1 Week	2 Years	–	–
7	Female	41	Casting	2	6 Months	18 Months	6 Months	18 Months
8	Female	56	Finishing, Repair	6	4 Years	2 Years	4 Years	2 Years
9	Male	50	Maintenance	14	3 Years	7 Years	–	–
10	Female	59	Casting	6	6 Months	2 Years	–	3 Years
11	Female	51	Casting	2	3 Months	9 Months	–	1 Year
12	Female	40	Casting	1	6 Months	6 Months	–	–

CA-ERs, cycloaliphatic epoxy resins; ER, epoxy resin

Table 3. Results of patch tests with epoxy resins

Case no.	Results									
	Araldit CY 184			Lekutherm X 100			Lekutherm X 287			Standard series epoxy resin 1%
	1%	0.3%	0.1%	1%	0.3%	0.1%	1%	0.3%	0.1%	
1	++	+ ?	–	+++	+	–	–	–	–	–
2	++++	++++	++++	++++	++++	++++	++++	++++	++++	–
3	+++	++	+	+++	+++	++	++	–	–	–
4	++	++	++	++	++	+	++	++	+	+++
5	++	+	–	++	+ ?	–	+	+ ?	–	–
6	++	++	–	+ ?	+ ?	+ ?	–	–	–	–
7	++	++	–	++	+	–	++	–	–	–
8	+++	+++	+++	++	++	++	+++	++	++	–
9	++	++	–	+++	+ ?	–	–	–	–	–
10	++	++	+ ?	+++	+	+ ?	++	+	–	–
11	+++	+++	+++	+++	+++	+	+++	++	+ ?	–
12	++	+	+ ?	++	+	+	+ ?	–	–	–

Table 4. Results of patch tests with epoxy-reactive diluents

Substance	Positive cases	Score
1,6-Hexanediol diglycidyl ether (Grilonit RV 1812)	2	+ + +
	11	+ +
	8, 10	+ ?
Neopentyl glycol diglycidyl ether (Grilonit RV 1815)	2	+ + +
	11	+ +
	10, 12	+ ?
Phenyl glycidyl ether	2	+ +
	8, 11	+
	10, 12	+ ?
Cresyl glycidyl ether	11	+
	10	+ ?

Of the 12 patients, 7 had no reactions to the epoxy-reactive diluents tested.

previous butanediol DGE-sensitized patients this patient did not react to hexanediol DGE [6].

On the basis of more than 2 years of follow-up, most of the patients sensitized to CA-ERs were able to continue their work. One reason is that the casting workers are not heavily exposed, as they do not handle liquid resins, but "oven-fresh", heat-cured insulators made of epoxy resins that still contain uncured monomers. Another reason is the minimization of exposure, after identification of the cause of contact dermatitis, by the following procedures [2]:

1. Improvements in housekeeping and the general cleanliness of the work site
2. Improvements in local ventilation in order to prevent exposure to evaporated vapors during the curing process
3. Instructions on how to clean and care for the skin
4. Immediate treatment of skin symptoms
5. Clean, thick terry-cloth gloves and arm cuffs
6. Instructions on the proper use of barrier cream
7. Education of the workers.

References

1. English JSC, Foulds I, White IR, Rycroft RJG (1986) Allergic contact sensitization to the glycidyl ester of hexahydrophthalic acid in a cutting oil. Contact Dermatitis 15: 66–68
2. Estlander T, Jolanki R (1988) How to protect the hands. Dermatol Clin 6: 105–114
3. Fregert S (1987) Contact dermatitis from epoxy resin systems. In: Maibach HI (ed) Occupational and industrial dermatology. Year Book medical, Chicago, pp 341–345
4. Gannon JA (1986) History and development of epoxy resins. Polymer Preprints 27: 188–190
5. Jolanki R, Estlander T, Henriks-Eckerman M-L, Kanerva L, Stjernvall T (1988) Skin protection and sensitizing epoxy compounds in electron microscopy laboratories. In: Mansdorf SZ, Sager

R, Nielsen AP (eds) Peformance of protective clothing: Second symposium, ASTM STP 989. American Society for Testing and Materials, Philadelphia, 1988: 389–395
6. Jolanki R, Estlander T, Kanerva L (1987) Contact allergy to an epoxy reactive diluent: 1,4-butanediol diglycidyl ether. Contact Dermatitis 16: 87–92
7. Jolanki R, Estlander T, Kanerva L (1987) Occupational contact dermatitis and contact urticaria caused by epoxy resins. Acta Derm Venereol (Stockh) [Suppl] 134: 99–94
8. Kanerva L, Estlander T, Jolanki R (1989) Allergic contact dermatitis from dental composite resins due to aromatic epoxy acrylates and aliphatic acrylates. Contact Dermatitis (in press)
9. Kanerva L, Tupasela O, Jolanki R, Vaheri E, Estlander T, Keskinen H (1988) Occupational allergic rhinitis from guar gum. Clin Allergy 18: 245–252
10. Thorgeirsson A (1978) Sensitization capacity of epoxy reactive diluents in the guinea pig. Acta Derm Venereol (Stockh) 58: 329–331

Addresses

R. Jolanki
Section of Dermatology, Institute of Occupational Health, Topeliuksenkatu 41 aA, SF-00250 Helsinki, Finland

M.-L. Sysilampi
Department of Dermatology, Vaasa Central Hospital, SF-65130 Vaasa, Finland

L. Kanerva
Section of Dermatology, Institute of Occupational Health, Topeliuksenkatu 41 aA, SF-00250 Helsinki, Finland

T. Estlander
Section of Dermatology, Institute of Occupational Health, Topeliuksenkatu 41 aA, SF-00250 Helsinki, Finland

Allergic Contact Dermatitis from Isocyanates

L. Kanerva, M.-T. Lähteenmäki, T. Estlander, R. Jolanki, and H. Keskinen

Summary

An allergological examination, including prick tests, scratch chamber tests, patch tests, and RAST tests, was performed in 83 consecutive patients exposed to isocyanates. Three cases of allergic contact dermatitis from isocyanates have been detected: the first patient was allergic to isophorone diisocyanate and trimethyl hexamethylene diisocyanate, the second to 4,4′-diphenylmethane diisocyanate (MDI) and toluene 2,4-diisocyanate (TDI), and the third to HDI and its prepolymer Desmodur-N. To our knowledge, this was the first patient reported to have allergic contact dermatitis from HDI. The optimal patch test concentrations were 2%–5% in petrolatum for TDI and MDI, and 0.1%–0.2% in petrolatum for HDI, whereas 0.5% was irritant.

Key words:

Epicutaneous test - Occupation - Allergic rhinitis - Asthma - Scratch chamber test

Introduction

Isocyanates are extensively used in the manufacture of foams, films, elastomeric fibers, and surface coatings. Exposure to isocyanate resins occurs among spray painters, manufacturing workers, lacquer and adhesive workers, insulation installers, and those accidentally exposed to the pyrolysis products. Pulmonary irritation and sensitization is the chief hazard. Obstructive lung disease may result from prolonged exposure to isocyanates. The chief pulmonary sensitizers are toluene 2,4-diisocyanate (TDI), 4,4′-diphenylmethane diisocyanate (MDI), and 1,6-hexamethylene diisocya-

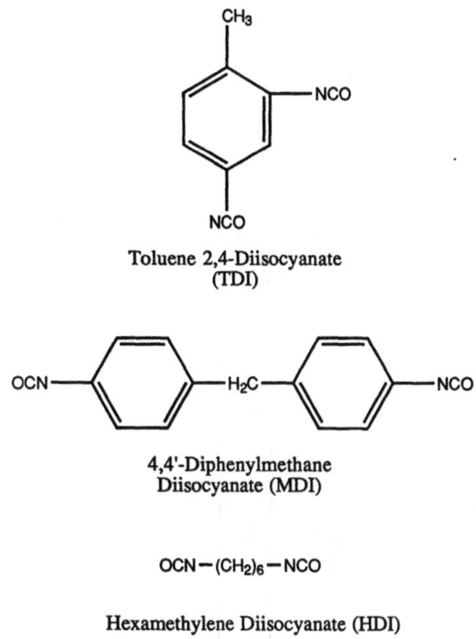

Fig. 1. The structural formulas of the most commonly used isocyanate resins

nate (HDI) (Fig. 1). Isocyanates are skin irritants, but only rare cases of allergic contact dermatitis have been reported. Here, we briefly review the previous cases of allergic contact dermatitis from isocyanates (Table 1, [1–12]) and present all our own cases ($n = 3$) detected thus far. We also present data on skin testing in order to detect immediate allergy to isocyanates.

Patients and Methods

Our first case of allergic contact dermatitis from isocyanates was detected in 1974. In 1983–1986, 83 consecutive patients with suspected occupational diseases caused by isocyanates were skin-tested. The symptoms were contact dermatitis ($n = 21$), urticaria and/or fever ($n = 5$), asthma ($n = 60$), rhinitis ($n = 17$), conjunctivitis ($n = 2$), and laryngitis ($n = 1$). All patients were patch- and scratch chamber-tested: the epicutaneous tests were read on removal (24-h occlusion) and 24, 48, and 96–120 h after removal (see [3]). The patch test concentrations in petrolatum (pet.) were as follows: TDI, MDI, and Desmodur-N (Bayer, FRG) 5%, 2%, and 1%; and HDI 0.5%, 0.2%, and 0.1%. In 20 unexposed control persons tested with these isocyanates at the above-mentioned concentrations, the results were negative. Scratch chamber tests [14] were performed with 1% TDI, MDI, HDI, and Desmodur-N in pet. The tests were read after 30 min. A reaction of 3 mm or more was considered positive. Specific IgE to isocyanates (MDI, HDI, and TDI) was determined with Phadezym RAST technique (see [14]) in some, but not all, cases.

Table 1. Patch test concentrations and reported cases of allergic contact dermatitis caused by isocyanates

Reference	Patch test concentration/vehicle (%)									Allergic contact dermatitis to isocyanates or hydralysis products of isocyanates *(n)*
	HDI	MDI	TDI	DMDI	IPDI	PAPI	TMDI	MDA	TDA	
[1]	–	1 Acet	–	–	–	–	–	–	–	1 MDI
[2]	–	–	Pure	–	–	–	–	–	–	–
[3]	–	–	1–3 Acet	–	–	–	–	–	–	1 TDI
[4]	–	–	0.5 Acet	–	–	–	0.5 Acet	–	–	1 TMDI
[5]	–	–	1 Pet	1 Oo	–	–	–	1 Oo	1 Oo	2 DMDI/MDA
[6]	–	2, 5 Acet	1 Acet	–	1 Acet	3, 5 Acet	–	0.5, 1 Acet	1 Pet	7 MDI/PAPI, 4 IPDI
[7]	–	1 Alc	1 Alc	1 Alc	1 Alc	–	–	–	–	1 DMDI
[8]	–	–	–	–	1 Alc	–	–	–	–	4 IPDI (cross-sensitivity between IPD and IPDI)
[9]	–	(30%–70% MDI) 2 Mek	–	–	–	–	–	0.5 Pet	–	1 MDI/MDA
[10]	–	–	–	1 Pet	–	–	–	–	–	2 DMDI
[11]	–	–	1 Pet	1 Pet	–	–	–	0.1 Oo	–	–
[12]	–	1, 2 Mek	–	–	–	–	–	0.5 Pet	–	1 MDA

Abbreviations: Mek, methyl ethyl ketone; Pet, petrolatum; Acet, acetone; Oo, olive oil; Alc, ethanol; HDI, 1,6-hexamethylene diisocyanate; MDI, 4,4′-diphenylmethane diisocyanate; TDI, toluene 2,4-diisocyanate; DMDI, dicyclohexylmethane 4,4′-diisocyanate; IPDI, isophorone diisocyanate; PAPI, polymethylene polyphenyl isocyanate; TMDI, trimethyl hexamethylene diisocyanate; MDA, 4,4′-diaminodiphenyl methane; TDA, toluene diamine; IPD, isophorone diamine

Results and Discussion

Of the 34 patients with isocyanate-induced asthma and/or rhinitis, only 1 was positive to isocyanates in scratch chamber tests [with TDI (3 mm) and HDI (3 mm), confirmed with positive RASTs]. Our first patient diagnosed (in 1974) as having allergic contact dermatitis due to isocyanates was a 30-year-old female laboratory technician, who had been exposed to isophorone diisocyanate (IPDI) and trimethyl hexamethylene diisocyanate (TMDI) for 1.5 years before she developed eczema on her thighs and chin. She had used protective gloves, and her hands were unaffected. In patch testing, she gave a 3+ reaction to 0.1% IPDI in pet. and a 2+ reaction to 0.1% and 0.2% TMDI in pet.

Of the 83 patients patch-tested, 2 had positive patch test reactions to isocyanates. Case 1 was a 28-year-old nonatopic woman, who, after 2 months of polyurethane spraying, developed a strongly itching dermatitis on her hands and respiratory symptoms soon afterwards. Patch tests with MDI (5%, 2%, and 1%) and TDI (5% and 2%) gave a 2+ to 3+ positive allergic reaction, while 1% TDI and HDI were negative. Diaminodiphenylmethane, a degradation product of isocyanate, was positive. MDI was positive in an open test. Inhalation provocation tests proved that she had MDI-induced asthma.

Table 2. Patch, scratch chamber, and prick test results in the patient allergic to 1,6-hexamethylene diisocyanate (HDI)

Test	Results		
	1st Session	2nd Session	3rd Session
Patch tests			
HDI			
0.5%	++		
0.2%	++	++	++
0.1%	+(+)	++	++
0.05%		++	++
0.02%		+	+
Desmodur-N			
20%	++		
10%	++		
5%	+		
2%	+		
1%			
TDI 5%, 2%, 1%	–		
MDI 5%, 2%, 1%	–		
Hardener[a]			
20%		++	
10%		+	
5%		(+)	
2%		–	
Standard series	–		
Scratch chamber tests (HDI, MDI, TDI)	–		
Prick tests (standard series)	–		

TDI, toluene 2,4-diisocyanate; MDI, 4,4′-diphenylmethane diisocyanate
[a] Containing 0.8% HDI.

Case 2 was a 50-year-old nonatopic male car painter, using paints containing HDI. After 6 months of exposure, he developed dermatitis on his hands; respiratory symptoms developed 2 years later. The patient was patch-tested three times to confirm the diagnosis (Table 2). HDI gave a positive patch test with 0.1% and later with 0.02%. Desmodur-N and the hardener (Z 50, Lesonal GmbH, Stuttgart, FRG) of the paint, containing 0.8% HDI, also gave positive reactions. The patient had HDI-induced asthma as well. HDI-, MDI-, and TDI-RASTs were negative. To our knowledge, this is the first reported case of allergic contact dermatitis caused by HDI.

The present study indicates that scratch chamber tests with isocyanate test substances in pet. are not useful in the diagnosis of isocyanate-induced respiratory diseases. Patch tests should be performed when allergic contact dermatitis is suspected. The commercial patch test substances TDI and MDI, 0.1% in pet. (Chemotechnique, Sweden), might be used at too low concentrations. Our TDI-allergic patient had a negative patch test with 1% TDI in pet.

References

1. Fregert S (1967) Allergic contact reaction to diphenyl-4,4'di-isocyanate. Contact Dermatitis Newsletter 2: 35
2. Wodniansky P (1967) Hautschäden bei der Erzeugung von Polyurethan-Kunststoffen. Berufsdermatosen 15: 81–92
3. Peschel H (1970) Hautveränderungen durch Isozyanate (Desmodur). Derm Monatsschr 156: 691–697
4. Hjorth N (1975) Dermatitis from trimethyl hexamethylene di-isocyanate. Contact Dermatitis 1: 59
5. Emmett E (1976) Allergic contact dermatitis in polyurethane plastic moulders. J Occup Med 18: 802–804
6. Rothe A (1976) Zur Frage arbeitsbedingter Hautschädigungen durch Polyurethanchemikalien. Berufsdermatosen 24: 7–24
7. Malten KE (1977) 4,4'-diisocyanato dicyclohexyl methane (Hylene W): a strong contact sensitizer. Contact Dermatitis 3: 344–346
8. LaChapelle JM, LaChapelle-Ketelaer MJ (1979) Cross-sensitivity between isopropone diamine (IPD) and isopropone diisocyanate (IPDI). Contact Dermatitis 5: 55
9. Lidén C (1980) Allergic contact dermatitis from 4,4'di-isocyanate-di-phenylmetane (MDI) in a molder. Contact Dermatitis 6: 301–302
10. White IR, Stewart JR, Rycroft RJG (1983) Allergic contact dermatitis from an organic di-isocyanate. Contact Dermatitis 9: 300–303
11. Fisher AA (1986) Contact dermatitis, 3rd edn. Lea and Febiger, Philadelphia, pp 562–565
12. Alomar A (1986) Contact dermatitis from a fashion watch. Contact Dermatitis 15: 44–45
13. Kanerva L, Estlander T, Jolanki R (1989) Allergic contact dermatitis from dental composite resins due to aromatic epoxy acrylates and aliphatic acrylates. Contact Dermatitis (in press)
14. Kanerva L, Tupasela O, Jolanki R, Vaheri E, Estlandet T, Keskinen H (1988) Occupational allergic rhinitis from guar gum. Clin Allergy 18: 245–252

Addresses

L. Kanerva
Section of Dermatology, Institute of Occupational Health, Topeliuksenkatu 41 a A, SF-00250 Helsinki, Finland

M.-T. Lähteenmäki
Section of Dermatology, Institute of Occupational Health, Topeliuksenkatu 41 a A, SF-00250 Helsinki, Finland

T. Estlander
Section of Dermatology, Institute of Occupational Health, Topeliuksenkatu 41 a A, SF-00250 Helsinki, Finland

R. Jolanki
Section of Dermatology, Institute of Occupational Health, Topeliuksenkatu 41 a A, SF-00250 Helsinki, Finland

H. Keskinen
Section of Dermatology, Institute of Occupational Health, Topeliuksenkatu 41 a A, SF-00250 Helsinki, Finland

Experiences of Contact Dermatitis Associated with Phenol Formaldehyde Resins

M. H. Beck

Summary

Ten cases of contact dermatitis (four irritant and six allergic) associated with the usage of phenol formaldehyde resins (PFR) are described. The affected subjects include six foundry workers, two aircraft construction workers and one analytical chemist. An additional patient, thought to have been sensitised from a hearing aid, is also described. It is concluded that persons with suspected dermatitis to PFR should be tested with their own resin. PFR 11-452 was also a reliable indicator of PFR allergy in our cases. PFRs supplied by Hermal for patch testing were poor indicators of sensitisation. There was no concomitant sensitivity with formaldehyde or cross-reactivity with PTBP formaldehyde resin.

Key words:

Phenol formaldehyde resins - Dermatitis - Irritant - Allergic

Introduction

Phenol formaldehyde resin (PFR) polymers are formed by a combination of formaldehyde and phenol or a mixture of phenols. The resins are particularly resistant to heat and good insulators against electricity. They are, therefore, widely utilised in electrical appliances and in the domestic environment. They are used as glues and laminates in the building, boat and aircraft construction industry. Their binding and adhesive properties result in their presence in foundry sand moulds, brake linings and clutch facings [1].

Case Reports

Dermatitis from Resinated Sand Affecting Moulders and Coremakers at a Foundry

Foundry sand itself contains PFR and furfuryl alcohol. It is hardened with phosphoric acid or sulphonic acid derivatives. Once used, it is broken up and recycled.

Irritant contact dermatitis was identified in four persons with hand dermatitis, all with negative patch tests to PFR. Recycling of the hardened sand may be contributory.

Two patients (cases 1 and 2) with *allergic contact dermatitis* were identified. Case 1, with dermatitis of the hands, was allergic to formaldehyde. Case 2, with an exposure pattern rash with generalised secondary spread, was shown to be allergic to his PFR.

Allergic Contact Dermatitis from Resinated Laminates

Two patients (cases 3 and 4), aircraft construction workers with hand dermatitis, were shown to be allergic to PFR which impregnated resinated laminates handled before they were hardened.

Allergic Contact Dermatitis from Chemicals Used in Brake Linings

One patient (case 5), an analytical chemist with an exposure pattern dermatitis, was allergic to a combination of PFR, cashew nut formaldehyde resin and cashew nut oil. He worked for a company producing brakes and handled these materials in his work.

Presumed Allergic Contact Dermatitis to a Hearing Aid

One patient (case 6) with chronic otitis externa confined to the ear where she wore a hearing aid was allergic to a combination of PFR and benzoyl peroxide; however, the clinical relevance was unproven.

The significant patch test results of this and the other five allergically sensitised subjects are described in Table 1.

Table 1. Results of patch tests in six allergic subjects

Test substance	Case					
	1	2	3	4	5	6
Formaldehyde (1%–2% aq)	++	Neg	Neg	Neg	Neg	Neg
Own resin (1%–5% pet)	Neg	++	++	++	++	++
Resin 11-452 (5% pet)	Neg	NT	++	++	++	++
PFR acid catalysed (5% pet)[a]	Neg	Neg	Neg	Neg	Neg	Neg
PFR alkali catalysed (5% pet)[a]	Neg	Neg	Neg	+	Neg	Neg
PTBP formaldehyde resin (1% pet)	Neg	Neg	Neg	Neg	Neg	Neg

aq, aqua; pet, petrolatum; Neg, negative
[a] Supplied by Hermal.

Discussion

Irritant contact dermatitis to PFR powder has been described [2], but I am not aware of previous reports of dermatitis to resinated sand. The affected subjects all indicated that they felt the recycling process may have been responsible at least in part.

Allergic contact dermatitis to PFR is well recognised and has been thoroughly reviewed by Bruze [1], who has identified several sensitising components within the resin. He has sent us a resin (PFR 11-452) which is clearly superior to those available from Hermal at tracing contact allergy: it has been successful in identifying all our PFR-sensitised patients tested with it. It would, nevertheless, seem wise in view of the heterogeneity of these resins that individuals should also be tested with their own resins. There has been no cross-reactivity between PFR and PTBP, and no concomitant sensitivity with formaldehyde.

Acknowledgements. I am grateful to Dr. Magnus Bruze of Lund, Sweden, for kindly supplying the PFR 11-452 with which to test our patients.

References

1. Bruze M (1985) Contact sensitisors in resins based on phenol and formaldehyde. Acta Derm Venereol [Suppl] 119: 1–83
2. Fregert S (1980) Irritant dermatitis from phenol formaldehyde resin powder. Contact Dermatitis 6: 493

Addresses

M. H. Beck
The Skin Hospital, Quay Street, Manchester M3 3HL, UK

Contact Dermatitis to Epoxy Resins in Composite Material

G. Lembo, N. Balato, F. Cusano, A. Baldo, and F. Ayala

Summary

An outbreak of allergic contact dermatitis in an aircraft factory where epoxy resin-impregnated materials were employed has been investigated. Of 30 operatives, 20 gave positive reactions to the composite material. In these patients, patch tests with epoxy resin 1% (Firma) gave a positive reaction in only four cases. Patch tests with diglycidyl ether of bisphenol A (DGEBA), tetraglycidyl-4-4′-methylene dianiline (TGMDA), triglycidyl derivative of *p*-aminophenol (TGPAP) and *o*-diglycidyl phthalate were performed in 18 of the patients. TGMDA, TGPAP and *o*-diglycidyl phthalate picked up all the 11 patients positive to the composite materials.

These data confirm that the composite materials must be used as is for patch testing due to the unreliability of the tests performed with common epoxy resin 1% in petrolatum. In addition, they indicate that TGMDA, TGPAP and *o*-diglycidyl phthalate, which are new constituents of carbon fibre epoxy resin system, can be used in order to reveal the sensitization.

Key words:

Contact dermatitis - Epoxy resin composite material - Aircraft industry - Triglycidyl derivative of *p*-aminophenol

Introduction

An outbreak of dermatitis which occurred in an aircraft factory using epoxy resin composite material has recently been reported by Burrows et al. [1]. The authors stressed that epoxy resins other than those of bisphenol A type are at present used in many factories producing materials characterized by great strength with lightness.

Carbon fibre impregnated with epoxy resin systems may contain potential sensitizers which are not included in routine patch test series. This report describes a series of contact dermatitis in an Italian aircraft industry where carbon fibre epoxy systems are used.

Materials and Methods

The aircraft factory concerned has about 2900 employees, 200 of whom handle carbon fibre impregnated with epoxy resins daily. The resins and other constituents are premixed and impregnated into the carbon fibre and supplied to the workers in the form of a slightly damp pliable cloth. Up to 1982, such materials were manually smeared on moulds for making light-aircraft components such as wings and rudders.

In this factory, an outbreak of dermatitis occurred in 1981 [3]; 20 workers developed rashes, mostly located on the hands and forearms, but also on the eyelids and face, and very occasionally also on genitalia and thighs. The severity of the symptoms varied widely from slight erythema to strong oedematovesicular lesions. These patients were patch-tested with the International Contact Dermatitis Research Group (ICDRG) standard battery, including epoxy resin 1% petrolatum (pet.) (Firma SpA, Florence, Italy), and with the composite materials handled in the factory. No positive reaction was obtained to the commercial haptens, but 13 patients strongly reacted to 3–11 composite materials. Composite materials not impregnated with epoxy resins gave no reactions; moreover, all raw materials were tested in 8 healthy volunteers, with negative results.

Since 1982, industrial processing of such materials has been automatized in part, and contact allergy has become rare in this particular factory. Nevertheless, ten more workers developed dermatitis. They were patch-tested with the above-mentioned haptens, and seven reacted only to the composite materials.

Recently, 11 of the 20 positive patients and 7 of the 10 negative ones have been available for retesting with single constituents of the carbon fibre epoxy system. In the composite material, diglycidyl ether of bisphenol A (DGEBA); diaminodiphenyl sulphone (DDS); dicyandiamide; boron trifluorine monoethylamine complex; hexamethylenetetramine; dichlorophenyl-1,1′-dimethyl urea; 1,1′-(2,4-toline)-bis-(3,3′-dimethyl urea); 1,1′-(1,2-phenylene)-bis-(3,3′-dimethyl urea); and 1-(*p*-chlorophenyl)-3,3′-dimethyl urea were known to be present. The last three substances mentioned were not available for testing; the other ones were all used for patch testing at a concentration of 1% (w/w) pet. Due to the presence of other unknown constituents, methylene dianiline (1% pet.); bisphenol A (0.5% pet.); epichloridrin (1% pet.); phthalic anhydride (1% pet.); dibutyl phthalate (5% pet.); and allyl-, butyl- and phenylglycidyl ether (each at 1% pet.) were also tested (all furnished by Firma SpA). Finally, in accordance with Burrows et al. [1], *o*-diglycidyl phthalate (1% acetone), tetraglycidyl-4,4′-methylene dianiline (TGMDA) (1.25% acetone) and triglycidyl derivative of *p*-aminophenol (TGPAP) (0.82% acetone) were also tested. Patch tests were performed with Al test on Scanpor following standard procedures.

Table 1. Patch test reactions in 11 subjects

Substance	Reactions										
	1	2	3	4	5	6	7	8	9	10	11
Epoxy resin	–	+	–	–	+	–	–	+	+	–	–
Diglycidyl ether of bisphenol A	+	+	+	+	+	–	–	+	+	–	–
Bisphenol A	–	–	–	–	–	–	–	+	–	–	–
o-Diglycidyl phthalate	–	+	–	+	+	+	–	–	+	–	+
Tetraglycidyl-4,4′-methylene dianiline	+	+	–	+	+	+	+	–	+	+	+
Triglycidyl derivative of *p*-aminophenol	+	+	+	+	+	+	+	+	+	+	–
Phenylglycidyl ether	–	+	+	+	+	–	–	–	+	–	–
Methylene dianiline	–	–	+	+	–	–	+	–	+	–	–
Composite epoxy material	+	+	+	+	+	+	+	+	+	+	–

Results

The results are summarized in Table 1. The seven patients who had not reacted to composite materials did not show any positive reactions; they are not included in Table 1. Of the 11 patients with positive reactions to composite materials, only 7 reacted to DGEBA, the molecular weight (MW) 340 oligomer of epoxy resin of bisphenol A type. Of these seven, four also reacted to epoxy resin, a mixture of oligomers with different MW, with an average MW lower than that of the epoxy resin used in standard patch tests in recent years. A patient who reacted to DGEBA and epoxy resin also reacted slightly (+) to bisphenol A. Of the other known constituents of the carbon fibre epoxy system, only methylene dianiline gave four positive reactions. Dichlorodiphenyl-1,1′-dimethyl urea gave strong irritative reactions in the first five patients and was no longer tested. TGPAP (10 positive reactions), TGMDA (9 positive reactions) and *o*-diglycidyl phthalate (6 positive reactions) picked up all the 11 patients, including the 4 DGEBA-negative ones. Finally, phenylglycidyl ether gave five positive reactions.

Discussion

The data obtained indicate that only the composite materials picked up the sensitivity in all the patients and can be used as is for patch testing. In our series, DGEBA picked up 7 (63.6%) of 11 sensitivities. Mixtures of oligomers with a higher MW have no role in patch tests, as well as bisphenol A and epichloridrin [2]. *o*-Diglycidyl phthalate, TGMDA and TGPAP together picked up all the epoxy resin sensitivities, even if they were not known as constituents of the carbon fibre epoxy resin system. According to the results of Burrows et al. [1], our data possibly indicate that the last three substances cross-react neither with each other nor with DGEBA.

This report stresses the role of patch testing with composite materials in epoxy resin systems; it also indicates that TGPAP, TGMDA and *o*-diglycidyl phthalate may be unknown constituents of such systems in the industry, especially within aerospace factories. To our knowledge, this report is the first that deals with the relationship between contact allergy and TGPAP.

Addendum

Thin-layer chromatography (TLC) was recently carried out in order to investigate the composition of the carbon fibre epoxy resin system. Using TGMDA, DDS and methylene dianiline as standards, we showed that these three substances were probably present in the composite materials. Further characterization is now being done.

Acknowledgements. The authors are indebted to Prof. S. Fregert for kindly supplying TGMDA, TGPAP and *o*-diglycidyl phthalate.

References

1. Burrows D, Fregert S, Campbell H, Trulsson L (1984) Contact dermatitis from the epoxy resins tetraglycidyl-4,4′-methylene dianiline and *o*-diglycidyl phthalate in composite material. Contact Dermatitis 11: 80–82
2. Fregert S, Thorgeirsson A (1977) Patch testing with low molecular oligomers of epoxy resins in humans. Contact Dermatitis 3: 301–303
3. Lembo G, Balato N, Cusano F, Ayala F (1983) Dermatiti da contatto da resine epossidiche in una industria aeronautica. Riv Med Lav Ig Ind 7: 57–64

Addresses

G. Lembo
Clinica Dermatologica, II Facoltà di Medicina, via S. Pansini 5, 80131 Naples, Italy

N. Balato
Clinica Dermatologica, II Facoltà di Medicina, via S. Pansini 5, 80131 Naples, Italy

F. Cusano
Clinica Dermatologica, II Facoltà di Medicina, via S. Pansini 5, 80131 Naples, Italy

A. Baldo
Clinica Dermatologica, II Facoltà di Medicina, via S. Pansini 5, 80131 Naples, Italy

F. Ayala
Clinica Dermatologica, II Facoltà di Medicina, via S. Pansini 5, 80131 Naples, Italy

Local Cutaneous Signs of Stainless Steel Hip Prosthesis Rejection in a Patient Sensitive to Hydroquinone (a Constituent of Implant Bone Cement)

F. Grimalt, J. Vilaplana, and C. Romaguera

A 71-year-old female patient underwent a metal-to-metal hip prosthesis implant for degenerative arthrosis 5 years ago. Subacute eczema appeared 1 year ago (20 cm by 8 cm, centred on the implant scar). Eczema improved with local treatment, only to reappear on cessation of treatment.

The patch test results were as follows:

1. Standard series showed positivity to only phenyl-*n*-cyclohexyl PPD, phenyl-*n*-isopropyl PPD, diphenyl PPD and hydroquinone (the four allergens gave a + +, + + response).
2. Allergens of plastic and glues series were negative.
3. Photographic products series showed only hydroquinone + +, + +.
4. Organic dyes series was negative.
5. Textile dyes series was negative.
6. Eleven acrylate derivative allergens for prostheses allergy tests were negative.

The bone cement used was CMW3 Bone Cement (CMW Laboratories Ltd., Exeter, Devon, UK). It is supplied as a packet of powder and one ampoule. The powder contains 88.18% polymethyl methacrylate, 2.72% residual peroxide and 9.10% barium sulphate. The ampoule contains 98.215% monomethyl methacrylate, 0.816% *N*: *N*-dimethyl-*p*-toluidine, 0.945% ethyl alcohol, 0.004% ascorbic acid and 0.002% hydroquinone.

The patient came on appointment 6 months later for further patch testing. Eczema persisted in spite of continued topical treatment with steroids. Apart from eczema, the implant was well tolerated. *p*-Toluidine patch test (2% petrolatum) was negative. Localization of the eczema on the implant scar and its persistence led us to suspect that the eczema was due to the implant. Usually, in allergy to implants many factors are to be considered. This patient does not react to patch tests, either to nickel or to acrylate allergens series. We have found allergy only to black-rubber allergens and to hydroquinone. Cross-reactions between black-rubber allergens, to which the patient is sensitized, and *p*-toluidine, a constituent of the bone cement liquid, can be accepted as possible. But the patient shows negative patch tests to both PPD and *p*-toluidine. There is no doubt that the patient is allergic to hydroquinone, as patch test positivity to this substance has been found twice: by standard series allergens and by photographic series ones.

Addresses

F. Grimalt
Department of Dermatology, University of Barcelona, Barcelona, Spain

J. Vilaplana
Department of Dermatology, University of Barcelona, Barcelona, Spain

C. Romaguera
Department of Dermatology, University of Barcelona, Barcelona, Spain

Part 4

Irritant Contact Dermatitis

Irritant Contact Dermatitis

P. J. Frosch

Summary

The current concept of irritant dermatitis and hyperirritable skin is reviewed. Irritant dermatitis is at least as frequent as allergic contact dermatitis, although reliable data are still very limited. Irritant contact dermatitis is a non-immunologic inflammatory reaction of the skin. The acute type usually only has a single cause, whereas chronic cumulative insult dermatitis is a multifactorial disease. Toxic chemicals (irritants) are the major cause, but mechanical, thermal, and climatic influences are important cofactors. Wet work, detergents and organic solvents are the major causes of irritation. The clinical spectrum of irritant contact dermatitis is much more variable than that of allergic contact dermatitis and ranges from drying and scaling of the stratum corneum to erythema, edema, whealing, papules, and pustules up to a full eczematous condition virtually indistinguishable from allergic contact dermatitis.

Individual susceptibility to irritants is extremely variable. Individuals with dry or hyperirritable skin, particularly atopics, are prone to develop a cumulative insult dermatitis. Subjects with hyperirritable skin have a thin and/or permeable stratum corneum with a small surface area of corneocytes. The effects of irritants on cutaneous targets are extremely variable and depend on the type of chemical, concentration, and mode of exposure. Inflammatory mechanisms include damage of cellular membranes, release of lysosomal enzymes, degranalution of mast cells, activation of polymorphonuclear leukocytes, and release of prostaglandins, leukotrienes, and kinins.

Useful techniques for the quantification of the irritant response are the measurement of transepidermal water loss by evaporimetry and the cutaneous blood flow by laser Doppler flowmetry.

Key words:

Irritation - Pathomechanisms - Hyperirritable skin - Noninvasive techniques - Stratum corneum

Definition

Irritant contact dermatitis may be defined as a nonimmunologic inflammatory reaction of the skin. The acute type, also called *irritant reaction*, usually has only a single cause, whereas the chronic form is a multifactorial disease. Toxic chemicals *(irritants)* are the major cause, but mechanical, thermal and climatic factors are important contributing cofactors. The clinical spectrum of irritant contact dermatitis is much more variable than that of allergic contact dermatitis and ranges from slight scaling of the stratum corneum to redness, whealing, and deep caustic burns, up to an eczematous condition indistinguishable from allergic contact dermatitis. Acute forms of irritant contact dermatitis may be painful and may be associated with sensations such as burning, stinging, or itching. Individual susceptibility to irritants is extremely variable.

Clinical Picture

The morphology of cutaneous lesions in irritant contact dermatitis is extremely variable and depends on the type and intensity of the irritant. Subtle changes in the form of scaling or drying may affect only the horny layer, but more intense reactions may involve redness, edema, and infiltration. Strong irritants such as caustic acids or alkalis produce blistering or ulcerative lesions with scar formation. In chronic forms of contact dermatitis such as hand eczema it is more or less characteristic that real polymorphism of allergic contact dermatitis is absent. There is rather pseudopolymorphism, which means that macules, papules, and vesicles are not present simultaneously but develop consecutively during the time course of inflammation. In chronic irritant hand eczema the skin is usually red and thickened and the stratum corneum shows scaling and fissuring in the most exposed regions, usually the thumb and index and ring fingers of the right hand in right-handed persons. Vesicles are usually absent but may be present, particularly in so-called *hybrids,* i.e., combined forms of irritant and allergic types, or in irritant and atopic hand eczema. These cases represent major problems in differential diagnosis.

Figure 1 illustrates the clinical spectrum of irritant contact dermatitis. Table 1 lists dermatoses where irritant factors play a major or contributing role.

Irritant reactions are most often to occupational materials, cosmetics, or dermatological therapeutics and are well known. Reactions to body excretions include diaper dermatitis and perianal dermatitis. Irritation by adhesive plaster is nonallergic in most cases. Textiles and fabrics frequently cause rashes that are thought to be allergic but later turn out to be of irritant nature. Dooms-Goossens et al. [6] and Lachapelle et al. [26] have collected a long list of airborne irritants that cause irritant dermatitis (Table 2).

A cold winter climate causes drying of the skin with pruritic patchy eczematous lesions, particularly in atopics. This condition is also frequently seen in persons who work in climatized rooms at high temperatures and low humidity (for example, manufacturing of electronic equipment) [50]. Eye lid eczema is frequently not aller-

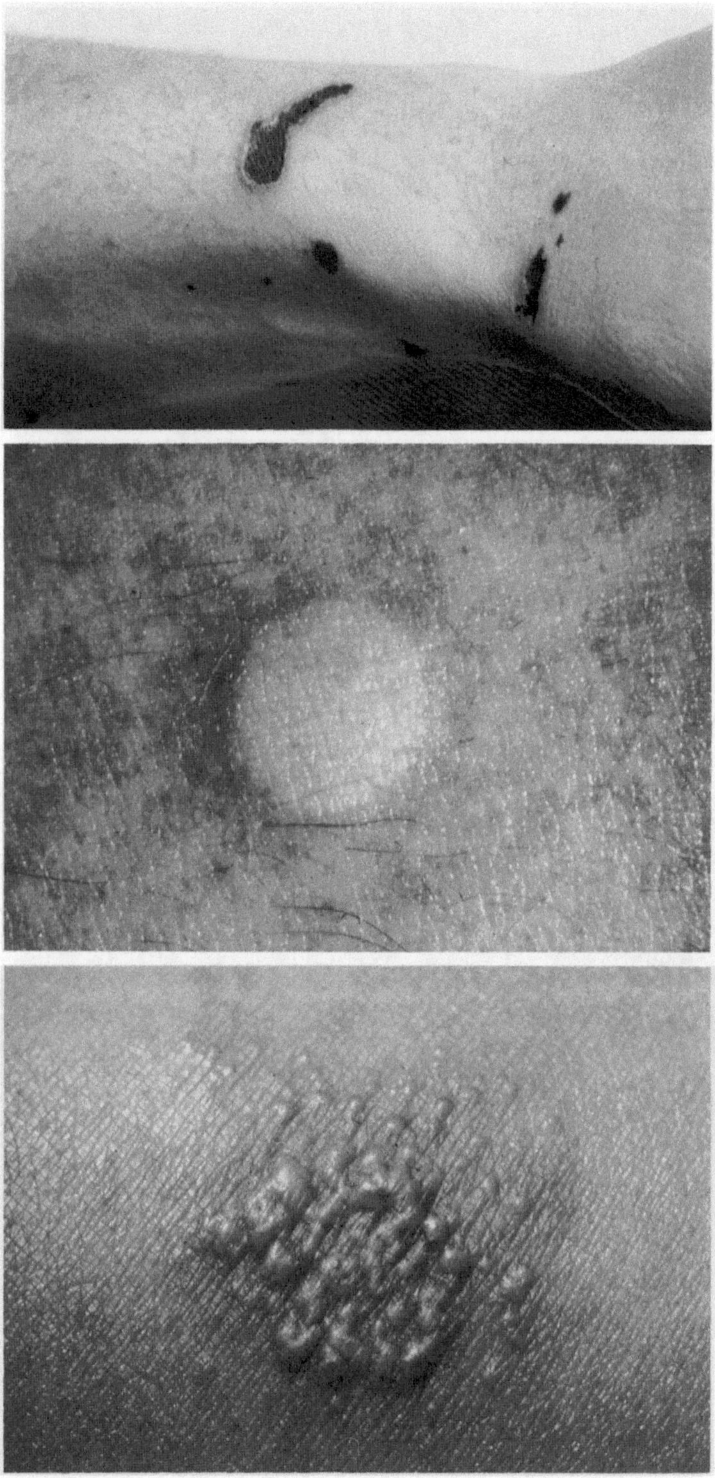

a b c

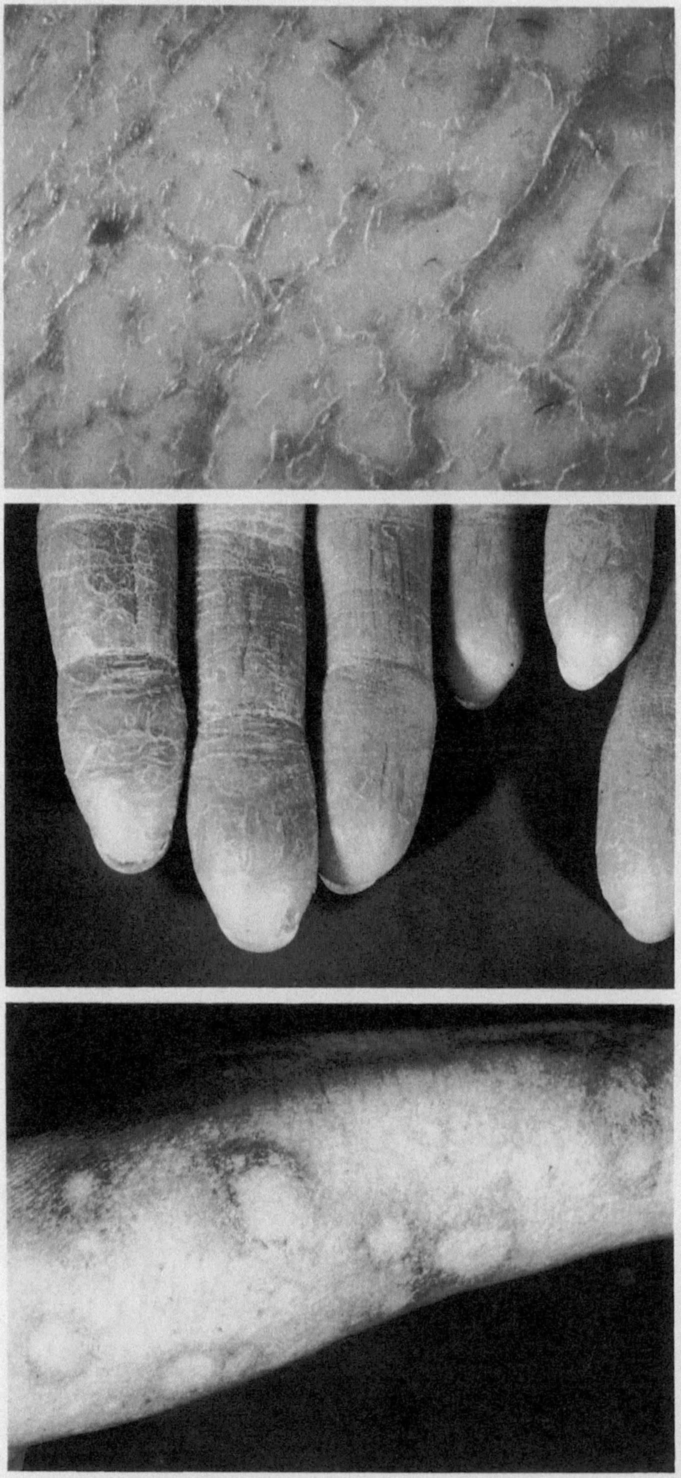

d

e

f

Table 1. Dermatoses where irritants play a major role in the pathogenesis

Hand eczema
Cosmetic dermatitis
Eyelid eczema
Reactions to therapeutics
Tape irritation
Diaper dermatitis
Perianal and stoma dermatitis
Asteatotic eczema
"Status eczematicus"
Juvenile plantar dermatosis
Photoirritation
Plant dermatitis
Reactions to wool and textiles
Contact urticaria
Subjective irritation ("stinging")
Airborne irritant dermatitis

Table 2. Causes of airborne irritant dermatitis (for references see [6])

Acids and alkalis
Aluminum
Ammonia
Anhydrous calcium sulfate
Arsenic
Bromacetoxy-2-butene
Calcium silicate
Cement
Diallylglycol carbonate monomer
Dichlorvos
Domestic products (e.g., cleaning products)
Epoxy resins
Formaldehyde
Glassfiber
Hexanediol diacrylate
Industrial solvents
Metallic oxide powders (slag)
Paper, no-carbon-required (NCR) paper
Phenol vapors
Phenolformaldehyde resins
Quinine dust
Sawdust from toxic woods
Sewage sludge
Silver
Sodium sesquicarbonate (trona)
Urea-formaldehyde insulating foam, dust from
Wool dust (in atopic individuals)

◁ **Fig. 1 a–f.** The clinical spectrum of irritant contact dermatitis. **a** Caustic burn by hydrochloric acid, **b** whealing and erythema by dimethylsulfoxide, **c** pustules by the cationic detergent Hyamine 3500, **d** scaling and fissuring by a harsh soap, **e** cumulative insult dermatitis in a housewife resulting from wet work and contact with numerous irritants, **f** iatrogenic acute irritant dermatitis by dithranol in a patient treated for psoriasis gic but irritant or due to atopy. Cosmetics are usually the precipitating factor. Subjective forms of irritation include stinging and burning of the skin caused by some sunscreens and cosmetics in hyperreactive individuals. Objective signs of irritation are frequently absent [15].

Epidemiology

There are very few solid data on the incidence of irritant contact dermatitis. One reason may be that most reactions are too slight and no medical advice is sought by the patient. In other cases the physician makes a diagnosis of "only irritation" and the problem is solved by eliminating the source. Chronic irritant contact dermatitis of the hands may affect nearly 100% of exposed persons in certain professions such as food handling, fishing, or veterinary medicine. In the metal industry at least 50% of dermatoses are of an irritant type. In Heidelberg a recent survey of 190 cases of hand eczema revealed the following distribution of diagnoses: atopy 40%, irritant dermatitis 27%, contact allergy 23%, and various diseases 10% [25].

The 50 patients with irritant hand eczema came from the typical high risk professions: nursing, housework, hairdressing and cleaning. In a large survey of reactions caused by cosmetics Eiermann et al. [8] found the share of irritancy to be 16%. They pointed out that irritation due to cosmetics is usually underestimated and is diagnosed much more frequently once the physician has been "sensitized" to this type of reaction.

The figures on the incidence of irritant contact dermatitis vary considerably with the population studied. We therefore need more precise data on irritative factors in the work place and home environment. Electronic processing of data from large populations is necessary to make accurate statements of general validity. The German Contact Dermatitis Research Group has started a multicenter study of this type. Initial results will be available in 1990.

Pathomechanisms

Today a number of factors have been identified as being involved in the pathogenesis of irritant dermatitis, particularly for the chronic cumulative type [30].

Exogenous Factors

Table 3 lists the numerous exogenous factors influencing the irritant response; these include the type of chemical, the concentration, the mode of exposure, and the body site. The inherent toxicity of the chemical for human skin and its penetration are the most important exogenous factors.

Table 3. Exogenous and endogenous factors influencing the irritant response of human skin

Exogenous factors
Type of irritant
Amount penetrated (solubility, vehicle, concentration, method and time of application)
Body site
Temperature
Endogenous factors
Individual susceptibility to irritant(s)
Primary hyperirritable ("sensitive") skin
Atopy
Inability to develop hardening
Secondary hyperirritability

Endogenous Factors

Relevant endogenous factors involve atopy and skin sensitivity. A number of excellent studies from Scandinavia have shown that previous or present atopic dermatitis is a high risk factor to develop hand eczema in professions involving wet work and irritants. The studies of Nilsson et al. [31], Rystedt [41], and Lammintausta and Kalimo [27] have confirmed this assumption of experienced clinicians. Recently, results of a large study on 1600 hand eczema patients in Erlangen (Federal Republic of Germany) were published [1, 2]. In essence, the authors came to the same conclusion.

Sensitive (Hyperirritable) Skin

Individuals with sensitive, hyperirritable skin do exist. This may be due to a genetic disposition, even without atopy. Racial differences in cutaneous irritability have been well documented [11, 14, 16, 47]. Blacks in general have less irritable skin than caucasoids of northern (Celtic) extraction. Our own group has shown that subjects with light skin complexions (types 1 and 2) not only have high UVB sensitivity but also have skin that is hyperirritable to chemicals in general [17]. Hyperirritable skin can also develop secondarily during the course of hand or leg eczema. Status eczematicus and "angry back syndrome" fall into this category.

The cause of hyperirritable skin is still unknown. There is good evidence so far that a thin and/or permeable stratum corneum plays a key role. Based on Fick's law for penetration, the thickness of stratum corneum influences the flux of the penetrating chemical. Weigand et al. [47] have shown that the stratum corneum of blacks has more cell layers on average than that of whites. This group also found an increased buoyant density of black stratum corneum, which may indicate a more compact barrier.

Marks' group was able to demonstrate a relationship between the minimal irritancy dose for dithranol and the mean corneocyte surface area; the smaller the corneocyte area, the lower the irritancy threshold [19]. They also found a positive correlation between the minimal blistering time with ammonium hydroxide and the skin surface contour and with various other irritants as well.

Regional variations in irritability are related to differences in keratinization and to the density of transepidermal shunts for penetration (sweat ducts, hair follicles).

The intercellular lipids of the stratum corneum play an important role in the barrier function of the skin. This has been shown by a number of investigators [7, 9, 10, 29, 48]. Based on recent reports, it seems that the ceramides and glucosylceramides may be the key elements in storage of water in the stratum corneum. In experiments on animals fed a diet free of essential fatty acids, the beneficial effect of externally or internally administered linoleic acid as regards an improved stratum corneum barrier has been demonstrated [9]. There is also some clinical evidence that this may have an effect in humans [36]. However, initial therapeutic trials with linoleic acid or ceramide-containing medicaments in atopic eczema and dry skin have not been very encouraging [3].

Individuals with hyperirritable skin are also more reactive when tested on scarified or stripped skin, i.e., after removal of the stratum corneum, major rate limiting factor for penetration [50]. This is also the basis for the assumption that these individuals may release more inflammatory mediators or may be more reactive to them in comparison to "normal" or "hyporeactive" subjects. At the moment, our group is focusing on this aspect by quantifying inflammatory mediators (prostaglandins, leukotrienes) in suction blisters from irritated skin. Initial results show marked individual variations. Intracutaneous injections of prostaglandins E_2 and D_2 revealed a decreased response in hyperirritable subjects (Stiegeler and Frosch, unpublished results). The dual action of prostaglandin E_2 with its antiinflammatory activity may be associated with this phenomenon [39, 40].

Diagnostic Tests

Diagnostic tests to determine a patient's susceptibility to irritants are listed in Table 4. None is really so simple and reliabe that it is used clinically on a wide scale. The diagnostic value of older tests such as the alkali resistance test of Burckhardt have been overestimated, particularly as regards their capacity to distinguish between allergic and irritant eczema. The diagnostic methods listed in Table 4, however, are very useful in determining threshold responses to various irritants. Subjects with an increased reactivity to one or more irritants can be identified and various influences such as the effect of repeated UVB exposure, cumulative effects of low-grade irritants, or protective effects of "barrier creams" can be quantified. Using these techniques we demonstrated that in a normal population with healthy skin the

Table 4. Diagnostic methods for the quantification of cutaneous irritability (for references see [11])

Alkali resistance (NaOH)
Ammonium hydroxide
DMSO
Threshold response to various irritants (SLS, benzalkonium chloride, kerosene, croton oil, anthralin)
Lactic acid stinging

proportion of subjects with hyperirritable skin was 14%; 25% were regarded as "hypoirritable" and 61% as "normal." The distinction between the three groups was made by use of cluster analysis, a statistical method which can compare and validate a number of criteria from one subject [11]. Although some individuals seem to have hyperirritable skin per se, one finds that the correlation between some irritants is rather weak, if a large number of irritants of very different chemical structure are used. In one study we found a good correlation between the response to sodium hydroxide, ammonium hydroxide, and water-soluble irritants, but a very weak and partially nonsignificant one to lipid-soluble irritants, such as croton oil and Kerosene [17]. In 1968, Björnberg had already shown that one may not necessarily be able to predict the reactivity to one irritant on the basis of reactivity to another irritant [4].

Action of Irritants

Irritants may affect the skin in various ways. Table 5 lists some targets of major irritants. Detergents have a very broad spectrum of attack. At low doses they affect primarily the horny layer and produce drying and scaling. At higher doses they dissolve membranes of cells and lysosomes. If applied repeatedly at low doses, signs of chronic inflammation develop, with acanthosis, increased DNA synthesis, and changes in cellular metabolism [35, 36]. We have shown that sodium laurylsulfate, an anionic detergent, and Hyamine 3500, a cationic detergent, are chemokinetic as well as chemotactic for polymorphonuclear leukocytes [13]. The motility of these cells is activated at low, nontoxic concentrations and they show a directional response towards the detergents at higher but still nontoxic doses. In this study marked individual differences were noted. Neutrophils from some donors barely reacted to the detergents and others showed a very strong response.

Organic solvents such as methanol or chloroform attack the blood vessels directly by causing hyperemia [22, 44]. Some irritants such as croton oil stimulate the migratory activity of polymorphonuclear leukocytes. The phorbol esters have been shown to be potent chemotactic attractants [18, 33]. Dimethyl sulfoxide (DMSO) is a very effective degranulator of mast cells [14].

Imokawa and other groups [21, 22, 38] have shown that detergents cause scaling of the skin by destroying the lysosomal enzymes in the uppermost horny layer. Keratohyaline granules release acid phosphatase. We recently developed a new assay

Table 5. Cellular targets of various irritants (for references see [11, 35])

Horny layer	Detergents, NaOH, DMSO
Cellular membranes	Detergents
DNA synthesis	Detergents, tretinoin
Epidermal metabolism	Detergents, tributyltin
Blood vessels	Organic solvents
Leukocytes	Croton oil, xylene, detergents
Mast cells	DMSO

using superficial stratum corneum biopsies to evaluate the damage to corneocytes both morphologically and by measuring the acid phosphatase [24]. The visible damage caused by detergents depends on the concentration and on the time of incubation. With SLS 2.5% for 24 h marked destruction of corneocytes was evident in most subjects. Alkylbenzene sulfonate and alkylether sulfate are also active in this assay. Marked individual differences in resistance to a group of detergents was found. Patients with atopic dermatitis reacted significantly more to SLS than subjects with normal skin. The measurement of acid phosphatase using a fluorescent technique based on umbillipherol phosphate has a potential for distinguishing between chemicals with high, moderate, and low capacity for damaging human stratum corneum.

Inflammatory Mediators in Irritated Skin

The future of research in the field of irritancy lies in studying inflammatory mediators and their inhibitors. Our understanding of the mechanisms of irritation must increase for us to be able to influence the irritant cutaneous response. The data obtained so far are fragments only. We know that prostaglandins, HETEs, and leukotrienes play a role in allergic and toxic reactions of the skin [43]. On the basis of the limited data available so far no pattern of irritant responses with this type of mediators seems to exist. However, Maibach's group [34] has performed a number of elegant experiments in animals using various inhibitors of inflammatory mediators such as antihistamines (cimetidin, mepyramine maleate), 5-hydroxytryptamine antagonists (methysergide maleate), inhibitors of prostaglandin synthesis (indamethacin) and kinins (aprotinin), complement-depleting agents (cobra venom factor) and neutropenia-inducing agents (mechlorethamine). They showed that these had very different effects on the responses to three irritants such as ethyl phenylpropiolate, croton oil, and methyl salicylate. Recently, the same group demonstrated using this model that those are important species-specific differences. It can be assumed that in the humans such differences might account for the marked racial and interindividual variations.

Our own group recently showed that α_2-macroglobulin, a nonspecific proteinase inhibitor, is involved in irritant skin reactions. This macroglobulin is known to be present in the skin and is thought to support the specific inhibitors after they are exhausted ("scavenger functions"). α_2-Macroglobulin can be quantified in suction blister fluids on the basis of an enzyme-linked immunosorbent assay with specific monoclonal antibodies [23]. Furthermore, by using of sodium dodecylsulfate polyacrylamide gel electrophoresis (SDS-PAGE) the free inhibitory form of α_2-macroglobulin can be differentiated from the activated α_2-macroglobulin protease complex type. Initial results show that in irritated skin (SLS and benzalkonium chloride) α_2-macroglobulin is converted completely from the native form to the active form after binding to proteases. This leads to the conclusion that in clinically inflamed skin, proteases are involved and inhibitory systems such as the α_2-macroglobulin are activated. Each irritant may have a specific pattern of inflammatory action and the individual's susceptibility as well as his capacity to counteract tissue destruction by mobilizing inhibitors of inflammation will determine the amount of clinically visible damage.

Quantification of the Irritant Response

Another very worthwhile approach in studying cutaneous toxicity is the use of non-invasive methods to quantify the irritant response. Many groups are now using evaporimeters to measure the transepidermal water loss [45, 46]. The Periflux laser flowmeter can quantify the blood flow using the Doppler principle [5, 32, 42]. Both instruments are quite sensitive and perform measurements in minutes without damaging the skin or requiring a biopsy. Limitations of these instruments have been demonstrated: very high rates of transepidermal water loss as well as very intense hyperemia due to venous stasis may be inaccurately evaluated by these instruments. However, they are very useful in our attempt to measure objectively the degree of skin damage. These methods have been successfully used in measuring the toxic effects of surfactants and organic solvents. Recently, the atrophogenicity of corticosteroids and the protective function of barrier creams have been assessed [12]. The combined measurement of transepidermal water loss and blood flow seems to have potential in differentiating between allergic and irritant reactions. In comparing weak or doubtful allergic reactions with clinically similar irritant reactions we found that in most irritant reactions there is a relatively large increase in transepidermal water loss with a slight or no change in blood flow. By contrast, in weak allergic reactions there is no change in transepidermal water loss but a relatively large increase in blood flow [42]. Lammintausta et al. [28] have shown that subjects with increased susceptibility to stinging have more vulnerable skin. After applying various irritants they found a slight increase in blood flow and transepidermal water loss in more susceptible subjects compared to less susceptible subjects. These differences in cutaneous reactivity were not detected on clinical grounds with the naked eye. This supports the view that the measurement of skin functions is worthwhile and should be promoted in future studies.

Therapy and Prevention

In the acute stage of irritant contact dermatitis topical corticosteroids are indicated. If there is deep tissue destruction or signs of bacterial infection antimicrobial agents may be added.

In all chronic cases of cumulative insult dermatitis a careful approach on a wide scale must be undertaken. Potential irritants in the work and home environment must be identified and whenever possible eliminated (replacement by other less irritant substances, reduction of exposure, protective gloves). Skin cleansing should be as mild as possible (liquid detergents based on alkylether sulfates or sulfosuccinate esters, avoiding organic solvents and hard brushes or other abrasives). Regular application of bland emollients to counteract desiccation should be encouraged. The use of barrier creams is still controversial as the clinical efficacy of the products available so far seems to be quite low. Long-term administration of potent corticosteroids is dangerous because of the risk of atrophogenicity and the further impairment of the stratum corneum barrier [12].

If all measures fail, the diagnosis of an irritant contact dermatitis must be reevaluated: atopy may be the dominant cause or a contact allergy (e.g., to the preservative or fragrance in a hand cream) may prevent recovery. As cumulative insult dermatitis is a multifactorial disease, psychological factors and lack of cooperation by the patient must also be kept in mind.

References

1. Bäurle G (1986) Handekzeme. Studie zum Einfluß von konstitutionellen und Umweltfaktoren auf die Genese. Schattauer, Stuttgart
2. Bäurle G, Hornstein OP, Diepgen TL (1985) Professionelle Handekzeme und Atopie. Dermatosen 33: 161–165
3. Bamford JTM, Gibson RW, Renier CM (1985) Atopic eczema unresponsive to evening primrose oil (linoleic and gammalinolenic acids). J Am Acad Dermatol 13: 959–965
4. Björnberg A (1968) Skin reactions to primary irritants in patients with hand eczema. Isacsons, Göteborg
5. Blanken R, van der Valk PGM, Nater JP (1986) Laser-Doppler flowmetry in the investigation of irritant compounds on human skin. Dermatosen 34: 5–9
6. Dooms-Goossens AE, Debusschere KM, Gevers DM, et al. (1986) Contact dermatitis caused by airborne agents. J Am Acad Dermatol 15: 1–10
7. Downing DT, Stewart ME, Wertz PW, Colton SW, Abraham W, Strauss JS (1987) Skin lipids: an update. J Invest Dermatol 88: 2s–6s
8. Eiermann HJ, Larsen W, Maibach HI, Taylor JS (1982) Prospective study of cosmetic reactions: 1977–1980. J Am Acad Dermatol 6: 909–917
9. Elias PM (1985) The essential fatty acid deficient rodent: evidence for a direct role for intercellular lipid in barrier function. Maibach HI, Lowe N (eds) Models in dermatology, vol. 1. Karger, Basel, pp 272–285
10. Elias PM, Brown BE, Ziboh VA (1980) The permeability barrier in essential fatty acid deficiency: evidence for a direct role for linoleic acid in barrier function. J Invest Dermatol 74: 230–233
11. Frosch P (1985) Hautirritation und empfindliche Haut. Grosse, Berlin
12. Frosch PJ (1985) Human models for quantification of corticosteroid adverse effects. In: Maibach HI, Lowe NJ (eds) Models in dermatology, vol. 2. Karger, Basel, pp 5–15
13. Frosch PJ, Czarnetzki BM (1987) Surfactants cause in vitro chemotaxis and chemokinesis of human neutrophils. J Invest Dermatol 88: 52s–55s
14. Frosch PJ, Duncan S, Kligman AM (1980) Cutaneous biometrics I: The DMSO test. Br J Dermatol 102: 263–274
15. Frosch PJ, Kligman AM (1977) A method for appraising the stinging capacity of topically applied substances. J Soc Cosm Chem 28: 197–209
16. Frosch PJ, Kligman AM (1977) Rapid blister formation in human skin with ammonium hydroxide. Br J Dermatol 96: 461–473
17. Frosch PJ, Wissing Ch (1982) Cutaneous sensitivity to ultraviolet light and chemical irritants. Arch Dermatol Res 272: 269–278
18. Goldstein IM, Hoffstein ST, Weissmann G (1975) Mechanism of lysosomal enzyme release from human polymorphonuclear leukocytes. J Cell Biol 66: 647–652
19. Hamami I, Marks R (1988) Structural determinants of the response of the skin to chemical irritants. Contact Dermatitis 18: 71–75
20. Hurley JV, Ham KN, Ryan GB (1967) Acute inflammation: a topographical and electron-microscope study of increased vascular permeability in bacterial and chemical pleurisy in the rat. J Pathol Bacteriol 93: 621–635
21. Imokawa G, Mishima Y (1979) Cumulative effect of surfactants on cutaneous horny layers: lysosome labilizing action. Contact Dermatitis 5: 151–162

22. Imokawa G, Mishima Y (1981) Cumulative effect of surfactants on cutaneous horny layers: lysosomal activity of human keratin layers in vivo. Contact Dermatitis 7: 65–71
23. Kramer MD, Justus C (1988) The antiproteolytic compound α_2-macroglobulin in human skin. Arch Dermatol Res 280: 93–96
24. Kunkel B (1989) Korneozytendestruktion und Freisetzung von saurer Phosphatase durch Irritantien. Thesis, Ruprecht-Karls-University, Heidelberg
25. Kühner-Piplack B (1987) Klinik und Differentialdiagnose des Handekzems. Eine retrospektive Studie am Krankengut der Universitäts-Hautklinik Heidelberg 1982–1985. Thesis, Ruprecht-Karls-University, Heidelberg
26. Lachapelle JM, Mahmoud G, Vanherle R (1984) Anhydrite dermatitis in coal miners. Contact Dermatitis 11: 188–189
27. Lammintausta K, Kalimo K (1981) Atopy and hand dermatitis in hospital wet work. Contact Dermatitis 7: 301–308
28. Lammintausta K, Maibach HI, Wilson D (1988) Mechanisms of subjective (sensory) irritation. Dermatosen 36: 45–49
29. Landmann L (1985) Permeabilitätsbarriere der Epidermis. In: Schirren C, Kreysel H-W (eds) Grosse, Berlin (Grosse scripta 9)
30. Malten KE (1981) Thoughts on irritant contact dermatitis. Contact Dermatitis 7: 238–247
31. Nilsson E, Mikaelsson B, Andersson S (1985) Atopy, occupation and domestic work as risk factors for hand eczema in hospital workers. Contact Dermatitis 13: 216–223
32. Nilsson GE, Otto U, Wahlberg JE (1982) Assessment of skin irritancy in man by laser Doppler flowmetry. Contact Dermatitis 8: 401–406
33. O'Flaherty JT et al. (1980) Phorbol myristate acetate: in vivo effects upon neutrophils, platelets and lungs. Am J Pathol 101: 79–92
34. Patrick E, Burkhalter A, Maibach HI (1987) Recent investigations of mechanisms of chemically induced skin irritation in laboratory mice. J Invest Dermatol 88: 24s–31s
35. Prottey C (1978) The molecular basis of skin irritation. In: Breuer MM (ed) Cosmetic science, vol 1. Academic, London, pp 275–349
36. Prottey C, Hartop PJ, Ferguson TFM (1973) The effect of soap upon certain aspects of skin biochemistry. J Soc Cosm Chem 24: 473–492
37. Prottey C, Hartop PJ, Press M (1975) Correction of the cutaneous manifestations of essential fatty acid deficiency in man by application of sunflower seed oil to the skin. J Invest Dermatol 64: 228–234
38. Prottey C, Oliver D, Coxon AC (1984) Prediction and measurement of surfactant action upon human skin under realistic conditions. Int J Cosm Sci 6: 263–273
39. Raud J, Dahlen SE, Sydbom A, Lindblom L, Hedqvist P (1988) Dual action of prostaglandin E2 in inflammation. Skin Pharmacol 1: 50
40. Ruzicka T, Burg G (1987) Effects of chronic intracutaneous administration of arachidonic acid and its metabolites. Induction of leukocytoclastic vasculitis by leukotriene B4 and 12-hydroxyeicosatetraenoic acid and its prevention by prostaglandin E2. J Invest Dermatol 88: 120–123
41. Rystedt I (1985) Atopic background in patients with occupational hand eczema. Contact Dermatitis 12: 247–254
42. Simons C (1988) Die Differenzierung von toxischen und allergischen Hautreaktionen durch kombinierte Messung von Hautdurchblutung und transepidermalem Wasserverlust. Thesis, Ruprecht-Karls-University, Heidelberg
43. Søndergaard J, Greaves MW, Jørgensen HP (1974) Recovery of prostaglandins in human primary irritant dermatitis. Arch Dermatol 110: 556–558
44. Steele RH, Wilhelm DL (1970) The inflammatory reaction in chemical injury. III. Leukocytosis and other histological changes induced by superficial injury. Br J Exp Pathol 51: 265–279
45. van der Valk PGM, Crijns MC, Nater JP, Bleumink E (1984) Skin irritancy of commercially available soap and detergent bars as measured by water vapour loss. Dermatosen 32: 87–90
46. Wahlberg JE (1984) Skin irritancy from alkaline solutions assessed by laser Doppler flowmetry. Contact Dermatitis 10: 111
47. Weigand DA, Haygood C, Gaylor JR (1974) Cell layers and density of negro and caucasian stratum corneum. J Invest Dermatol 62: 563–568
48. Wertz PW, Miethke MC, Long SA, Strauss JS, Downing DT (1985) The composition of the ceramides from human stratum corneum and from comedones. J Invest Dermatol 84: 410–412

49. White I, Rycroft RJG (1982) Low humidity occupational dermatosis – an epidemic. Contact Dermatitis 8: 287–290
50. Willers P (1984) Die Bedeutung der Hornschicht für die Irritabilität der Haut. Thesis, Wilhelms University, Münster

Addresses

P. J. Frosch
Department of Dermatology, University of Heidelberg, 6900 Heidelberg, FRG

Comparison of the Time Course, Dose Response, and Mediators of Chemically Induced Skin Irritation in Three Species

E. Patrick and H. I. Maibach

Summary

Following topical application to the skin of mice, methyl salicylate, croton oil, and ethyl phenylpropiolate (EPP) produce irritant inflammation by different mechanisms. The time course, dose response, and mediator involvement in responses to methyl salicylate, croton oil, and EPP in mice, rats, and rabbits were compared. Solutions of the irritants in acetone were applied to one ear of ICR mice and Sprague-Dawley rats and to the shaved back of New Zealand white rabbits. Ear thickness measurements in mice and rats were used to quantitate the degree of inflammation; reactions in rabbits were evaluated visually for erythema and edema. Both qualitative and quantitative species differences in response were observed. Rats were less reactive to methyl salicylate and EPP than mice or rabbits. EPP-induced inflammation was maximum at 8 h after application to rabbits, at 1–2 h in rats, and was biphasic in mice with peaks at 1 and 8 h. Comparison of histologic sections of mouse and rat ears dosed with EPP showed that rats do not develop the cellular infiltrate characteristic of the 8-h response in mice. The degree of suppression of inflammation produced by antagonists, synthesis inhibitors, and depleting agents used to study mediator involvement varied by species. These results suggest that differences in potency of irritants in different species are due in part to amplification of differences in mechanisms of inflammation.

Key words:

Irritation - Mechanisms - Mice - Rats - Rabbits

Introduction

Historically, animal models have been used to predict the potential of chemicals to produce skin irritation and to screen drugs for antiinflammatory activity. One problem associated with the use of animals is the lack of agreement between studies conducted using different species. For instance, Davis et al. [1] studied the responses to eight chemicals in seven species of laboratory animals and in man, and reported agreement between the evaluation in man and other species in only 50% of cases. These differences have been attributed to species differences in skin structure and barrier function.

We reported that in mice, chemicals produce skin irritation by multiple mechanisms and that they activate different inflammatory pathways [3, 4]. We conducted a series of studies to determine if a given chemical produces irritation by the same mechanism in different species.

Methods

The time course, dose–response relationship, and effect of pharmacologic interventions on the responses to methyl salicylate, croton oil, and ethyl phenylpropiolate in female ICR mice, female Sprague-Dawley rats, and New Zealand white rabbits was evaluated. Solutions of the irritants in acetone were applied to one ear of mice and rats, and to the shaved back of rabbits. The volumes applied were 10 µl, 30 µl, and 0.3 ml, respectively. The degree of inflammation was quantified as change in ear thickness measured with a micrometer in mice and rats, and visually using the dual grading scales of Draize et al. [2]. Doses of cimetidine, pyrilamine maleate, methysergide maleate, indomethacin, aprotinin, cobra venom factor, and mechloramine which have been reported to be effective in suppression of other types of inflammation in each species tested (Table 1) were administered to separate groups of animals. The severity of responses of the groups were compared by analysis of variance, followed by *t* tests to determine which treatments resulted in significantly less intense responses than controls.

Table 1. Antiinflammatory drugs administered

	Dosage	Putative mediator blocked
Cimetidine	1 mg/kg s.c.; −30, 3, 6 h	Histamine
Pyrilamine maleate	1.5 mg/kg s.c.; −30, 3, 6 h	
Methysergide maleate	1.5 mg/kg s.c.; −30, 3, 6 h	5-hydroxytryptamine
Indomethacin	1 mg/kg p.o.; −30, 6 h	Prostaglandins, leukotrienes
Aprotinin	mice 22 mg/kg i.v.; −15, 2, 4, 6 h	Kinins
	rats/rabbits 100000 KIU/kg; −15, 2, 4, 6 h	
Cobra venom factor	mice 12 µg/30 gm mouse i.p. −46 h	Complement
	rats/rabbits 20 I.U./100 gm i.v. −24 h	
Mechlorethamine	mouse 60 µg/kg i.v.; −96 h	Neutrophil products
	rats 0.9 mg/kg i.v.; −96 h	
	rabbits 1.2 mg/kg i.v.; −96 h	

Results

Croton oil-induced inflammation was most intense 6 h after application in all three species. Responses to methyl salicylate were maximum 15 min after application to mice and rats, and at 30 min in rabbits. Ethyl phenylpropiolate produced a biphasic response in mice with peaks at 1 and 8 h. The response to ethyl phenylpropiolate was maximum at 1–2 h in rats, and at 8 h in rabbits.

The maximum responses and log doses (mg/cm^2) for croton oil at 6 h, methyl salicylate at 15 or 30 min, and ethyl phenylpropiolate at 1 and at 8 h were plotted. Changes in ear thickness of 0.7 mm in mice and 0.8 mm in rats, or in rabbits a primary irritation index of 8 as calculated by Draize, were used as maximum responses. The dose required to produce 50% of the maximal response (ID_{50}) to each chemical in each species was calculated. It was not possible to calculate an ID_{50} for methyl salicylate in rats, or for ethyl phenylpropiolate at 1 h in rabbits, because values were below 10% of the maximum (Table 2).

Table 2. Doses required to produce 50% of the maximum response

	Mice	Rats	Rabbits
Croton oil	0.02	0.07	0.06
Methyl salicylate	8	–	200
1-h ethyl phenylpropiolate	7	0.2	–
8-h ethyl phenylpropiolate	0.5	–	2.0

Table 3. Summary of effect of pharmacologic agents on the irritant response

	Mice		Rats		Rabbits	
Croton oil						
Dose applied (mg/cm^2)	0.02		0.08		0.53	
Indomethacin	<0.005		<0.001		<0.001	
Aprotinin	<0.002		<0.001		<0.02	
Mechlorethamine	<0.005		<0.001		<0.01	
Methyl salicylate						
Dose applied (mg/cm^2)	1.8		4.7		79	
Indomethacin	<0.005		<0.001		N.S.	
Aprotinin	<0.002		<0.001		N.S.	
Ethyl phenylpropiolate						
Dose applied (mg/cm$_2$)	0.7		1.0		21	
	1 h	8 h	1 h	8 h	1 h	8 h
Antihistamines	N.S.	<0.005	N.S.	N.S.	N.S.	<0.02
Methysergide maleate	N.S.	<0.005	N.S.	N.S.	N.S.	N.S.
Indomethacin	<0.002	<0.001	<0.05	<0.05	N.S.	0.001
Aprotinin	<0.002	<0.005	<0.001	N.S.	N.S.	<0.001
Cobra venom factor	N.S.	<0.02	N.S.	N.S.	N.S.	<0.001
Mechlorethamine	<0.002	<0.001	N.S.	<0.01	N.S.	<0.01

A summary of the statistical evaluation of the effects of the pharmacologic agents is presented in Table 3. The intensity of the response to croton oil was significantly reduced by indomethacin, aprotinin, and mechlorethamine in all three species. The response to methyl salicylate was significantly less intense in mice and rats given either aprotinin or indomethacin. The response of rabbits to methyl salicylate was not significantly altered by any of the pharmacologic agents. The 1-h response to ethyl phenylpropiolate was significantly less intense in mice and rats given either indomethacin or aprotinin; the 1-h response in rabbits was not significantly altered by any agent. The 8-h response to ethyl phenylpropiolate in mice was inhibited by all pharmacologic agents, and in rabbits only methysergide maleate failed to supress the response. This was in great contrast to the 8-h response of rats which was partially suppressed by only two agents: indomethacin and mechlorethamine.

Discussion

The inflammatory time course and dose response to croton oil was similar in mice, rats, and rabbits, and the response in each animal was suppressed by the same pharmacologic interventions. The time course of the response to methyl salicylate was also similar in all three species. However, potency varied by more than 25-fold. The pharmacologic interventions produced similar effects in mice and rats, but had no effect in rabbits. The apparent lack of effect of the drugs on the response may be due in part to the number of animals tested. Calculations using power equations show that to detect a 50% suppression of the response as being statistically significant, 20 rabbits per group would need to be tested.

Differences in the responses to ethyl phenylpropiolate were striking. Mice developed a biphasic response with an early peak similar to the response of rats and a later peak similar to the response of rabbits. The 8-h response in mice was partially suppressed by all the pharmacologic agents, and in rabbits only the 5-hydroxytryptamine (5-HT) antagonist failed to suppress the response. However, the platelets of rabbits do not contain 5-HT, and only mice and rats develop increases in permeability following injection of 5-HT [5].

Ethyl phenylpropiolate was more potent in producing the 1-h response in rats than in mice (ID_{50} 0.2 vs 7 mg/cm^2). The response was partially suppressed by indomethacin and aprotinin in both species, but mechlorethamine also suppressed the response in mice. This suggests that there are common components of the response to ethyl phenylpropiolate in mice and rats, but the processes are not identical. In additional unreported studies, we found that rats fail to develop increases in vascular permeability and blood flow after between 4 and 6 h, and that the number of neutrophils present late in the response is reduced. Leukotriene B_4 (LTB_4) is produced following application of ethyl phenylpropiolate to ears of mice (unpublished data), and probably contributes to the late phase of the response. LTB_4 is not a strong chemotactic agent for the neutrophils of rats, and this may account in part for differences in response of rats and mice.

While these studies have provided strong evidence for common mechanisms of inflammation in different species following exposure to some chemicals, important differences in the responses to other chemicals were noted. Future studies will determine if these differences are due to differences in sensitivity to specific mediators, or differences in the ability to generate the mediators of a specific inflammatory pathway.

References

1. Davies RE, Harper KH, Kynoch SR (1972) Interspecies variation in dermal reactivity. J Soc Cosmet Chem 23: 371–381
2. Draize JH, Woodard G, Calvery HO (1944) Methods for the study of irritation and toxicity of substances applied topically to the skin and mucous membrane. J Pharmacol Exp Ther 82: 377–390
3. Patrick E, Burkhalter A, Maibach H (1987) Recent investigations of mechanisms of chemically induced skin irritation in laboratory mice. J Invest Dermatol 88: 24s–31s
4. Patrick E, Burkhalter A, Maibach H (1987) Mouse ear assays as models for studying mechanisms of chemically induced irritation. In: Maibach H, Lowe N (eds) Models in dermatology. Karger, Basel, pp 86–92
5. Douglas WW (1975) Histamine and anti-histamines; 5 hydroxytryptamine and antagonists. In: Goodman LS, Gilman A, Gilman AG, Koelle GB (eds) The pharmacologic basis of therapeutics. Macmillan, New York, pp 590–629

Addresses

E. Patrick
Department of Dermatology, University of California, San Francisco, CA 94143, USA

H. I. Maibach
Department of Dermatology, University of California, San Francisco, CA 94143, USA

Comparison of Expression of Human Lymphocyte Class II Antigens by Cutaneous Langerhans Cells and Keratinocytes Between Patients with Allergic, Irritant and Atopic Dermatitis

K. McKenna, D. Burrows, and M. Walsh

Summary

Cutaneous Langerhans and keratocyte cell expression of class II human lymphocyte antigens was compared in allergic, irritant and atopic dermatitis groups using monoclonal antibodies. Similar expression of class II antigens occurred in allergic and irritant contact dermatitis groups. A small number of patients with atopic dermatitis weakly expressed class II antigens on keratinocytes.

Key words:

Langerhans cells - Class II antigens - Keratinocytes

Antigens of the major histocompatibility complex are divided into two classes. Class I, human lymphocyte antigens (HLA) -A, -B and -C are present on most tissues; while class II antigens, the HLA-D series which have a more limited tissue distribution, are found only on certain immunologically active cells. HLA-D has three distinct and antigenically different subregions: DP, DQ and DR.

In normal human skin, only Langerhans cells express HLA-D antigens [1]. However, in many skin diseases including allergic contact dermatitis, HLA-DR antigens are also expressed by keratinocytes [2].

This study had two main objectives. The first was to discover whether HLA-D antigen expression on Langerhans cells and keratinocytes can distinguish allergic contact from irritant contact dermatitis. The second was to confirm that HLA-D antigens are not expressed on keratinocytes in atopic dermatitis [3].

HLA-D antigen expression on epidermal cells was examined in experimentally-induced allergic and irritant reactions in patients with allergic and irritant contact dermatitis. Epidermal cell HLA-D expression was also examined in eczematous atopic skin.

HLA-D antigen expression was determined using monoclonal antibodies [4]. Dithranol was used to provoke an irritant reaction. Dithranol was chosen as reactions to this substance were highly consistent.

Material and methods

Patients

This study involved three groups of patients.

Group 1. The allergic contact dermatitis group consisted of 15 patients (age range 15–76 years). All had typical history and distribution of rash. There was no personal or family history of atopy. Allergy was confirmed by patch test.

Group 2. The irritant contact dermatitis group consisted of 13 patients (age range 22–59 years). All patients had negative patch tests to European battery. There was no personal or family history of atopy.

Group 3. The atopic dermatitis group consisted of 13 patients (age range 18–37 years). All had characteristic rash of atopic eczema, with associated personal or family history of atopy. No patch testing was performed.

Methods

Epicutaneous Patch Tests. Patch tests were applied to the patient's back. In addition to the standard battery of patch tests each patient in the allergic and irritant groups had an irritant reaction provoked with dithranol 0.2% in petrolatum.

In the allergic group, positive patch tests included reactions to one or more of the following: nickel sulphate 5%, potassium dichromate 0.5%, paraphenylenediamine (PPD) 0.5%, cobalt chloride 1%, framycetin mixture 8%, and thiuram mixture 1%.

Biopsies. Biopsies were performed using a 3-mm punch biopsy under local anaesthesia. In the allergic group, biopsy specimens of respective allergic patch test and irritant patch test reactions were taken. In the irritant group the irritant patch test reaction was biopsied. The biopsy specimens were taken between 72–96 h after application of patch tests.

In the atopic group all patients had a biopsy specimen of affected eczematous skin; topical corticosteroid therapy had not been withdrawn.

Immunocytochemistry. The biopsy specimens were snap-frozen in liquid nitrogen. Serial sections 5 μm thick were cut on a cryostat at $-20°$ C. The sections were dried and incubated with a panel of monoclonal antibodies, labelling class II human lymphocyte antigens HLA-DR, DQ, DP (produced by Becton-Dickinson, Rutherford, NJ). Afterwards a polyclonal fluorescein labelled antibody was incubated with the skin. The skin sections were mounted on aqueous medium and viewed using a fluorescent microscope.

Statistical Analysis. Fisher's exact probability test and the binomial test were used. A significance level of <0.05 was used.

Results

In the allergic and irritant groups the HLA-DR subregion was expressed more than the DP and DQ subregions on both Langerhans cells and keratinocytes (Figs. 1, 2).

On comparing each HLA-D subregion response to allergic and irritant reactions within the allergic group, there was a statistically significant difference in the expression of the HLA-DR subregion on keratinocytes. The greater response occurred with the irritant reaction (Figs. 3–5).

There was no difference in expression of HLA-D subregions to dithranol between the allergic and irritant groups (Figs. 7, 8).

In the atopic dermatitis group, Langerhans cells maximally expressed the HLA-DR subregion. A very small number of patients expressed HLA-D antigens on keratinocytes. This expression was weak and focal and was significantly less than in both allergic and irritant contact dermatitis groups (Fig. 6).

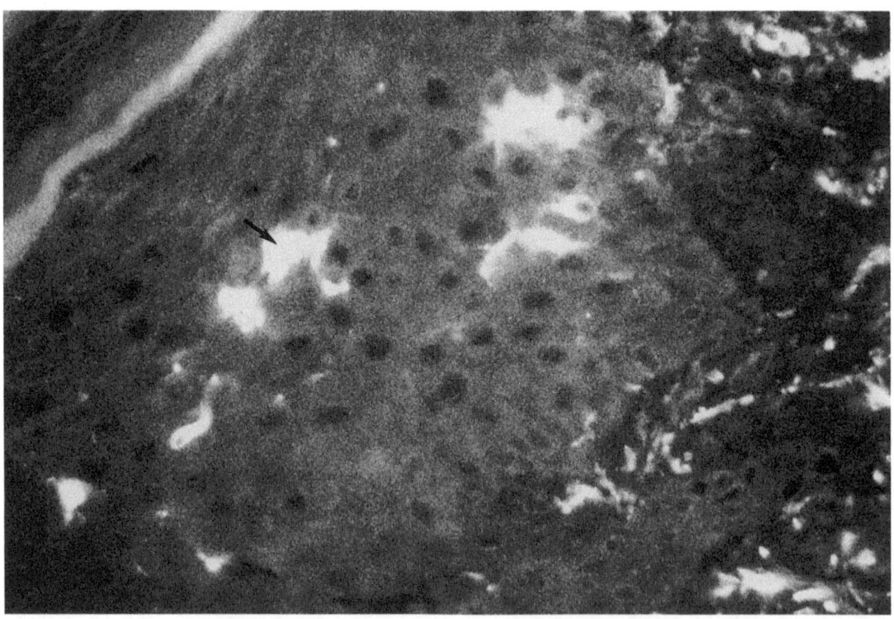

Fig. 1. Epidermal staining of Langerhans cells *(arrow)* using anti-HLA-DQ monoclonal antibody. (×400)

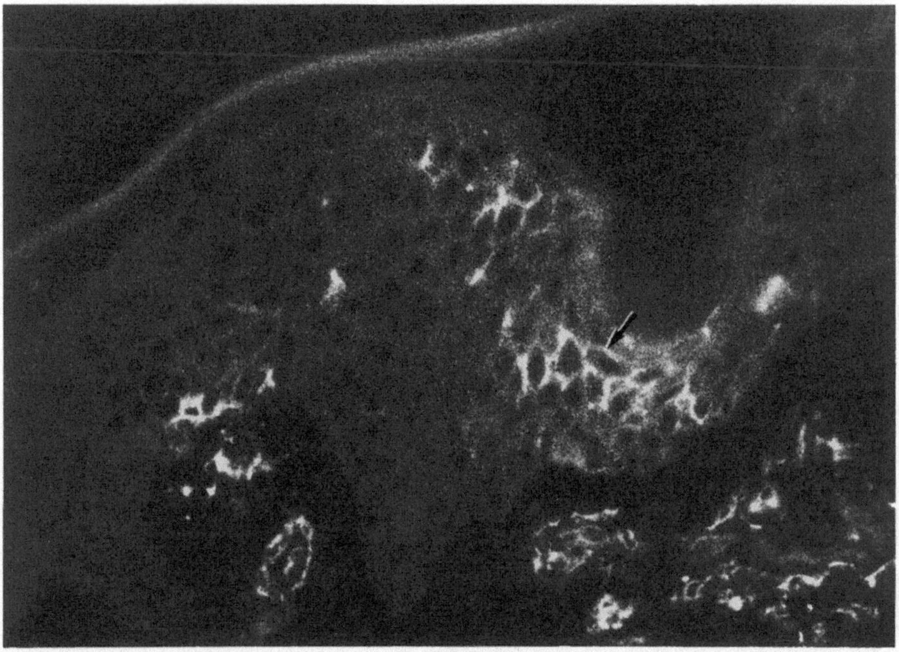

Fig. 2. Epidermal staining of keratinocytes *(arrow)* using anti-HLA-DR monoclonal antibody. (×400)

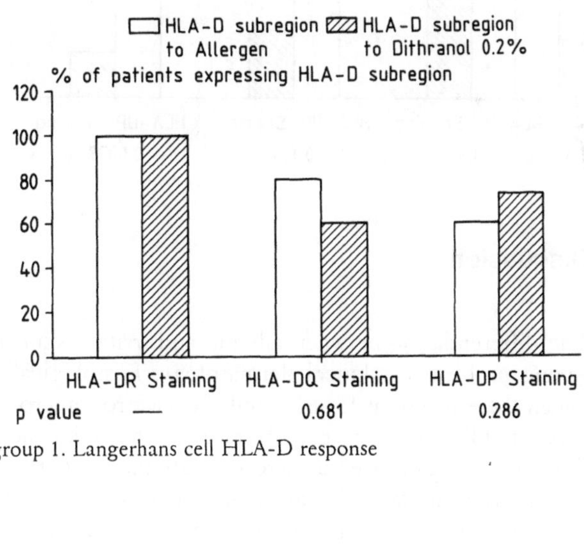

Fig. 3. Allergic contact dermatitis group 1. Langerhans cell HLA-D response

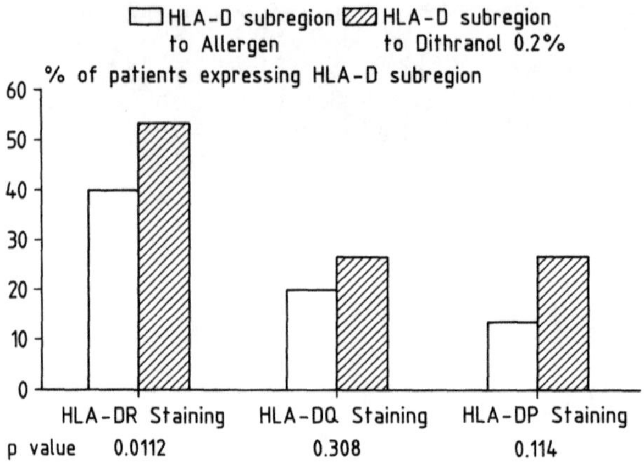

Fig. 4. Allergic contact dermatitis group 1. Keratinocyte cell HLA-D response

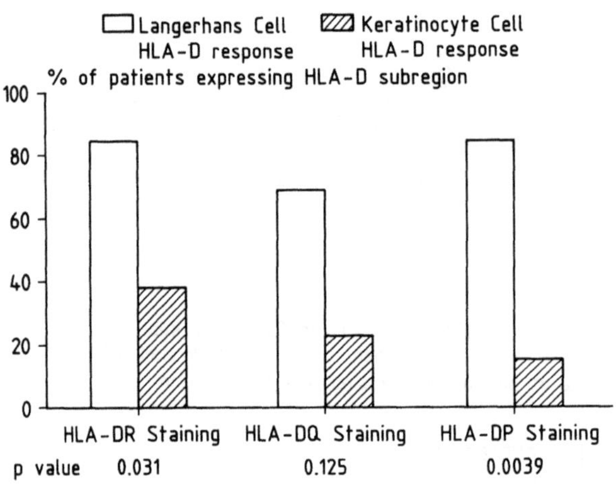

Fig. 5. Irritant contact dermatitis group 2

Discussion

The differentiation between allergic and irritant skin reactions has for long been a vexing problem in clinical dermatology. Histologically there is no difference between these reactions [5, 6]. Similarly, electron microscopy and immunohistochemistry of inflammatory cell infiltrate has been inconclusive [7, 8]. Laser Doppler flowmetry has also been used to separate these two types of reaction without success [9]. It has been claimed that these reactions can be differentiated by means of skin thickening using high frequency ultrasound [10] or by differences in transepidermal water loss [11]. However, it is unlikely that such techniques will have feasible clinical application.

There was no striking difference in the expression of HLA-D subregions between patients with allergic contact dermatitis and irritant contact dermatitis. However,

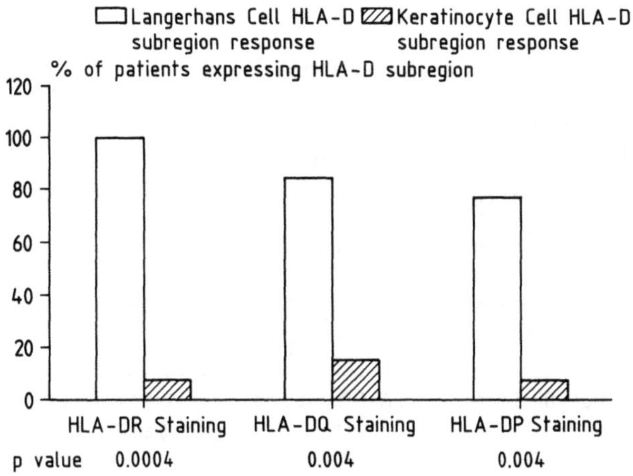

Fig. 6. Atopic dermatitis group 3

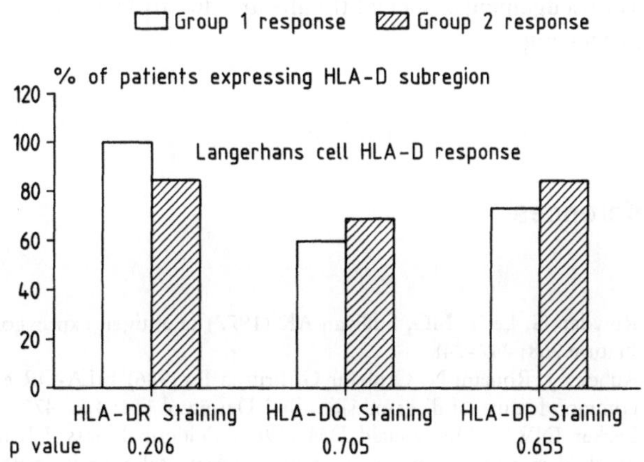

Fig. 7. Comparison of expression of HLA-D subregions to dithranol 0.2% (groups 1 and 2)

when patients with allergic contact dermatitis also had an irritant reaction induced, comparison of allergic and irritant reactions within these individuals did show a significant difference in expression of the HLA-DR subregion. The greater response occurred for the irritant reaction. However, with the number of patients involved and without further study this cannot be regarded as a marker in distinguishing these two reactions.

This study also showed that some patients with atopic dermatitis do express HLA-D subregions on keratinocytes. This expression was certainly less compared with the contact dermatitis groups. Thus, the expression of HLA-D subregion antigens on keratinocytes may prove to be a useful diagnostic tool in distinguishing atopic dermatitis from contact dermatitis.

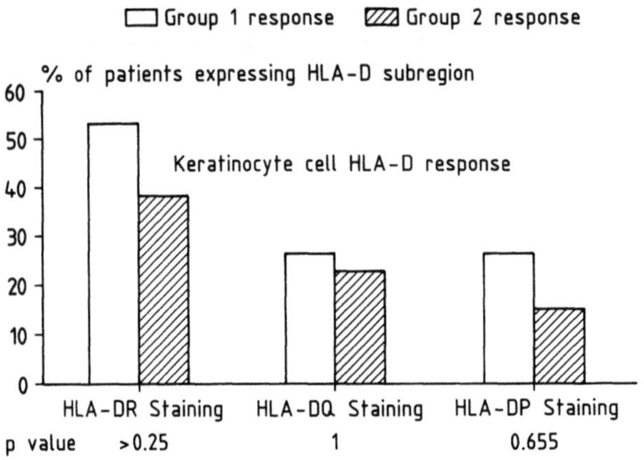

Fig. 8. Comparison of expression of HLA-D subregions to dithranol 0.2% (groups 1 and 2)

Acknowledgements. Special thanks are due to Mr. J. C. Sandford for help with biopsy processing.

References

1. Rowden G, Lewis MG, Sullivan AK (1977) Ia antigen expression on human Langerhans' cells. Nature 268: 247–248
2. Aubock J, Romani N, Grubaur G, Fritsch P (1986) HLA-DR expression on keratinocytes is a common feature of diseased skin. Br J Dermatol 114: 465–472
3. Barker JNWN, MacDonald DM (1987) Epidermal class II lymphocyte antigen expression in atopic dermatitis: a comparison with experimental allergic contact dermatitis. J Am Acad Dermatol 16: 1175–1179
4. Bodmer JG, Bodmer WF (1984) Monoclonal antibodies to HLA-determinants. Br Med Bull 40: 267–275
5. Lever WF, Schaumburg-Lever G (1975) Non-infectious vesicular and bullous diseases. In: Histopathology of the skin, 5th edn. Lippincott, Philadelphia, p 95
6. Nater JP, Hoedemaeker PHJ (1976) Histological differences between irritant and allergic patch test reactions in man. Contact Dermatitis 2: 247
7. Ranki A, et al. (1983) T and B lymphocytes, macrophages and Langerhans' cells during the course of contact allergic and irritant reactions in man. Acta Derm Venereol (Stockh) 63: 376–383
8. Willis CM, et al. (1986) Immunopathological and ultrastructural findings in human allergic and irritant contact dermatitis. Br J Dermatol 115: 305–316
9. Staberg B, Serup B (1988) Allergic and irritant skin reactions evaluated by laser Doppler flowmetry. Contact Dermatitis 18: 40–45
10. Serup J, Staberg B (1987) Ultrasound for assessment of allergic and irritant patch test reactions. Contact Dermatitis 17: 80–84
11. Serup J, Staberg B (1987) Differentiation of allergic and irritant reactions by transepidermal water loss. Contact Dermatitis 16: 129–132

Addresses

K. McKenna
Departments of Dermatology and Pathology, Royal Victoria Hospital, Belfast BT12 6BA, UK

D. Burrows
Departments of Dermatology and Pathology, Royal Victoria Hospital, Belfast BT12 6BA, UK

M. Walsh
Departments of Dermatology and Pathology, Royal Victoria Hospital, Belfast BT12 6BA, UK

Cumulative Skin Irritancy from Heat-Decomposed Polyethylene Plastic

K. Thestrup-Pedersen, J. B. Madsen, and K. Rasmussen

Summary

Six female workers complained of itching skin eruptions on hands, arms, neck and face after skin contact with repeatedly heated polyethylene plastic. Extensive patch testing did not reveal an underlying cell-mediated immune reaction. However, user test with daily application of the heat-decomposed polyethylene plastic led to an itching papulous eruption in patients and control persons. The eruption occurred 5 days after starting the application and spread beyond the application area. One patient experienced a severe attack of Quincke's oedema. The study indicates that substances from heat-decomposed polyethylene plastic have a cumulative skin irritant property, which can mimic a true allergic reaction. The chemical nature of these substances is not known.

Key words:

Patch testing - Quincke's oedema

Introduction

Plastic products are ubiquitous. Plastic consists of polymers, which are long chains of repetitive, simple compounds such as ($-CH_2-CH_2-$) in polyethylene, and additives. Additives are used to stabilize, soften, colour or "lubricate" the plastic product. A review concerning plastic and toxicology has been prepared by Malten and Zielhuis [1]. Plastic is considered inert and polyethylene plastic has apparently not given cause for allergic or irritant skin reactions. It is easily burned and the breakage of the polymer leads to many volatile compounds. The best-known side effect of heating plastic is meat-wrappers asthma [2].

This report describes skin irritant symptoms from contact with heated polyethylene plastic.

Description of Exposure

Employees at a plant producing various plastic products had for some time complained of itching on their hands, lower arms, neck and face, when working at a package machine. The plastic used for wrapping was polyethylene without colour. The machine performed the cutting of plastic with a heated steel string (approximately 180°–220° C), which was pressed towards the plastic for a few seconds. This procedure took place approximately every fifth second. It left a sticky yellow plastic decay around the string, which had to be cleaned several times during the day. The waste material was very sticky and the employees felt that even though they washed their hands, the plastic material was left on the skin.

Of nine employees, six complained of itching and an intermittent red, papulous eruption on hands, lower arms, neck and face. The symptoms were clearly related to exposure to heated plastic. One woman had previously experienced difficulty in breathing, but this had not been related to her occupation.

Methods

Testing. We used the European Standard Series, and the plastic and glue series I and II for patch testing (Hermal-Chemie, Reinbek, FRG). Plastic dust and plastic decay were used as is. Chloroform and alcohol extracts of the plastic decay (10% and 1% in petrolatum) were made for further patch testing. We also tested with a series of allergens provided by Professor Sigfrid Fregert and Lena Trulson, University of Lund, Sweden (Table 1). The testing procedure and reading followed internationally accepted guidelines.

User Test. A user test was performed in which the participants were asked to apply the sticky plastic decay twice daily to the skin in the left elbow in an area 5 cm in diameter. Four volunteers served as control persons.

Table 1. Some of the allergens used for patch testing. All tests were negative

1. Dimethyl Thiourea 1% in water
2. Ethanol extract of heat-decomposed plastic 10% in ethanol
3. Ethanol extract of polyethylene plastic 1% in ethanol
4. Ethanol extract of heat-decomposed plastic 1% in ethanol
5. Dietylftalat 2% in petrolatum
6. Diphenylthiourea 1% in petrolatum
7. Dibutylthiourea 2% in petrolatum
8. Dialfolftalat 2% in petrolatum
9. Diethylthiourea 1% in petrolatum
10. Diisodecylftalat 2% in petrolatum
11. Di-2-ethylhexylftalat 2% in petrolatum
12. Di-n-butylftalat 2% in petrolatum
13. Dimethylftalat 2% in petrolatum

Results

When visiting the plant on a Monday, none of the employees had signs of skin eruption. Six of the employees with skin complaints participated in extensive patch testing. We found nickel allergy in 4/6, cobalt allergy in 2/6, and one subject with primula allergy. Two had negative reactions. None had allergy towards formalin or formaldehyde resin. Testing was negative using the plastic and glue series I and II. The plastic extracts showed negative reactions in all persons, but one person developed a lichenoid reaction after 3 weeks, which clinically and histologically did not resemble allergic sensitization.

Scratch tests with the plastic decay were negative, and our standard prick test series was negative in all six persons.

Five employees and five volunteers performed the user test. All employees and four of five volunteers experienced an itching, papulous eruption on day 4 or 5 consisting of solitary 1- to 2-mm large conical papules (Fig. 1). It was remarkable that the eruption was not confined to the application area, but extended to the lower arm and in some to the opposite arm. The manifestation of the skin symptoms was most pronounced 5 to 8 days following the start of the user test. Two of five subjects complained of itching in the face, and the person, who had previously experienced an attack of asthma during work, developed a strong papulous eruption in the face

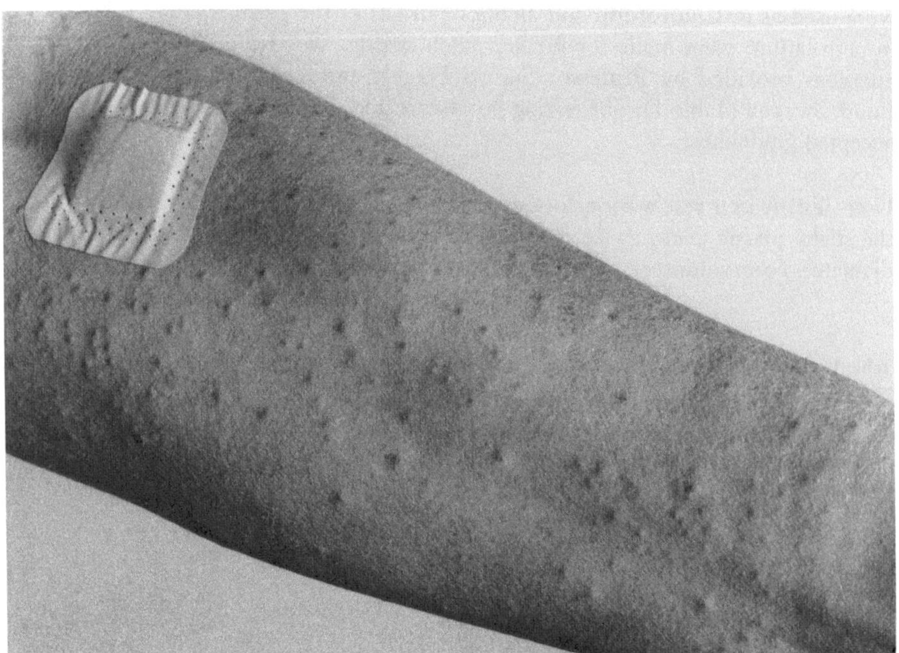

Fig. 1. Papulous eruption on the left lower arm 5 days after user test with heat-decomposed plastic. The next day this patient experienced an anaphylactoid reaction

and on the arms (Fig. 1), Quincke's oedema and shortness of breath. She was given 30 mg prednisolone systemically, but despite that she was admitted to the intensive care unit in the local hospital with severe Quincke's oedema, which disappeared within 24 h after treatment with methyl prednisone 100 mg intravenously and antihistamine.

Discussion

The mechanisms behind the described symptoms are most likely due to intolerance. Cutaneous testing with the plastic was negative. The lichenoid dermatitis-like reaction does not resemble true sensitization. The user test confirms that persons not previously exposed to the plastic developed similar skin symptoms. The person showing an anaphylactoid reaction demonstrates that the cumulative irritant effect may be severe and can give rise to symptoms from the skin and the airways.

Preliminary studies at the chemical laboratory of the Institute for Occupational Health in Copenhagen have shown that the heat-decomposed plastic contained at least 57 chemical substances, many of which could not be identified.

This report draws attention towards a very common occupational procedure of plastic wrapping. If, during the process, plastic is heated repeatedly to 200° C or above, irritant compounds may arise.

Acknowledgments. We want to thank Professor Sigfrid Fregert and Lena Trulson, Ph. D., for their help for supplying additional material for patch testing and for suggestions during the study.

References

1. Malten KE, Zielhuis RL (1964) Industrial toxicilogy and dermatology in the production and processing of plastics. Elsevier, Amsterdam
2. Sokol WN, Adony Y, Beall GN (1973) Meat-wrappers asthma. A new syndrome? JAMA 226: 639–641

Addresses

K. Thestrup-Pedersen
Department of Occupational Dermatology and Department of Occupational Medicine, University of Aarhus, 8000 Aarhus C, Denmark

J. B. Madsen
Department of Occupational Dermatology and Department of Occupational Medicine, University of Aarhus, 8000 Aarhus C, Denmark

K. Rasmussen
Department of Occupational Dermatology and Department of Occupational Medicine, University of Aarhus, 8000 Aarhus C, Denmark

Acute Irritant Contact Folliculitis in a Galvanizer

K. E. Andersen, K. E. Sjølin, and P. Solgaard

Metal compounds and halogens (e.g., nickel, chromium, mercury, arsenic, iodide, and fluoride) may provoke pustular patch test reactions in man [2, 3]. Such reactions are more common in patients with atopic dermatitis. The pustular reaction pattern is often not reproducible on repetition in the clinical situation [1]. Wahlberg and Maibach [4] developed an animal model (the rabbit) which in a reproducible way could identify contact pustulogens (e.g., sodium lauryl sulfate and mercuric chloride). For some chemicals (e.g., nickel sulfate, potassium iodide, and sodium arsenate) it was necessary to damage the skin to obtain pustules.

We present a case of presumed contact pustular folliculitis in a galvanizer.

Case Report

A 31-year-old male galvanizer presented with acute folliculitis on the back. It developed in 2 days. Previous and family history were negative.

He had been working for the same company for the past 3 years. After working on a hot humid summer day he suddenly developed a rash on the back. Examination showed numerous follicular pustules surrounded by a red halo distributed over both scapular regions. The erythema surrounding the pustules was partially confluent. The elements were of the same stage of development; some had a black necrotic center or a central umbo formation. His general health was not affected.

Microscopy of the pus stained with methylene blue showed cellular debris and leukocytes but no microorganisms. Routine bacterial culture showed no pathogens and a culture for herpes simplex virus was negative.

A skin biopsy specimen showed an abscess, without eosinophilic elastic fibers, in reticular dermis in relation to a hair follicle. The overlying infundibulum was acanthotic, dilated by keratin. A few neutrocytes were seen near the surrounding preserved follicles, and a few yeast cells were seen in stratum corneum and in the abscess. There were perivascular lymphohistiocytic infiltrates, and no specific inflammation or foreign bodies in polarized light. The histologic picture was not compatible with folliculites perforans nor with acne aestivalis.

The patient was treated with a topical corticosteroid and the folliculitis healed within a few weeks leaving no scars. The patient continued work without recurrence.

Elemental Analysis

Tissue from the biopsy specimen embedded in paraffin, normal cadaver skin prepared in the same way, and neat paraffin were investigated for the content of Zn and other elements by inductive coupled plasma mass spectrometry using a PlasmaQuad from VG Elemental. Prior to the measurements the samples were dry ashed using excited oxygen in a low temperature asher thereby avoiding loss of Zn. The ashes were dissolved in pure nitric acid. There was no significant difference in the ppm content of Zn and other trace elements when the two biopsy specimens were compared.

Comments

The galvanization method consists of dipping the metal in molten zinc at a temperature of 475° C. The metal is cleaned in a 5%–10% HCl solution and zinc chloride and ammonium chloride are used as fluxes.

The cause of the pustular folliculitis in this case was not determined. Was it provoked by acid fumes trapped in the man's sweaty moist shirt where they had intimate skin contact, or was it an irritant reaction related to zinc chloride? However, the history and the course of the folliculitis point to an occupational origin of the skin disease. The follicular reaction pattern seems to be dependent not only on the substance but also on the subject and the exposure circumstances.

References

1. Andersen KE, Petri M (1982) Occupational irritant contact folliculitis associated with triphenyl tin fluoride (TPTF) exposure. Contact Dermatitis 8: 173–177
2. Becker SW, O'Brian MP (1959) Value of patch tests in dermatology. Arch Dermatol 79: 569–577
3. Björnberg A (1968) Skin reactions to primary irritants in patients with hand eczema. O. Isacsons, Göteborg
4. Wahlberg JE, Maibach HI (1982) Sterile cutaneous pustules: a manifestation of primary irritancy? Identification of contact pustulogens. J Invest Dermatol 76: 381–383

Addresses

K. E. Andersen
Dermatology Clinic, Algade 33, Roskilde, Denmark

K. E. Sjølin
Laboratory of Pathology, Saltværksvej 168, Kastrup, Denmark

P. Solgaard
Risø National Laboratory, Roskilde, Denmark

Influence of Repeated Exposure to Surfactants and Solubilizers on the Human Skin, Evaluated by Transepidermal Water Loss and Visual Scoring

R. A. Tupker, J. Pinnagoda, P.-J. Coenraads, and J. P. Nater

Summary

The purpose of this study was to develop a new model for the induction of chronic irritant dermatitis. Such a model enables us to test the irritating potency of various weak toxic agents and to study the interindividual variation in susceptibility to these agents. Also, by this model, it should be possible to determine the sensitivity of transepidermal water loss (TEWL) measurements compared with visual scoring in respect of the detection of early skin changes. Therefore, 11 widely used surfactants and solubilizers were applied to the skin of the forearms of healthy volunteers in aqueous solutions of 12.5 mmol per liter for 45 min twice daily for 3 weeks. The effect on the skin was evaluated daily by means of TEWL measurements and by a visual scoring system. Each solution caused an increase in TEWL value over time due to the cumulative irritating action on the epidermal barrier. This increase in TEWL was different for the various solutions. Thus, it was possible to rank the agents according to irritating potency. This ranking order was the same in each individual and remained constant during the 3 weeks. There was a large interindividual variation in susceptibility to the agents. The TEWL value after 4 days of exposure to sodium laurylsulphate is highly correlated to the baseline TEWL value ($r = 0.71$). In comparison with the visual scoring system, the TEWL measurements were more sensitive in the detection of early changes in the skin.

Key words:

Surfactants - Repeated exposure - Chronic irritant dermatitis - Susceptibility to irritants - Transepidermal water loss

Introduction

Some investigators have repeatedly exposed the skin to surfactants as a model for the induction of irritant dermatitis [3, 4, 12]. They observed an increasingly damaging clinical effect [3, 4] accompanied by an increasing transepidermal water loss (TEWL) [12]. Many investigators have noted a great interindividual variation in intensity of reaction after application of sodium laurylsulphate (SLS) to the skin of healthy volunteers [1–3, 6, 11]. The aim of our study was to refine the above-mentioned repeated-exposure models, in order to obtain a new model which yields a better reflection of the conditions in daily practice. Such a model allows a good comparison between different surfactants and solubilizers and also it can give insight into the variation in subjects' susceptibility to these agents. Furthermore, it is possible to determine the sensitivity of TEWL compared with visual scoring in detecting early skin changes.

Material and Methods

A series of 11 surfactants and solubilizers was tested on the forearms of a group of 33 healthy volunteers, ranging in age from 19 to 47 years and without any skin ailments in their medical history. In addition to an unexposed control site, one control site was exposed to water and one to sodium laurylsulphate (SLS). Since in one individual only six solutions could be tested on the area of the forearm suitable for testing, two groups were necessary: one comprised of 18 (10 women and 8 men) and the other of 15 (6 women and 9 men) volunteers.

The experiments were performed from the end of March until the beginning of June and in September, 1987.

All agents (see Table 1) have the same mean alkyl chain length (12 carbon atoms), with the exception of nonylphenol 9-ethoxylate, which has nine carbon atoms in its aliphatic part. They were tested in an aqueous solution of 12.5 mmol per liter (for SLS, this is equivalent to a concentration of ± 0.5 g/v%). The pH of the solutions was in the range of 5.5 to 8.6.

Table 1. Surfactants and solubilizers tested on two groups of volunteers

Group A	Group B
Distilled water	Distilled water
Sodium laurylsulphate (SLS)	Sodium laurylsulphate (SLS)
Sodium dodecylbenzenesulphonate (DBS)	Shellsol K (SOL)
Sodium secondary docecansulphonate (SDS)	Nonylphenol 9-ethoxylate (NPEO9)
Unexposed skin	Unexposed skin
Sodium lauryl 3-ethoxysulphate (EO3S)	Dodecylalcohol 8-9-ethoxylate (DAEO9)
Disodium lauryl 3-ethoxy sulphosuccinate (EO3SUC)	Lauramide-DEA (DEA)
Sodium laurate (LAU)	Cocamidopropylbetaine (COCO)

Of each solution 0.3 ml was applied to a disc of absorbing Whatman paper of a diameter of 20 mm (Schleicher and Schuell, no. 258 gC, 's-Hertogenbosch, The Netherlands). This disc fitted into a round flat plastic chamber (Agfa Bayer, Leverkusen, FRG) with an inside diameter of 22 mm. Four chambers were fixed to the volar side of each forearm by means of nonadhesive bandages. Two applications lasting for 45 min each were made on each working day for 3 weeks. The mean time interval between these two applications was 3 h. After their removal, the skin was cleaned with running water and gently dried with a cotton towel. Each day before the solutions were applied, the effects on the skin were judged by TEWL measurements and by a visual scoring system. For the TEWL measurements, use was made of the ServoMed Evaporimeter (ServoMed, Vallingby/Stockholm, Sweden). The operating principle of this instrument is described in detail by Nilsson [9]. The measurements were performed in an air-conditioned room at a constant temperature of 20° C and a relative humidity of 45% ± 5%. After an acclimatization period of 5 to 10 min, the probe was applied parallel to the skin surface. Results were read after stabilization of the displayed values was achieved (about 1 min). Clinical changes at the exposure sites were graded according to Frosch and Kligman [3].

Results

Figure 1 shows the group means with the standard error of the mean of the TEWL values for three anionic surfactants on each day of measurement. Each solution caused a different increase in TEWL, resulting in different mean TEWL values on the last day of the experiment. These differences were significant in most cases (*t*-test). Thus, it was possible to rank the solutions according to irritating potency. In each individual, this ranking order was the same. SLS was clearly the most irritating to the skin. In some sensitive individuals, SLS caused a steep initial increase in the

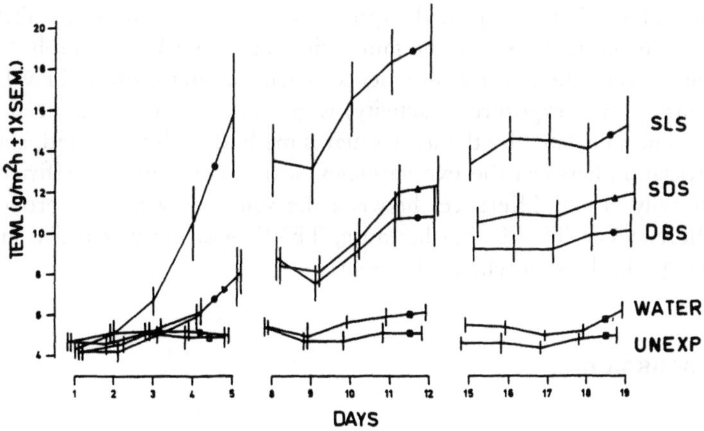

Fig. 1. Mean ± 1 SE of the mean of transepidermal water loss *(TEWL)* values for exposure during 3 weeks to three anionic surfactants and two controls. *SLS*, sodium laurylsulphate; *SDS*, sodium secondary dodecansulphonate; *DBS*, sodium dodecylbenzenesulphonate; *UNEXP*, unexposed site

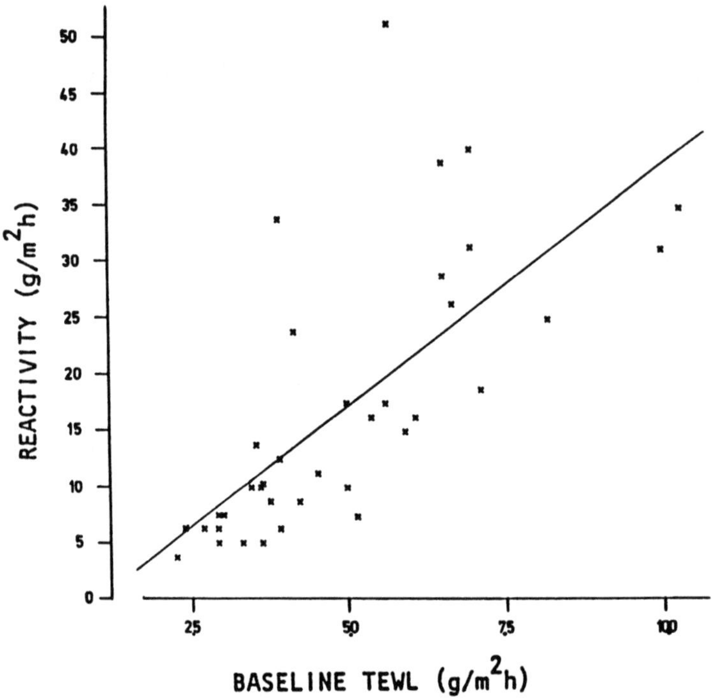

Fig. 2. Relationship between the preexposure baseline TEWL value and the reactivity (TEWL value after 4 days of exposure to SLS). Fitted regression line ($r = 0.71$)

first week followed by a decrease in the following weeks. Relatively large interindividual variations in the baseline TEWL level (i.e., before the first application) were found (mean, 4.9; SD, 1.90). In all individuals, this baseline TEWL level remained constant during all measurement days. Figure 2 represents the plots of each individual's TEWL before repeated exposure to SLS (X axis) versus TEWL on the fifth day of exposure to SLS at the same skin area (Y axis). The graph shows the association between the two measurements: when the preexposure TEWL is high, the response to SLS exposure (reactivity) is generally more pronounced. A fitted regression line calculated by the least-squares method is also depicted, showing the linear association between the two variables, with a correlation coefficient r of 0.71. The clinically visible differences between the solutions were less pronounced than the differences in TEWL. Furthermore, TEWL was more sensitive in detecting early changes in the skin (chi-square test).

Discussion

The repeated-exposure scheme offers a realistic model for the induction of chronic irritant dermatitis. It also makes it possible to detect toxic qualities of solutions which would escape attention when tested in a one-time application [4, 5, 9]. TEWL measurements are a reliable method for comparing the damaging influence of surfactants and solubilizers on the epidermal barrier and are more sensitive and accurate than clinical evaluation [7]. Some surfactants (such as EO3S, EO3SUC, NPEO9 and DAEO9) are shown to be more safe to the skin than others.

The interindividual variation in baseline TEWL was related to the overall sensitivity to surfactants but did not affect the ranking order of irritancy of the tested solutions. Thus, the observed variation in the group means of TEWL values for the solutions on each day of measurement is due to an interindividual variation in reactivity to surfactants in general and not to a variation in the ranking order of irritancy of the solutions between the individuals.

The observed decrease in TEWL in the third week can be explained as an adaptation phenomenon. It apparently occurs only after a certain irritation level. The sooner this irritation level is reached, the sooner the adaptation process will start.

The TEWL depends on the integrity of the stratum corneum as a barrier against diffusional water loss [9]. SLS damages the stratum corneum and consequently increases the TEWL value [6, 10, 12]. In our study, the degree of barrier damage (reactivity) is strongly related to the barrier function before exposure (baseline TEWL). In persons with a high preexposure baseline TEWL, the barrier function of the stratum corneum is apparently impaired from the start. This allows SLS to penetrate and damage the skin more easily, resulting in a high reactivity. The relation between the degree of inflammation caused by SLS and an increase in TEWL is still under discussion [9]. It is tempting to assume that individuals with a high reactivity are at increased risk of irritant contact dermatitis when exposed to weak toxic substances in the occupational environment. The use of TEWL as a parameter for recognizing the chemically vulnerable skin might be of great practical importance.

References

1. Bjornberg A (1968) Skin reactions to primary irritants in patients with hand eczema. An investigation with matched controls. Thesis. Oscar Isacsons, Gotenburg
2. Frosch PJ, Kligman AM (1977) Rapid blister formation in human skin with ammonium hydroxide. Br J Dermatol 96: 461–473
3. Frosch PJ, Kligman AM (1979) The soap chamber test. J AM Acad Dermatol 1: 35–41
4. Kligman AM, Wooding WM (1967) A method for the measurement and evaluation of irritants on human skin. J Invest Dermatol 49: 78–94
5. Kligman AM (1980) Assessment of mild irritants in humans. Current concepts. In: Drill VA, Lazar P (eds) Cutaneous toxicity. Academic Press, New York, pp 69–94
6. Lammintausta K, Maibach HI, Wilson D (1987) Irritant reactivity in males and females. Contact Dermatitis 17: 276–280
7. Malten KE (1981) Thoughts on irritant contact dermatitis. Contact Dermatitis 7: 238–247
8. Murahata RI, Crowe DM, Roheim JR (1986) The use of transepidermal water loss to measure and predict the irritation response to surfactants. Int J Cosmetic Sci 8: 225–231
9. Nilsson GE (1977) Measurement of water exchange through the skin. Med Biol Eng Comput 15: 209–218
10. Scheuplein R, Ross L (1970) Effects of surfactants and solubilizers on the permeability of the epidermis. J Soc Cosm Chem 21: 853–870

11. Valk v d PGM, Nater JP, Bleumink E (1984) Skin irritancy of surfactants as assessed by water vapor loss measurements. J Invest Dermatol 82: 291–293
12. Valk v d PGM (1984) Skin vapor loss measurements on human skin. Thesis. State University of Groningen, The Netherlands

Addresses

R. A. Tupker
Occupational Dermatology Unit, State University Hospital, 9700 RB Groningen, The Netherlands

J. Pinnagoda
Occupational Dermatology Unit, State University Hospital, 9700 RB Groningen, The Netherlands

P.-J. Coenraads
Occupational Dermatology Unit, State University Hospital, 9700 RB Groningen, The Netherlands

J. P. Nater
Occupational Dermatology Unit, State University Hospital, 9700 RB Groningen, The Netherlands

DMSO Irritancy Assessed Using Noninvasive Methods

T. Agner and J. Serup

Summary

The dimethylsulfoxide (DMSO) test is a quick and reliable test of the barrier function of the skin. In this study, in order to quantify the response, the physiological components of the DMSO response are investigated using noninvasive methods.

Key words:

Dimethylsulfoxide - Electrical conductance - Transepidermal water loss - Laser Doppler flowmetry - Ultrasound A scan

When investigating irritant dermatitis, lack of quantitative skin tests has been a practical problem. The dimethylsulfoxide (DMSO) test has been suggested by Frosch et al. [1] as a quick and simple test of the barrier function of the skin. When strong concentrations of DMSO are applied to the skin a wealing response of the skin is provoked. The purpose of this study was to investigate the physiological components that determine the magnitude of the DMSO response, and to attempt to quantify the response using noninvasive methods.

Material and Methods

Six healthy volunteers participated in the study (age 31–45 years). Informed consent was obtained, and the study was approved by the local ethics committee. DMSO 100% (analytical grade) was applied to the skin on the flexor side of the upper arm by means of a plastic block with circular holes 8 mm in diameter [2]. Petrolatum was smeared around the holes to avoid having the fluid spread away from the test area.

Table 1. Grading of the clinical response of the dimethylsulfoxide (DMSO) test

0	– No reaction
1	– Follicular weal
2	– Slightly elevated, solid weal
3	– Elevated, solid, tense weal

On each person two holes were filled up with DMSO. One test area was used to determine the skin thickness, the other test area was used for all other measurements (i.e., when measuring skin thickness water is applied to the skin, which may influence other measurements). After 5 min DMSO was carefully wiped off. For comparison, measurements were performed on normal adjacent skin.

The clinical grading was performed according to criteria given in Table 1. The skin response to DMSO was evaluated, using noninvasive methods, 5, 15, 30, 45, and 60 min after removal of DMSO. The hydration state of the superficial epidermis was evaluated using the Skicon-100 hydrometer which registers the electrical conductance of the skin surface [3, 4]. The recording time is 3 s, and the conductance is expressed as reciprocal impedance (1/μohm).

Transepidermal water loss (TEWL) was measured with an evaporimeter, Servo Med EP1. The relative humidity and temperature in a cylindrical chamber placed upon the skin is thus calculated automatically and expressed in g/m^2 h [5]. Reading was performed 25–30 s after application of the chamber onto the skin.

Cutaneous blood flow was measured by the Periflux Pf2 laser Doppler flowmeter [6]. Reading was performed when the level was stabilized, and expressed in arbitrary units.

Skin thickness was measured using a 20 MHz ultrasound A-scan apparatus, Dermascan A [7]. For calculation of skin thickness an acoustic velocity of 1580 m/s was used.

All values were recorded as the median of three measurements. Subjects were brought to relax before the examination, and the measurements were taken with the arm on a level with the heart. The environmental temperature was in the range 19°–21° C.

Statistics

Wilcoxon's matched-pairs test was used when comparing values of provoked skin with basic values. The chosen level of significance was 5% (two-tailed).

Results

All persons responded clinically to DMSO (median grade 3, range 1–3). Values of hydration state, transepidermal water loss, blood flow, and skin thickness, are shown in Table 2. Five minutes after removal of DMSO values of electrical conductance were increased by 7.9, transepidermal water loss by 3.6, blood flow by 9.4, and skin thickness by 1.3 compared with basic values.

Table 2. Median values of hydration state of the superficial epidermis (1/μohm), transepidermal water loss (TEWL, g/m² h), blood flow (a. u.), and skin thickness (mm). Measurements were performed 5, 15, 30, 45, and 60 min after removal of DMSO, applied for 5 min to the skin. Basic values were obtained from adjacent unexposed skin

Time (min)	Basic	5	15	30	45	60
Hydration state	25	198	134	83	44	33
TEWL	6.4	23.6	17.5	16.1	14.0	13.2
Blood flow	7	66	50	42	46	37
Skin thickness	0.92	1.16	1.33	1.30	1.24	1.10

Parameters of hydration (as evaluated by electrical conductance and measurement of TEWL), as well as parameters of inflammation (blood flow and skin thickness) were all significantly increased after 5 min, compared with basic values. After 60 min, TEWL, blood flow, and skin thickness were still significantly increased. With respect to the hydration state of the epidermis, no significant difference could be demonstrated in 60-min values compared with basic values.

Discussion

The present clinical grading of the DMSO responses was in accordance with earlier findings [1].

Increase in the hydration state of the epidermis as well as increased TEWL has earlier been reported [1, 8]. To our knowledge measurement of blood flow and skin thickness of the DMSO response has hitherto not been performed.

In this study we found that the increased hydration of the epidermis was rapidly restored to normal values, while the increase in parameters of inflammation was more persistent during the observation period. Thus, the DMSO test is more than just a test of the barrier function of the skin. The test also reflects the reactivity of cutaneous vessels to stimuli inducing vasodilatation and edema, the main effects of physiological mediators of inflammation. The DMSO test is therefore most relevant for testing skin irritancy in man.

References

1. Frosch P (1985) Hautirritation und empfindliche Haut. Grosse-Verlag, Berlin
2. Frosch P, Duncan S, Kligman AM (1980) Cutaneous biometrics I. The response of human skin to dimethyl sulfoxide. Br J Dermatol 102: 263–274
3. Blichmann CW, Serup J (1988) Assessment of skin moisture. Measurement of electrical conductance, capacitance and transepidermal water loss. Acta Derm Venereol (Stockh) (in press)
4. Tagami H, Yoshikuni K (1980) Evaluation of the hydration state of the stratum corneum in vivo by electrical measurement. J Invest Dermatol 75: 500–507

5. Blichmann C, Serup J (1987) Reproducibility and variability of transepidermal water loss measurement. Acta Derm Venereol (Stockh) 67: 206–210
6. Tenland T (1982) On laser Doppler flowmetry. Linköping University medical dissertations no 136
7. Serup J (1984) Localized scleroderma (Morphoea): thickness of sclerotic plaques as measured by 15 MHz pulsed ultrasound. Acta Derm Venereol (Stockh) 64: 214–219
8. Malten KE (1978) Topical toxicity of various concentrations of DMSO recorded with impedance measurements and water vapour loss measurements. Contact Dermatitis 4: 80–92

Addresses

T. Agner
Department of Dermatology, Rigshospitalet, 9 Blegdamsvej, DK-2100 Copenhagen, Denmark

J. Serup
Department of Dermatology, Rigshospitalet, 9 Blegdamsvej, DK-2100 Copenhagen, Denmark

Persistent Maleic Acid Irritant Dermatitis in the Guinea Pig*

R. L. Rietschel

Summary

Repeated exposure of guinea pig skin to maleic acid over a period of 8 months did not result in substantial irritant accommodation. Induction of dinitrochlorobenzene sensitivity was not facilitated by maleic acid irritant dermatitis but rather diminished. Chronically irritated guinea pig skin was acanthotic and showed hypergranulosis. Langerhans cell morphology was slightly altered with shorter and less numerous dendrites.

Key words:

Maleic acid - Irritant - Guinea pig

Introduction

Repeated exposure to irritants and allergens results in either a sustained level of inflammation, hyperresponsiveness, or hyporesponsiveness. The hyporesponsive state is known as accommodation with irritants and as immunologic tolerance with allergens. In an attempt to further understand the accommodation phenomena to irritant insult, studies were undertaken to establish a guinea pig model of this reaction and evaluate the response of accommodated skin to immunologic challenge.

* Based on work done at Emory University School of Medicine, Atlanta, GA, under NIOSH grant #R01-0H01124

Methods

Female, Hartley strain, albino guinea pigs weighing 350 g or more were selected for study. Pilot studies in guinea pigs using 20% maleic acid solution as had been studied in man [7, 8] led to an excoriated dermatitis when applied five times per week, and decreasing applications to twice weekly failed to decrease the excoriations. Further, no signs of hyporesponsiveness were noted after several months. Thirty animals were then exposed to five different programs of irritant exposure to one-half of the animal's flank on a five times per week challenge. Five animals were exposed to 5%, 5 to 1%, and 10 to 0.5% maleic acid. Two additional groups of 5 animals each were exposed once to 20% and 5% maleic acid, rested 2 weeks, then exposed 5 times weekly to 5% and 1% maleic acid, respectively. These latter groups were an attempt to mimic the tolerance scheme of Lowney [4]. One additional group of 5 animals was exposed to 20% maleic acid once, 1% for 2 months, and 0.5% thereafter. This group is included only in the immunologic studies reported here. Irritants were applied over an 8-month time interval.

Clipping and epilating with barium sulfide was performed at 1- to 2-week intervals or as infrequently as possible based on hair growth. Prior to irritant or allergen challenge, animals were epilated and rested 1 day. Irritant challenges were applied as 4-h occlusive patch tests with 20 µl irritant on Finn chambers premounted on Scanpor tape at 2 months, 4 months, and 7 months of irritant challenge. A 24-h irritant challenge was used at 8 months. Patch test readings were taken at the time of patch removal and 24 h later. Irritants studied varied but included maleic acid at concentrations of 20%, 5%, 1%, 0.1%, and 0.01% as well as 17% and 3% benzalkonium chloride, 5% sodium laurylsulfate, 20% and 5% malonic acid, 5% acrylic acid, and 10% citric acid.

Dinitrochlorobenzene (DNCB) sensitization was accomplished by applying 2000 µg in 50 µl acetone to a circular 2-cm diameter area of skin near the shoulder blade on either treated (irritated) skin only or on both treated and normal skin simultaneously. Three weeks later, elicitation of sensitivity was performed with 100 µg, 50 µg, and 5 µg of DNCB in 20 µl acetone as open patch tests to 1-cm diameters of both normal and treated guinea pig skin. The DNCB induction and elicitation occurred during the fifth month of irritant exposure.

Irritant patch test readings were graded as follows: 0, no reaction; 0.5, faint macular erythema; 1, definite macular erythema; 2, palpable erythema; 3, erythema with some glazing or early erosion; 4, severe, eroded reaction.

Skin biopsy specimens were taken from treated and normal skin during the sixth month of challenge and studied by routine hematoxylin and eosin (H&E) staining and ATPase staining for Langerhans cells [9].

Results

The irritants chosen for study and the average patch test reactions at each study period are seen in Tables 1–5. After 4 months of exposure no evidence of hyporesponsiveness was seen with 20% maleic acid 4-h challenge. The opposite, hyperrespon-

Table 1. Average 24-h reading to 4-h patch tests to maleic acid after 2 months of treatment

Treatment (%)	Animals (*n*)	Maleic acid concentration (%)				
		20	5	1.0	0.1	0.01
5	4	2.0	0.1	0	0.2	0.2
1	5	1.6	0.4	0	0	0.8
0.5	8	0.6	0.3	0	0	0
20→5	5	2.2	1.7	0.8	0.2	0.2
5→1	4	1.0	0.1	0	0.2	0.2

Table 2. Average 24-h reading to 4-h patch tests after 4 months of treatment

Treatment (%)	Animals (*n*)	20% Maleic acid		17% Benzalkonium chloride		5% Sodium lauryl-sulfate	
		Normal	Treated	Normal	Treated	Normal	Treated
5	4	0.6	1.6	0.7	0.7	0.1	0.7
1	5	0.6	1.1	1.0	0.6	0	0
0.5	6	0.2	0.9	1.3	0.7	0	0
20→5	5	0.3	1.0	1.0	1.2	0	0
5→1	4	0.4	1.0	0.7	1.5	0.9	0.4

Table 3. Average 24-h reading to 4-h patch tests after 7 months of treatment

Treatment (%)	Animals (*n*)	5% Maleic acid		5% Malonic acid		5% Acrylic acid		10% Citric acid	
		Normal	Treated	Normal	Treated	Normal	Treated	Normal	Treated
5	4	0.6	0.1	0.5	0	0.5	0	0.2	0.1
1	3	0.3	0	0	0.2	0	0.5	0	0
0.5	8	0.1	0.2	0	0.1	0.3	0.4	0	0.1
20→5	5	0.1	0	0.3	0	0.4	0.1	0.1	0
5→1	4	0.1	0	0	0.1	0.5	0.2	0	0

Table 4. Average 48-h patch test reading to 24-h closed patch tests after 8 months of treatment

Treatment (%)	20% Maleic acid		5% Maleic acid		20% Malonic acid		5% Acrylic acid		3% Benzalkonium chloride		5% Sodium laurylsulfate	
	Normal	Treated	Normal	Treated	Normal	Treated	Normal	Treated	Normal	Treated	Normal	Treated
5 (4)	0.7	1.2	0.5	0.9	0.5	0.5	0.5	0.5	0.2	0.6	0.2	0.4
1 (5)	1.3	1.1	0.6	0.5	0.8	0.3	1.2	0.3	0.3	0.4	0.7	0.3
0.5 (8)	0.7	0.7	0.6	0.4	0.3	0.1	0.3	0	0.4	0.1	0.2	0.1
20→5 (5)	1.2	0.4	0.4	0.4	0.6	0.1	0.1	0.1	0.3	0.2	0.4	0.1
5→1 (4)	1.2	0.2	0.7	0.5	0.2	0.2	0.4	0.2	0.6	0.7	0.7	1.1

Table 5. Patch test reactions (24 h of occlusion) read at 48 h in all 26 animals

Skin status	20% Maleic acid	5% Maleic acid	20% Malonic acid	5% Acrylic acid	3% Benzalkonium chloride	5% Sodium lauryl-sulfate
Normal	1.0	0.4	0.6	0.4	0.4	0.4
Treated	0.9	0.2	0.5	0.2	0.3	0.3

Table 6. DNCB response on normal skin with 50-μg challenge

2000-μg DNCB induction on	Animals sensitized	Not sensitized
Treated skin only	6	13
Treated and normal skin	11	4

Table 7. DNCB response on treated skin with 50-μg challenge

2000-μg DNCB induction on	Animals sensitized	Not sensitized
Treated skin only	7	12
Treated and normal skin	14	1

siveness, was the rule. A lower concentration of maleic acid (5%) was studied at 7 months and seemed to show a slight (but insignificant) decrease in reactivity on treated skin. At 8 months a more comprehensive challenge showed some suggestions of hyporesponsiveness which extended to some degree to other related irritants (Table 4). Since no significant difference was seen among the five different treatments, the data were combined in Table 5 which shows a consistent trend for decreased response to all irritants on treated skin, but none of the differences are statistically significant.

The histology by H&E examination showed only acanthosis and hypergranulosis as the main changes in treated skin with a variable degree of cellular infiltration.

Sensitization to DNCB was manifest in only one animal of 34 at the 5-μg challenge (and that reaction only occurred on treated skin). At the 100-μg challenge, all but one animal reacted on normal skin. The 50-μg challenge was discriminatory in the sense that many animals would not be deemed sensitized by this response. At this elicitation dose there was a significant difference in the number of animals sensitized by induction on treated skin compared with induction on both treated and normal skin (Tables 6, 7). If positive DNCB reactions on normal skin only are used to determine whether sensitization is present, then $\chi^2 = 5.84$ and the results are significant at the 5% level. If DNCB responses on treated skin are used as the determinant, then $\chi^2 = 11.32$ and the results are significant at the 1% level.

Langerhans cells were observed on both normal and treated skin, but dendrites were shorter and less numerous on treated skin.

Discussion

Maleic acid did not prove to be a good irritant for accommodation studies in the guinea pig. The 20% concentration which produced a modest, tolerable dermatitis in man [7] was too strong, and lower concentrations produced insignificant degrees of accommodation even after prolonged administration. The histologic features of acanthosis and hypergranulosis are similar to the findings of McOsker and Beck with surfactant accommodation in the guinea pig [6].

In man, the presence of dermatitis or strongly positive patch tests can result in an increase in the nonspecific reactivity of skin: the excited skin syndrome [1]. In the guinea pig, Maurer points out that multiple positive tests actually result in a lower degree of reactivity as compared with reactivity when tested singly [5]. This would be the opposite of excited skin syndrome. Uehara and Ofuji showed that dermatitis on one side of the guinea pig can lead to a decrease in delayed hypersensitivity on the opposite side, the opposite of excited skin syndrome [10]. Some types of inflammation will facilitate induction of delayed hypersensitivity, while others actually decrease induction [3]. The observations with 50-μg elicitation doses of DNCB are in keeping with the concept that inflammation interferes with induction as was observed with maleic acid and DNCB in man [7].

Since all animals studied with DNCB had been subjected to months of irritation which may have altered reactivity to both induction and elicitation concentrations of DNCB, it is hard to be absolute about which concentrations discriminate irritant from allergic phenomena. Immunologically naive animals of this strain were previously found to universally respond to a concentration of 75 μg; i.e., 75 μg or more would be an irritant concentration [2]. However, with the decreased reactivity due to multiple tests and existent inflammation, 100 μg may or may not be an irritant and could conceivably represent true sensitization. The 2000-μg induction dose was also previously found to sensitize all animals [2]. It could reasonably be argued that higher concentrations of DNCB would be needed to sensitize animals with existent inflammation. The increased number of animals elicited with a 50-μg challenge when both normal and treated skin were induced would then reflect nothing more than the doubled (4000 μg) induction dose producing higher degrees of sensitivity. If the 100-μg dose is seen as irritant, then the 50-μg data would be used to discuss the number of animals with induced allergy. But if the 100-μg data are viewed as showing sensitization, then the 50-μg data would indicate the degree of sensitization. Either point of view is consistent with the concept that the presence of maleic acid inflammation in the guinea pig may dampen or hamper the induction and subsequent elicitation of delayed hypersensitivity. None of the findings support the concept that maleic acid irritant dermatitis will enhance the degree of sensitization to a strong allergen.

If the 50-μg dose is viewed as the discriminator between the presence or absence of true allergy, then sensitization has indeed been disturbed by maleic acid pretreatment. However, this difference in sensitivity could still be a result of the higher induction concentration, viz., 4000 μg vs 2000 μg. Had the induction dose been applied only on normal skin, the issue would be resolved, but the design of this study was set to mimic the human study already completed [7].

The ATPase stains of epidermal sheets from treated skin showed the presence of Langerhans cells which were only slightly decreased in number. Dendrites were present but decreased in number compared with normal skin specimens. Dendrites were shorter and the ends tended to be rounded as compared with tapered and slender in normal skin. These changes could conceivably reflect damage to antigen-binding sites that could diminish immunologic function.

Based on the studies reported here, the guinea pig would not be anticipated to be a suitable model for maleic acid accommodation or for the excited skin syndrome.

References

1. Bruynzeel DP, Maibach HI (1986) Excited skin syndrome (angry back). Arch Dermatol 122: 323–328
2. Colby SL, Artis WM, Rietschel RL (1983) Liposomes containing 3-n-pentadecylcatechol induce tolerance to toxicodendron. J Invest Dermatol 80: 145–149
3. Friedlaender MH, Chisari FV, Baer H (1973) The role of the inflammatory response of skin and lymph nodes in the induction of sensitization to simple chemicals. J Immunol 111: 164–170
4. Lowney ED (1964) Topical hyposensitization of allergic contact sensitivity in the guinea pig. J Invest Dermatol 43: 487–490
5. Maurer T (1983) Contact and photocontact allergens. Marcel Dekker, New York, pp 51–52
6. McOsker DE, Beck LW (1967) Characteristics of accommodated (hardened) skin. J Invest Dermatol 48: 372–383
7. Rietschel RL, Klemm J, Jones HE (1982) Chronic irritant dermatitis interferes with induction of dinitrochlorobenzene (DNCB) sensitization. Clin Res 30: 915A
8. Rietschel RL, Klemm J, Thompson M (1982) The influence of accommodation (hardening) on the response to irritants, allergens, and mediators of inflammation in humans. Clin Res 30: 605A
9. Robins PG, Brandon DR (1981) A modification of the adenosine triphosphatase method to demonstrate epidermal Langerhans cells. Stain Technol 56: 87–89
10. Uehara M, Ofuji S (1977) Suppressed cell-mediated immunity associated with eczematous inflammation. Acta Derm Venereol (Stockh) 57: 137–139

Addresses

R. L. Rietschel
Department of Dermatology, Ochsner Clinic and Alton Ochsner Medical Foundation, New Orleans, LA 70121, USA

Degradation of Human Epidermal Keratin and Induction of Inflammation by Proteolytic Enzymes from Fish

G. Volden and S. Bjelland

Summary

After developing an in vitro assay system, we found that fish stomach and intestinal homogenates as well as purified fish pepsin and trypsin effect significant degradation of human epidermal keratin. The activity of trypsin and pepsin of five different fish species was studied. All the fish species had pepsin pH optimum around pH 3.3–3.4 and trypsin pH optimum between pH 8.5 and 9.5. Boiled homogenates and boiled enzymes caused no degradation. Specific inhibitors of pepsin and trypsin significantly inhibited the keratin-degradation process. Intracutaneous injection of trypsin and pepsin induced inflammation. Repeated percutaneous application of stomach and intestinal homogenates and purified trypsin and pepsin caused a slight degradation of the keratin layer and a slight inflammation was also observed. These results together may explain irritative contact hand eczema following continuous handling of stomach and intestinal contents of fish.

Key words:

Human epidermal keratin - Fish pepsin - Fish trypsin - Hand eczema

We have observed that irritative contact eczema is often caused by exposure to fish. Accordingly, fish tissues may contain substances capable of destroying the epidermal barrier function of stratum corneum and inducing an inflammatory reaction. Since the main structural element of epidermis is keratin, proteolytic enzymes are suspected as etiological agents.

Materials and Methods

From each fish species (cod *Gadus morhua*, Atlantic herring *Clupea harengus*, Atlantic salmon *Salmo salar*, redfish *Sebastes marinus*, and plaice *Pleuronectes platessa*) intestines and stomach with its content were homogenized with water followed by centrifugation and filtration [1].

Pepsins were purified from cod viscera [3], and trypsin was purified from cod intestines [4]. These enzymes were used to study keratin degradation. The preparation of keratin from human plantar callus and the assay procedure for determining keratin degradation in vitro are described elsewhere [2].

Cod intestinal and stomach homogenates and purified fish pepsin and bovine trypsin as well as heat-inactivated homogenates and enzymes were applied in closed chambers on intact human skin of some volunteers every 2nd h for 48 h (except during the night). Active and heat-inactivated trypsin and pepsin were also injected intracutaneously.

Results

Stomach extract degraded human epidermal keratin effectively in vitro at a pH optimum around 3.3–3.4. The keratin-degrading activity of pepsin I and pepsin II purified from cod showed a pH optimum of 3.7 and 3.1, respectively. Extracts of intestines and fish trypsin degraded human keratin effectively in vitro with pH optima between 8.5 and 9.5.

Boiled homogenates and enzymes caused no degradation, indicating an enzymatic mechanism. Specific inhibitors also significantly inhibited the keratin-degradation process.

Percutaneous treatment with stomach and intestinal homogenates as well as with trypsin and pepsin resulted in a slight erythematous reaction. Histology revealed more thinning of stratum corneum and a slightly more pronounced inflammatory reaction at the test sites treated with active enzymes and homogenates containing active enzymes than at the test sites treated with heat-inactivated materials. Intracutaneous injection of trypsin and pepsin induced significantly stronger inflammatory reactions than did heat-inactivated enzymes.

Discussion

The digestive organs are the major source of proteases in fish, and in the present investigation it is demonstrated that pepsin and trypsin are highly effective in degrading human epidemal keratin in vitro. However, because of the neutral pH of fish tissue and seawater, pepsin should be of minor importance compared with trypsin in causing destruction of stratum corneum during exposure to fish, although this may not be true when direct contact with stomach contents is achieved. In the case of pepsin, handling of acidified fish material, e.g. fish silage, in the fish-processing industry, should be of far more practical importance.

The degradation of human epidermal keratin by fish trypsin and pepsin and the induction of inflammation may together explain irritative contact hand eczema following continuous handling of intestinal and stomach contents of fish.

Acknowledgements. This work is part of a project (No III 406.001) supported by the Norwegian Fisheries Research Council (NFFR).

References

1. Bjelland S, Gildberg A, Volden G (1988) Degradation of human epidermal keratin by fish pepsin. Arch Dermatol Res 280: 119–123
2. Bjelland S, Volden G, Raa J (1988) A simple assay for determining keratin and collagen degradation in vitro. Arch Dermatol Res 280: 50–53
3. Gildberg A, Almås KA (1986) Utilization of fish viscera. In: LeMaguer M, Jelen P (eds) Food engineering and process applications, vol 2 (Unit operations). Elsevier Applied Science, London, pp 383–393
4. Hjelmeland K, Raa J (1982) Characteristics of two trypsin type isozymes isolated from the Arctic fish capelin *(Mallotus villosus)*. Comp Biochem Physiol 71B: 557–562

Addresses

G. Volden

Department of Dermatology, University of Trondheim, N-7006 Trondheim, Norway

S. Bjelland

Norwegian Defence Research Establishment, Division for Environmental Toxicology, P.O. Box 25, N-2007 Kjeller, Norway

Part 5

Contact Urticaria

Effects of Capsaicin and Topical Anesthesia on Nonimmunologic Immediate Contact Reactions to Benzoic Acid and Methyl Nicotinate

E. Larmi, A. Lahti, and M. Hannuksela

Summary

The effects of topical capsaicin (a liberator of substance P) and topical anesthesia were studied in order to obtain information about the role of sensory nerves and substance P in the pathophysiology of nonimmunologic immediate contact reactions (NIICRs) induced by benzoic acid (BA) and methyl nicotinate (MN) in human skin. BA 500, 250, 125, 62, and 31 m*M* and MN 50, 25, 13, 7, 3, 1.5, and 0.75 m*M* in petrolatum were tested on the skin areas pretreated with capsaicin solution in 13 test subjects. BA 500, 125, 62, and 31 m*M* and MN 25, 10, 2, and 0.5 m*M* in petrolatum were tested on skin areas of 15 test subjects, anesthesized with a topical anesthetic cream (lidocaine 25 mg/g, prilocaine 25 mg/g). Prick tests with histamine dihydrochloride (10 mg/ml) were also performed on test and reference areas. Reactions were monitored 40 min after application with laser-Doppler flowmetry, and the sizes of erythema and edema reactions were measured. Capsaicin treatment inhibited erythema reactions to histamine, but did not inhibit erythema or edema from BA and MN. Topical anesthesia inhibited erythema and edema reactions to histamine as well as to BA and MN. These results suggest that neither erythema nor edema reactions to BA and MN are mediated by mechanisms sensitive to capsaicin (substance P). The mechanism by which a topical anesthetic inhibits skin reactions may result from its effect on cutaneous nerves, or it may have general antiinflammatory properties.

Key words:

Capsaicin - Topical anesthesia - Nonimmunologic immediate contact reactions - Contact urticaria - Benzoic acid - Methyl nicotinate - Substance P

Introduction

The pathophysiological factors involved in nonimmunologic immediate contact reactions (NIICRs) are poorly understood. The possible mechanisms include a release of histamine, prostaglandins, leukotrienes, substance P or other inflammatory mediators, or a direct effect on dermal vessel walls [6, 11–13].

Capsaicin (trans-8-methyl-*N*-vanillyl-6-nonenamide), the most abundant of the pungent principles of the red pepper (Capsicum) is known to induce vasodilatation and protein extravasation caused by the specific release of a bioactive peptide, substance P, from axons of unmyelinated C-fibers of sensory nerves [2, 4, 5, 7]. Systemic administration of capsaicin to guinea pigs and rats results in insensitivity of the skin to some chemical irritants, lasting from weeks to months [4, 8]. In man, capsaicin pretreatment has been found to inhibit erythema reactions in histamine skin tests [1].

Sensory nerves are a modulating factor in various inflammatory processes of the skin [9, 10]. In earlier studies, the effect of local anesthesia and the role of sensory nerves in the pathophysiology of NIICRs have been controversial [11].

The present study investigated the effects of topical capsaicin treatment and topical anesthesia on the skin reactions induced by benzoic acid (BA), methyl nicotinate (MN), and histamine dihydrochloride.

Material and Methods

Test Subjects. The capsaicin group comprised 13 (8 women, 5 men; mean age, 23 years), and the topical anesthesia group 15 healthy medical students (10 women, 5 men; mean age, 23 years). They received no antiinflammatory analgesic or antihistaminic drugs for 3 days before testing or during the tests.

Capsaicin Treatment. On the first day, a skin area of 6 × 16 cm of the upper back was treated twice and on the second day once with 1 ml capsaicin solution, 1 mg/ml in 94% ethyl alcohol (10 μl/cm^2). On the second day, 6 hours after the third application, one more application of capsaicin solution, 10 mg/ml, was performed on the same area. A reference area on the contralateral side of the back was treated correspondingly with ethyl alcohol. Untreated normal skin was another reference area. After each application, both areas were covered with a polyethylene film (Lapin Muovi, Rovaniemi, Finland) and the edges were sealed with Scanpor surgical tape (Norgesplaster, Oslo, Norway). The occlusive wrap was removed after 2 h unless intolerable burning led to an earlier removal. The occlusion time was, on average, 94 min (10–120 min).

Topical Anesthesia. Four 6 × 16 cm areas were marked on the upper back. One area was treated with 9.6 ml (1 ml/10 cm^2) [3] of an anesthetic cream (lidocaine 25 mg/g, prilocaine 25 mg/g, Emla®, Astra Läkemedel, Södertälje, Sweden) and on the contralateral side of the back with the vehicle for the cream. Nothing was applied to the remaining two areas. Areas treated with the topical anesthetic and its vehicle as well as one of the two control areas were covered for 2 h with the occlusive wrap, in a manner similar to the capsaicin treatment. After occlusion, the creams were wiped off with blotting paper and dermal analgesia was confirmed with a lancet (1 mm peak, Prick-Lancett, Dome/Hollister-Stier, Miles Laboratories, Great Britain) and confirmed again after the NIICR tests [3].

Histamine Prick Tests. Prick tests were performed with histamine dihydrochloride, 10 mg/ml (Allergologisk Laboratorium, Copenhagen, Denmark) on the test areas in the capsaicin group about 23 h after the last capsaicin application, and in the topical anesthesia group after removal of the anesthetic cream. For erythema and edema reactions, the sum of the maximal diameter and the maximal diameter perpendicular to it were recorded 15 min after application, and the blood flow was measured using laser-Doppler flowmetry (LDF).

NIICR Tests. In the capsaicin group ten microliter doses of benzoic acid, 500, 250, 125, 62, and 31 m*M*, and methyl nicotinate, 50, 25, 13, 7, 3, 1.5, and 0.75 m*M*, (Sigma Chemical, St. Louis, MO, USA) in petrolatum were applied without occlusion to 1×1 cm areas of the upper back skin, 2 cm apart from each other, 23 h (18–27 h) after the last capsaicin treatment. There were two 1×1 cm reference sites on the areas treated with capsaicin solution and ethyl alcohol: one treated with petrolatum, and another site left untreated.

In the topical anesthesia group, BA 500, 125, 62, and 31 m*M*, and MN 25, 10, 2, and 0.5 m*M* were correspondingly applied to the test areas after removal of the cream. Erythema and edema reactions were graded visually 40 min after the application of the test substances as follows: −, no reaction; +, faint; + +, moderate; + + +, strong, and the blood flow was measured.

Blood Flow Measurements. The blood flow measurements were performed by one person using the LDF device (Periflux PF1, Perimed, Stockholm, Sweden) according to the manufacturer's recommendations. The instrument was equipped with a special multifiber probe (Perimed, Stockholm, Sweden) which has seven fiber triplets, one in the middle and six around forming a circle, 8 mm in diameter, in the probehead. Thus, the blood flow value is the mean of the seven spots. The values were recorded with a pen recorder for a period of about 30 s, and the average blood flow was calculated. The final results were expressed as changes in the blood flow, which were calculated by subtracting the reference value from the value of the corresponding test site. The test subjects were in a sitting position in a room with a temperature of $24° \pm 1$ °C.

Statistical Tests. The Student's *t*-test for paired observations was used for the results of LDF measurements and measurements of histamine reactions, and the Wilcoxon signed-rank test for paired observations for the visual observations of NIICRs.

Results

Histamine Prick Tests. Erythema reactions were reduced in size on anesthesized and on capsaicin-treated skin areas ($P<0.001$) as compared with the normal untreated skin (Fig. 1 a and b). In the topical anesthesia group, the edema reactions induced by histamine were smaller ($P<0.001$) on anesthesized skin as compared with the normal skin (Fig. 1 b). Blood flow in the histamine reactions was diminished in the capsaicin-treated area as compared with the area treated with ethyl alcohol ($P<0.05$) or to the untreated nonoccluded reference area ($P<0.001$). Also, the topical anes-

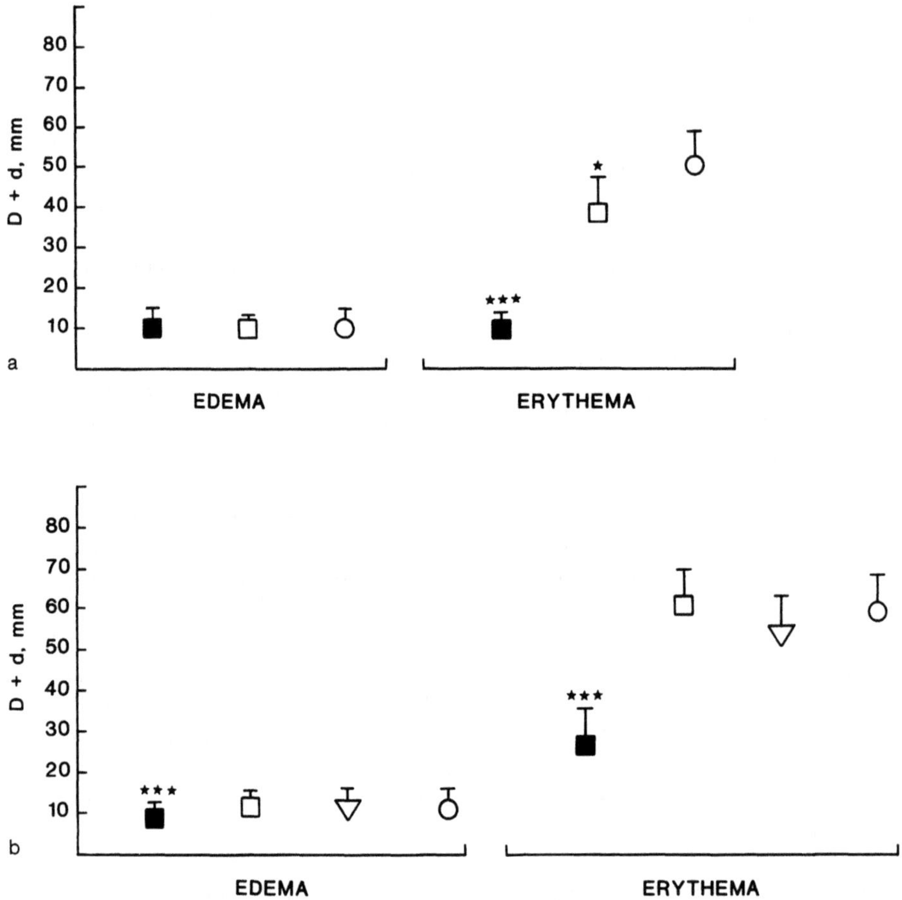

Fig. 1 a, b. Edema and erythema reactions to histamine dihydrochloride (10 mg/ml) in prick test on the back skin; **a** treated with capsaicin solution *(black square)* or with ethyl alcohol *(open square)*, as compared with histamine reactions on the normal, untreated, nonoccluded skin *(open circle; n* = 13); **b** treated with anesthetic cream *(black square)*, placebo cream *(open square)*, or occlusion *(open triangle)*, as compared with histamine reactions on the normal, untreated skin *(open circle; n* = 15). The sizes of the reactions are expressed as the sum of the maximal diameter and the maximal diameter peripendicular to it *(D+d)* in mm. $^{*}P<0.05$; $^{***}P<0.001$ in paired *t*-test

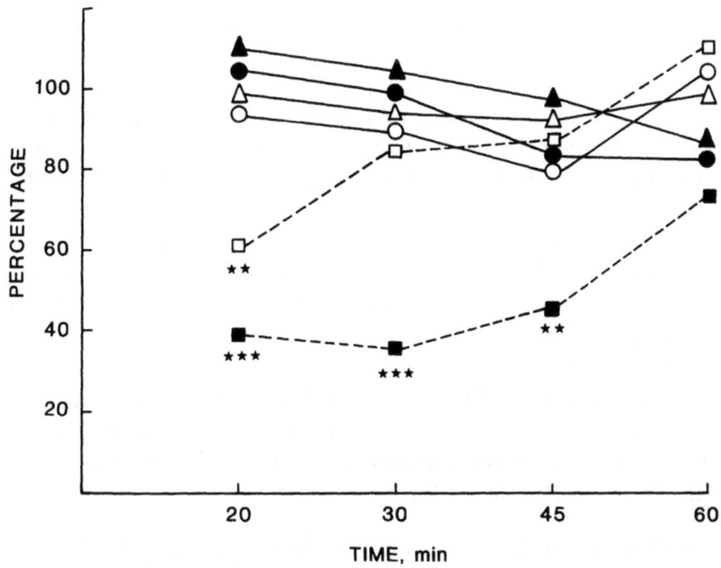

Fig. 2. Erythema reactions induced by 500 m*M* benzoic acid *(black symbols)* and 25 m*M* methyl nicotinate *(open symbols)* measured with laser-Doppler flowmetry on the upper back skin treated with anesthetic cream *(square)*, placebo *(circle)*, and occlusion *(triangle)*. Percentage of the flow values on the test site compared with values on the normal untreated skin (100%). ** $P<0.01$; *** $P<0.001$ in paired *t*-test

thetic cream diminished blood flow in the histamine reactions as compared with untreated skin ($P<0.01$).

NIICR Tests. Topical anesthesia, but not capsaicin pretreatment, diminished blood flow in the NIICRs to all concentrations of BA and MN ($P<0.01$–0.001) when measured at 20 min after application of the substances (Fig. 2).

In the visual assessment, no differences in erythema or edema reactions to BA and MN were seen between capsaicin and control areas. In the topical anesthesia group, both erythema and edema reactions to BA and MN ($P<0.05$–0.01) were weaker on the anesthesized than on the untreated control area.

Discussion

In the present study, topical capsaicin treatment did not have any distinct effect on erythema caused by topical BA and MN, suggesting that mechanisms sensitive to capsaicin (substance P) are not substantially involved in the NIICRs to these substances. Capsaicin treatment and depletion of substance P from sensory nerves interfere with certain irritant reactions in the skin (also called neurogenic edema and erythema). For example, parenteral capsaicin pretreatment or a substance P antagonist blocks erythema reactions induced by vanillyl-*n*-decoyl-amide, diminishes edema reactions to undecylenoyl-piperidine, methyl salicylate and vanillyl-ethyl-*n*-hexylketone [8] and inhibits skin edema from heat in rat skin [14].

In human skin, topical capsaicin pretreatment inhibits erythema in histamine prick test [1], which was confirmed and used as a sign of capsaicin effect also in the present study. Erythema reactions to a dilute ammonia solution [8] and erythema after a small skin injury from heat also seem to be reactions in human skin which can be inhibited by capsaicin pretreatment [2].

In the present study, topical anesthesia inhibited both erythema and edema reactions induced by BA, MN and histamine, but it is not known whether the inhibitory effect was due to the influence of lidocaine and prilocaine on the sensory nerves of the skin only, or if they also affect other cell types or regulatory mechanisms of immediate type skin inflammation [9, 10].

The mechanisms of NIICRs are still obscure, but the results of the present study suggest that pathways sensitive to capsaicin are not substantally involved in NIICRs to BA and MN. What the explanation for the inhibitory effect of topical anesthetic cream is remains a topic for further research.

Acknowledgements. This study has been financially supported by the Foundation for Allergy Research in Finland. Emla cream and its vehicle were generously supplied by Astra Läkemedel, Södertälje, Sweden.

References

1. Bernstein JE, Swift RM, Keyoumars S, Lorincz AL (1981) Inhibition of axon reflex vasodilatation by topically applied capsaicin. J Invest Dermatol 76: 394–395
2. Carpenter SE, Lynn B (1981) Vascular and sensory responses of human skin to mild injury after topical treatment of capsaicin. Br J Pharmacol 73: 755–758
3. Danielson K, Evers H (1987) Dermal analgesia after epicutaneous application of lidocaine/prilocaine cream. In: 17th world congress of dermatology, Berlin.
4. Fitzgerald M (1983) Capsaicin and sensory neurones – a review. Pain 15: 109–130
5. Foreman JC (1986) Neuropeptides and the pathogenesis of allergy. Allergy 42: 1–11
6. Gollhausen R, Kligman AM (1985) Human assay for identifying substances which induce non-allergic contact urticaria: the NICU-test. Contact Dermatitis 13: 98–106
7. Hägermark Ö, Hökfelt T, Pernow B (1978) Flare and itch induced by substance P in human skin. J Invest Dermatol 71: 233–235
8. Jancso N (1960) Role of the nerve terminals in the mechanism of inflammatory reactions. Bull Buffalo 7: 53–77
9. Johnson HG, Miller MD (1979) Inhibition of histamine release and ionophore-induced calcium flux in rat mast cells by lidocaine and chlorpromazine. Agents Actions 9: 239–243
10. Kazimierczak W, Peret M, Maslinski C (1976) The action of local anesthetics on histamine release. Biochem Pharmacol 25: 1747–1750
11. Lahti A (1980) Non-immunologic contact urticaria. Acta Derm Venereol [Suppl 91] (Stockh) 60: 1–49
12. Lahti A, McDonald DM, Tammi R, Maibach HI (1986) Pharmacological studies on non-immunologic contact urticaria in guinea pigs. Arch Dermatol Res 279: 44–49
13. Lahti A, Oikarinen A, Viinikka L, Ylikorkala O, Hannuksela M (1983) Prostaglandins in contact urticaria induced by benzoic acid. Acta Derm Venereol (Stockh) 63: 425–427
14. Lundberg JM, Saria A, Rosell S, Folkers K (1984) A substance P antagonist inhibits heat-induced oedema in the rat skin. Acta Physiol Scand 120: 145–146

Addresses

E. Larmi
University of Oulu, Department of Dermatology, SF-90220 Oulu, Finland

A. Lahti
University of Oulu, Department of Dermatology, SF-90220 Oulu, Finland

M. Hannuksela
University of Oulu, Department of Dermatology, SF-90220 Oulu, Finland

Nonimmunologic Immediate Contact Reactions to Three Isomers of Pyridine Carboxaldehyde

A. Hannuksela, A. Lahti, and M. Hannuksela

Summary

Pyridine carboxaldehyde (PCA) has recently been found to be one of the many substances able to produce nonimmunologic immediate contact reactions (NIICRs). This study investigated the ability of three isomers of PCA, 2-, 3- and 4-PCA, all in ethyl alcohol, to produce NIICRs in the guinea pig and man. In the guinea pig ear swelling test, five animals were used for each concentration of each test substance. 2-PCA did not cause swelling of the ear, 50 m*M* 4-PCA produced slight and 1 *M* moderate swelling, whereas 3-PCA was the most active in inducing slight to moderate swelling at a concentration as low as 1.6 m*M*. The results of the NIICR test (open application) on the upper back skin of ten healthy untanned Caucasians agreed with those of the guinea pig ear swelling test. The results indicate marked differences between the three isomers of PCA in the ability to produce NIICRs in both man and the guinea pig.

Key words:

Nonimmunologic immediate contact reaction - Contact urticaria - Guinea pig ear swelling test - Laser-Doppler flowmetry - Pyridine carboxaldehyde isomers

Introduction

The number of known substances producing nonimmunologic immediate contact reactions (NIICRs) continues to increase. Archer and Cronin [1] found that pyridine carboxaldehyde (PCA) was the cause of nonimmunologic contact urticaria in a

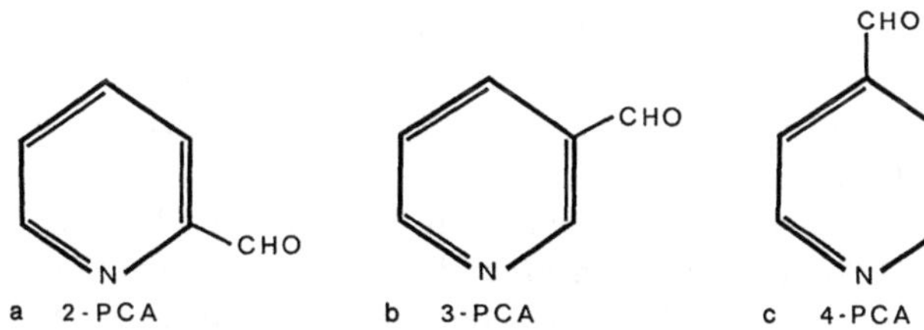

Fig. 1. Molecular structures of the three isomers of pyridine carboxaldehyde (PCA)

23-year-old female postgraduate chemistry laboratory student. These authors did not, however, state which one of the three isomers of PCA (Fig. 1) was the causative agent in the case of their patient. The purpose of this study was to investigate possible differences in the ability of 2-, 3- and 4-PCA to elicit NIICRs in guinea pig and human skin.

Materials and Methods

Guinea Pig Ear Swelling Test. Hartley strain guinea pigs of both sexes weighing from 650 g to 1000 g were fed with pellet animal diet (Ewos, Södertälje, Sweden), fresh cabbage and carrots, and water was given ad libitum. Two to ten animals were housed per cage in an artificially illuminated (12 h/day) environment with a temperature of 23° ± 1 °C and a relative humidity of around 60%.

Groups of five animals were used in the ear swelling test [2] for each concentration of the isomers of PCA (Sigma Chemical, St. Louis, MO, USA) dissolved in absolute ethyl alcohol. The concentrations of the isomers for the guinea pig and human tests were selected after performing a pilot study using 100 m*M* PCAs in open application tests on the upper back (10 μl to 1 × 1 cm area) in eight test subjects. These were 2-PCA, as is and 1 *M;* 3-PCA, 100 m*M,* 50 m*M,* 25 m*M,* 12.5 m*M,* 1.6 m*M* and 0.4 m*M;* 4-PCA, 1 *M,* 500 m*M,* 250 m*M,* 100 m*M,* 50 m*M,* 25 m*M* and 12.5 m*M.* Doses of 50 μl were applied to both sides of the animal's right earlobe. The left ear was treated in a similar way with absolute ethyl alcohol as a reference substance.

The thickness of the earlobe was measured with a micrometer (Model 7309, Mitutoyo, Tokyo, Japan) at the midpart of the ear 0.5 cm from the outer rim. The measurement was conducted twice before the application of the substance, and twice every 15 min during the first hour and every 30 min during the second hour; the mean of each pair of measurements was then recorded. The thickness prior to the application was subtracted from the maximum value, usually occurring 30 min after application, and this change in ear thickness was used for final calculations.

NIICR Test in Man. Ten healthy untanned Caucasians, two men and eight women, four of whom were atopics, participated as volunteers in this part of the study. The mean age was 26.6 years (range, 20 to 49 years). The subjects refrained from taking acetylsalicylic acid or other prostaglandin inhibitors for 5 days, or antihistamines for 3 days, and they had not been subjected to ultraviolet light irradation for at least 2 weeks before the test.

The following were applied in 10-μl doses: 2-PCA, as is and 1 *M;* 3-PCA, 50 m*M,* 1.6 m*M* and 0.4 m*M;* and 4-PCA, 1 *M,* 50 m*M* and 1.6 m*M.* Together with absolute ethyl alcohol as the vehicle these substances were applied without occlusion to 1 × 1 cm areas of the upper back skin.

The reactions were observed visually, and the blood flow was measured at 20, 40 and 60 min after application. Four grades were used in the visual assessment: −, no reaction; +, slight; + +, moderate; and + + +, intense erythema or edema.

Blood flow was measured with a laser-Doppler flowmetry (LDF) device (Periflux PF1, Perimed, Stockholm, Sweden) according to the manufacturer's recommendations. The difference in blood flow values between each NIICR test site and a reference site treated with ethyl alcohol was calculated.

During testing, the test subjects were in a sitting position in a room with a temperature of 25° ±2 °C.

Results

In the guinea pig ear swelling test, 3-PCA caused stronger reactions than the other two isomers (Fig. 2). 4-PCA was next in order and 2-PCA induced no reactions at all.

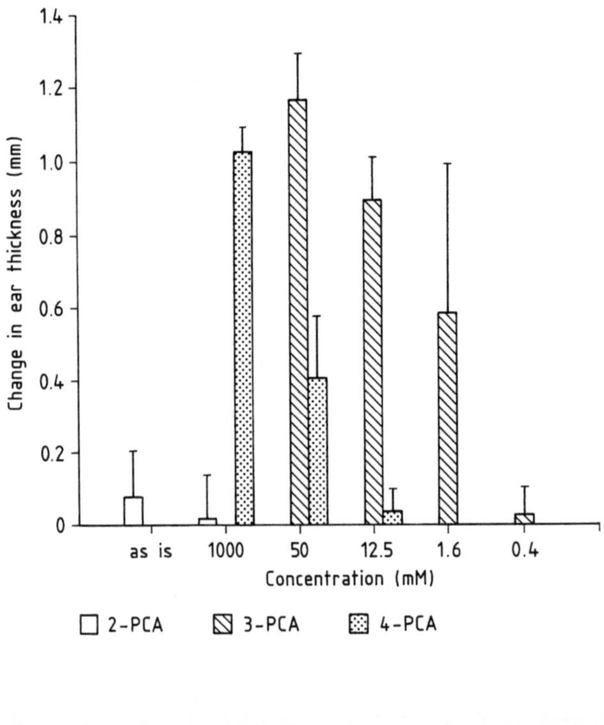

Fig. 2. The results of the guinea pig ear swelling test with the three isomers of pyridine carboxaldehyde (PCA; 50 μl on both sides of the ear lobe) expressed as change in the ear thickness (mean, SD, $n = 5$)

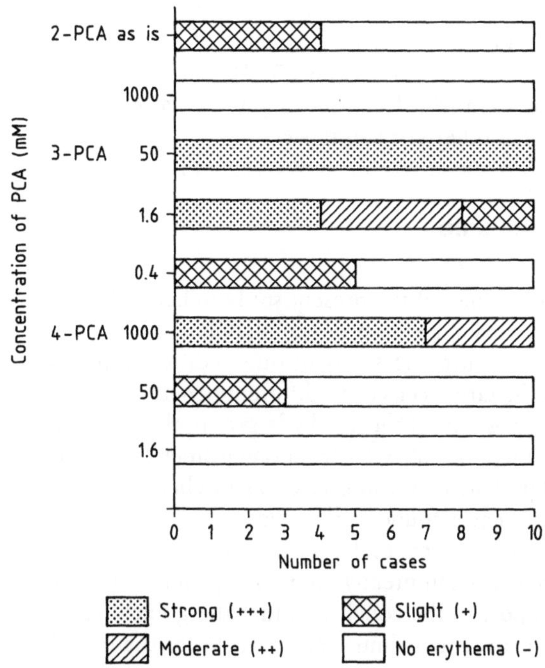

Fig. 3. Erythema induced by the three isomers of pyridine carboxaldehyde (PCA) on human back skin ($n = 10$) at 20 min after application

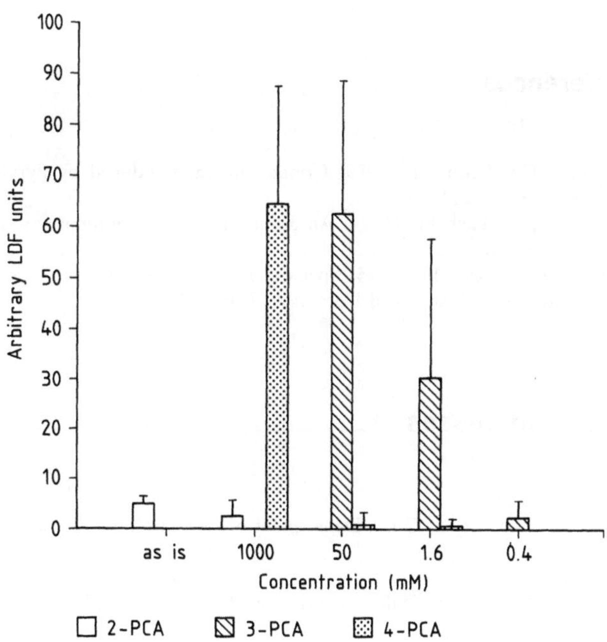

Fig. 4. Changes in blood flow measured with laser-Doppler flowmetry (LDF) at 20 min after application of the three isomers of pyridine carboxaldehyde (PCA) to the human upper back skin ($n = 10$)

In human skin, the same order of NIICR-eliciting potency was found as in guinea pig skin. The visual assessments of erythema correlated well with the results of the LDF measurements (Figs. 3, 4). Slight to marked edema was produced by 50 m*M* and 1.6 m*M* 3-PCA and slight edema by 1 *M* 4-PCA, but no edema was produced by the other test substances.

Discussion

The results of the present study indicate that the three isomers of PCA have different capabilities to produce NIICRs.

The differences may be due to different physicochemical properties of the isomers in the target cells or to different penetration rates through intact skin. Depending on the position of the aldehyde group, the three-dimensional structure and the polarity of the molecule vary from one isomer to another. 2-PCA is less polar than the other two. This may cause changes in chemical activity, and may be one reason for the differences found in the study.

The present results show that only a slight change in the molecular structure of a chemical can greatly alter its capability to produce NIICRs. Our findings also give support to the conclusion that the guinea pig ear swelling test and the NIICR tests in man render similar results as far as the NIICR-producing ability of a substance is concerned [3].

References

1. Archer CB, Cronin E (1986) Contact urticaria induced by pyridine carboxaldehyde. Contact Dermatitis 15: 308–309
2. Lahti A, Maibach HI (1984) An animal model for nonimmunologic contact urticaria. Toxicol Appl Pharmacol 76: 219–224
3. Lahti A, Maibach HI (1985) Species specifity of nonimmunologic contact urticaria: guinea pig, rat and mouse. J Am Acad Dermatol 13: 68–69

Addresses

A. Hannuksela
University of Oulu, Department of Dermatology, SF-90220 Oulu, Finland

A. Lahti
University of Oulu, Department of Dermatology, SF-90220 Oulu, Finland

M. Hannuksela
University of Oulu, Department of Dermatology, SF-90220 Oulu, Finland

Immediate Type Dermatitis, Contact Urticaria, and Rhinitis from Carbonless Copy Paper: Report of Four Cases

M. Hannuksela and F. Björksten

Summary

Carbonless copy paper (CCP) has been reported to be able to cause type I immediate reactions, especially in the airways. Within a 2-year period, four female patients were seen with chronic dermatitis on their palms, resembling dermatitis known as infectious or chronic dermatitis of unknown origin. One of them also had rhinitis. All four were office-workers and handled CCP for several hours per day. In contact urticaria tests with the upper CCP sheet and the back side towards the patients' skin, tiny wheals and erythema appeared in all four cases. RASTs were performed with the sera of three patients, using four different CCP brands. The RAST value was slightly greater (1.5 kU/l) in one patient's serum than in any of three control sera (maximum 0.6 kU/l). All four patients were able to continue their work by reducing contact with the paper. The present findings suggest that immediate-type skin reactions appearing as contact urticaria and chronic hand dermatitis may be more common than has been assumed.

Key words:

Carbonless copy paper - Contact urticaria - Immediate contact reaction - Allergic rhinitis

Introduction

Two types of reactions to carbonless copy paper (CCP) have been reported. Delayed-type allergy to the chemical colouring previously expressed as allergic contact dermatitis, is an uncommon reaction [2]. Immediate-type reactions in the skin and mucous membranes – including redness of the skin, contact urticaria, hoarseness and airway obstruction (as objective symptoms) and fatigue, nausea, headache, and burning of the nose, eyes, mouth and chest, as well as itching, chest tightness and pain, breathing difficulty, and rapid heart beat (as subjective symptoms) – have been reported in a number of office-workers [1, 3, 4]. The mechanism responsible for the immediate reactions has not, however, been found.

This is a report of a study of contact urticaria from CCP, expressed as chronic dermatitis on the palms of four female patients, one of whom also complained of rhinitis when handling CCP.

Case Reports

Four female office-workers with chronic dermatitis on the palms, resembling nonspecific "infectious" hand dermatitis, were seen in Oulu within 18 months (in 1986–1987). All of them handled various types of CCP for 4–7 h daily, and had suffered from itchy hand dermatitis for 10 months to 5 years (Table 1). They had noticed that the dermatitis improved during weekends and usually disappeared during summer holidays, but worsened clearly already on Mondays. One patient (KR) also suffered from a runny nose and sneezes at her workplace.

The contact urticaria test with the back side of the upper sheet of CCP was clearly positive in all four cases, and the front side of the lower sheet elicited a positive reaction in two cases (Table 1).

RAST tests with sera of three patients and with three control sera from patients without signs of hypersensitivity to self-copying paper were performed in the Allergy Hospital, Helsinki, using pieces of the upper sheets of four brands of CCP as RAST discs. The results are recorded in Table 2.

Patient TO reacted positively to nickel, formaldehyde and fragrance mix in the European standard patch test series. These reactions were allergic but irrelevant to the present dermatitis. All four patients continued their work as office-workers, reducing the handling of CCP as much as possible. Dermatitis improved in every case within 1 or 2 months.

Table 1. Clinical data of four cases of immediate-type hypersensitivity to carbonless copy paper (CCP) and results of a contact urticaria test with the back side of the upper sheet [1] and with the front side of the lower sheet [2] of CCP

Patient	Age years	Personal history of atopy	Duration of		Contact-urticaria test	
			Hand dermatitis	Rhinitis	1	2
PK	30	No atopy	2 Years	–	++	–
TO	32	No atopy	5 Years	–	++	+
KR	25	(Atopic?) Dermatitis on buttocks	10 Months	10 Months	++	++
TV	34	Asthma and rhinitis in childhood, active dermatitis at present	1 Year	–	++	–

++, Wheals and flare; +, redness only; –, no reaction

Table 2. RAST test results with the upper sheet of four brands of carbonless copy paper (CCP) in sera of three patients with contact urticaria and chronic hand dermatitis from CCP, and of three control patients

	Total serum IgE (kU/l)	RAST results with four brands of CCP (kU/l)			
		A	B	C	D[a]
Patients					
PK	26	0.4	0.0	0.5	0.5
TO	30	0.4	0.0	0.4	0.5
TV	820	1.2	0.0	0.6	1.5
Controls					
1	100	0.1	0.0	0.1	0.2
2	590	0.4	0.0	0.3	0.5
3	2700	0.5	0.1	0.4	0.6

[a] Recipe form

Discussion

Especially in the 1970s, office-workers attributed their many skin and mucous membrane symptoms to CCP. Calnan [1] patch-tested 18 office-workers and collators, with negative results. Patch tests with 17 constituents of CCP were also negative in 25 employees of the Copenhagen Telephone Company subjected to skin testing because of their skin symptoms, which had been suspected to be caused by the paper [4]. Nor were immediate open-test reactions with the paper or its constituents observed in eight people tested. Eleven of 26 reacted to CCP in prick tests but the meaning of this finding remained obscure [4].

In a plant survey of a factory engaged in printing, cutting and collating business forms, 10 of 59 employees complained of throat irritation, skin itching, rash, headache, hoarseness, breathing difficulty and other indefinite symptoms [3]. One of them, a 27-year-old woman, was investigated thoroughly. She showed contact urticaria and airway obstruction from CCP, and both appeared in provocation tests. The plasma throboxane B_2 and prostaglandin PGF_2 levels increased during the provocation, suggesting that the symptoms may be mediated by prostaglandins.

In the present study, a contact urticaria test was clearly positive in four patients with chronic-type dermatitis of the palms. Results in RASTs were inconclusive. Immediate reactions to CCP, allergic or not, are obviously more common than is generally assumed.

References

1. Calnan CD (1979) Carbon and carbonless copy paper. Acta Derm Venereol [Suppl 85] (Stockh) 59: 27–32
2. Marks JG (1981) Allergic contact dermatitis from carbonless copy paper. JAMA 245: 2331–2332

3. Marks JG Jr, Trautlein JJ, Zwillich CW, Demers LM (1984) Contact urticaria and airway obstruction from carbonless copy paper. JAMA 252: 1038–1040
4. Menné T, Asnaes G, Hjorth N (1981) Skin and mucous membrane problems from "no carbon required" paper. Contact Dermatitis 7: 72–76

Addresses

M. Hannuksela
Department of Dermatology, University of Oulu, SF-90220 Oulu, Finland

F. Björksten
Allergy Hospital, Helsinki University Central Hospital, Helsinki, Finland

Immediate and Late Type Allergy to Latex: Contact Urticaria, Asthma and Contact Dermatitis

J. Görtz and M. Goos

Summary

A growing number of case reports of IgE-mediated contact urticaria to rubber latex are being published. The present case concerns a combined immediate and late type allergy to latex: an 8-year-old boy with atopic background (eczema of the flexures 6 months previously) developed generalized urticaria after contact with rubber balloons. Upon blowing up a rubber balloon, once, asthma occurred. A scratch test showed an immediate wheal and flare response (20 min) with ruber balloons and latex gloves, but not with vinyl gloves. Latex RAST ELISA was positive. Patch tests with rubber latex pieces showed no immediate reaction (20 min), but a marked eczema (+ + +) after 48 and 72 h. Patch testing with a rubber ingredients test series was negative. Possible pathomechanisms are discussed.

Key words:

Latex allergy - Contact urticaria - Asthma - Contact dermatitis - Specific IgE

Contact dermatitis to rubber is common and is usually due to the ingredients of rubber. In contrast, reports of sensitivity to rubber latex itself did not appear before 1979 [7]. Recently, allergy, especially contact urticaria, to rubber latex has been reported by several authors [1, 2, 5, 6, 8, 9].

In the reports of immunological contact urticaria, there are a few observations concerning consecutive eczema after previous contact urticaria [5, 7].

Case Report

For 2 years an 8-year-old boy with atopic background (eczema of the flexures 6 months previously) developed generalized urticaria after contact with rubber balloons or with rubber mats during sports. Upon blowing up a rubber balloon, once, asthma occurred.

A rubbing test with rubber balloons and latex gloves was negative after 20 min.

A scratch test showed an immediate wheal and flare response (20 min) with rubber balloons (+ + +) and latex gloves (+ + +), but not with vinyl gloves, balloon or glove powder (NaCl negative, 1% histamine, + + +).

Patch tests with rubber latex pieces showed no immediate reaction (20 min), but a marked eczema (+ + +) after 48 and 72 h. There was no difference in reaction between the inner or outer surface of the gloves or after removal of the powder. Patch testing with the standard series of the ICDRG, rubber ingredients, rubber balloon powder and glove powder was negative. Latex RAST was positive (class 2).

Discussion

Recent publications have demonstrated that latex contact allergy is more frequent than initially assumed: Turjanmaa [9] reported 15 (3%) persons with immediate latex glove allergy among 512 glove-using hospital employees.

Studies by Meding and Fregert showed that the antigen in latex contact urticaria is a water-soluble protein [6]. The antigen seems to have a molecular weight higher than 30000 Daltons and is trypsin-sensitive [1]. Turjanmaa [9] also found a water solubility of the latex allergen.

Several studies have shown latex contact urticaria to be IgE-mediated [2, 8]: circulating IgE antibodies against natural latex have been detected by positive passive transfer, radioimmunoassay, histamine release assay and immunoenzymatic assay [1].

The latex allergy can lead to a generalized urticaria and to respiratory reactions like rhinitis or even asthma or, rarely, anaphylactic reactions [8].

A latex contact urticaria is especially frequent in the medical professions (nurses, dentists and surgeons). In most publications the high prevalence of atopic diathesis is noticed: Turjanmaa [9] found an atopic disease in 2/3 of the persons with latex contact urticaria. Atopic individuals often suffer from irritant hand eczema and hence must use rubber or vinyl gloves for hand protection. Continuous wearing of rubber gloves on eczematous hands may be one predisposing factor for the development of either delayed or immediate rubber allergy.

Surgeons with a latex contact allergy seem to work successfully by wearing (cotton or vinyl) undergloves or using a brand of latex glove reportedly causing fewer symptoms [9].

In our case, oral therapy with terfenadine had a beneficial effect on the boy's pruritus and whealing when given prior to contact with rubber.

In the reports of immunological contact urticaria, there are a few observations concerning a consecutive eczema after previous contact urticaria [5, 7]. Nutter [7] states that it is uncertain whether the combination of positive prick test and patch tests represents a double hypersensitivity; alternatively, a positive patch test may be produced by a type I reaction in a patient with atopic dermatitis if persistent antigen challenge is maintained for 3 days.

Some authors regard eczematous dermatitis in contact urticaria patients as a late phase reaction after a type I reaction [3, 5] and, hence, the dermatitis might be classified as protein-contact dermatitis [4, 5].

References

1. Carrillo T, Cuevas M, Munoz T, Hinojosa M, Moneo I (1986) Contact urticaria and rhinitis from latex surgical gloves. Contact Dermatitis 15: 69–72
2. Frosch PJ, Wahl R, Bahmer FA, Maasch HJ (1986) Contact urticaria to rubber gloves is IgE-mediated. Contact Dermatitis 14: 241–245
3. Gleich GJ (1982) The late phase of the immunoglobulin E-mediated reaction: a link between anaphylaxis and common allergic disease? J Allergy Clin Immunol 70: 160–169
4. Hjorth N, Roed-Petersen J (1976) Occupational protein contact dermatitis in food handlers. Contact Dermatitis 2: 28–42
5. Kleinhans D (1984) Soforttyp-Allergie gegen Latex: Kontakt-Urtikaria und Ekzem. Akt Dermatol 10: 227–228
6. Meding B, Fregert S (1984) Contact urticaria from natural latex gloves. Contact Dermatitis 10: 52–53
7. Nutter AF (1979) Contact urticaria to rubber. Br J Dermatol 101: 597–598
8. Seifert HU, Seifert B, Wahl R, Vocks E, Borelli S, Maasch HJ (1987) Immunglobulin E-vermittelte Kontakturtikaria bzw. Asthma bronchiale durch Latex enthaltende Haushaltsgummihandschuhe. Derm Beruf Umwelt 35: 137–139
9. Turjanmaa K (1987) Incidence of immediate allergy to latex gloves in hospital personnel. Contact Dermatitis 17: 270–275

Addresses

J. Görtz

Department of Dermatology, University of Essen, Hufelandstrasse 55, 4300 Essen 1, FRG

M. Goos

Department of Dermatology, University of Essen, Hufelandstrasse 55, 4300 Essen 1, FRG

Latex-Contact Urticaria Associated with Delayed Allergy to Rubber Chemicals

K. Turjanmaa and T. Reunala

Summary

Fifty-three glove-allergic patients, 35 with immediate allergy to latex (natural rubber) and 18 with previously verified delayed allergy to rubber chemicals, were examined in order to determine the concomitant occurrence of these allergies. Of latex-allergic patients, 5/35 (14%) showed positive patch tests to thiurams and 1/18 (6%) patients with delayed allergy to rubber chemicals had positive prick test to latex. In addition, 3/53 (6%) patients showed urticarial reactions to rubber chemicals in scratch-chamber tests. These results indicate that the coexistence of immediate and delayed rubber-glove allergies is not infrequent.

Key words:

Latex - Rubber - Prick tests - Patch tests

Introduction

Rubber chemicals in gloves are a well-known cause of contact dermatitis [2]. Recently, latex protein persisting in rubber gloves after manufacture has also been recognized as an allergen causing contact urticaria. The frequency of this immediate allergy was as high as 3% among personnel using gloves in our hospital [8]. In contrast, the simultaneous occurrence of immediate and delayed rubber-glove allergies has rarely been reported [6]. For this reason we examined more thoroughly 53 patients allergic to rubber gloves. All were patch or scratch-chamber (S-C) tested using various rubber chemicals, and prick tests were performed using latex protein eluted from the rubber gloves.

Table 1. Clinical history of 35 patients with immediate and 18 patients with delayed rubber-glove allergy

Patients	Sex		Mean age years (range)	Personal atopy[a], n (%)	Hand eczema[a], n (%)	Sensitizing glove	
	F	M				Surgical (n)	Cleaning (n)
With immediate latex allergy (n=35)	30	5	36 (20–69)	29 (83%)	34 (97%)	23	12
With delayed rubber chemical allergy (n=18)	13	5	40 (21–57)	7 (39%)	16 (89%)	2	16

[a] Past or present symptoms

Patients and Methods

The first group consisted of 35 glove-using patients with previously diagnosed latex-contact urticaria (Table 1). These were patch-tested using ICDRG standard series (Epicon, Finland) and 29 of them also with a rubber series including 13 chemicals: N-cyclohexylbenzothiazyl sulphenamide (CBS), N-cyclohexyl-N′-phenyl-para-phenylenediamine (CPPD), 1,3-diphenylguanidine (DPG), phenyl-β-naphthylamine (PBN), hexamethylene tetramine, tetramethylthiuram monosulphide (TMTM), diphenyl-p-phenylenediamine (DPPD), 2,2′-dibenzothiazyl disulphide (MBTS), morpholinylmercaptobenzothiazole (MOR), tetraethylthiuram disulphide (TETD), dipentamethylenethiuram disulphide (PTD), zinc dibutyldithiocarbamate (ZBC), all 1% in petrolatum and 4,4′-dihydroxydiphenyl (DOD) 0.2% in petrolatum. The patch tests were applied for 24 h using Finn chambers on Scanpor and read on days 1 and 3 or 4.

The second group consisted of 18 patients with previously diagnosed rubber-glove contact dermatitis (Table 1). Seventeen of these patients had had positive patch tests to thiurams and one to naphthyl mix. Moreover, eight of these had positive tests to carba mix and five to components of mercapto mix.

Latex prick, RAST and use tests were carried out as described earlier [8, 9]. Prick tests were also performed using solutions from vinyl-glove and corn-starch glove powder (Biosorb, Johnsson and Johnsson, Arlington, Texas, USA). S-C tests with thiuram-, mercapto- and PPD mixes and ZBC in petrolatum were performed on the volar side of the forearm and were read after 15 min. The test was regarded as positive if the size of test reaction was at least half of that for histamine (10 mg/ml).

Results

Table 2 shows the prick, S-C and patch test results of 53 patients. Five (14%) of the latex-allergic patients (nos. 1–5, Table 2) had positive patch tests to thiurams and one of the 18 patients with delayed allergy to rubber chemicals (no. 6, Table 2) gave

Table 2. Prick, scratch-chamber and patch test results in seven patients with immediate and delayed rubber-glove allergy

Patient no.	Occupation	Age/Sex	Latex tests			Rubber chemicals	
			Prick	RAST score (0–4)	Use test with glove	Patch tests[a]	S-C tests
1.	Charwoman	60/F	+	1	+	Thiuram mix, carba mix TMTM, TMTD, PTD	–
2.	Cutter	39/F	+	2	+	TMTM, CPPD	–
3.	Saw mill worker	28/F	+	0	+	Thiuram mix, TETD	–
4.	Instrument cleaner	42/F	+	2	+	Thiuram mix, TMTM, PTD	Thiuram mix, mercapto mix, PPD
5.	Laboratory nurse	30/F	+	0	+	Thiuram mix, TETD, MBTS	–
6.	Bakery worker	55/F	+	3	+	Naphthyl mix[b]	Thiuram mix, MBT
7.	Housewife	29/F	–	0	+	TETD, MOR, MBT, CBS, MBTS, DPG	MBT

[a] With ICDRG routine and rubber series
[b] Rubber series not tested

a positive latex prick test result. The latter patient also had a clearly positive latex use test and RAST. She had experienced hand eczema, and facial and lid oedema when using rubber gloves in her work. Three of the 53 patients showed urticarial reactions to rubber chemicals in S-C tests. All three had positve patch tests to rubber chemicals and positive glove use test, but one of these three (no. 7, Table 2) was not allergic to latex. None of the 53 patients showed positive prick tests to glove powder or vinyl gloves.

Discussion

Several recent reports have described patients with contact urticaria and even systemic immediate symptoms when surgical or cleaning latex gloves are used [1, 3, 6, 12]. Several of these patients have had, in addition to contact urticaria, hand eczema, which disappeared when the use of rubber gloves was avoided [9, 12]. Such an eczema may represent true "protein-contact dermatitis" from the latex in the gloves or may be due to other mechanisms [5]. In the present study we examined 35 latex-allergic patients of whom 97% had a past history of hand eczema and 74% suffered from it at present. Patch tests disclosed that five of these were allergic to thiurams. Therefore, the concomitant delayed allergy to rubber chemicals may explain hand eczema in some of these latex-allergic people, but the remaining patients could have either irritant dermatitis or true "protein-contact dermatitis" caused by the rubber gloves. Latex proteins originate from the rubber tree *(Hevea brasiliensis)* and, interestingly, a recent report has shown that at least in experimental conditions plant protein such as birch pollen can produce eczematous patch test reactions in sensitized subjects [7].

In the literature concomitant delayed and immediate allergy to rubber gloves seems rare. Kleinhans [6] has described one male nurse who had positive patch tests to mercapto mix, TETD and ZDC (zinc diethyldithiocarbamate) and was allergic to latex. In the present study we examined 18 patients who had been previously diagnosed as having rubber-glove contact dermatitis. Prick testing disclosed one patient, a bakery worker, who had clearly positive latex prick test, and both the use test and RAST confirmed her latex allergy. Therefore, patients with delayed allergy to rubber chemicals may also have undetected coexistent latex allergy. Conversely, latex allergy may be accompanied by undetected, delayed allergy to rubber chemicals. In addition to allergy to latex, some recent reports have described a few patients with an immediate allergy to rubber chemicals. Helander [4] found that one kitchen worker developed contact urticaria when using cleaning gloves. She had positive S-C tests in response to ZDC and to the outer and inner surface of the glove, but unfortunately no latex prick test was performed. Wrangsjö et al. [12] reported one latex-allergic patient with positive scratch tests to ZPD (zinc pentamethylene dithiocarbamate) and ZDBC (zinc dibutyl dithiocarbamate). We performed S-C tests using several rubber chemicals and found three (6%) patients with immediate reactions. Two of these were latex-allergic and all three also had a delayed allergy to several rubber chemicals. The patient not allergic to latex developed contact urticaria when a rubber-glove use test was performed and also showed immediate urticarial reactions in the MBT patch test area. However, the S-C test reactions in this patient and the other two patients were smaller than the size of histamine, suggesting that S-C tests using rubber chemicals in petrolatum should be interpreted carefully.

The coexistent immediate latex and delayed rubber-chemical allergy in 11% of the present patients deserves practical consideration. Patients for whom the delayed allergy to rubber chemicals is verified with patch tests, while an immediate allergy to latex remains undetected, may even be at risk of developing anaphylaxis as a result of the contact with surgical latex gloves during operations or deliveries [10]. The latex allergy can be easily confirmed using a latex prick test [11]. Therefore, the simultaneous patch testing with rubber chemicals and prick testing with latex are recommended, even if a patient using rubber gloves has only hand-eczema symptoms and especially when a patient is atopic.

Acknowledgements. The excellent assistance of Mrs. Leena Petman in allergological testing is acknowledged. This study was supported by a grant from Tampere University Central Hospital.

References

1. Axelsson JGK, Johansson SGO, Wrangsjö K (1987) IgE-mediated anaphylactoid reactions to rubber. Allergy 42: 46–50
2. Cronin E (1980) Contact dermatitis. Churchill Livingstone, Edinburgh London New York, pp 734–747
3. Frosch PJ, Wahl R, Bahmer FA, Maasch HJ (1986) Contact urticaria to rubber gloves is IgE-mediated. Contact Dermatitis 14: 241–245
4. Helander I, Mäkelä A (1983) Contact urticaria to zinc diethyldithiocarbamate (ZDC). Contact Dermatitis 9: 327–328
5. Hjorth N, Roed-Petersen J (1976) Occupational protein contact dermatitis in food handlers. Contact Dermatitis 2: 28–42
6. Kleinhans D (1984) Contact urticaria to rubber gloves. Contact Dermatitis 10: 124–125
7. Reitamo S, Visa K, Kähönen K, Käyhkö K, Stubb S, Salo OP (1986) Eczematous reactions in atopic patients caused by epicutaneous testing with inhalant allergens. Br J Dermatol 114: 303–309
8. Turjanmaa K (1987) Incidence of immediate allergy to latex gloves in hospital personnel. Contact Dermatitis 17: 270–275
9. Turjanmaa K, Reunala T (1988) Contact urticaria from rubber gloves. Dermatologic Clin 6: 47–51
10. Turjanmaa K, Reunala T, Tuimala R, Kärkkäinen T (1988) Latex glove allergy – an unusual complication during delivery. BMJ 297–1029
11. Turjanmaa K, Reunala T, Räsänen L (1988) Comparison of diagnostic methods in latex surgical glove contact urticaria. Contact Dermatitis 19: 241–247
12. Wrangsjö K, Mellström G, Axelsson G (1986) Discomfort from rubber gloves indicating contact urticaria. Contact Dermatitis 15: 79–84

Addresses

K. Turjanmaa

Department of Dermatology, Tampere University Central Hospital, SF 33520 Tampere, Finland

T. Reunala

Department of Clinical Sciences, University of Tampere, SF 33520 Tampere, Finland

Contact Urticaria and Allergic Contact Dermatitis to Constituents of Human Seminal Fluid

H.-G. Schimkat, M. Andary, J. Clot, C. Humeau, B. Descomps, A. Dieng, B. Previero, C. Sultan, M. Robinet-Levy, G. Barneon, J. M. Meynadier, and J. Meynadier

Summary

We describe a woman who suffered from coital vaginal burning and pain, rarely accompanied by genital and facial swelling. Six hours later genital erythema appeared. Fifteen hours after intercourse she observed painful vulvar erosions. Histology showed eczema. Local provocation with her partner's fresh whole semen produced an erythemato-vesiculous eruption, which on histology showed eczema. Patch tests, scratch test and RAST for antibodies to human seminal plasma were negative. Lymphocyte transformation tests were positive with some fractions of her partner's seminal fluid. History, clinical observation and test results favor the conclusion that there can be a coexistence of contact urticaria and allergic contact dermatitis to constituents of human semen.

Key words:

Contact urticaria - Allergic contact dermatitis - Seminal fluid

Introduction

From the time of the first report on anaphylactic allergy to a glycoprotein present in human seminal fluid [5], observations of a variety of allergic reactions - mainly localized and generalized anaphylactic reactions - to human semen and its constituents have been published (for review see [2, 3]), but also the association of a local reaction with a rash [1] and recently the association of allergy to human semen and sweat have been described [4]. We observed a patient who suffered from coital vaginal burning and postcoital vulvar and perivulvar erythemato-vesiculous eruptions, which, to the best of our knowledge, have no published precedent.

Case Report

A 25-year-old woman consulted for symptoms during and after intercourse. She had been living with the same man for 6 years. Contact with other partners and nonvaginal sexual practices were denied. Condoms and spermicides had not been used prior to consultation. Intercourse was limited owing to the frequent professional absences of her partner. In the first 4 years of their partnership, no sexual problems appeared other than painful penetration in the first 2 weeks. Two years ago she observed for the first time postcoital genital erosions (Fig. 1). Symptoms then progressively evolved to their present state: despite extensive use of lubricants, not employed before, she has the sensation that her partner becomes jammed. Vaginal burning and pain irregularly appear during intercourse, subsiding completely within 1 h after it's end, and obliging her sometimes to stop lovemaking. Burning and pain were also present on the few occasions when the couple used condoms. When ejaculation in the vagina occurs, she feels the vaginal entry becoming "wrinkled and as contracted" at 15 min, rendering the first micturition "difficult but not painful". At 6 to 8 h erythema appears on the genitalia, accompanied at 15 h by vesicles which develop into painful erosions covered by a white-yellowish coating (Figs. 2 and 3). Healing without scarring takes 3 weeks. Episodes were accompanied by infectious colpitis (candida, streptococci, staphylococci) and urethritis. She also reported rare postcoital genital and facial swelling. An episode of hand eczema was well controlled by emollients and the wearing of cotton gloves beneath the plastic gloves used for wet work. The patient was aware that she had "sensitive skin". The family history revealed psoriasis in her mother and asthma in a nephew. The patient did not take medications with the exception of an oral contraceptive. For skin test see Fig. 4. Total IgE was in the normal range. The commercial RAST for IgE antibodies to human seminal fluid was negative. Different fractions from seminal plasma were obtained by gel chromatography (G-200) and added at various dilutions to peripheral blood mononuclear cells from the patient; preliminary data showed lymphoproliferative responses in the presence of some fractions already reported as immunogenic; further studies are in progress. Assay plate sperm agglutination for serum and cervi-

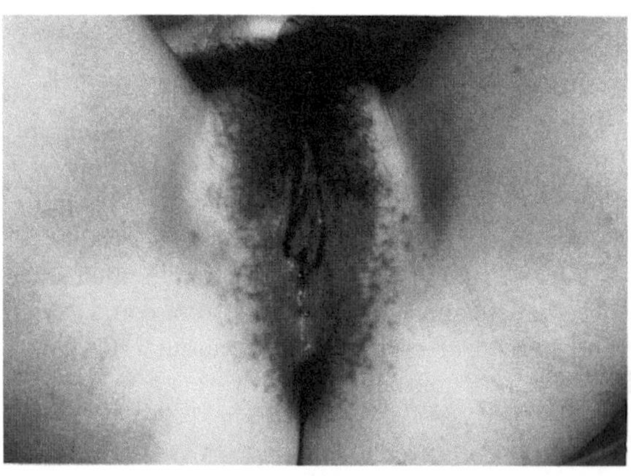

Fig. 1. Provoked eruption of the vulva and perivulvar erythema, swelling of the right minor labium; vesicles can not be recognized here, but were clinically evident

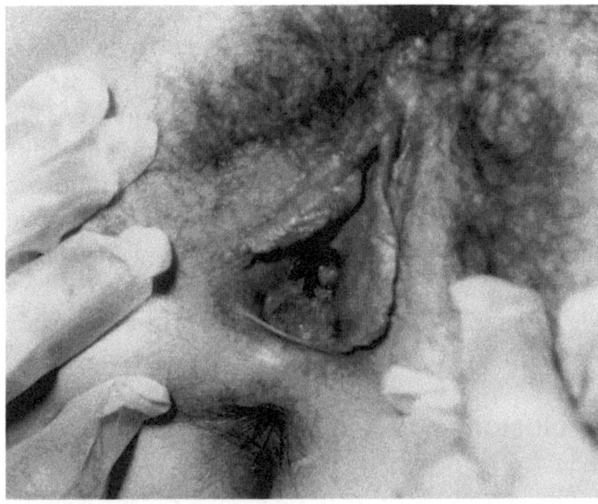

Fig. 2. Postcoital erythema and erosions of the vulva. Erosions are covered by a white-yellowish coating

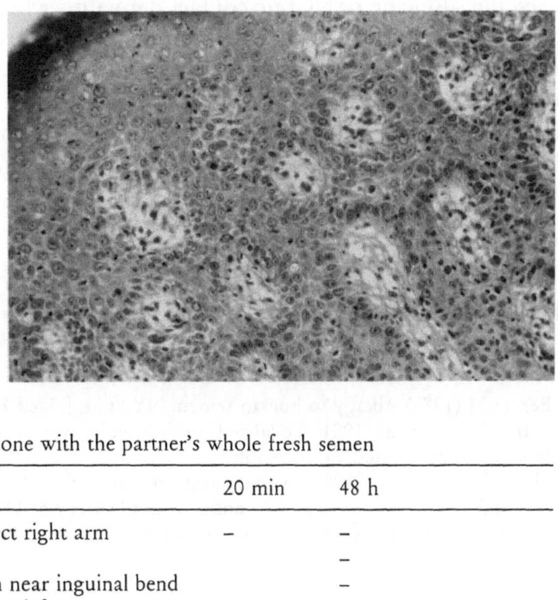

Fig. 3. Histology of a postcoital eruption showing parakeratosis and spongiosis of the horny layer, spongiosis and lymphocytic exocytosis of the basal cell and squamous cell layer, and oedema and perivascular lymphocytic infiltrate of the dermis

Fig. 4. Skin tests. All skin tests were done with the partner's whole fresh semen

		20 min	48 h
– Open	Volar aspect right arm	–	–
– Patch	Back		–
	Righ thigh near inguinal bend		–
– Scratch	Volar aspect left arm	–	
	➧ Covered by chamber		–
– Intradermal	ND		
– Provocative testing	Vulvar and perivulvar	–	+ + + Erythemato-vesiculous

cal mucus antispermatozoid antibodies were negative. Cell cultures for herpes simplex virus were repeatedly negative.

The patient refused long-term condom use. She was therefore advised to take diphenhydramine 0.06 g 30 min before exposure and to have a vaginal shower immediately after ejaculation. This combination proved completely effective in prevention of delayed erythemato-vesiculous eruptions and also alleviated burning and pain. One night she fell asleep after problem-free intercourse without having had a vaginal shower, and experienced a complete relapse on waking up the next morning (painful vulva, erythemato-vesiculous eruption; Fig. 2). Since then she associates regular use of a spermicide (benzalkonium chloride), diphenhydramine and a postcoital vaginal shower with complete prevention of vesicles and erosions. Burning and pain during and shortly after intercourse, however, persist to varying degrees, from "no complaints" to "severe enough to stop lovemaking". Erythema and increased sensitivity of her vulva persist for 4 to 5 days, in effect allowing for one episode of intercourse per week. Leukorrhea has become rare.

Conclusions

Some authors have found evidence of cell-mediated hypersensitivity to human semen in the laboratory work-up of their patients. In our case, the clinical picture raised the suspicion of allergic contact dermatitis which was confirmed by local provocative testing. Preliminary data of lymphoblastic proliferation tests favour the hypothesis that the eliciting agent(s) can be found in fractions of human seminal plasma. Concomitant contact urticaria to human semen has been diagnosed on clinical grounds. Negativity of the skin tests with regard to immediate reactions may be explained by differences in sensitivity between the test sites and the vagina.

References

1. Berger H (1975) Allergy to human semen. NY State J Med 75: 1072–1073
2. Bernstein IL, et al. (1981) Localized and systemic hypersensitivity reactions to human seminal fluid. Ann Intern Med 94: 459–465
3. Blair H, Parish WE (1985) Asthma and urticaria induced by seminal plasma in a woman with IgE-antibody to a seminal plasma antigen. Clin Allergy 5: 117–130
4. Freeman S (1986) Woman allergic to husband's sweat and semen. Contact Dermatitis 14: 110–112
5. Halpern BN, et al. (1967) Clinical and immunological study of an exceptional case of reaginic type sensitization to human seminal fluid. Immunology 12: 247–258

Addresses

H.-G. Schimkat
Service de Dermatologie, Hôpital Saint Charles, Montpellier, France

M. Andary
Laboratoire d'Immunologie, Hôpital Saint Eloi, Montpellier, France

J. Clot
Laboratoire d'Immunologie, Hôpital Saint Eloi, Montpellier, France

C. Humeau
Laboratoire de Fécondation In Vitro Maternité, Montpellier, France

B. Descomps
Laboratoire de Biochimie D, Montpellier, France

A. Dieng
Laboratoire des Stéroïdes, R. I. A. Hôpital Lapeyronie, Montpellier, France

B. Previero
Laboratoire des Stéroïdes, R. I. A., Hôpital Lapeyronie, Montpellier, France

C. Sultan
Laboratoire des Stéroïdes, R. I. A. Hôpital Lapeyronie, Montpellier, France

M. Robinet-Levy
Centre de Transfusions Sanguines, Montpellier, France

G. Barneon
Laboratoire d'Anatomie Pathologique Gui de Chauliac, Montpellier, France

J. M. Meynadier
Service de Dermatologie, Hôpital Saint Charles, Montpellier, France

J. Meynadier
Service de Dermatologie, Hôpital Saint Charles, Montpellier, France

Part 6

Photosensitizers

Basic Mechanisms of Photosensitization

P. Thune

Summary

To the dermatologist photosensitization means cutaneous photosensitive responses to an added chemical and includes photoallergic or phototoxic reactions; several substances are capable of producing both types. Many of the compounds that cause photoallergy are halogenated, aromatic hydrocarbons which can generate free radicals as a result of homolysis of the photolabile carbon-halogen bond. Most of the photosensitizers function in the presence of oxygen and the intra-cellular reaction site has been established with certainty in several compounds. Definite proof has been provided that in mice contact photosensitivity is a highly specific delayed-type hypersensitive (DTH) reaction which is effected by T-cell subsets.

Key words:

Photosensitization - Phototoxicity - Photoallergy

To the dermatologist photosensitization means cutaneous photosensitive responses to an added chemical and includes photoallergic or phototoxic reactions. The former involve immunologic mechanisms resulting from the formation of an antigen in the skin by the light-induced reaction of the photosensitizer. Thus, immunologic reactivity can arise as the result of a reaction(s) initiated by the absorption of radiation by (a) the chemical or a complex containing the chemical, (b) a biotransformation product of the chemical, or (c) a host molecule altered by the chemical. Photoallergy has features in common with ordinary contact allergy and histologically the reactions are quite similar. Cellular metabolism may convert several compounds into the actual photoallergic molecules, but this aspect has not been studied in detail. Other steps in the photosensitizing process are also very complex and only partly understood. Initially it was postulated that stable photoproducts from the photosensitizer were involved, but recent reports suggest that this may not always be the case. Instead reactive, short-lived molecules produced by UV irradiation may be involved [2, 8, 11].

The pathogenesis of phototoxicity does not involve the immune system, although several agents are capable of producing both phototoxic and photoallergic reactions in the skin. To biologists photosensitization means phototoxic reactions in cells. Usually the studies concern the kinetics of cell death/destruction. Since cell death is a rather non-specific end-product for assessing a cellular response, much recent research has been directed toward a more refined elucidation of the mechanism of different kinds of cell damage (Table 1) using different model systems, including membrane photomodification, different kinds of cells and isolation of subcellular structures [3, 15, 18].

Photosensitization occurs after absorption of radiant energy and the majority of the reactions occur after UV irradiation, although sometimes longer wavelengths can also be involved. Some sensitizers are natural compounds but most are synthetic. A photosensitizer may be defined as a chemical which, on activation by radiation, causes another component of a cellular system to react. Thus, the first step in a photosensitization process requires the absorption of non-ionizing radiation by molecules. The light-absorbing molecule is referred to as a chromophore and specific chromophores exist for each photobiologic response. During the process the electromagnetic energy of a photon is converted to chemical bonding energy that is contained within the molecule. Absorption of a photon promotes electron changes within the molecule which is then promoted to an excited singlet state. The molecules remain in electronically excited states until they undergo a chemical change to form a photoproduct, or transfer the energy to another molecule or shed their excess energy as either light or heat. When the chromophore is chemically changed during the reaction, a direct photochemical or free radical reaction (type 1), is said to be involved. The chromophore alone may be chemically changed or it may react with another molecule. When the chromophore is not changed, the reaction is called a pho-

Table 1. The subcellular site of photosensitization

Plasma membrane
- Xanthine derivatives, fluorescein class (rose bengal, erythrosine B)
- NSAIDs (indomethacin, piroxicam, benoxaprofen)
- Phenothiazines (chlorpromazine, promethazine)
- Amiodarone (cordarone, desethylamiodarone)
- Quinidine (?)
- Porphyrins
- Lichen acids (atranorin, evernin, usnic acid)
- Secondary plant metabolites (phenylheptatriyne (PHT), alphaterthienyl)

DNA
- Psoralens
- Phenothiazines (chlorpromazine, promethazine)
- Tetracyclines
- Sulphanilamide
- Coal-tar extracts, anthracene

Mitochondria
- Tetracyclines

tosensitized reaction and the chromophore is called a photosensitizer. When oxygen is required for the reaction to occur, the reaction is often called photodynamic (type II) and most of the photosensitizers function only in the presence of oxygen. The chemicals are triplet sensitizers which help convert molecular oxygen into its first electronically excited singlet state, a powerful oxidant capable of inducing a variety of deleterious effects.

Photochemical reactions can be classified by the types of molecular changes which occur in molecular bonding such as isomerization, cycloaddition, intramolecular rearrangement, photosensitization, etc. A typical example is furocoumarin (psoralen species) photosensitization, well known from PUVA therapy. The psoralens photosensitize the modification of DNA through monofunctional and bifunctional (cross-linked) adducts, but the side effects of PUVA therapy may involve membrane damage. It was originally believed that the cytotoxic effects were derived from type I photochemistry, but there is now mounting evidence that $^1O_2$-mediated reaction are also important [3, 5, 15].

Other natural photosensitizers from plants are the polyacetylenes and their thiophene dervatives from the Asteracea (Composita) family, including alpha-terthienyl and phenyl-heptatriyne. These compounds photoreact with membranes either by generation of singlet oxygen or by reaction in a free radical mechanism or by both [17]. Some derivatives may also react with cellular DNA. However, evidence for the participation of these substances in the photosensitivity reactions of human skin to Compositae is still lacking.

In vitro photochemical experiments have indicated that reactive intermediates (free radicals) are formed upon irradiation of photoallergic compounds. The structures of some of these free radicals have been established. These include the radicals formed from halogenated salicylanilides, chlorpromazine, Jadit, Musk ambrette and p-aminobenzoic acid (PABA).

Many of the compounds that cause photoallergy are halogenated aromatic hydrocarbons [1, 2, 6, 8, 11]. Upon UV irradiation they can generate free radicals as a result of homolysis of the photolabile carbon-halogen bond. Some studies support the theory that free radicals are involved during photodehalogenation of several compounds which cause photosensitive reaction. Examples of haloaromatic compounds which are known to generate aryl radicals and free halogen atoms upon UV photolysis include amiodarone, chlorpromazine and benoxazoles [1, 5–7, 11]. Recently this mechanism has also been postulated for salicylanilides such as bithionol and fentichlor [8]. Furthermore, bithionol has been reported to consume oxygen upon irradiation and it is probable that the free hydroxyl radical is derived from a photolysis product formed by the reaction of irradiated bithionol with molecular oxygen:

$$ArCl \xrightarrow{h\nu} ArR' + Cl$$

$$Ar' + O^2 \longrightarrow ArOO'$$

$$ArOO' \xrightarrow{'H} ArOOH$$

$$ArOOH \xrightarrow{h\nu} ArO' + 'OH$$

Aryl radicals are highly reactive chemical molecules which readily abstract hydrogen atoms from suitable chemical donors. In vivo these radicals may initiative lipid peroxidation and they may also react with secondary free radicals formed from macromolecules to form covalent complexes which can act as antigens.

Another hypothesis which has been proven is that photoproducts are formed which in some cases can act as contact allergens. Upon absorption of a photon the photosensitizing compound is chemically altered to form another stable compound, the hapten. The hapten then combines with protein without further absorption of radiation and the hapten-protein conjugate is the antigen as in ordinary contact allergy. The potentials of several such photoproducts have been evaluated and although several products can act as contact allergens this one mechanism cannot explain all cases. Thus, both this and the previous mechanism may apply in different cases [2, 11].

A third hypothesis which has been proposed is that the photosensitizing compound absorbs radiation and then photochemically alters a protein which then becomes the antigen. This mechanism requires further investigation. It can be considered to be a possible explanation for persistent light reactivity in that the antigenicity of some normal constituent of the body is altered during the photoallergic reaction. The initial photochemical reaction produces a photoproduct that is antigenic and induces an immune response. Subsequent exposure to radiation triggers the immune response by formation of the same or closely related "normal" photoproducts from an endogenous substance. Evidence for photochemical alteration of the carrier protein in an in vitro system involving TCSA has been established; thus, this mechanism is at least theoretically possible [11].

There are a few examples of industrial outbreaks of persistent light reactivity (PLR) following air-borne contact with photoactive compounds from epoxy polyester resin used as electrostatic painting powder [12]. The products developed during pyrolysis at temperatures of 400°–500° C were spread from the painting room throughout the factory via the ventilation system. Many patients suffered an extreme limitation of their working capacity and social life for years afterwards. GC-MS analysis of the decomposition products from bisphenol A indicated a semiquinone structure to be the offending agent. The ESR spectra confirmed the yield of free radicals. Photoallergy has not been proved in this connection and the clinical picture is likely to be more in favour of a phototoxin reaction initiating PLR.

Although several data suggest a cell-mediated immune pathogenesis for contact photosensitivity, the mechanisms of cellular regulation have not been fully elucidated. Contact photosensitivity to TCSA in mice has been demonstrated to be a T-cell-mediated DTH reaction [16]. Both the kinetics of the reaction and the histologic picture were indistinguishable from those of ordinary contact sensitivity. The photosensitivity could also be transferred with lymph-node T cells to MHC-compatible naive recipients. In addition, peritoneal exudate cells of sensitized guinea pigs which contain cellular immune effector T-cells in large numbers, can be used to accomplish passive transfer of TCSA contact photosensitivity.

Clinical photoallergic reactions induced by systemic drugs are less common and less understood than cutaneous reactions induced by topical photoallergens. Until recently there has been no evidence to support an immune pathogenesis for reactions described as systemic photoallergy. Experimentally induced systemic photoallergy to sulphanilamide and chlorpromazine in mice by i.p. administration of the drug followed by UV irradiation of the skin has now been demonstrated [4]. The specific, acquired altered reactivity was adoptively transferred to naive mice with lymph-node cells taken from photosensitized donors.

Most studies on drug photosensitization, following systemic administration, involve phototoxicity. The non-steroidal anti-inflammatory drugs (NSAIDs) and the antidysrhythmic drug amiodarone have been particularly under focus. The propionic, acid-derived NSAIDs were more likely to be phototoxic than other classes tested [9, 10]. Photochemical studies using flash photolysis and electron spin resonance (ESR; spin trap) experiments, have shown that the substances undergo decarboxylation and that the photoproducts are capable of singlet oxygen generation and initiation of free radical reactions. The different reactivities of the decarboxy radicals probably would influence the extent to which naproxen and benoxaprofen might be incorporated into biological membranes or DNA following in vivo photoactivation.

The photolysis of amiodarone and its major metabolite mono-*N*-desethylamiodarone has been studied by absorption spectroscopy, ESR spectroscopy (spin trapping) and oxygraph measurements [7]. The studies indicate that drugs undergo deiodination and an aryl radical from amiodarone is formed during UV irradiation. The aryl radical abstracted a hydrogen atom from suitable chemical donors, among them the unsaturated fatty acid linoleic acid. Reaction of the dienyl radical derived from linoleic acid could yield the corresponding peroxyradical, thereby initiating lipid peroxidation. This would explain the deposition of lipoprotein, lipofuscin, a pigment formed from the products of lipid peroxidation in the skin of patients receiving amiodarone.

The systemic use of phenothiazines causes phototoxic reactions, but topically they can cause photoallergy as well as phototoxicity. Some studies with phenothiazine derivatives in mice suggest that photoallergy may also occur [9]. In man CPZ is metabolized to several derivatives and photodechlorination seems to be directly related to the degree of phototoxicity. Several derivatives photosensitize cleavage of DNA and form covalent photoadducts with DNA and nucleotide bases. A non-singlet oxygen pathway has been demonstrated for CPZ-induced photohemolysis (membrane damage). However, it would appear that promazine-induced phototoxicity may result in part from the generation of superoxide (O_2^-). Hydroxyl radicals and some unknown peroxy intermediate are involved [1].

Photochemistry of porphyrins has attracted much interest in recent years [13, 14]. It is likely that porphyrin-sensitized reactive oxygen molecules cause subsequent photooxidative damage to target biomolecules by singlet excited oxygen. The pathomechanisms include peroxidation of cell-membrane lipids, cross-linking of cell membrane and intercellular proteins, inhibition of cell-membrane-associated cytosolic, mitochondrial and microsomal enzymes, and disruption of intracellular organelles. Relative affinities of different porphyrins for subcellular structures are dependent on solubility properties, protoporphyrin being more toxic to lipophilic structures (erythrocyte membrane, mitochondria, membrane-bound enzyme activity), while uroporphyrin was most toxic to water-soluble targets (tryptophan, cytosolic enzymes). The hydroscopicity correlates with sensitizing potency, suggesting a key role for membrane association as seen with the tumor photosensitizer hematoporphyrin derivative responsible for photosensitized cell killing. Intramembranous location of porphyrin has been suggested with protoporphyrin inserted into the membrane bilayer with its charged groups at the interface. The location in the cell membrane is known for several photosensitizers (Table 1).

References

1. Chignell CF, Motten AG, Buettner GR (1985) Photoinduced free radicals from chlorpromazine and related phenothiazines: relationship to phenothiazine-induced photosensitization. Environ Hlth Persp 64: 103–110
2. Epling GA, Wells JL, Ung Chan Yoon (1988) Photochemical transformations in salicylanilide photoallergy. Photochem Photobiol 47: 167–171
3. Girotti AW (1983) Mechanisms of photosensitization. Photochem Photobiol 38: 745–751
4. Guidici PA, Maguire HC (1985) Experimental photoallergy to systemic drugs. J Invest Dermatol 85: 207–211
5. Kochevar IE (1987) Mechanisms of drug photosensitization. Photochem Photobiol 45: 891–895
6. Li ASW, Chignell CF (1987) Spectroscopic studies of cutaneous photosensitizing agents. XI. Photolysis of chlorpromazine metabolites: a spin-trapping study. Photochem Photobiol 45: 695–701
7. Li ASW, Chignell CF (1987) Spectroscopic studies of cutaneous photosensitizing agents. IX. A spin-trapping study of the photolysis of amiodarone and desethylemiodarone. Photochem Photobiol 45: 191–197
8. Li ASW, Chignell CF (1987) Spectroscopic studies of cutaneous photosensitizing agents. XII. A spin-trapping study of the free radicals generated during the photolysis of photoallergens bithionol and fentichlor. Photochem Photobiol 46: 445–452
9. Ljunggren B, Bjellerup M (1986) Systemic drug photosensitivity. Photodermatol 3: 26–35
10. Moore DE, Chappnis PP (1988) A comparative study of the photochemistry of the non-steroidal anti-inflammatory drugs, naproxen, benoxaprophen and indomethazin. Photochem Photobiol 47: 173–180
11. Morison WL, Kochevar IE (1983) Photoallergy. In: Parrish JA, Kripke M, Morison WL (eds) Photoimmunology. Plenum, New York, pp 227–253
12. Peltonen K, Zitting A, Koskinen H, Itkonen A (1986) Free radicals from photodecomposition of bisphenol-A. Photchem Photobiol 43: 481–484
13. Poh-Fitzpatrick MB (1986) Molecular and cellular mechanisms of porphyrin photosensitization. Photodermatol 3: 148–157
14. Sandberg S, Romslo I (1981) Porphyrin-induced photodamage at the cellular and the sub-cellular level as related to the solubility of the porphyrin. Clin Chem Acta 109: 193–201
15. Spikes JD (1983) Photosensitization in mammalian cells. In: Parrish JA, Kripke M, Morison WL (eds) Photoimmunology. Plenum, New York pp 23–49
16. Takigawa M, Miyachi Y (1982) Mechanisms of contact photosensitivity in mice: T-cell regulation of contact photosensitivity to tetra-chlorosalicylanilide under the genetic restrictions of the major histocompatibility complex. J Invest Dermatol 78: 108–115
17. Towers GHN, Hudson JB (1987) Potentially useful antimicrobial and antiviral phototoxins from plants. Photochem Photobiol 46: 61–66
18. Valenzeno DP (1987) Photomodification of biological membranes with emphasis on singlet oxygen mechanism. Photochem Photobiol 46: 147–160

Addresses

P. Thune
Department of Dermatology, Ullevaal Hospital, 0407 Oslo 4, Norway

Clinical Aspects of Photosensitizers

I. R. White

Summary

The changing importance of contact photoallergens is emphasized with respect to variations in the degree of population exposure to them. Ways in which photosensitivity can coexist or be masked by contact sensitivity are discussed. The usefulness of a new indicator of compositae allergy in the investigation of individuals with eczema on light-exposed areas is mentioned.

Key words:

Photosensitivity - Sunscreens - UV absorbers - Compositae

Photosensitivity reactions caused by exposure to external factors are of four types: topical photoallergic, topical phototoxic, systemic photoallergic and systemic phototoxic. The first two types occur when photoreactivity is caused by topical (contact) exposure to an agent and the latter two types by systemic absorption of an agent. Systemic reactivity is most commonly attributable to drug ingestion and topical phototoxicity to plants (phytophototoxic). Aspects of photoallergic contact reactions are considered here.

In discussing external causes of photosensitivity the importance of distinguishing between two other types of photosensitivity has to be appreciated. Chronic actinic dermatitis (CAD) and persistent light reactivity (PLR) are morphologically indistinguishable conditions which present with chronic eczematous changes on light-exposed areas with or without spread elsewhere. In both conditions abnormal monochromator tests occur along the ultraviolet (UV) light spectrum. The difference between the two is that in CAD there is no apparent relevant (photo)allergen and in PLR there is evidence of hypersensitivity to a relevant (photo)allergen.

Numerous topical photoallergens have been described, but in most instances reports of such photoallergens are sporadic and rare. In the decade before 1975 the halogenated salicylanilides, used as antibacterial agents in soaps, for instance, caused an epidemic of photosensitivity reactions. The problem was first identified by Wilkinson, who described the clinical sign of sparing of a small area of skin behind the ears in those photosensitive individuals with eczematous changes on their faces; this sign is known as "Wilkinson's triangle" [13]. Once halogenated salicylanilides had been removed from the domestic environment the epidemic settled, although a very few affected individuals have remained with PLR. In 1978 musk ambrette, used primarily as a fragrance enhancer in toiletries, was identified as a photoallergen by Larsen. During the next few years musk ambrette became an important photoallergen with simple allergic contact dermatitis also occurring. Again, following the identification of the problem and the lowering of the quantities of musk ambrette used in toiletries the incidence of new cases of musk ambrette photosensitivity has fallen dramatically. During the last few years there has been appreciably greater population exposure to a number of sunscreening agents brought about by the greater awareness of the carcinogenic potential of sunlight and its effect of causing premature ageing of the skin. Contact and photocontact sensitivity to these sunscreens is now starting to become a problem.

Musk Ambrette

Musk ambrette has been used extensively as a fragrance enhancer in many perfumed toiletries and in high concentrations (up to 4%) in aftershaves. It is also found in other products such as soaps, hair sprays, furniture polish and in fruity flavoured edibles such as yoghurts and sweets. These various consumables may still contain musk ambrette but under the recommendations of the IFRA the concentrations used, and especially in male toiletries, have been reduced. Paralleling this reduction in population exposure there has been a reduced incidence of musk ambrette photosensitivity. Other musk substances, tibetine, xylene, ketone and moskene do not seem to be as photosensitising as musk ambrette and cross reactions are not the norm.

Musk ambrette typically causes photosensitivity in males. Three clinical types of photosensitivity occur [2]. The majority of affected males presented with daubs of eczema on their faces in the areas on which their aftershaves were patted onto the cheeks and chin. Fewer individuals presented with a more widespread eczematous reaction with a distribution on the light-exposed areas which mimicked CAD. Although the majority of affected subjects have had complete clearing of their skin, in a few cases, even after carefully removing known sources of musk ambrette from their environment, there has been persistence of photoreactivity which is PLR. These PLRs have been treated with photoprotection but also by PUVA [8], azathiaprine [1] and cyclosporin.

Sunscreens

The use of UV light absorbers has increased considerably recently and with the consequent increase in skin contact there has been an increase of reports of adverse reactions [10]. The global campaign warning of the association of excessive sunlight exposure and the development of malignant melanoma has been one reason for the increased use of these agents. A second reason has been the more frequent incorporation of UV light absorbers into facial toiletries and cosmetics, and especially those which have an antiwrinkle claim, because of the public's awareness that excessive sunlight exposure is a potent cause of premature ageing of the skin. The third reason has been the incorporation of UV absorbers into toiletries to increase the shelf-life of the product by protecting against photodegregation [3].

The main groups of UV absorbers are PABA and its derivatives, cinnamates, benzophenones and dibenzoylmethanes. The latter, with excellent long-wave UV absorbing properties, are being increasingly used in Europe [4].

UV absorbers can cause an allergic contact dermatitis which may present acutely and have features of an allergic contact dermatitis similar to those of any cosmetic allergen such as lanolin. However, because the UV-screening toiletries will generally be applied liberally before exposure to sunlight, simple allergy or photoallergy to the screens may be misinterpreted as an idiopathic light sensitivity. Additionally, some subjects using sunscreens to treat photodermatoses may acquire allergy or photoallergy which may exacerbate the pre-existing condition. Such an example has been demonstrated with photoallergy to 2-ethoxy-p-methoxycinnamate in an Asian using the screen, who had CAD with negative previous photopatch tests [9]. In such cases the sunscreen may appear to cause "persistence" of the light-related dermatosis.

Diagnostic Difficulties

Chronic eczema on the light-exposed areas may be due to true "idiopathic" light sensitivity and also to other factors. It has been mentioned that musk ambrette can present as a pattern of photosensitivity identical to such idiopathic sensitivity. More commonly, however, chronic eczema on the exposed areas is not due to photosensitivity but is the result of air-borne contact allergy. In the UK this is seen with phosphorus sesquisulphide, but more globally it occurs with compositae dermatitis. Although air-borne allergic contact dermatitis characteristically involves the eyelids and extends to involve the skin under the chin and behind the ears, this is not always so, and in CAD/PLR there may be involvement of these areas which are typically spared in these conditions.

Compositae

Allergic contact dermatitis to compositae can mimic CAD morphologically [5] and, in addition, both are worse in the summer months when there is increased sunlight exposure and exposure to compositae allergens. Patch testing with leaves or flowers of compositae will not always detect compositae dermatitis because of huge ranges in species content of the allergens and seasonal variation. Occlusive patch tests performed with oleoresin extracts which have been commercially available have caused false-positive irritant reactions which were often interpreted as true allergies. Open tests with the commercially available oleoresins may have given false-negative results in compositae-sensitive subjects. Use of a sesquiterpene lactone mix developed by Ducombs and Benezra has given more promising reliability in the detection of compositae dermatitis. This mixture does not seem to be an irritant and in a consecutive series of 1128 subjects there were 33 reactions which tended to occur in elderly individuals who were either florists, gardeners or did gardening as a hobby. Ten of the sensitive individuals were being investigated for possible light sensitivity and of these four had abnormal monochromator light tests in addition to being sesquiterpene-lactone sensitive. This has supported the observation that compositae sensitivity may be associated with light sensitivity.

Photopatch Testing

It is clear that there can be diagnostic difficulties between allergic contact dermatitis, photoallergic contact dermatitis and idiopathic photodermatitis (CAD). The purpose of a protocol of photopatch testing is, therefore, to give an adequate screen of those allergens which can mimic photoallergic reactions as well as being able to detect true photoallergens. There is both temporal and geographical variation in those photoallergens to which an individual is likely to be exposed. New cases of halogenated salicylanilide photosensitivity among the UK general population are unlikely to be found as it has not been exposed for nearly two decades. Photoallergy to musk ambrette is rapidly decreasing as population exposure has been reduced. Reactions from sunscreening compounds is increasing as population exposure is increasing. In the UK, photocontact dermatitis to fentichlor has not been reported from domestic exposure to it for more than a decade while more recent domestic use in Scandinavia has meant more recent reports of photoallergy to it in these countries. Because of these factors there is no single "simple" series of allergens which is going to be a good screen for photoallergy in all countries while an excessively comprehensive series may be used on a few subjects at specialist centres but not on the majority of patients elsewhere.

The Scandinavians have agreed upon a photopatch test series which suits their circumstances [6] and results from this series have been published [11]. In the UK, at St John's Hospital the "photopatch test series" is reviewed regularly and is changed at intervals. The series presently used appears to suit the UK domestic exposure to photoallergens as well as detecting those allergens which mimic photosensitivity (Table 1).

Table 1. St John's Hospital "Light" Series 1988

Not for irradiation
- Enhanced "standard" European series of contact allergens
- A face series of contact allergens, including
  - Sesquiterpene lactone mix (Ducombs, Benezra)
  - Phosphorus sesquisulphide
  - "Photo" series

For irradiation ("photo" series)
- Musk ambrette
- PABA
- Octyl dimethyl PABA
- Hydroxy methoxy methyl benzophenone
- Ethoxy ethyl-p-methoxy cinnamate
- Isopropyl dibenzoylmethane
- Butyl methoxy dibenzoylmethane
- Phenyl methoxy benzoxazol
- Ethyl hexyl methoxycinnamate
- Benzocaine
- Chlorpromazine
- Promethazine

Although one may expect that there are regional differences in those photoallergens which are important, is it reasonable to expect diverse differences in amounts of UV-A used in irradiating photopatch tests? In Scandinavia 5 J/cm^2 UV-A is recommended or ½ MED (minimal erythema dose) UV-A, whichever is the smaller, for routine irradiation of patch test during photopatch testing. The general dermatologist who may undertake photopatch testing probably does not know the MED of his patients. Exposing an unselected series of patients for photopatch testing to 5 J UV-A can give a very severe reaction to the exposed area. In the series reported by Cronin [2] the photoallergic reactions to musk ambrette were elicited by 1 J UV-A. The photoallergic contact reaction to 2-ethoxy-p-methoxycinnamate [9] in an Asian was to 2 J UV-A. Wennersten et al. [12] have commented that many of the reactions obtained to phenothiazines during photopatch testing in their clinics may be phototoxic. Before a regimen either of 5 J of ½ MED UV-A is adopted for photopatch testing there should be a thorough investigation of the actual amount of UV-A needed to elicit allergic photocontact reactions in sensitive individuals.

Environmental exposure to photoallergens changes. A European forum will help to monitor continental exposure to photoallergens. As we move to a "unified" Europe, geographical national differences will become less evident and the importance of a unified approach to photopatch testing will become more important.

References

1. Cirne de Castro JL, Pereira MA, Prates Nunes F, Pereira dos Santos A (1986) Successful treatment of a musk ambrette sensitive persistent light reactor with azathiaprine. Photodermatology 3: 241–242

2. Cronin E (1984) Photosensitivity to musk ambrette. Contact Dermatitis 11: 88–92
3. English JSC, White IR, Cronin E (1987) Sensitivity to sunscreens. Contact Dermatitis 17: 159–162
4. English JSC, White IR (1986) Allergic contact dermatitis from isopropyl dibenzoylmethane. Contact Dermatitis 15: 94
5. Hjorth N, Roed-Petersen J, Thomsen K (1976) Airborne contact dermatitis from compositae oleoresins stimulates photodermatitis. Br J Dermatol 95: 613–620
6. Jansen CJ, Wennersten G, Rystedt I, Thune P, Brodthagen H (1982) The Scandinavian standard photopatch test procedure. Contact Dermatitis 2: 155–158
7. Larsen W (1978) Photoallergy to musk ambrette found in aftershave lotion. Presented at the American Academy of Dermatology meeting, San Francisco, 1978
8. Lindberg L, Larkö O, Roupe G (1986) Successful PUVA treatment for musk ambrette induced persistent light reaction. Photodermatology 3: 111–112
9. Murphy GM, White IR (1987) Photoallergic contact dermatitis for 2-ethoxy-p-methoxycinnamate. Contact Dermatitis 16: 296
10. Thune P (1984) Contact and photocontact allergy to sunscreens. Photodermatology 1: 5–9
11. Wennersten G, Thune P, Brodthagen H, Jansen C, Rystedt I (1984) The Scandinavian multicenter photopatch study – preliminary results. Contact Dermatitis 10: 305–309
12. Wennersten G, Thune P, Jansen CT, Brodthagen H (1986) Photocontact dermatitis: current status with emphasis on allergic contact photosensitivity (CPS) occurrence, allergens, and practical phototesting. Sem Dermatol 5: 277–289
13. Wilkinson DS (1962) Patch test reactions to certain halogenated salicylanilides. Br J Dermatol 74: 302–306

Addresses

I. R. White
St. John's Hospital for Diseases of the Skin, Lisle Street, London WC2H 7BJ, UK

The Scandinavian Multicenter Photopatch Study 1980–1985*

P. Thune, N. McFadden, C. Jansén, I. Rystedt, G. Wennersten, and H. Brodthagen

Summary

The results of photopatch testing of 1993 patients with suspected photodermatoses at 16 Scandinavian university dermatology departments, from 1980–1985, are described. The aim of the study was to establish the incidence and causes of photocontact dermatitis and the occurrence of other sun-related skin diseases in this group. Patch testing with the SPDRG standard battery showed a total of 369 positive test reactions and photopatch testing gave 274. The highest incidence of patch and photopatch test responses occurred in the plant derivatives/cosmetics ingredients (73%) and therapeutic agents (41%) subgroups respectively. Subdivision of the sensitizers into three groups, antimicrobials, plant derivatives/cosmetics ingredients and therapeutic agents, showed fentichlor, musk ambrette, and paraaminobenzoic (PABA) to be the most frequent photosensitizers in the respective groups. Perfume mixture (consisting of six different ingredients), balsam of Peru and lichen mixture (eight different species) were found to be the likeliest causes of a contact dermatitis. Polymorphous light eruption was the commonest photodermatosis (38%), while solar urticaria, persistent light reaction, and actinic reticuloid were infrequent diagnoses and combined, occurred in only 6.4% of the group. Secondary aggravation by sunlight of preexisting skin diseases, such as atopic dermatitis and psoriasis, was established in 309 patients (16%), while 169 patients (9%) were not found to be light sensitive at all.

* The following also participated in this multicenter study: M. Cramers, Marselisborg Hospital, Aarhus, Denmark; L. Emtestan, Södersjukhuset, Stockholm, Sweden; T. Fischer, University Hospital, Uppsala, Sweden; M. Forsbeck, Södersjukhuset, Stockholm, Sweden; L. Förström, University Hospital, Helsinki, Finland; K. Hamman, Gentofte Hospital, Hellerup, Denmark; K. Kalimo, University Hospital, Turku, Finland; J. Karvonen, University Hospital, Oulu, Finland; E. A. Knudsen, Hvidore Hospital, Hvidore, Denmark; B. Ljunggren, General Hospital, Malmö, Sweden; B. Meding, Sahlgrenska Hospital, Gothenburg, Sweden; M. Skogh, University Hospital, Linköping, Sweden; H.-C. Wulff, Finsen Institute, Copenhagen, Denmark; P. Ø. Larsen, Marselisborg Hospital, Aarhus, Denmark; O. Laskö, Sahlgrenska Hospital, Gothenburg, Sweden; B. Berne, University Hospital, Uppsala, Sweden; A. Waerstedt, Gentofte Hospital, Hellerup, Denmark; S. Ullman, Rigshospitalet, Copenhagen, Denmark; G. Kavli, Tromsö Hospital, Tromsö, Norway.

Key words:

Photopatch testing - Contact allergy - Photocontact allergy - Photodermatosis

The Scandinavian Photodermatology Research Group (SPDRG), representing 16 different university dermatology departments in Denmark, Finland, Norway, and Sweden, designed a standard photopatch test procedure which has been in use since January 1980 [5]. In a coordinated effort to determine the pattern and frequency of photocontact allergy in Scandinavia and to assess the efficacy of the test substances, the results of photopatch testing of 745 patients during 1980–1981 were presented in a preliminary report in 1984 [10]. The present study examines the results of photopatch testing of 1993 patients during the period 1980–1985, and includes the original group of 745 patients. While determining the incidence and causes of photocontact sensitivity, the study was also used to establish the frequency of the occurrence of other sun-related skin diseases in Scandinavia.

Materials and Methods

A total of 1993 patients with a clinical history and features suggesting a photosensitivity were photopatch-tested using the SPDRG standard photopatch tray, which includes 19 test substances. Concentrations of the test substances and the appropriate vehicles are described in a previous report [5], which also includes the details of the test procedures and guidelines for interpretation of the skin reactions. Where indicated, other test substances were used in addition to those of the standard SPDRG tray, particularly in suspected cases of sunscreen and cosmetic photosensitivity. In addition to routine laboratory examination, blood and urinary porphyrin estimations and minimal erythema dose (MED) testing, photoprovocation testing, and histologic examination of lesional skin biopsy specimens were also performed, when indicated. The clinical diagnosis was established after consideration of the history, clinical findings, and test results.

Results

Polymorphic light eruption (PLE) was the commonest photodermatosis (749 patients), followed by secondary light sensitivity (309 patients) and photocontact dermatitis (217 patients). Plain contact dermatitis was observed in 190 patients, while 169 patients were not light sensitive and 108 had unclassified light sensitivity.

Table 1. Number of positive reactions in the Scandinavian standard photopatch tray (1993 patients)

Substance	Concentration	Positive reactions (total)	
		Photocontact	Contact
Antimicrobial agents			
Trichlorcarbanilide (TCC)	1% pet.	0	1
Tribromsalicylanilide (TBS)	1% pet.	9	2
Tetrachlorsalicylanilide (TCS)	0.1% pet.	12	3
Bithinol	1% pet.	11	3
Hexachlorophene	1% pet.	6	5
Fentichlor	1% pet.	25	3
Triclosan (irgasan, DP 300)	2% pet.	3	7
Chlorhexidine gluconate	0.5% pet.	2	6
Plant derivatives and cosmetic ingredients			
Balsam of Peru	25% pet.	13	84
Wood mix[a]	20% pet.	2	20
Lichen mix[b]	16% pet.	7	64
Musk ambrette	1% pet.	54	12
6-Methylcoumarin (6-MC)	1% alc.	4	1
Perfume mix[c]	6% pet.	10	88
Therapeutic agents			
Promethazine	1% pet.	37	13
Chlorpromazine HCl	0.1% pet.	33	11
p-Aminobenzoic acid (PABA)	5% alc.	43	44
Others			
Diphenhydramine chloride[d]	1% pet.	1	2
Thiourea[d]	0.01% aq.	2	0

[a] Pine, spruce, birch and teak, 5% each
[b] A mixture of *Parmelia, Hypogymnia, Pseudovernia, Cladonia, Plasmatica, Physcia, Umbilicaria,* and *Cetraria* species, 2% each
[c] Cinnamic alc., cinnamic aldehyde, hydroxy-citronellal, eugenol, isoeugenol, and geraniol, 1% each
[d] Tested in 1572 patients
pet., petrolatum; aq., water

Patch testing with the SPDRG standard battery showed a totol of 369 positive test reactions, while photopatch testing showed 274 (Table 1). The diagnosis of PLE (38%) and photosensitive dermatoses (16%; secondary aggravation by sunlight of preexisting skin diseases) accounted for more than one-half of the total diagnoses. Positive patch tests (77) and photopatch tests (50) were secondary findings in 120/749 PLE patients (Table 2). Persistent light reaction (PLR), actinic reticuloid (AR), porphyria and solar urticaria were relatively rare diagnoses and had a combined group incidence of only 6%. Of the 63 patients with PLR/AR, 27 patients had a positive patch and/or photopatch response on testing (Table 3). A photodermatitis due to systemic drugs was noted in 5%, while extensive phototesting failed to establish the cause in 108 patients (5.4%) presenting with a suspected photosensitive rash.

Table 2. Positive patch and photopatch tests in 120 out of 749 patients with PLE

	Positive reactions	
	Photocontact	Contact
Trichlorcarbanilide (TCC)	–	–
Tribromsalicylanilide (TBS)	2	–
Tetrachlorsalicylanilide (TCS)	2	2
Bithionol	–	-
Hexachlorophene	1	1
Chlorhexidine gluconate	–	4
Triclosan	–	1
Fentichlor	5	1
Promethazine	13	3
Chlorpromazine HCI	6	8
Diphenhydramine chloride	–	–
Balsam of Peru	–	14
Wood mix	–	–
Lichen mix	–	5
Musk ambrette	3	3
6-Methylcoumarine (6-MC)	–	1
Perfume mix	–	14
Para-aminobenzoic acid (PABA)	12	9
Thiourea	–	–
Compositae	–	3
Sunscreens other than PABA	6	8

Table 3. Positive patch and photopatch tests in 27 out of 63 patients with PLR/AR

	Positive reactions	
	Photocontact	Contact
Trichlorcarbanilide (TCC)	0	1
Tribromsalicylanilide (TBS)	6	–
Tetrachlorsalicylanilide (TCS)	5	–
Bithionol	4	–
Hexachlorophene	3	–
Chlorhexidine gluconate	–	–
Triclosan	1	–
Fentichlor	3	2
Promethazine	5	5
Chlorpromazine HCI	8	–
Diphenhydramine chloride	–	–
Balsam of Peru	–	11
Wood mix	–	8
Lichen mix	–	17
Musk ambrette	1	2
6-Methylcoumarine (6-MC)	–	–
Perfume mix	1	11
Para-aminobenzoic acid (PABA)	8	2
Thiourea	1	0
Compositae	–	13
Sunscreens other than PABA	6	4

Discussion

With an estimated incidence of 11% in the general population [6], it was not unexpected that PLE was the predominant photodermatosis in the group. On photopatch testing, 1 in 6 PLE patients were shown to have either a photocontact (50 reactions) or a contact sensitivity (77 reactions). Among these sunscreens were responsible for 18 photocontact reactions and 17 contact allergic reactions (Table 2). Photopatch testing is therefore especially recommended in the PLE patient group, where the use of sunscreens is often extensive. A contact allergy was a more frequent finding than a photocontact allergy in PLE patients, and perfume mixture and balsam of Peru together were responsible for more than one-third of all reactions in PLE patients with a coincident contact dermatitis. The PLR/AR patient group showed a remarkably similar trend to the PLE patients, with contact allergic reactions outnumbering photocontact reactions and sunscreen ingredients being responsible for ¼ of all photopatch test responses, while plant derivatives including perfume mixture and balsam of Peru accounted for 75% of the implicated contact sensitizers. The salicylanilides were still the most frequent photosensitizers in the PLR/AR patient group. Contact allergy to plant compounds, compositae oleoresins, and lichens has previously been reported as frequent in PLR/AR patients [9]. Plant extracts were, on the other hand, a rare cause of photocontact allergy in both PLR/AR and PLE patient groups. Musk ambrette, in the present study, in contrast to previous reports [1, 3], was an infrequent sensitizer in the PLR/AR patient group.

In the total group, the leading cause of a photoallergic response was musk ambrette, closely followed by para-aminobenzoic acid (PABA), both together accounting for more than a ⅓ of all positive photocontact reactions (Table 1). In the 4-year period, 1982–1985, following the preliminary report of the SPDRG [10], musk ambrette and PABA have replaced promethazine and chlorpromazine as the main photosensitizers. PABA, the leading sunscreen-ingredient sensitizer, was almost as fre-

Table 4. Reactions to other sunscreen ingredients; the total no. of patients tested is not known

Substance	Reactions	
	Photocontact	Contact
Oxybenzone 3%	8	2
Octyl dimethyl PABA 2%	0	5
Amyl dimethyl PABA 2%	0	3
Glyceryl PABA 2%	3[a]	1[a]
4-Isopropyl-dibenzoylmethane 10%	1	0
2-Phenyl-benzimidazole-5		
Sulfonic acid sodium salt 10%	1	1
3-(4-Methylbenzlidene) camphor 10%	0	1
2-Ethylhexyl-4-methoxycinnamate 1%	0	0
Ethoxyethyl-p-methoxycinnamate 1%	2	1
Alpha-amyl cinnamic acid 1%	0	2
Benzocaine	2	1

[a] Reported cases due to contaminants

quently implicated as a cause of a photocontact sensitivity as it was of a plain contact sensitivity. PABA esters, octyl dimethyl- and amyl dimethyl-PABA, showed no photosensitizing capacity, but were responsible for eight cases of a contact dermatitis. There have been several recent reports of contact and photocontact sensitivity to various new non-PABA sunscreens [2, 4, 7, 8], including substituted benzophenones and dibenzoyl-methanes. Similar reactions were observed in the present group (Table 4), but the total number of patients tested for these substances is unknown, and it is therefore impossible to estimate the incidence. The most frequent contact sensitizers in the total group were perfume mixture and balsam of Peru, together responsible for 47% of all positive contact reactions. Since the preliminary report, in 1981, perfumes have become the principal contact sensitizer, in the total patient group, at the expense of balsam of Peru. The incidence of a contact dermatitis due to the latter substance has only marginally increased, while that due to perfume sensitivity has tripled.

It is also interesting, in comparing our two studies, to note that the proportional distribution of the photodermatoses here is otherwise remarkably similar to the 1980–1981 findings.

References

1. Barber KA, Cronin E (1984) Patch and photopatch testing in chronic actinic dermatitis. Contact Dermatitis 10: 69–73
2. Davies MG, Hawk JLM, Rycroft RJG (1982) A case of photosensitivity from the sunscreen 2-ethyoxyethyl-p-methoxy-cinnamate. Contact Dermatitis 8: 190–192
3. Giovinnazo VJ, Harber LC, Armstrong RB, Kochevar IE (1980) Photoallergic contact dermatitis to musk ambrette: clinical report of 2 patients with persistent light reactor patterns. J Am Acad Dermatol 3: 384–393
4. Hölzle E, Plewig G (1982) Photoallergische Kontaktdermatitis durch benzophenonhaltige Sonnenschutzpräparate. Hautarzt 33: 391–393
5. Jansén CT, Wennersten G, Rystedt I, Thune P, Brodthagen H (1982) The Scandinavian standard photopatch test procedure. Contact Dermatitis 8: 155–158
6. Morison WL, Stern RS (1982) Polymorphous light eruption: a common reaction uncommonly recognized. Acta Derm Venereol (Stockh) 62: 237–240
7. Schauder S, Ippen H (1986) Photoallergic and allergic contact dermatitis from dibenzoyl-methanes. Photodermatology 3: 140–147
8. Thune P (1984) Contact and photocontact allergy to sunscreens. Photodermatology 1: 5–9
9. Thune P, Eeg Larsen T (1984) Contact and photocontact allergy in persistent light reactivity. Contact Dermatitis 11: 98–107
10. Wennersten G, Thune P, Brodthagen H, Jansen C, Rystedt I (1984) The Scandinavian multicenter photopatch study: preliminary results. Contact Dermatitis 10: 305–309

Addresses

P. Thune
Department of Dermatology, Ullevaal Hospital, 0407 Oslo 4, Norway

N. McFadden
Department of Dermatology, Ullevaal Hospital, 0407 Oslo 4, Norway

C. Jansén
University Hospital, Turku, Finland

I. Rystedt
Karolinska Hospital, Stockholm, Sweden

G. Wennersten
Karolinska Hospital, Stockholm, Sweden

H. Brodthagen
Finsen Institute, Copenhagen, Denmark

Reproducibility of Contact and Photocontact Tests with Photoallergens

T. Hasan and C. T. Jansén

Summary

We retested 24 patients, who initially had been diagnosed to be either contact or photocontact allergic to one or more allergens in our photoepicutaneous test series. The interval from the initial test was 1–63 months, with an average of 23 months. Using a standard allergen concentration and a standard UVA dose (5 J/cm), 21% of previously significant (+ +/+ + +) photocontact reactions and 54% of significant contact reactions were reproduced. Reactions to paraaminobenzoic acid could be reproduced in two-thirds of the cases.

Key words:

Contact allergy - Photocontact allergy - Allergy reproducibility

Introduction

Recent follow-up studies of allergic contact reactivity have shown a 50%–59% persistence of the sensitivity to various allergens [2–4].

To the best of our knowledge there are no previous publications on the reproducibility of photocontact allergic test reactions. We now report data on the reproducibility of allergic contact and of photocontact reactions to 13 allergens of our routine photocontact test battery.

Patients and Methods

The study included 24 patients (9 men, 15 women; age 32–74 years; mean 55 years at the time of the follow-up test), who during the years 1980–1985 had been investigated for possible photocontact allergy and had reacted with at least one significant (++/+++) contact or photocontact allergic reaction in our standard photo-epicutaneous test series. Most of the initial test reactions had been purely of either photocontact or contact nature. There were, however, five borderline cases with a 2+ reaction on the irradiated side and a 1+ reaction on the covered side.

Both the initial and the follow-up tests were performed in accordance with the standardized Scandinavian photopatch-test protocol [1]. Briefly, two test series were applied on each side of the back or on each arm. Test substances were applied onto Finn chamber aluminium discs (Epitest) attached to Scanpor tape (Norgeplaster). The patches were removed after 24 h in dim light and the test sites inspected for any reactions. One of the series was immediatly convered with light-proof black plastic. The uncovered test series was exposed to 5 J/cm UVA light with the Uvasun 5000 equipment [5] emitting in the 340 to 450 nm range. As an exception, however, five of the earliest primary tests (performed in 1980–1981) had been irradiated with a bank of Airam LUA fluorescent tubes, emitting in the 315–410 nm range, with a maximum at 360 nm. Forty-eight hours after the irradiation, both the irradiated and light-covered series were inspected. The reactions were recorded and interpreted as follows: plain erythema (1+) was considered insignificant, while erythema and oedema as well as erythema, oedema and vesicles (3+) were considered significant reactions. If a significant reaction was recorded only on the light-exposed side, it was interpreted as photocontact allergy, while a reaction on both sides signified plain contact allergic reaction.

The chemicals and concentrations used in the follow-up test are summarized in Table 1.

Table 1. List of the allergens and concentrations of the follow-up test

	%		%
Alantolactone	0.1	Fragrance-mix	7
Atranorin	1	Hexachlorophene	1
Balsam of Peru	25	Lichen mix	16
Blancophor	1	PABA	5
Chlorhexidine	1	Trichlorcarbanilide	1
Chlorpromazine	0.1[a]	Usnic acid	1
Fentichlor	1		

[a] In the initial test three out of five tests were made with an allergen concentration of 1%

Results

Of the significant (+ +/+ + +) contact allergic reactions 54% were reproduced after a mean interval of 18 months (Table 2), while only 21% of the photocontact allergic reactions were reproducible, after an average interval of 31 months (Table 3). Table 4 lists results from patients who in the initial testing had reacted with a questionable, mixed photocontact (+ +)/contact (+) reaction. Three of the previous + +/+ reactions had turned negative (−/−). One balsam of Peru reaction had turned into a (+ +/−) photocontact reaction and an other initially + +/+ balsam of Peru reaction had turned into an insignificant (+/+) reaction.

Taken together, any kind of PABA reaction was reproducible in eight out of 13 cases, after a mean interval of 19 months. Two contact allergy reactions had changed to photocontact allergy and two photocontact reactions had changed to contact allergy, while three contact allergic reactions and one photocontact allergic reaction remained unchanged. The remaining contact and photocontact allergies had faded.

Table 2. Reproducibility of contact allergic reactions

	Initial test	Follow-up test	Interval (months)
PABA	+ + +	+ + +	12
	+ +	+ +	7
	+ +	+ +	2
	+ +	−	1
	+ +	−	15
	+ +	− [a]	56
	+ +	− [a]	5
Lichen substances			
Lichen-mix	+ + +	+ +	16
	+ + +	−	11
	+ +	+ + +	12
	+ +	+ +	28
	+ +	+ +	1
	+ +	+ +	34
Atranorin	+ +	+ + +	12
	+ +	+ +	34
	+ +	−	11
Usnic acid	+ + +	+ +	54
Alantolactone	+ + +	−	34
Fragrances			
Fragrance-mix	+ + +	+ + +	16
	+ + +	+ + +	3
Balsam of Peru	+ + +	+ + +	3
	+ +	−	27
	+ +	−	39
Others			
Blancophor	+ +	−	15
Chlorhexidine	+ +	+	1
Trichlorcarbanilide	+ +	−	28

[a] Changed to photocontact allergic reactions

Table 3. Reproducibility of photocontact allergic reactions

	Initial test	Follow-up test	Interval (months)
PABA	++	++	49
	++	++	3[a]
	++	++	2[a]
	++	−	47
	++	−	8
Chlorpromazine	+++	+++	17
	++	++	12
	++	−	56[b]
	+++	−	49[b]
	++	−	47[b]
Balsam of Peru	++	+	63
	++	−	15
Chlorhexidine	++	−	17
Fentichlor	++	−	47

[a] Changed to plain contact allergic reactions (identical reaction recorded on the irradiated and non-irradiated test side)
[b] Initial test made with 10 × concentration of allergen (1%)

Table 4. Reproducibility of questionable mixed photocontact (+ +) and contact (+) reactionts

	Initial test		Follow-up test		Interval (months)
	Irradiated	Covered	Irradiated	Covered	
PABA	++	+	−	−	34
Chlorhexidine	++	+	−	−	1
Hexachlorofen	++	+	−	−	10
Balsam of Peru	++	+	++	−	1
	++	+	+	+	28

Lichen-mix contact allergy was reproducible in five out of six cases and the lichen-related chemicals atranorin, alantolactone and usnic acid gave a positive follow-up reaction in three out of five cases.

None of the three initial chlorpromazine photocontact ractions, which had been produced by 1% allergen concentration, could be reproduced, while two photocontact reactions produced by 0.1% concentration evoked an equipotent photocontact reaction in the follow-up test. Neither of these two patients, however, had any history of taking or handling chlorpromazine drugs.

Discussion

Our 54% contact allergy reproducibility rate is rather similar to the results of three larger series published over the past 15 years [2–4]. The time interval between the two tests in our series is much shorter, only 18 months, compared with 3–10 years of those three studies. Interestingly, however, te Lintum and Nater did not find any clear influence of time on the persistence of positive patch tests. It could therefore be assumed, that either a true contact allery can disappear very quickly when the sensitizing chemical can be avoided or the original test result has been a false-positive reaction and only a true allergic contact sensitivity, once acquired, is lifelong. A third theoretical explanation is that the contact between the chemical and the skin in some tests would not have been good enough in the follow-up test, resulting in false-negative reactions.

Also controversial is the influence of the degree of allergen exposure on the persistence of contact test reactivity. Keczkes et al. [2] noticed that some easily avoided allergens turned negative when retested, but, on the other hand, a large number of patients still produced positive reactions on re-patch testing to allergens they had probably not been exposed to since their original sensitization. Nielsen and Jörgensen [6] showed that 75% of ethylenediamine contact allery reactions still persisted after 10 years, in spite of avoidance of the chemical. te Lintum and Nater [3] came to the conclusion that avoidance of the allergen could not be proved to have a decisive influence on the persistence of the sensitivity. In our series lichen-mix and related chemicals, fragrance-mix and PABA could be reproduced in quite a high percentage of cases. The lichen-mix allergic patients often came from agricultural environments and thus the avoidance of the chemical was rather difficult. Also total elimination of the fragrances has proved to be impossible. On the other hand, all the patients being contact allergic to PABA asserted that they had not used it since the original test. The relatively high reproducibility rate of PABA could be explained by the high sensitizing potential: two of our patients reported the first side effects after having used PABA only a couple of times.

All photocontact reactions to chlorpromazine that had been initially obtained with a 1% allergen concentration turned negative when retested with a 0.1% concentration. It is obvious that the primary reactions were phototoxic, because it has been shown (e.g. [7]) that an appropriate test concentration of chlorpromazine is 0.1%.

References

1. Jansen CT, Wennersten G, Rystedt I, Thune P, Brodthagen H (1982) The Scandinavian standard photopatch test procedure. Contact Dermatitis 8: 155–158
2. Keczkes K, Basheer AM, Wyatt EH (1982) The persistence of allergic contact sensitivity: a 10-year follow-up in 100 patients. Br J Dermatol 107: 461–465
3. te Lintum JCA, Nater JP (1973) On the persistence of positive patch test reactions to balsam of Peru, turpentine and nickel. Br J Dermatol 89: 629–634
4. Meneghini CL, Angelini G (1977) Behaviour of contact allergy and new sensitivities on subsequent patch tests. Contact Dermatitis 3: 138–142
5. Mutzhas MF, Hölzle E, Hofmann C, Plewig G (1981) A new apparatus with high radiation energy between 320–460 nm, physical description and dermatological applications. J Invest Dermatol 76: 42–47
6. Nielsen M, Jörgensen J (1987) Persistence of contact sensitivity to ethylenediamine. Contact Dermatitis 16: 275–276
7. Schauder S (1985) How to avoid phototoxic reactions in photopatch testing with chlorpromazine. Photodermatology 2: 95–100

Addresses

T. Hasan
Department of Dermatology, University of Turku, SF-20520 Turku, Finland

C. T. Jansén
Department of Dermatology, University of Turku, SF-20520 Turku, Finland

Contact and Photoallergic Dermatitis to Topical Nonsteroidal Antiinflammatory Drugs (Propionic Acid Derivatives): A Study of Eight Cases

N. Mozzanica, M. Pucci, and P. D. Pigatto

Summary

Many new nonsteroidal antiinflammatory drugs (NSAIDs) have been introduced into topical preparations for treatment of inflammatory or posttraumatic musculoskeletal disorders. Those NSAIDs, which are propionic acid derivatives, include ibuproxam, ibuprofen, naproxen, ketoprofen, fenoprofen, indoprofen, flurbiprofen and tiaprofenic acid, all of similar use, action, and toxicity. Cases of contact dermatitis and photodermatitis are rare and have been reported only anecdotally. We have seen eight patients with contact and photocontact dermatitis due to a single compound of this group of NSAIDs. All patients underwent ordinary patch and photopatch tests with standard series and all compounds of the aryl propionic group. Five patients had contact dermatitis: four to ibuproxam and one to ketoprofen, without any cross-reactivity, in spite of the marked chemical similarity in this group of NSAIDs. One case was a photodermatitis of an allergic type to tiaprofenic acid. The other two patients, negative for contact dermatitis, showed a typical photocontact allergy to ketoprofen, without any cross-reactivity. Other reports stated that cross-reactivity may happen, but we feel that this phenomenon is rare within this group of antigens, since the immune response, whether allergic or photoallergic, seems to be highly specific. Perhaps instead of cross-reactivity it would be better to speak of a concomitant allergy following several successive applications of topical preparations, each with a different one of these compounds.

Key words:

Contact dermatitis – Photoallergy – Arylpropionic acid derivatives – Nonsteroidal antiinflammatory drugs

Introduction

Allergic contact dermatitis is the most frequent cutaneous side effect to drugs. Nonsteroidal antiinflammatory drugs (NSAIDs), especially aryl propionic acid derivatives, are important in the development of allergic contact dermatitis, particularly in countries like those bordering the Mediterranean, where the use of topical antiinflammatory drugs is widespread and exposure to light is very great. Photosensitivity is also a well-recognized cutaneous side effect of some of these drugs. Immunological mechanisms are involved, but the reactions are rarely classified with precision. The molecular basis of photoallergy remains to be established, and even less is understood about why the same compound can cause contact allergy in some patients and photocontact allergy in others. Prior to 1978, allergy and photoallergy to aryl-propionic NSAIDs were unknown. Since then, these NSAIDs have been reported to cause skin allergological problems [1–3, 5–7, 9–11]. We have studied eight patients with allergic or photoallergic reactions to this group of compounds, investigating their allergological potential and the possibility of cross-reactivity among those drugs presently marketed in topical or suppository form.

Materials and Methods

Patch Tests

All patients were patch-tested with standard Italian Contact Dermatitis Research Group (GIRDCA) series [4], NSAID propionic acid derivatives and the commercial creams, that are sold in Italy, suspected to cause sensitization. The patch tests were applied to the backs of patients with Finn chambers on Scanpor (Norgeplaster, Oslo, Norway) and left there for 48 h. Results were read at 48, 72, and 96 h, according to international standards.

Table 1. Patch test results in eight patients

Substance	Case 1[a]			Case 2[a, c]			Case 3		
	48 h	72 h	96 h	48 h	72 h	96 h	48 h	72 h	96 h
GIRDCA series	–	–	–	++[d]	++[d]	++[d]	–	–	–
Ibudros cream	+++	+++	+++	–	+++	+++	+++	+++	+++
Deflogon cream	NT	NT	NT	NT	NT	NT	NT	NT	NT
Fastum gel	NT	NT	NT	NT	NT	NT	NT	NT	NT
Ibuproxam 5% pet.	+++	+++	+++	–	+++	+++	+++	+++	+++
Ibuprofen 5% pet.	–	–	–	–	–	–	–	–	–
Ketoprofen 2.5% pet.	–	–	–	–	–	–	–	–	–
Naproxen 5% pet.	–	–	–	–	–	–	–	–	–
Flurbiprofen 5% pet.	–	–	–	–	–	–	–	–	–
Fenoprofen 5% pet.	–	–	–	–	–	–	–	–	–
Tiaprofen ac. 5% pet.	NT	NT	NT	NT	NT	NT	NT	NT	NT

[a] see Ref. [1] [b] see Ref. [2] [c] see photopatch tests [d] Fragrance mix (Hermal)

Photopatch Tests

Test substances were applied for 24 h and then irradiated with 10 J/cm^2 from UVA Philips TLK 40 W 09/N fluorescent bulbs. Sites were examined 24 h and 48 h after irradiation. Black control patches (b.c.) were applied for 48 h and were examined 24 and 48 h later, to exclude simple contact sensitization. A photo-challenge test was done for one patient, with a therapeutical oral dose of tiaprofenic acid. Her back had been irradiated with sun-simulating radiation (1000 W Oriel Solar Simulator) of 0.75 MED (6.5 J/cm^2), repeated thrice every 2 h. The reactions were read after 30 and 90 min and on 3 successive days.

Case Reports

Cases 1, 2, and 5 have been published in part as "Short Communications" in *Contact Dermatitis* [6, 7].

Case 1 (Ibuproxam): A 19-year-old man applied a cream containing ibuproxam (Ibudros) for pain of the right knee. After 2 weeks of constant application, he noticed an eczematous eruption with erythema, edema, and vesicular lesions, extremely itchy, at the site of application, later extending towards both right leg and thigh. The site of the eczematous dermatitis had never been photoexposed, neither before nor after application of Ibudros cream. The patient said that no one in his family had any history of contact dermatitis or of atopy. Forty-eight hours after patch tests with standard GIRDCA series, Ibudros cream (as is) and NSAID propionic acid derivatives, there were intensely positive reactions to Ibudros cream and to ibuproxam 5% pet. (Table 1). The patch tests with standard GIRDCA series and the remaining NSAID propionic acid derivatives were negative. Results were the same after 72 and 96 h. No phototests nor photopatch tests were done.

Case 4			Case 5[b, c]			Case 6[c]			Case 7[c]			Case 8[c]		
48 h	72 h	96 h	48 h	72 h	96 h	48 h	72 h	96 h	48 h	72 h	96 h	48 h	72 h	96 h
–	–	–	–	–	–	–	–	–	–	–	–	–	–	–
NT	NT	NT	NT	NT	NT	NT	NT	NT	NT	NT	NT	NT	NT	NT
+++	+++	+++	NT	NT	NT	NT	NT	NT	NT	NT	NT	NT	NT	NT
NT	NT	NT	++	+++	+++	+	+	+	–	–	–	NT	NT	NT
+++	+++	+++	–	–	–	–	–	–	–	–	–	–	–	–
–	–	–	–	–	–	–	–	–	–	–	–	–	–	–
–	–	–	++	+++	+++	+	+	+	–	–	–	–	–	–
–	–	–	–	–	–	–	–	–	–	–	–	–	–	–
–	–	–	–	–	–	–	–	–	–	–	–	–	–	–
–	–	–	–	–	–	–	–	–	–	–	–	–	–	–
NT	NT	NT	NT	NT	NT	NT	NT	NT	NT	NT	NT	–	–	–

Case 2 (Ibuproxam): A 49-year-old woman used a cream containing ibuproxam (Ibudros) for pain of right elbow and shoulder. After about 10 days she stopped applying the cream, because, at the site of application she had developed an eczematous dermatitis with erythema, edema, and vesiculation, with severe itching. The patient did not remember whether the site of application had been exposed to sunlight or not, but she said that neither she nor her family had any history of contact dermatitis or of atopy. Forty-eight hours after patch tests with the same antigens as for case 1, there was a positive reaction (+ +) to fragrance mix (hermal) in the standard GIRDCA series, but the patch tests with Ibudros cream and propionic acid derivatives were negative. After 72 h she had intense positive reactions (+ + +) to Ibudros cream and to ibuproxam 5% pet., but the patch tests to other NSAID propionic acid derivatives were still negative (Table 1). The reactions were the same after 96 h. We did photopatch tests with our standard photopatch test series, Ibudros cream, and NSAID propionic acid derivatives; readings were made after 24 and 48 h revealing a positive reaction (+ +) to fragrance mix and intense positive reaction (+ + +) to Ibudros cream and to ibuproxam 5% pet. The remaining standard photopatch tests and other NSAID propionic acid derivatives were negative (Table 2). Photostimulation did not increase the intensity of the allergic reaction to the antigen.

Case 3 (Ibuproxam): A 32-year-old woman used a cream containing ibuproxam (Ibudros) for left knee pain, after a musculoskeletal trauma. After 2 weeks of application she noticed an eczematous eruption with severe itching at the site of application. The patient said that she had never photoexposed her lower limbs, before or after application of Ibudros cream. There was no personal or family history of contact dermatitis or of atopy. Forty-eight hours after patch tests with the same antigens as for case 1, there were intensely positive reactions to Ibudros cream and to ibuproxam 5% pet. (Table 1). The remaining patch tests were all negative. The results were the same after 72 and 96 h. Photopatch tests were not done.

Table 2. Photopatch test results in five patients

Substance	Case 2		Case 5		Case 6		Case 7		Case 8	
	48 h	72 h	48 h	72 h	48 h	72 h	48 h	72 h	48 h	72 h
Standard series	+ +[a]	+ +[a]	–	–	–	–	–	–	–	–
Ibudros cream	+ +	+ + +	NT	NT	NT	NT	NT	NT	NT	NT
Fastum gel	NT	NT	+ +	+ + +	NT	NT	+ +	+ +	NT	NT
Ibuproxam 5% pet.	+ +	+ + +	–	–	–	–	–	–	–	–
Ibuprofen 5% pet.	–	–	–	–	–	–	–	–	–	–
Ketoprofen 2.5% pet.	–	–	+ +	+ + +	+ + +	+ + +	+ +	+ +	–	–
Naproxen 5% pet.	–	–	–	–	–	–	–	–	–	–
Flurbiprofen 5% pet.	–	–	–	–	–	–	–	–	–	–
Fenoprofen 5% pet.	–	–	–	–	–	–	–	–	–	–
Tiaprofen ac. 5% pet.	NT	NT	NT	NT	NT	NT	NT	NT	–	–

[a] Fragrance mix (Hermal)
NT, not tested

Case 4 (Ibuproxam): A 22-year-old man used a cream containing ibuproxam (Deflogon) for right elbow pain. After 15 days he stopped the treatment because of an eczematous eruption with vesiculation and itching at the site of application, extending toward the arm. The patient said he had never exposed that area to sunlight, before or after application of Deflogon cream. Forty-eight hours after patch tests with the standard GIRDCA series, Deflogon cream (as is) and NSAID propionic acid derivatives there were intensely positive reactions to Deflogon cream and to ibuproxam 5% pet. (Table 1). The remaining patch tests were negative. Results were the same after 72 and 96 h. Photopatch tests were not done.

Case 5 (Ketoprofen): A 49-year-old man with "tennis elbow" (right epicondylitis) applied a cream containing ketoprofen (Fastum Gel) for 2 weeks. He stopped treatment because of a typical eczematous dermatitis at the site of drug application. The site of eczematous reaction had been photoexposed before and after topical treatment with Fastum Gel. Neither he nor his family had any previous history of contact dermatitis or of atopy. Forty-eight hours after patch tests with standard GIRDCA series, Fastum Gel (as is) and NSAID propionic acid derivatives there were positive reactions (+ +) to Fastum Gel and to ketoprofen 2.5% pet.; readings made at 72 and 96 h were more intensely positive to the same two products; the remaining patch tests were always negative (Table 1). At 24 and 48 h after irradiation of photopatch tests with our standard photopatch test series, Fastum Gel and NSAID propionic acid derivatives with long-wave UVA-light, there were positive reactions (+ + +) to Fastum Gel and ketoprofen 2.5% pet. (Table 2), comparable to those in the patch tests at 48 and 72 h.

Case 6 (Ketoprofen): A 41-year-old woman was seen with an acute eczematous rash on the right knee. The rash appeared within 12 days after having applied a cream containing ketoprofen (Fastum Gel) for a sport injury after solar exposure. She improved with a steroid cream and avoidance of light exposure. Patch tests with the standard series and propionic acid derivatives elicited only mild (+) reactions at 48, 72, and 96 h to Fastum Gel and to ketoprofen 2.5% pet. After 2 weeks she was photopatch tested with our standard photopatch series and the same NSAID propionic acid derivatives series, with strong positive reaction (+ + +) to ketoprofen, after irradiation with 10 J/cm^2 UVA. The reaction was proportional both to concentration of ketoprofen and intensity of light (Table 3).

Table 3. Photopatch tests results in case 6 with descending concentration of ketoprofen and decreasing intensity of light

Case 6	Photopatch Tests (UVA)		
	10 J/cm^2	6 J/cm^2	3 J/cm^2
Ketoprofen			
2% pet.	+ + +	+ + +	+ +
1% pet.	+ + +	+ +	+
0.5% pet.	+ +	+ +	−
0.2% pet.	+	+	−
0.1% pet.	+	−	−

Case 7 (Ketoprofen): A 33-year-old woman had been using a gel containing ketoprofen (Fastum Gel) as topical treatment for a rheumatic pain of the left elbow, during her summer holidays at the seaside. After a short time, she noticed a red swollen area with vesiculation where she had applied the gel. Patch tests with GIRDCA standard series, Fastum Gel, and NSAID propionic acid derivatives were negative; whereas, 24 h after 10 J/cm^2 UVA irradiation, Fastum Gel, and ketoprofen 2.5% pet. were positive (+ +). A reading 24 h later confirmed the same results (Table 2).

Case 8 (Tiaprofenic Acid): A 22-year-old woman was seen in July 1987 with acute dermatitis of the face and suprasternal area; borders were sharp, defining the shaded area of her head. She had mild rheumatoid arthritis, treated with tiaprofenic acid per os, staring 2 weeks before the dermatitis developed. She improved after stopping the drug and with topical treatment with steroids. A severe relapse appeared on taking the drug again. Patch tests and photopatch tests with our standard series were negative (Tables 1 and 2). A photochallenge test, made in the winter 1987, 6 h after taking tiaprofenic acid, irradiating an area on her shoulders with sun-simulating radiation, elicited a clear eczematous reaction after 24 h, that lasted for 4 days and itched violently.

Results

Cases 1, 3, and 4 were diagnosed as contact dermatitis, because of history and the positivity to patch tests. We did not think it necessary to do photopatch tests, for these patients. Cases 2 and 5 had similar responses to patch and photopatch tests. This, plus the clinical history, suggests a diagnosis of simple contact dermatitis. Case 6 was diagnosed as photocontact dermatitis. The patch tests were only mildly positive (+), while the photopatch tests were intensely positive (+ + +). This case might be only photoenhancement of a contact allergy, but this was ruled out by the later tests with various concentrations of ketoprofen and exposure to light (Table 3). The final diagnosis was photocontact allergic dermatitis. Case 7 was a classical example of photocontact dermatitis with positive photopatch tests and negative patch tests. Case 8, in our opinion, was a photodermatitis of an allergic type. We think that it was not a toxic reaction, because (a) the clinical aspect of the dermatitis was eczematous, with erythema, vesiculation, and intense itching; and (b) the time required to induce a positive photochallenge test (24 h after irradiation) is typical for allergic reactions, whereas toxic reactions appear after a shorter time (30–90 min).

Discussion

In our experience, ibuproxam is the most frequently responsible aryl propionic compound for contact dermatitis, whereas it seems never to be responsible for photocontact dermatitis. In the past 2 years we have observed four cases of contact dermatitis to ibuproxam and another two cases have been recently published by others

[10, 11]. In these latter two cases, patch tests with Ibudros cream and with ibuprofen 5% pet. were both positive, indicating cross-reactivity between the two drugs or else allergy to both drugs. Since none of our four patients showed any cross-reactions with ibuprofen (in spite of the considerable chemical similarity of these compounds), nor with other NSAID propionic acid derivatives, we think that cross-reactivity among aryl propionic derivatives is very uncommon. It is more likely that the two patients with positive patch test to Ibudros cream and ibuprofen 5% pet. had concomitant allergies to both, following application of several preparations containing these two compounds.

In the literature, ketoprofen is the most frequently responsible for allergic dermatitis. A certain number of case reports of patients with contact dermatitis [2, 3, 5, 7, 9] and photodermatitis [1, 5] due to ketoprofen have been published and our three cases confirmed that ketoprofen can induce both contact and photocontact dermatitis, without any cross-reactivity with the tested NSAID propionic acid derivatives series.

Although the ketoprofen photosensitivity index is experimentally very low [3], photoallergic sensitization to this drug seems to be quite common, after topical use. Two of our three cases had photocontact dermatitis. Besides, in a recent publication, Cusano et al. [5] observed that six in a series of eight patients with allergic dermatitis to ketoprofen had photocontact dermatitis, and only two cases were simple contact dermatitis. Only one of our cases showed a photosensitivity reaction to tiaprofenic acid. This is in agreement with the results of Przybilla [8] and von Kries [12], who found no cross-reactions, but a high incidence in the photosensitive population.

Many NSAID propionic acid derivatives have been recently introduced as topical preparations. It is our impression that adverse reactions to the topical use of these drugs could become a problem in countries where products containing them are popular remedies. However, although cross-reactivity may occur, we think that it does so rarely within this group of antigens, since the immunoresponse, whether allergic or photoallergic, is highly specific.

References

1. Alomar A (1985) Ketoprofen photodermatitis. Contact Dermatitis 12: 112–113
2. Angelini G, Vena G (1983) Contact allergy to ketoprofen. Contact Dermatitis 9: 234
3. Camarasa GC (1986) Contact dermatitis to ketoprofen. Contact Dermatitis 14: 120–122
4. Contact dermatitis announcement (1984) The Italian Contact Dermatitis and Environment Research Group (GIRDCA). Contact Dermatitis 11: 117
5. Cusano F, Rafanelli A, Bacchilega R, Ettico G (1987) Photocontact dermatitis from ketoprofen. Contact Dermatitis 17: 108–109
6. Mozzanica N, Pucci M, Negri M, Pigatto PD (1987) Contact dermatitis to ibuproxam. Contact Dermatitis 16: 281–282
7. Mozzanica N, Pucci M, Pigatto PD (1987) Contact allergy from ketoprofen. Contact Dermatitis 17: 325–326
8. Przybilla B, Ring J, Schwab U, Galosi A, Dorn M, Braun-Falco O (1987) Photo-sensibilisierende Eigenschaften nichtsteroidaler Antirheumatika in Photo-patch-tests. Hautarzt 38: 18–25

9. Valsecchi R, Falgheri G, Cainelli T (1983) Contact dermatitis from ketoprofen. Contact Dermatitis 9: 163–164
10. Valsecchi R, Cainelli T (1985) Contact dermatitis from ibuprofen. Contact Dermatitis 12: 286–287
11. Veronesi S, De Padova MP, Bardazzi F, Melino M (1986) Contact dermatitis to ibuprofen. Contact Dermatitis 15: 103–104
12. Von Kries R, Hoelzle E, Lehmann P, Plewig G (1987) Routine photopatch tesing with tiaprofenic acid. Photodermatology 4: 306–307

Addresses

N. Mozzanica
Second Department of Dermatology, University of Milan, 20122 Milan, Italy

M. Pucci
Second Department of Dermatology, University of Milan, 20122 Milan, Italy

P. D. Pigatto
Second Department of Dermatology, University of Milan, 20122 Milan, Italy

Photocontact Allergy from Photocopy Paper: A Report of Two Cases

A. Niinimäki

Summary

Two patients, a plumbing and central heating designer and a master builder, contracted photocontact dermatitis from handling photocopies of construction designs in their work. The course of the dermatitis was somewhat misleading in both cases: the dermatitis of one was not consistent with photoaggravated dermatitis, and in the other case a typical photodermatitis developed only 1½ years after the first signs of the dermatitis. The actual cause of the dermatitis in both patients was thiourea + UV-A. Thiourea, which is used to coat some photocopy papers in order to protect them from turning yellow, should be borne in mind as a possible photoallergen.

Key words:

Photocontact allergy - Thiourea

Introduction

Thiourea and its derivatives may cause both contact and photocontact allergies. In a recent report that included a review of the literature on the subject [2], rubber, adhesive tapes, and photocopy papers were the source of thiourea cited in most reports on contact allergy, and photocopy papers in reports on photocontact allergy.

The following describes two patients who contracted photocontact dermatitis from thiourea in photocopy papers. The course of the dermatitis was somewhat misleading in both patients.

Case Reports

Patient 1. A 36-year-old male plumbing and central heating designer contracted dermatitis on the ulnar side of his left hand in the beginning of summer 1986. The patient himself suspected photocopy papers to be the cause of the dermatitis, because the diseased area was in contact with photocopy papers while he drew and corrected construction designs. Patch tests with the European standard patch test series and with the photocopy papers were negative.

During the summer his dermatitis spread to the dorsal sides of both hands, and during the following autumn to the upper back, chest, upper arms and to both sides of the neck. At the same time the hand dermatitis healed with the exception of the wrists. Clothes, shampoos, and soaps were suspected to be the cause of the rash. In January 1987 patch tests with ingredients of personal hygiene products and with clothing series remained negative. In the photopatch tests, made in spring 1987, 0.1% thiourea, irradiated with 5 J/cm^2 UV-A, produced a positive reaction, while the nonirradiated test remained negative. According to the manufacturer, the photocopy papers used by the patient have a thiourea content below 1%. The patient changed jobs, and has been healthy ever since.

Patient 2. A 40-year-old master builder without any previous skin complaints contracted dermatitis on his hands in summer 1985. Both sides of the hands were affected first. In the autumn the dermatitis spread to his arms, flanks, thighs, legs, and soles. The dorsal sides of the hands were the worst affected. In February 1986 patch testing with the European standard patch test series revealed formaldehyde allergy, which was considered to be nonrelevant or only an additional cause of his dermatitis. During the winter most of the dermatitis healed, but still remained on his palms and soles. The sunny days of spring 1987 produced dermatitis on all areas exposed to the sun. Tests with ultraviolet light B and A were negative, but in the photopatch test series, thiourea was clearly positive on the irradiated side but negative on the nonirradiated side. The patient handled photocopy papers several times a day, and these particular papers were finished with a solution containing 4%–5% thiourea. The patient was advised to handle the papers with gloves and, consequently, his dermatitis cleared up everywhere except on his palms and soles, which met the criteria for chronic "infectious" dermatitis.

Discussion

The distribution and course of the first patient's dermatitis was not typical of photocontact eczema. In the second case the diagnosis was easier to establish. Thiourea and its derivatives are used in photocopy papers, rubber, adhesive tapes, photography, and in the manufacture of resins [1, 2] as well as in a variety of other areas [3]. Thiourea should obviously be included in the photocontact test series, because it seems to be an important allergen and hypersensitivity to it is rather unpredictable. Cross-reactivity between thiourea and its derivatives should also be established.

References

1. Cronin E (1980) Contact dermatitis. Churchill Livingstone, Edinburgh
2. Dooms-Goossens A, Chrispeels MT, De Veylder H, Roelandts R, Willems, L, Degreef H (1987) Contact and photocontact sensitivity problems associated with thiourea and its derivatives: a review of the literature and case reports. Br J Dermatol 116: 573–579
3. Merck Index, 10th edn (1983) Merck, Rathway, New Jersey

Addresses

A. Niinimäki
Department of Dermatology, University Central Hospital of Oulu, 90220 Oulu, Finland

Part 7

Diagnostic Methods

Patch Testing

Patch Test Standardization

T. Fischer

Summary

Patch test standardization is presently in a stage of rapid evolution and it is time to set rules and to come to agreements not only concerning the allergen concentration in the test material, but also other areas of test standardization. Guidelines are suggested concerning allergen analysis, validation of the test material, choice of vehicle, and the control of the function and the stability of the test material.

Key words:

Contact allergy - Patch testing - Standardization - Test technique

Background

Contact allergy, a cell-mediated type IV reaction, is verified by the application of the allergen to the skin of the patient. In case of sensitization, an area of contact dermatitis appears at the site of application. The standardization of patch-test material has been a step-by-step development since Jadassohn's first "modern" test application 90 years ago. Until recently, little has changed in the area of vehicle choice and pharmaceutical preparation, since petrolatum was accepted as standard vehicle about 30 years ago.

Present Standardization

Standardization is presently accomplished to various degrees of sophistication dependent on how frequent and interesting the allergen is, and how much problems it causes (Table 1). The standardization may include the following steps: A patient

Table 1. Present standardization of patch test material

Suspicion of allergic contact dermatitis
Application of suspected material
• On patient
• In vehicle
• In different concentrations
• On nonallergic control patients
Identification of allergen
Control of purity
Population frequency studies

Table 2. Proposed standardization of patch test material

• Development of analytical methods
• Validation of raw material
• Choice of vehicle
• Pharmaceutical preparation
• Choice of application method
• In vitro standardization of allergen dose
• In vivo standardization of allergen dose
• Packaging of test material
• Stability control
• Batch-to-batch control
• Clinical validation

demonstrates dermatitis, suspected to be caused by a new allergen. This allergen is then applied to the skin of the upper back of the patient. The allergen is usually mixed in petrolatum vehicle. The investigator may decide to use different concentrations of allergen. A positive reaction is controlled by applying the same test to at least 20 control patients who should demonstrate negative reactions. Furthermore attempts may be made to control the identity and purity of the allergen. If the test material is a mixture or a biological material the allergen identification may be difficult or even impossible.

Population studies will indicate the frequency of sensitization in the population.

If the allergen proves to be frequent, it is eventually included in test panels, suggested by national and international contact dermatitis research groups.

Proposed Standardization of Frequent Allergens

Common contact allergens ought to be standardized in a systematic way. The standardization should include the steps included in Table 2.

Development of Analytical Methods. Quantitative and qualitative analytical methods are necessary tools in the control of identity, homogeneity, dosage, and stability of the test material. Such methods should also detect impurities and interference between allergens in mixtures and evaluate possible interactions between the allergens, the vehicle, the test device, and the packing material.

Validation of Raw Material. Allergens which are known to be distinct chemical compounds must be as pure as possible. Biological materials with allergens of more or less unknown structure, should conform to identification criteria which can be used in the analysis, until the chemical background of the true allergens is identified.

The Vehicle. The vehicle must be nonallergenic, nonirritant, compatible with the allergens, institute an adequate allergen release to the skin, and be easy to handle. Petrolatum as presently used functions well with many allergens, but it is far from optimal with others and the application implies a tedious procedure. With the gels used in the TRUE Test it has been possible to optimize the incorporation of the allergen into the vehicle [1].

Pharmaceutical Preparation. Many allergens are difficult to incorporate homogeneously in petrolatum although present petrolatum mixed test materials are significantly better than those used just a few years ago, when droplets and particles of a size of up to 0.5 mm could be observed [2]. No sensitizing additives should be permitted. The allergens of the TRUE Test are homogeneously incorporated into a dry cellulose film. On contact with the skin, this film hydrates and the allergen is released [1].

Application Method. The occlusive patch is the present standard of application. The Al test uses filter paper patch on an aluminum-plastic backing. Most popular at present are different aluminum and plastic chambers. The TRUE Test is printed on occlusive polyester backing. It should be emphasized, that the allergen concentration/dose should be accomodated to the individual application method. Ease of application is essential to stimulate patch testing, and readymade test panels like the TRUE Test are expected to be used increasingly in the future.

In Vitro Verification of Allergen Dose. The determination of the accurate allergen dose is best started in vitro by certifying the amount of allergen in the test material, the release of allergen from this material, and the compatibility between allergen, vehicle, device, and packing material.

Diffusion chamber studies of allergen uptake and penetration through skin and various membranes are of value in the selection of correct vehicle and in the standardization of such difficult allergens as formaldehyde, fragrances, parabens, and caines.

In Vivo Standardization of Allergen Dose. The in vivo determination is performed on patients sensitive to the actual allergen and in nonsensitized controls using serial dilution technique. Two test series applied with different methods at the same time will give necessary information concerning the optimal, the minimal, and the irritant dose intervals for different allergens. The standard dose should detect contact allergy in patients with low sensitivity, but avoid irritation and sensitization. The choice of test dose is a compromise for many allergens, since they irritate at a concentration optimal for patch testing.

The Packaging. The packaging is an often-disregarded part of the standardization procedure. The package should protect the test mechanically, against atmosphere, humidity, light, and UV radiation. The packaging should be inert, which means impermeable to the allergens, not interfere with them and be nonsensitizing.

Stability and Quality Control. We ought not to accept test material which is uncontrolled and undeclared concerning stability. Test material kept at different temperatures for different time intervals should be investigated accordingly, and visual and microscopic inspection, chemical analysis of the allergen amount, microbiological control, and clinical function tests should all be undertaken. The clinical function is controlled by applying aged test material on sensitive patients. The quality control should also include a chemical verification that different batches of test material conform to given criteria.

Clinical Verification (Multicenter Studies). The ultimate verification of the test material is the clinical verification of high performance, which includes the validation of a good function and a control of the side effects. Several clinics with long experience in patch testing should be included in this test. Adequate function means, that the test indicates allergy accurately, has high technical quality and good patient compliance. The evaluation of side effects should include irritation, influence on the skin disease and sensitization risk.

References

1. Fischer T, Maibach HI (1988) Easier patch testing. J Am Acad Dermatol (in press)
2. Fischer T, Maibach HI (1984) Patch test allergens in petrolatum: a reappraisal. Contact Dermatitis 11: 224–228

Addresses

T. Fischer
Department of Occupational Dermatology, University Hospital, S-75185 Uppsala, Sweden

Swedish Multicenter Study with TRUE Test, Panel 2

B. Stenberg, K. Billberg, T. Fischer, L. Nordin, L. Pettersson, M. Ruhnek-Forsbeck, K. Sundberg, G. Swanbeck, L. Svensson, J. E. Wahlberg, L. Widström, and K. Wrangsjö

Summary

Using panel 2 of a new patch test, the TRUE Test (TT), 369 consecutive patients with contact dermatitis and 37 healthy controls were patch tested with 11 different allergens (or allergen mixes). For control, the same allergens in standard concentrations in petrolatum (except Kathon CG in water) were applied using the Finn chamber (FC) technique. The allergen doses of TT were chosen according to the results of a previous serial dilution patch-test study. In the population tested, there were reactors to all the 11 allergens or allergen mixes. The concordance of positive reactions was 60% between the TT and the FC technique, 28% were indicated only with TT and 12% only with FC. The frequency of questionable and irritant reactions was about the same for the two tests and was recorded in less than 1% of all test patches. In 2 of 37 healthy volunteers tested, late reactions after 5–7 days appeared. The study indicates that TT is a well-standardized technique and gives a good accuracy.

Key words:

Patch testing - Contact dermatitis - TRUE Test - Vehicle

The precision of patch test methods used in the clinic today is not sufficient, and irritant reactions are not uncommon [1–4]. A new test technique, the TRUE Test (TT) was developed with the aim to simplify the test procedure and to minimize nonspecific, irritant reactions [5]. TT is a ready-to-use patch test which at present includes a full standard panel except for formaldehyde. The accuracy of the first 12 allergens has been confirmed clinically [6, 7].

The aim of this study was to investigate the reliability of the second part of the TT standard panel (see Table 1) and to ascertain the allergen doses.

Table 1. The dosage/concentration of the panel 2 allergens of TRUE Test (mg/cm^2) and petrolatum test material (%)

Allergens	TRUE Test (mg/cm^2)	Concentration in petrolatum (%)
13. p-t-Butylphenol formaldehyde	0.040	1.0
14. Parabens[a]	1.00 (5 × 0.20)	3.0 (5 × 0.60)
15. Carba mix[b]	0.25 (3 × 0.080)	1.0 (3 × 0.33)
16. Black rubber mix[c]	0.075 (2 × 0.030 + 0.012)	0.60 (2 × 0.25 + 0.10)
17. Kathon CG	0.0040	0.02
18. Quaternium 15	0.10	1.0
19. Mercaptobenzothiazole	0.075	2.0
20. Wool alcohols	1.00	30
21. Negative control		
22. Mercapto mix[d]	0.075 (3 × 0.025)	0.75 (3 × 0.25)
23. Thiomersal[e]	0.012	0.1
24. Quinoline mix[f]	0.20 (2 × 0.10)	3.0 (2 × 1.50)

[a] Methyl parahydroxybenzoate; ethyl parahydroxybenzoate; propyl parahydroxybenzoate; butyl parahydroxybenzoate; benzyl parahydroxybenzoate
[b] 1,3-Diphenylguanidine; zinc diethyldithiocarbamate; zinc dibutyldithiocarbamate
[c] N-Cyclohexyl-N′-phenyl-paraphenylenediamine; N-Isopropyl-N′-phenyl-paraphenylenediamine; N,N′-Diphenyl-paraphenylenediamine
[d] Morpholinylmercapto-benzothiazole; n-cyclohexylbenzothiazylsulphenamide; dibenzothiazyl disulphide
[e] The dose hase been adjusted to 0.008 mg/cm^2
[f] Clioquinol; Chlorquinaldol

Material and Methods

The study was carried out at eight different departments of dermatology in Sweden during August–October 1987.

Test Material. TT (Pharmacia, Sweden) is manufactured by incorporating the allergen in different hydrophilic gels, commonly hydroxypropylcellulose. A thin layer of the allergen/gel mix is printed on a plastic film, dried, and cut into 9 × 9 mm patches, which are mounted on an acrylic tape (Cederroths, Solna, Sweden). The tape strip is protected with a siliconized plastic cover and packed in a laminated airtight, light-impermeable envelope.

The allergen doses of the patches have been calibrated in a clinical dose-response study and controlled by in vitro analysis [8].

The reference test material was standard allergens in petrolatum, Kathon CG in water (Chemotechnique Diagnostics, Malmö, Sweden or Hermal Chemie, Reinbek b. Hamburg, FRG), in concentrations recommended by the ICDRG and applied in Finn chambers on Scanpor (Epicon, Helsinki, Finland).

Patients. A total of 369 consecutive patients (232 women and 137 men) with suspected contact dermatitis and 37 healthy volunteers (30 women and 7 men) were tested.

Trial Design. A controlled, nonblind, within-patient design was used. The patients were allocated consecutively. The two test strips were applied symmetrically on the upper back. A strip with the vehicle-gels served as placebo. Left/right application of the respective test varied at random. The tests were removed at 48 h and evaluated at 72, 96, or 120 h according to generally accepted recommendations [9]. Responsiveness, quality, i.e., size of positive reactions, adhesiveness, and side effects were recorded.

Test Results

Although 2 dropped out and are not included, 367 patients completed the study. No patient left the study due to side effects. Evaluation of 329 patients was made at 72 h, of 39 at 96 h, and of 1 at 120 h.

Responsiveness. Each of the 11 allergens had reactors in the test population, see Fig. 1. In either or both of the tests 77 pairs of tests resulted in positive (+ to + + +) reactions; 46 were indicated in both tests, thus the concordance was 60%. Another 22 (28%) were indicated only with TT and 9 (2%) only with FC. Of the 22 solitary positive TT test reactions, 9 were caused by thiomersal.

Thiomersal was found to be significantly more often causing irritant or questionable reactions in TT than in FC (Fisher's exact test, $P<0.05$). For all other substances the frequency of such reactions was similar or lower for TT than for FC (see Fig. 2). Four irritant/questionable vehicle reactions were noted.

A history raising suspicion of contact allergy to allergens in panel 2, was verified by TT in 33% and by FC test in 28% of the patients. Of 11 previously positive reactions to allergens in panel 2, 8 were reproduced in TT and 9 in the FC test.

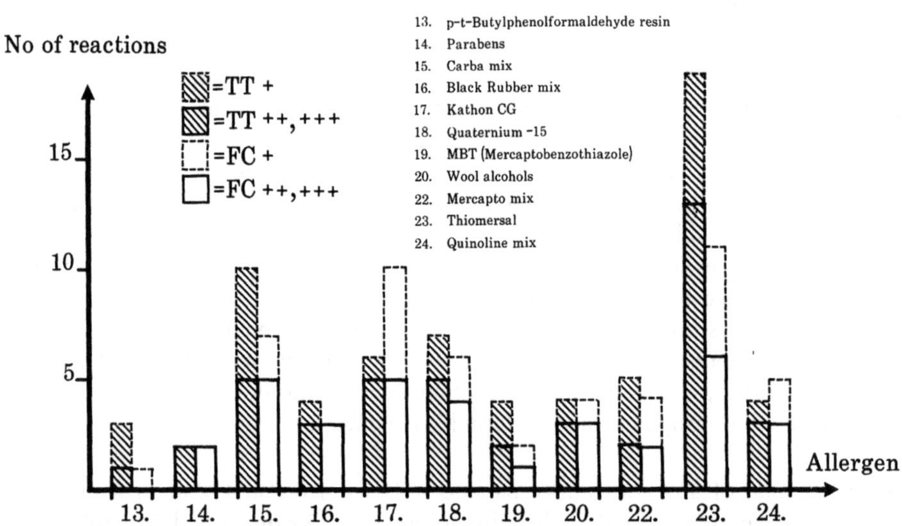

Fig. 1. Positive reactions in 369 patients

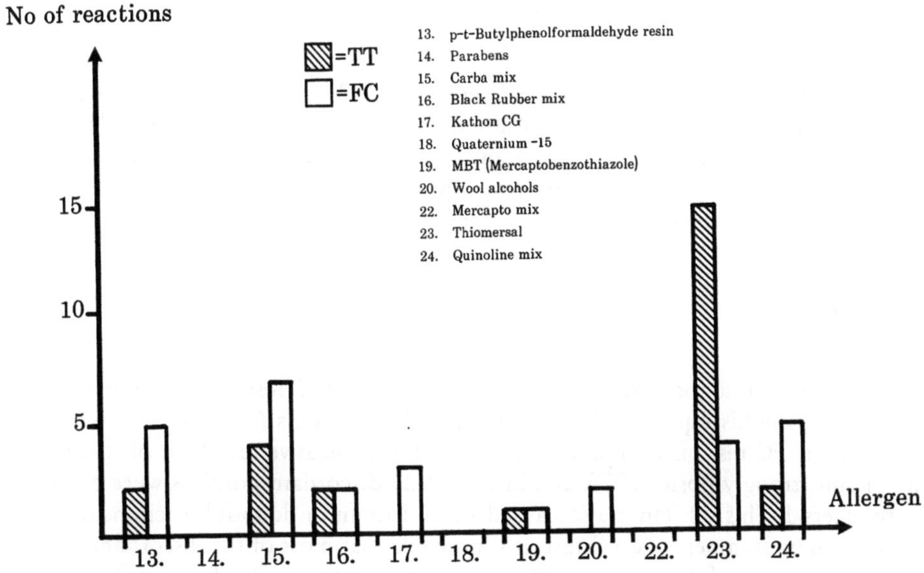

Fig. 2. Irritant and questionable test reactions in 369 patients

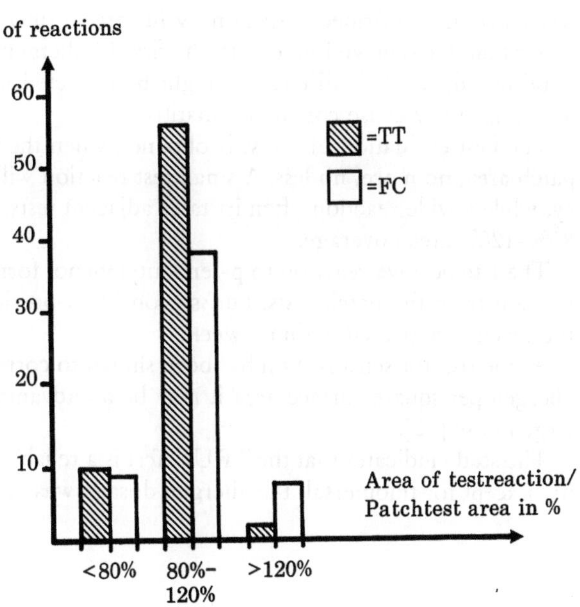

Fig. 3. The area of positive (+, ++ and +++) reactions compared to the patch area, per test method

Quality. There was no statistical difference in the quality scores between TT and FC tests (Fisher's exact test; Fig. 3).

Adhesiveness. The tape adhesiveness was significantly better (Chi^2 test, $P < 0.01$) for TT, where 344 strips adhered perfectly. The figure for the FC test was 321.

Side Effects. Irritation from tape rarely occurred. No difference was noted between the test methods.

Healthy Volunteers. Of 37 healthy volunteers tested, 2 had positive reactions to p-tert-butylphenol formaldehyde, 1 to Kathon CG, and 5 to thiomersal at 72 h. Two reported late reactions appearing at 5 and 7 days respectively. They were retested and one of them had positive (+ +) reactions with both FC and TT method to p-tert-butylphenol formaldehyde, whereas the other was negative.

Discussion

In general there is a good concordance between the TRUE Test and the Finn chamber test. This holds especially for strongly positive reactions (+ + to + + +). Six TTs and one FC test of this grade corresponded to a negative test. Four of these six discordant strongly positive TTs and in total 9/22 discordant positives were caused by thiomersal. This substance also caused 12/17 irritant or doubtful reactions to TT corresponding to a negative FC test. It is probable that most of the discordant positive reactions were false positives. The dose of thiomersal in TT has now been reduced from 0.012 mg/cm^2 to 0.008 mg/cm^2.

It is difficult to identify the causative allergen by patient history. In this study the test reactions confirmed suspicion by history in only about 30%. This frequency is lower than the one we found with the first 12 allergens of the TRUE Test (52%, unpublished data). This difference might be expected as the substances of this panel less frequenctly cause contact dermatitis.

The best evaluation of a test is obtained when the test reaction covers the entire patch area, no more, no less. A small test reaction will raise the suspicion of irritancy, while a wide reaction often irritates adjacent tests. TT gave a high proportion of 80%–120% area coverage.

The late positive reaction to p-tert-butylphenol formaldehyde may indicate sensitization from the patch tests, but is probably a previously established sensitivity as the reaction appeared within 1 week.

As the risk for sensitization has been shown to correlate with the concentration of allergen per square surface area it may be an advantage to use TT with its low allergen dose [10].

The study indicates that the TRUE Test is a reliable test technique with high quality. Except for thiomersal, the allergen dosage was confirmed to be adequate.

References

1. Fischer T, Rystedt I (1985) False-positive, follicular and irritant patch test reactions to metal salts. Contact Dermatitis 12: 93–98
2. Kalimo K, Lammintausta K (1984) 24 and 48 h allergen exposure in patch testing. Contact Dermatitis 10: 25–29

3. Schmidt H, Schultz Larsen F, Ølholm Larsen P, Søgaard H (1980) Petechial reaction following patch testing with cobalt. Contact Dermatitis 6: 91–94
4. Fischer T, Maibach HI (1984) Amount of nickel applied with a standard patch test. Contact Dermatitis 11: 285–287
5. Fischer T, Maibach HI (1985) The thin layer rapid use epicutaneous test (TRUE-test), a new patch test method with high accuracy. Br J Dermatol 112: 63–68
6. Lachapelle J-M, et al. (1988) European multicenter study of the TRUE Test. Contact Dermatitis 11: 91–97
7. Ruhnek-Forsbeck M, et al. (1988) Comparative multi-center study with TRUE Test and Finn Chamber patch test methods in eight Swedisch hospitals. Acta Derm Venereol (Stockh) 68: 123–128
8. Fischer T, Maibach HI (1989) The science of patch test standardization. Immunology and Allergy Clinics. Saunders, Philadelphia (in press)
9. Fregert S (1981) Manual of contact dermatitis, 2nd edn. Munksgaard, Copenhagen
10. White SI, Friedmann PS, Moss C, Simpson JM (1986) The effect of altering area of application and dose per unit area on sensitization by DNCB. Br J Dermatol 115: 663–668

Addresses

B. Stenberg
Department of Dermatology, University Hospital, S-90185 Umeå, Sweden

K. Billberg
Pharmacia AB, Uppsala, Sweden

T. Fischer
Department of Dermatology, University Hospital, Uppsala, Sweden

L. Nordin
Department of Dermatology, Sahlgrenska Hospital, Gothenburg, Sweden

L. Pettersson
Department of Dermatology, Gävle Hospital, Gävle, Sweden

M.Ruhnek-Forsbeck
Department of Dermatology, Södersjukhuset, Stockholm, Sweden

K. Sundberg
Department of Dermatology, Regional Hospital, Linköping, Sweden

G. Swanbeck
Department of Dermatology, Sahlgrenska Hospital, Gothenburg, Sweden

L. Svensson
Department of Dermatology, Gävle Hospital, Gävle, Sweden

J. E. Wahlberg
Department of Occupational Dermatology, Karolinska Hospital, Stockholm, Sweden

L. Widström
Regional Hospital, Örebro, Sweden

K. Wrangsjö
Department of Occupational Dermatology, Karolinska Hospital, Stockholm, Sweden

Reproducibility of Patch Test Results: Comparison of TRUE Test and Finn Chamber Test

R. Gollhausen, B. Przybilla, and J. Ring

Summary

For evaluation of reproducibility duplicate patch test series comprising 12 allergens were applied to either side of the back in a total of 139 patients. The reproducibility of a newly developed patch test system, the TRUE Test, was compared with that of the Finn chamber test. In the TRUE Test 20 of 63 patients had at least one positive reaction, the total number of positive reactions being 28. Five of these 28 reactions (17.9%) were found on only one side of the back, i.e. they were nonreproducible. In the Finn chamber test 33 of 76 patients had at least one positive reaction, and 22 of 58 positive reactions (37.9%) were nonreproducible. The percentage of nonreproducible positive results was more than twice as high in the Finn chamber test as in the TRUE Test. However, due to the low number this difference in reproducibility between the two test systems was not statistically significant using the chi-square test ($P=0.1$).

Key words:

Patch test - Reproducibility - False-positive reactions - False-negative reactions - TRUE Test - Finn chamber test

In the evaluation of any test system the reproducibility of its results is of crucial importance. Recently it has been shown for the Finn chamber test that the reproducibility of patch test results is rather low [8]. Now a newly developed patch test design, the TRUE Test (Pharmacia, Uppsala, Sweden), has been introduced in the United States and several European countries [5]. Thus, we examined the reproducibility of the TRUE Test in comparison with the Finn chamber test.

In the manufacture of the TRUE Test, the allergens are incorporated into a gel, which is dried and attached to the test tape. Thus, the set is ready to use: the test

Table 1. The concentrations of the allergens in the TRUE Test (mg/cm^2) and in the Finn chamber test (%)

Allergens	TRUE Test (mg/cm^2)	Concentration in petrolatum (%)
Nickel sulphate	0.2	5.0
p-Phenylenediamine[a]	0.05	1.0
Neomycin sulphate	0.2	20.0
Potassium dichromate	0.025	0.5
Caine mix	0.7	8.0
Fragrance mix	0.6	16.0
Colophony	1.5	20.0
Epoxy resin	0.05	1.0
Thiuram mix	0.025	1.0
Balsam of Peru	0.8	25.0
Ethylenediamine[a]	0.05	1.0
Cobalt chloride	0.02	1.0

[a] In the TRUE Test as dihydrochloride salt, in the Finn chamber test as base

tape with the allergens can be applied to the skin of the upper back without further manipulations. The Finn chamber test is widely used and well known. Due to the different manufacture of the TRUE Test, the test concentrations of the various allergens differ from the concentrations used in the Finn chamber test (Table 1).

Patients and Methods

After giving informed consent, 139 patients of both sexes (69 women, 70 men) between the ages of 19 and 86 years participated in the investigation. They were in- and outpatients at our clinic referred for patch testing at least 3 weeks after skin lesions of dermatitis had cleared. The skin of the test site, i.e. the upper back had to be free of any sign of irritation like scratch marks, was not shaved and not subjected to any form of treatment. Of course, no systemic steroid treatment was performed. Test materials were supplied by Pharmacia, Uppsala, Sweden (TRUE Test) or by Maser, Herne, FRG, Hermal-Chemie, Reinbek, FRG and by the pharmacy of the clinic (allergens in petrolatum, Finn chambers on Scanpor).

For evaluation of the reproducibility of a patch-test system, the test set was applied in duplicate each to either side of the upper back of the patients.

Exposure time was 2 days. Semiquantitative reading was done 2 and 3 days after application by the responsible physician of the allergy service, according to Bandmann and Dohn [1] and as shown in Table 2. Only reactions exhibiting at least an infiltrated erythema (+ reaction) were regarded as positive. For evaluation of the reproducibility, the grade of reactivity was neglected and questionable or irritant reactions were taken as negative. When an allergen showed up either at both sides or only at one side of the back, it was regarded as yielding one positive reaction. If at test reaction was positive only at one side, this result was regarded as nonreproducible. The quotient of nonreproducible positive results to the overall number of

Table 2. Evaluation of patch test results [1]

0	No visible reaction
IR	Irritative reaction
(+)	Erythema
+	Infiltrated erythema
++	Infiltrated erythema with scattered papules/vesicles
+++	Infiltrated erythema with dense papules/vesicles
++++	Bullous reaction

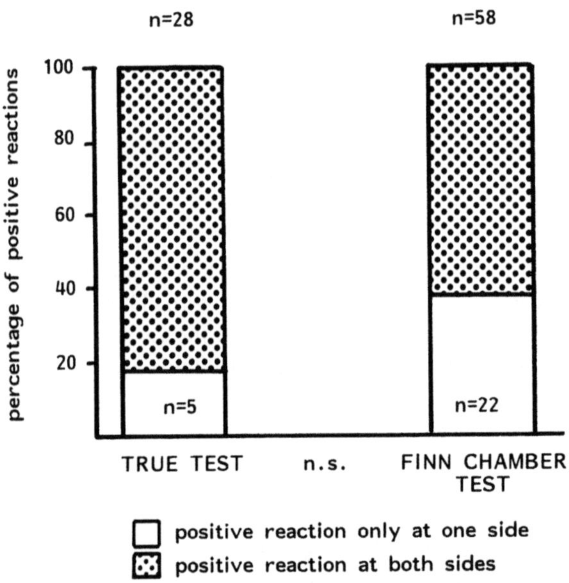

Fig. 1. Reproducibility of TRUE-Test and Finn chamber test

positive reactions was calculated in percent and taken as an inverse measure of reproducibility.

Only the 12 allergens available in panel 1 of the TRUE Test (Table 1) were included in the study.

In 63 patients a TRUE Test was applied in duplicate each to either side of the back and in 76 patients a Finn chamber test was performed in the same manner.

The reproducibility of the TRUE and the Finn chamber test was compared using the chi-square test.

Results

In the TRUE Test, 20 of 63 patients had at least one positive reaction, for a total of 28 positive reactions. The average and the standard deviation of positive reactions per person were 0.4 ± 0.7 (28/63). Five of the 28 positive reactions (17.9%) were nonreproducible (Fig. 1).

In the Finn chamber test, 33 of 76 patients had at least one positive reaction, the average and the standard deviation of positive reactions per person being 0.8 ± 1.1 (58/76). Of 58 positive reactions 22 (37.9%) were nonreproducible (Fig. 1). Weakly positive reactions were significantly less reproducible than marked positive reactions (Fig. 2).

The positive (reproducible and nonreproducible) allergens are listed in Table 3.

The percentage of nonreproducible positive results was more than twice as high in the Finn chamber test as in the TRUE Test (Fig. 1). However, this difference of reproducibility of the two test systems was not significant using the chi-square test ($P < 0.05$).

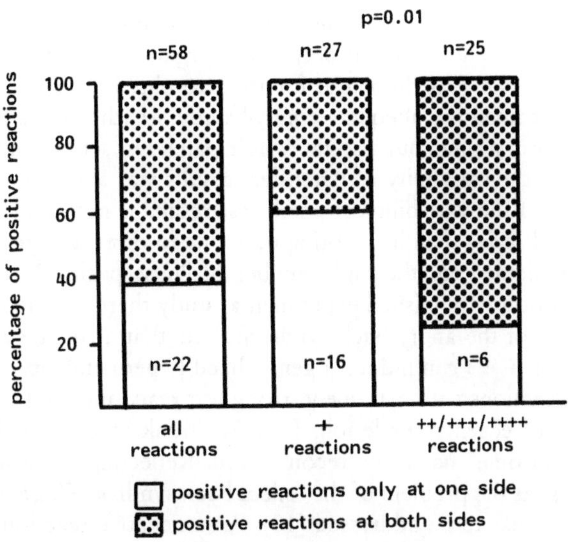

Fig. 2. Reproducibility of weakly and strongly positive reactions (Finn chamber)

Table 3. List of allergens exhibiting positive results in the TRUE Test and in the Finn chamber test

	Nonreproducible/all positive reactions	
	TRUE Test	Finn chamber test
Nickel sulphate	1/10	3/9
p-Phenylenediamine[a]	1/1	2/6
Neomycin sulphate	0/3	2/10
Potasium dichromate	0/0	1/2
Caine mix	0/0	3/7
Fragrance Mix	0/3	2/4
Colophony	1/4	0/3
Epoxy resin	0/0	1/1
Thiuram mix	0/0	3/4
Balsam of Peru	1/4	3/7
Ethylendiamine[a]	0/1	0/1
Cobalt chloride	1/2	2/4
Total	5/28	22/58

[a] In the TRUE Test as dihydrochloride salt, in the Finn chamber test as base

Discussion

Many positive reactions were not reproducible in this study. In accordance with other authors the reproducibility of one plus reaction was especially low [3, 13]. At this congress the reproducibility of photopatch testing has also been reported to be very low [9].

The problem of variability of patch test results is seldom directly addressed. However, if one is aware of this problem, one will find a low reproducibility in many published studies. Quite a number of investigators reported the loss of about 40% of positive reactions at retesting patch tests and they published this low reproducibility under the headings of the "angry back syndrome" or "excited skin syndrome" [3, 4, 11–13]. They retested only one allergen at a time, and therefore claimed concomitant testing as the cause for their results. However, only Bandmann and Agathos performed the adequate control study, i.e. they retested not only one to three allergens at a time, but also the whole patch test set including 26 substances. They found that the variability of patch-test results was about in the same range in both retests [2]. If the variability of patch-test results is not greater in retesting the whole standard series than in retesting only one to three allergens, concomitant testing cannot be blamed for the high number of "false positive" reactions. Furthermore, in one previously published experimental study there was no evidence in favour of the concept of the angry back syndrome, i.e. that a single strongly positive reaction (+ + to + + +) can induce a generalized hyperirritability of the skin [10]. There may be exceptions with extremely strong test reactions (> + + +) inducing a general flare-up of eczematous lesions [12]. We think that the pathogenesis of the "angry back syndrome" has to be reconsidered. Reflecting the low reproducibility of patch test results the problem of the "silent back syndrome", i.e. of false negative patch-test results has to be addressed [10]. False negative reactions are as important a pitfall of patch testing as false positive ones [7].

In order to evaluate the accuracy of a test system, it is necessary to examine the reproducibility of its results. In this study the reproducibility of positive reactions was better in the TRUE Test than in the Finn chamber test, indicating a higher accuracy of the TRUE Test; however, this difference was not significant. The indicated higher accuracy of the TRUE Test may be explained by a better surface distribution of the allergen in the vehicle [5]. Further studies of the reproducibility of patch-test reactions will help in judging the accuracy of the different test systems.

References

1. Bandmann HJ, Dohn W (1967) Die Epikutantestung. Bergmann, München
2. Bandmann HJ, Agathos M (1981) Das 'Angry Back Syndrome'. Untersuchungsergebnisse mit Sequenztestungen, Wiederholungstestungen und dem Cocarden-(Target-)Test. Hautarzt [Suppl V] 32: 97–104
3. Bruynzeel DP (1983) Angry back or excited skin syndrome. Thesis. Kripps Repro Mettel, Amsterdam

4. Bruynzeel DP, Maibach HI (1986) Excited skin syndrome (angry back). Arch Dermatol 122: 323–328
5. Lachapelle JM, Bruynzeel DP, Ducombs G, Hannuksela M, Ring J, White IR, Wilkinson J, Fisher T, Billberg K (1988) European multicenter study of the TRUE test. Contact Dermatitis 19: 91–97
6. Fischer T, Maibach HI (1985) The thin layer rapid use epicutaneous test (TRUE-test), a new patch method with high accuracy. Br J Dermatol 112: 63–68
7. Fischer T, Maibach HI (1986) Patch testing in allergic contact dermatitis: an update. Sem Dermatol 5: 214–224
8. Gollhausen R, Przybilla B, Ring J (1987) Reproducibility of patch testing. Proceedings of the XVII Congressus Mundi Dermatologiae, 24–29 May, 1987. Volume of abstracts. University of Steglitz, Berlin, p 59
9. Hasan T, Jansen CT (1988) Reproducibility and dosaging in photocontact testing. (This volume)
10. Kligman AM, Gollhausen R (1986) The "angry back". A new concept or old confusion? Br J Dermatol [Suppl 31] 115: 93–100
11. Maibach HI, Fregert S, Magnusson B, Pirilä V, Hjorth N, Wilkinson D, Malten K, Meneghini C, Lachapelle JM, Calnan C, Cronin E (1982) Quantification of the excited skin syndrome (the 'angry back'). Retesting one patch at a time. Contact Dermatitis 8: 78
12. Luderschmidt C, Heilgemeier G, Ring J, Burg G (1982) Polyvalente Kontaktallergie versus 'Angry Back': Zur Problematik falsch positiver Epikutantestreaktionen. Allergologie 5: 262–264
13. Mitchell JC (1977) Multiple concomitant positive patch test reactions. Contact Dermatitis 3: 315–320

Addresses

R. Gollhausen
Dermatologische Klinik und Poliklinik der Ludwig-Maximilians-Universität, 8000 Munich 2, FRG

B. Przybilla
Dermatologische Klinik und Poliklinik der Ludwig-Maximilians-Universität, 8000 Munich 2, FRG

J. Ring
Dermatologische Klinik und Poliklinik der Ludwig-Maximilians-Universität, 8000 Munich 2, FRG

Chemical and Pharmaceutical Standardization of Fragrance Mix for Patch Testing

A.-M. Svensson, S. Enström, L. Thurell, and H. Swanberg

Summary

A selective gas chromatographic method was developed for the determination of fragrance mix, one of the allergens in the standard panel of the TRUE Test. The method was used in the pharmaceutical development to establish a stable formulation of fragrance mix. A formulation with beta-cyclodextrin and hydroxypropyl cellulose had the best stability of the formulations tested.

Key words:

Patch test - Fragrance mix - Gas chromatography - Beta-cyclodextrin - Stability

Introduction

Many parameters secure accuracy and reliability of a patch test, such as an equal and correct concentration from batch to batch, a good stability of the allergen, an optimal release of the allergen form the patch. These parameters are controlled by standardized production, sufficient quality control and a relevant stability program.

The fragrance mix is one of 12 allergens in the standard panel 1 of the TRUE Test. The mix consists of eight perfumes: geraniol, cinnamaldehyde, hydroxycitronellal, cinnamyl alcohol, eugenol, isoeugenol, alfa-amyl cinnamaldehyde and oak moss. All perfumes except for oak moss are chemically well-defined. Oak moss is an extract from a lichen and contains a great number of compounds [1].

All the perfumes have a volatile character and evaporate easily, therefore studies to find a formulation with good stability properties were necessary.

Materials and Methods

The fragrance mix was incorporated in different dry films:

1. Hydroxypropyl cellulose (Klucel GF)
2. Polyethylene glycol 600 (PEG 600) and hydroxypropyl cellulose
3. Polyvinylpyrrolidone (PVP 90)
4. Beta-cyclodextrin and hydroxypropyl cellulose

All films were printed on a polyester backing.

Gas chromatography was done with a Hewlett-Packard 5700 equipped with a split/splitless injector, a flame ionization detector (FID) and a Shimadzu Chromatopac CR3A integrator. We used a BP10 bonded phase column (12 m × 0.22 mm I.D.) from S.G.E, Australia. The chromatographic conditions were as follows: detector , 250 °C; injector, 250 °C; column, 110°–200 °C, 8 °C/min, 2 min at 200 °C; and carrier gas, helium. The gas flow parameters were: column, 1.3 ml/min; split, 33 ml/min; septum, 3 ml/min; and auxiliary, 27 ml/min. The chemicals used were ethanol, 99,5% and eugenol, reinst (Merck).

Sample and Standard Preparation

A patch, 9 × 9 mm, was transferred into a 3-ml injection flask and 1.0 ml ethanol was added. The flask was placed in an ultrasonic bath for 30 min. The sample solution was transferred to an Eppendorf tube and centrifugated for 2–3 min.

Standard solutions were prepared corresponding to 5, 10, 30, 60 and 80 μg of eugenol/ml ethanol.

Procedure

Standard and sample solutions, each 3 μl, were injected and the peak areas were integrated. The concentration of each perfume was calculated from a standard graph with the concentration of eugenol versus peak area. The value of oak moss was multiplied by a factor of 8 due to the low response for oak moss in relation to the other perfumes. The results are reported as the sum of the individual perfumes. Figure 1 shows a chromatogram of fragrance mix.

Results and Discussion

The stability of the fragrance mix in a pre-formulation with hydroxypropyl cellulose was found to be less than 2 weeks at 8 °C. This is either due to the relatively high vapour pressure of the perfumes or chemical degradation. Accordingly the perfumes ought to be stabilized. Three different types of formulations were tested under accelerated conditions in a stability study.

The vapour pressure of volatile substances can be decreased by the addition of an inert compound with high vapour pressure, i.e. polyethylene glycol. A formulation with polyethylene glycol 600 was tested.

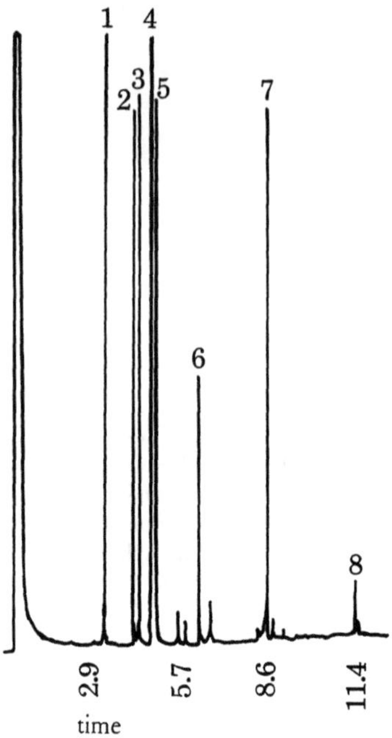

Fig. 1. Chromatogram of fragrance mix. *1*, geraniol; *2*, cinnamaldehyde; *3*, hydroxicitronellall; *4*, cinnamyl alcohol; *5*, eugenol; *6*, isoeugenol; *7*, α-amyl cinnamaldehyde; *8*, oak moss

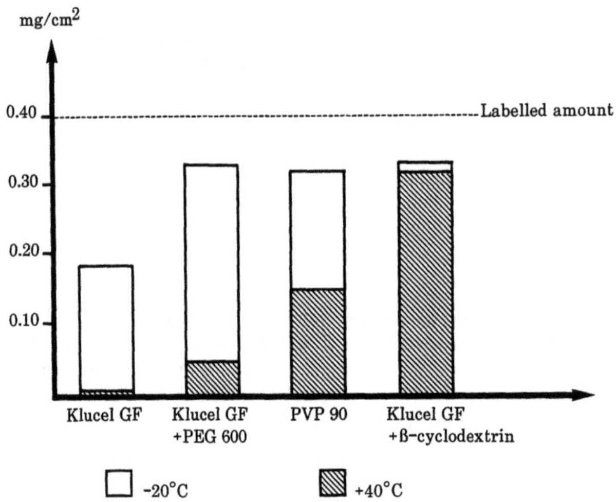

Fig. 2. Stability of different formulations at 1 month

Another way to stabilize the perfumes is by complex binding. One formulation with polyvinylpyrrolidone, which acts both as film- and complex-forming agent, and one with beta-cyclodextrin was evaluated. Beta-cyclodextrin is a cyclic, non-reducing oligosaccaride built up from seven glycopyranose units. The cyclodextrin molecule acts as a "host" molecule and forms an inclusion complex with the "guest" molecule. Only physical forces are involved in the complex formation, i.e. no covalent bonding [2].

The formulation with beta-cyclodextrin and hydroxypropyl cellulose was more stable than the other formulations (Fig. 2).

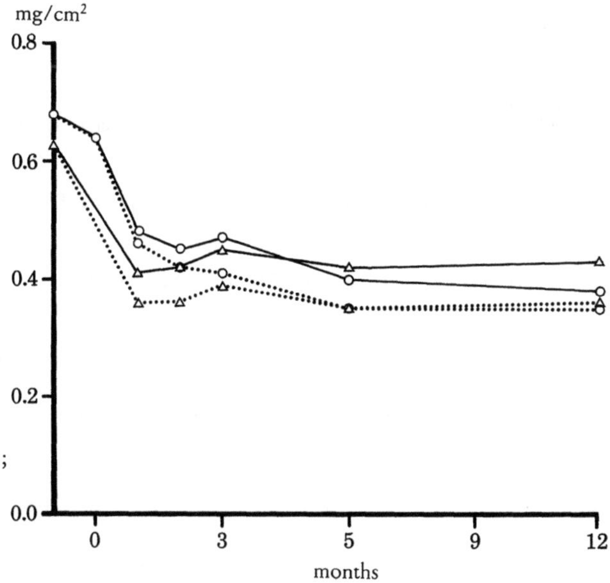

Fig. 3. Stability of fragrance mix. *Vertical axis,* amount mg/cm^2; *horizontal axis,* months *(n)*;
—O—, MM 81087, +8 °C;
···O···, MM 81087, +25 °C;
—△—, NB 81551, +8 °C;
···△···, NB 81551, +25 °C

The chosen formulation was tested clinically by using a serial dilution technique on patients sensitive to perfumes. A concentration of 0.6 mg/cm^2 was found to be the dose of choice.

A stability program was started on patches with the established concentration, including both research and production batches. They were stored at three temperatures: +8 °C, +25 °C and +40 °C. Samples were analyzed after 1, 2, 3, 6, 12, 18 and 24 months. Patches stored at +40 °C were analyzed up to 6 months. In Fig. 3 the stability of two batches at +8 °C and +25 °C is illustrated. Figure 3 shows an initial decrease in concentration but after about 1 month the concentration reaches a plateau on which it is stable for at least 18 months. The initial decrease in concentration is probably a result of an excess of perfumes in relation to beta-cyclodextrin.

The chemical results have been verified by in vivo function tests, where sensitized patients have been tested with patches stored for 6 and 12 months, with positive results.

References

1. Heide R et al. (1975) Qualitative Analysis of the Odoriferous Fraction of Oakmoss (Evernia prunastri (L) Ach). J Agric Food Chem 23: 950–957
2. Szejtli J (1982) Cyclodextrins and their inclusion complexes. Akadémiai Kiado, Budapest

Addresses

A.-M. Svensson
Pharmacia LEO Therapeutics AB, S-751 82 Uppsala, Sweden

S. Enström
Pharmacia LEO Therapeutics AB, S-751 82 Uppsala, Sweden

L. Thurell
Pharmacia LEO Therapeutics AB, S-751 82 Uppsala, Sweden

H. Swanberg
Pharmacia LEO Therapeutics AB, S-751 82 Uppsala, Sweden

β-Cyclodextrin Formaldehyde Complex in Patch Testing of Formaldehyde Contact Allergy

S. Albrechtsen, J. Hansen, and K. Hedegaard

Summary

The aim of this work was to introduce a formaldehyde patch to the Pharmacia TRUE Test panel for testing for formaldehyde contact allergy. The work was complicated by the volatile character of formaldehyde. Therefore, we synthesized a complex between β-cyclodextrin and formaldehyde. The ability of the complex to release formaldehyde in a manner similar to standard methods used in the clinic today was investigated. The in vitro release of formaldehyde from the complex as a function of pH showed an independent release between pH 4 and 7. Thus, the formaldehyde is released from the patch by the transdermal sweat secretions. Furthermore, in vitro penetration studies through human warm separated epidermis showed a formaldehyde release and penetration from the complex similar to that with a 1% formaldehyde solution. In vivo experiments performed on formaldehyde-sensitized guinea pigs using the guinea pig maximimazation test method confirmed the results. Over a 29-week period at different temperatures, the complex showed a satisfactory stability.

Key words:

Formaldehyde - Patch testing - TRUE Test - β-Cyclodextrin formaldehyde complex

Introduction

The standard method for patch testing in the clinic today is the Finn chamber or related systems. Pharmacia has developed the TRUE Test system consisting of allergens incorporated into a solid dry matrix. Although 23 allergens have been incorporated into the test system, so far a patch containing formaldehyde has been impossible due to its volatile character.

To overcome this problem a complex between β-cyclodextrin and formaldehyde was synthesized. Its ability to release formaldehyde was investigated in different in vitro and in vivo models and compared with the standard methods used in the clinic today. In addition, the stability of the complex was evaluated over a 29-week period.

Materials and Methods

Quantitative Determination of Formaldehyde

Stability Determinations. The content of formaldehyde on the patches was determined using a colometric procedure. After extraction at 30 °C with 10.00 ml 0.1 *M* carbonate buffer (pH 9) for 30 min, a 200-μl sample was diluted with 1800 μl water; 2.00 ml reagent (ammonium acetate (15.4%), acetyl acetone 2×10^{-3}%, acetic acid 3×10^{-3}% in water) was added, and the solution was placed at 60 °C for 10 min. The absorption was determined at 412 nm against a reagent blank.

In Vitro Penetration Studies. The amount of formaldehyde penetrated was determined by the same method as described for the stability determinations, except for the extraction procedure.

Release of Formaldehyde as a Function of pH

The release of formaldehyde as a function of pH was investigated by the use of semicarbazide as a model protein. A 10^{-2} *M* solution of semicarbazide HCl in phosphate buffer (0.05 *M*) was prepared. The pH was adjusted to different values ranging from 4 to 7. β-Cyclodextrin formaldehyde complex was added in concentrations of approximately 2×10^{-4} *M*. The binding of formaldehyde to semicarbazide was determined spectrophotometrically at 235 nm against a reagent blank.

In Vitro Penetration Studies

Human skin was obtained by surgical excision of excess skin from either the abdomen or the mammae. The epidermis was warm separated from the dermis in physiological saline at 60 °C for 1 min, and mounted in static diffusion cells. The epidermal membrane was exposed to ambient laboratory conditions, while the lower half contained water thermostated at 30 °C. Aliquots were taken from the receptor medium in a scheduled manner. Quantitation of the penetrated formaldehyde was determined as described.

Guinea Pig Maximization Test (GPM Test)

The GPM test was performed as described by Magnusson and Kligmann [1] and Andersen et al. [2] who evaluated the optimum formaldehyde concentrations to be used for sensitization. The intradermal injections were performed with 0.3% (v/v) formaldehyde. Topical induction was with 10% (v/v) formaldehyde solution and challenge with a formaldehyde solution in a Finn chamber corresponding to 0.78 mg/cm^2. The β-cyclodextrin formaldehyde complex was tested in two concentrations, namely 0.3 and 1.0 mg/cm^2 with respect to formaldehyde in a dried in hydroxypropylcellulose vehicle. The challenge response was read 48 and 72 h after application of the test substances.

Results

The formation of a complex between formaldehyde and β-cyclodextrin results in a 2:1 (molar ratio) complex. The release of formaldehyde from this complex as a function of pH showed that in the pH range between 4 and 7 the release was pH-independent.

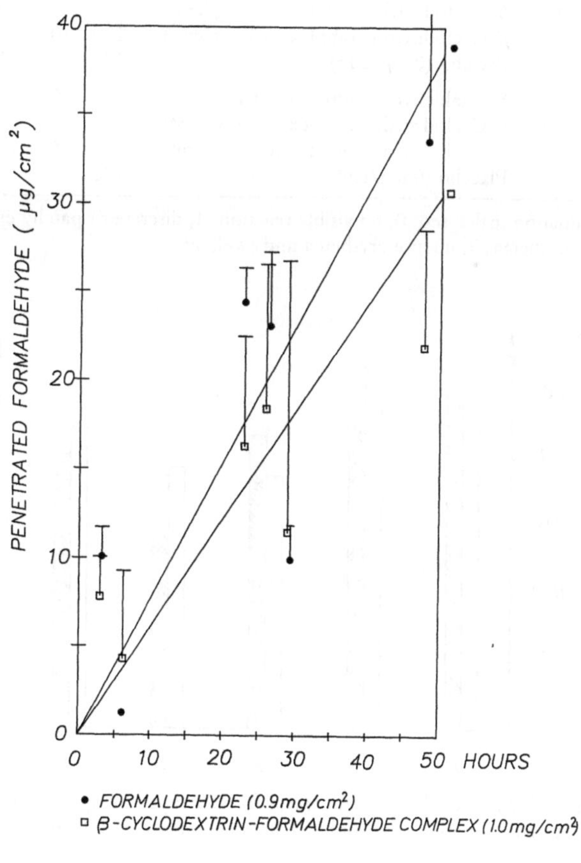

Fig. 1. In vitro penetration of formaldehyde through human epidermis from β-cyclodextrin formaldehyde complex (1.0 mg/cm^2) and formaldehyde solutions (0.9 mg/cm^2). Values indicate mean plus standard deviation. Regression lines are placed by eye

The in vitro studies showed that the release and penetration of formaldehyde from the complex was in the same order of magnitude as the penetration of formaldehyde from a 1% formaldehyde solution in a Finn chamber (Fig. 1).

The in vivo penetration and release of formaldehyde from the complex was investigated in guinea pigs sensitized to formaldehyde by the GPM-test method. In the experiments the animals were challenged with two concentrations of β-cyclodextrin formaldehyde, namely 0.3 and 1.0 mg/cm^2 with respect to formaldehyde. The challenge response 24 and 48 h after removal of the challenge patches was identical for the two concentrations tested as for the control vehicle, 1% formaldehyde in a Finn chamber (Table 1).

Table 1. Challenge response 48 and 72 h after application of β-cyclodextrin formaldehyde complex and formaldehyde solution in guinea pigs sensitized to formaldehyde (GPM test)

Application		Postapplication reading							
		48-h response (% of total)				72-h response (% of total)			
		0	1	2	3	0	1	2	3
Control	Formaldehyde solution (0.78 mg/cm^2)	90	10	0	0	60	40	0	0
($n=10$)	β-Cyclodextrin complex (1.0 mg/cm^2)	70	30	0	0	70	20	10	0
	β-Cyclodextrin complex (0.3 mg/cm^2)	100	0	0	0	70	30	0	0
	Placebo (0 mg/cm^2)	100	0	0	0	100	0	0	0
Test	Formaldehyde solution (0.78 mg/cm^2)	0	0	0	100	0	0	0	100
($n=20$)	β-Cyclodextrin complex (1.0 mg/cm^2)	0	10	16	74	0	5	0	95
	β-Cyclodextrin complex (0.3 mg/cm^2)	0	16	10	74	0	0	0	100
	Placebo (0 mg/cm^2)	100	0	0	0	100	0	0	0

Evaluation scale used: 0, no visible reaction; 1, discrete or patchy erythema; 2, moderate or confluent erythema; 3, intense erythema and swelling

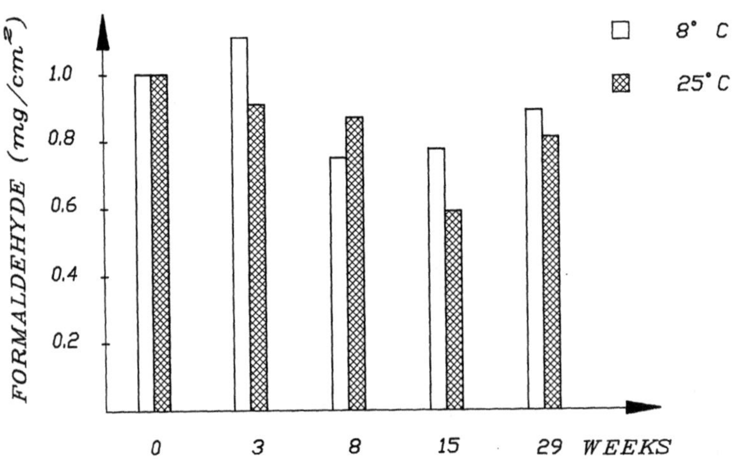

Fig. 2. Stability of the β-cyclodextrin formaldehyde complex as a function of time. The complexes are stored in light- and air-tight packaging material at 8 °C and 25 °C

The stability of the complex was evaluated by storing the patches under different temperatures in light- and air-tight packaging material. For temperatures up to 25 °C the stability was acceptable for a period up to 29 weeks (Fig. 2).

Conclusion

The β-cyclodextrin formaldehyde complex is a useful concept in patch testing of formaldehyde contact allergy. Both in vitro and in vivo studies have shown that the release pattern is similar to standard methods used in the clinic today.

References

1. Magnusson B, Kligman AM (1969) The identification of contact allergens by animal assay. The guinea pig maximization test. J Invest Dermatol 52: 268–276
2. Andersen KE, Boman A, Vølund A, Wahlberg JE (1985) Induction of formaldehyde contact sensitivity: dose-response relationship in the guinea pig maximization test. Acta Derm Venereol (Stockh) 65: 472–478

Addresses

S. Albrechtsen
Pharmacia AS, Herredsvejen 2, DK-3400 Hillerød, Denmark

J. Hansen
Pharmacia AS, Herredsvejen 2, DK-3400 Hillerød, Denmark

K. Hedegaard
Pharmacia AS, Herredsvejen 2, DK-3400 Hillerød, Denmark

Nickel Bioavailability from Patch Tests: Comparison Between Nickel Sulphate and Nickel Chloride Using TRUE Test

K. Kalimo, and K. Lammintausta

Summary

The development of local allergic skin reactions in nickel-sensitive individuals was examined with the TRUE Test, using various application times and different test concentrations of nickel sulphate and nickel chloride. The positive reactions seen with standard nickel sulphate concentration in the TRUE Test were comparable with those seen with the Finn chamber method. For both tests 48-h occlusion was needed for the optimal result. Three times higher nickel sulphate concentrations did not improve the results. Nickel chloride in the new vehicle of the TRUE Test penetrated the skin more effectively to trigger the immune system, since positive results comparable to the above-mentioned nickel sulphate tests were seen already after 3–6 h patch application when the actual nickel concentrations were comparable.

Key words:

TRUE Test - Finn chamber test - Nickel sulphate - Nickel chloride

Introduction

Under normal circumstances 48-h occlusion time is needed for adequate absorption of allergens for the widely used standard patch tests [6, 7]. Shorter application time would be more convenient for the patients and recently Bruze [1] showed that application time for nickel sulphate could be shorter if the allergen was diluted in water in fivefold concentration. Wahlberg [9] and Mendelow et al. [8] have studied various vehicles for patch testing and found considerable differencies between them. In this study we wanted to compare the standard Finn chamber method with the TRUE Test [6], using different nickel sulphate and nickel chloride concentrations and various application times to see whether these would allow shorter occlusion times.

Patients and Methods

A total of 51 patients with a history of nickel contact allergy and a previous positive nickel patch-test reaction participated. The patch testing was carried out using the TRUE Test (Pharmacia, Uppsala, Sweden) with nickel sulphate and nickel chloride. The nickel concentration in the patches was 0.043 (concentration also in standard TRUE) and 0.123 mg/cm^2. The tests were applied to the upper arms of the patients and removed after 1, 3, 6, and 12 h application. Nickel sulphate as in the standard TRUE was kept occluded also for 24 and 48 h. For one patient one concentration of both nickel sulphate and nickel chloride was tested with varying application times. For comparison a simultaneous test with 5% nickel sulphate in petrolatum (Chemotechnique Diagnostics, Malmö, Sweden) with Finn chamber (Epitest, Helsinki, Finland) with 48-h occlusion was carried out. The test reactions were recorded after 96 h and the reaction was considered positive if induration and/or papules and/or vesicles were present at the test site. Plain erythema and/or follicular reactions were registered separately.

Results and Discussion

It was evident that with the standard nickel sulphate concentration either in Finn chamber or in the TRUE Test, the number of positive reactions were reciprocal and dependent on occlusion time, as reported earlier [7]. Only 6/14 of the patients were

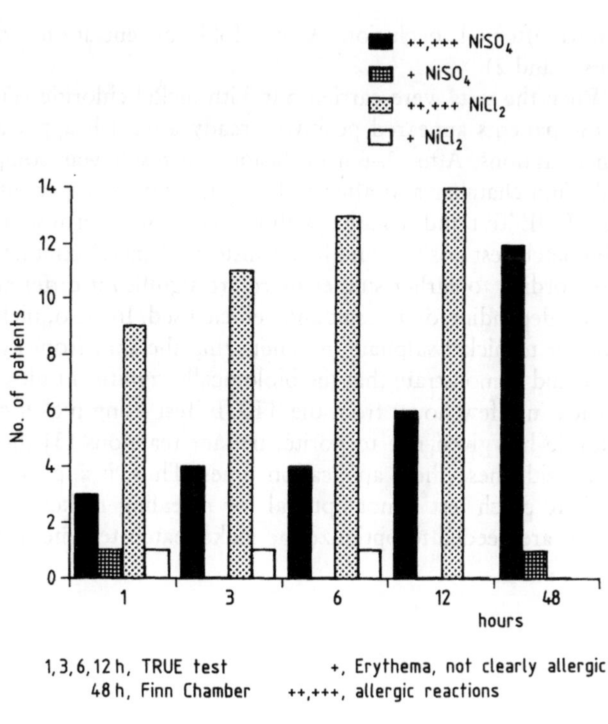

Fig. 1. The number of positive patch test reactions in 14 patients tested with standard concentration of nickel sulphate and nickel chloride with different application times

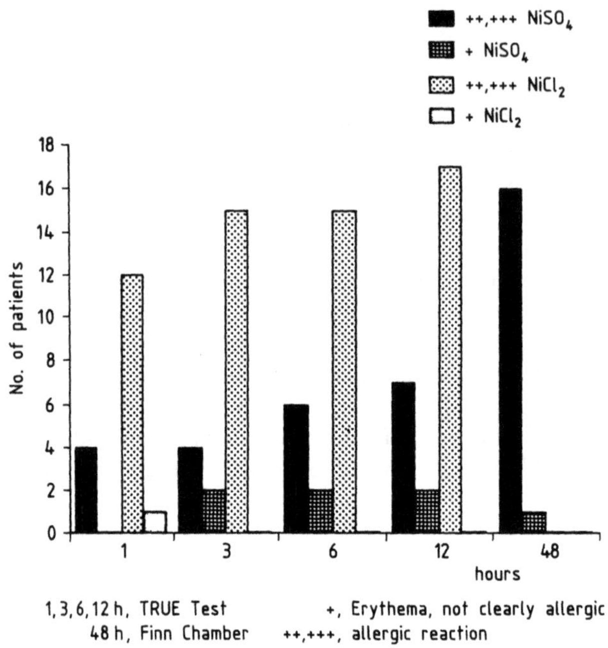

Fig. 2. The number of positive patch test reactions in 18 patients tested with threefold concentration of nickel sulphate and nickel chloride with different application times

positive after 6 h occlusion. A threefold concentration did not improve the result (Figs. 1 and 2).

When the tests were carried out with nickel chloride (Figs. 1 and 2) the majority of the patients appeared positive already after 1 h application time with both test concentrations. After 3–6 h occlusion the result was comparable to that obtained with Finn chamber and after 12 h application three patients appeared positive with the TRUE Test and negative with the Finn chamber test. These patients had earlier been patch-test positive and had a history of metal-contact allergy.

According to earlier studies there are significant differencies in nickel skin penetration depending on the salt and vehicle used. In vitro, nickel chloride has appeared superior to nickel sulphate in penetrating the skin from hydrophilic vehicles [4, 5]. We could demonstrate that the biologically significant nickel penetration took place already in a few hours from the TRUE Test using nickel chloride. Although nickel chloride has given rise to porite, irritant reactions [3] these were not seen in our study with these short application times. Thus, it appears that our standard nickel sulphate patch test is not optimal for revealing nickel contact allergy, but further studies are needed to optimize the nickel patch-test method.

References

1. Bruze M (1988) Patch testing with nickel sulphate under occlusion for 5 hours. Acta Derm Venereol (Stockh) 68: 361–364
2. Fischer TI, Maibach HI (1985) The thin layer rapid use epicutaneous test (True test), a new patch test method with high accuracy. Br J Dermatol 112: 63–68
3. Fischer T, Rystedt I (1985) False-positive, follicular and irritant patch test reactions to metal salts. Contact Dermatitis 12: 93–98
4. Fullerton A, Andersen JR, Hoelgaard A, Menne T (1986) Permeation of nickel salts through human skin in vitro. Contact Dermatitis 15: 173–177
5. Fullerton A, Andersen JR, Hoelgaard A (1988) Permeation of nickel through human skin in vitro effect of vehicles. Br J Dermatol 118: 509–516
6. Kalimo K, Lammintausta K (1984) 24 and 48 h allergen exposure in patch testing. Contact Dermatitis 10: 25–29
7. Kalimo K, Lammintausta K, Maki J, Teuho J, Jansen CT (1985) Nickel penetration in allergic individuals: bioavailability versus X-ray microanalysis detection. Contact Dermatitis 12: 255–257
8. Mendelow AY, Forsyth A, Florence T, Baille A (1985) Patch testing for nickel allergy. The influence of the vehicle on the response rate to topical nickel sulphate. Contact Dermatitis 3: 29–33
9. Wahlberg J (1980) Petrolatum – a realiable vehicle for metal allergens. Contact Dermatitis 6: 134–136

Addresses

K. Kalimo

Department of Dermatology, University of Turku, 20520 Turku, Finland

K. Lammintausta

Department of Dermatology, University of Turku, 20520 Turku, Finland

Subspecification of Allergens (Type I): Testing by Anionic/Cationic Iontophoresis in Humans

W. Remy, J. Rakoski, H.-U. Voigt, and O. Mielcke

Summary

Common inhalant allergens (commercial allergen extracts "Hollister-Stier") were applied to intact skin in atopic subjects with allergic rhinitis by percutaneous iontophoresis. The skin reactions were judged in comparison with the conventional skin-prick test. An allergic reaction of varying intensity was observed beneath the anode, the cathode, or both electrodes in all cases. Thus, using this method a further subspecification of allergies into anionic and cationic allergens is possible for individual patients. Furthermore, these results challenge the question of the molecular size of the allergens and/or the possible routes for their penetrant entry through the skin, e.g. "leaks" in the stratum corneum, and open discussion of whether atopic dermatitis might be a protein-contact dermatitis.

Key words:

Allergens, anionic - Allergens, cationic - Allergens, grass pollen - Iontophoresis - Skin absorption

Current concepts are in favour of application of drugs or test substances by transdermal delivery systems. The iontophoretic application of grass pollen allergens was evaluated again in this context [1].

Patients and Methods

Sixteen volunteer subjects were enrolled in the study. Twelve had allergic rhinitis, positive prick-test reactions to grass pollen allergens (wheal >50% of histamine control), and a positive RAST (>class 2). The four healthy volunteers without allergies served as controls (age 22 to 46 years; 8 men and 7 women).

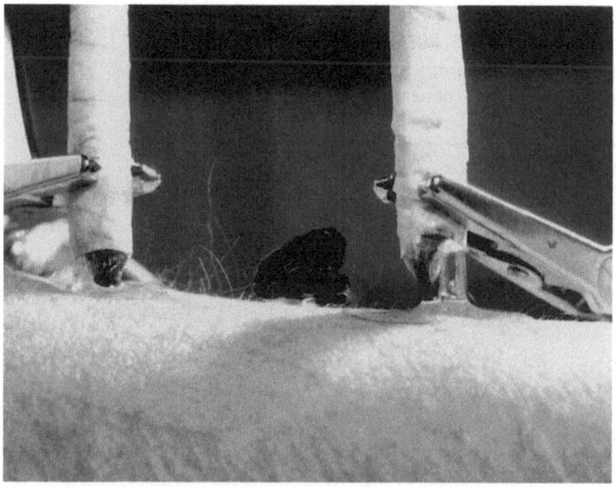

Fig. 1. Percutaneous iontophoresis of grass pollen allergens beneath the anode and the cathode simultaneously. Electric current is delivered by small graphite electrodes to the top of the drops

Twelve allergic and four healthy subjects underwent skin-prick tests with a grass pollen extract (Gräser IV, 2.20, pollen 1:20 G/V, Tropon). Skin-prick tests were performed in the usual way on the flexor surfaces of the forearms. Three additional sites were covered with a drop (about 0.05 ml) of these prick-test solutions. One drop was allowed to diffuse passively, while electric current delivered by small graphite electrodes was applied both anodically and cathodically to the top (no skin contact, Fig. 1) of the two other drops.

A constant amperage of 0.2 mA/drop (about 0.3 cm^2) for 10 min was applied by a device consisting of three batteries (3 × 9 V), regulated by a potentiometer.

Evaluation of the skin reactions was performed 10 min after iontophoresis, i. e. 20 min after application of the drops. The criterion was size of the wheal. Additionally, all 12 allergic subjects underwent testing skin-prick test with a pollen extract (for example, tree pollen), against which no sensitivity was expected.

Results

The skin reactions of the 12 allergic persons tested with skin-prick test and anodic and cathodic iontophoresis are shown in Table 1. It was possible in all cases to achieve penetration and absorption of the grass pollen extracts through intact skin by percutaneous iontophoresis. The intensity of reactions (skin-prick test, anodic or cathodic iontophoresis) differed in each patient (Table 1).

Table 1 shows furthermore that the allergic skin reactions produced by iontophoresis occurred nearly always under both electrodes. Passive diffusion of the pollen extract through intact skin led to no allergic reaction at all. The four nonallergic controls showed only a circumscribed erythema under both cathode and anode.

Table 1. Skin reactions (wheal in mm) to grass pollen allergens in 12 allergic subjects 20 min after testing with skin-prick test (pr) and percutaneous iontophoresis (pi), beneath the anode (a) and the cathode (c)

Patient	pr	pi	
		a	c
1	12	14	2
2	8	4	0
3	12	8	8
4	8	0	8
5	6	2	8
6	10	14	20
7	10	8	14
8	8	0	10
9	6	8	0
10	4	8	0
11	12	10	8
12	8	8	4

Discussion

We were able to show that the absorption of allergens occurs beneath the anode, the cathode, or both electrodes at the same time. Similar results were obtained studying other common/inhalant allergens (e.g. house dust, house dust mite, moulds, animal hair) [4]. Thus, this method improves the specificity of the allergens for the individual patient.

Furthermore, these results give rise to questions about the molecular size of the allergens and the possible routes for their penetrant entry through the skin, via the hair follicles, the sweat glands or across "leaks" in the stratum corneum. New insights into the structure of the stratum corneum and the anatomical basis of its barrier function make the percutaneous penetration and absorption of molecules of this size unlikely [3]. Grass pollen allergen extracts are today believed to form a mixture of heterogeneous proteins and glycoproteins with molecular weights of 11 000 and 31 000 Daltons [2]. These results invite discussion of whether atopic dermatitis might be a protein contact dermatitis [5]. If these molecules are able to cross the horny layer using iontophoresis this should be possible also by passive diffusion: iontophoresis only enhances their penetration through the stratum corneum.

References

1. Abramson HA (1941) Skin reactions. X. Preseasonal treatment of hay fever by electrophoresis of ragweed pollen extracts into the skin: preliminary report. J Allergy 12: 169–175
2. Cottam GP, Moran DM, Standring R (1986) Physicochemical and immunochemical character-

ization of allergenic proteins from rye-grass *(Lolium perenne)* pollen prepared by a rapid and efficient purification method. Biochem J 234: 305–310
3. Orfanos CE (1981) Aufbau der Hornschicht im Hinblick auf ihre Funktion. In: Klaschka F (eds) Stratum corneum. Struktur und Funktion. Grosse, Berlin, pp 29–30
4. Remy W, Rakoski J (1988) Testung von Allergenen (Typ I) mittels perkutaner Jontophorese beim Menschen. Akt Dermatol 14 (in press)
5. Seifert B, Seifert H-U, Wollemann G, Borelli S (1987) Neurodermitis – eine Proteinkontaktdermatitis? Dtsch Dermatol 32: 1200–1210

Addresses

W. Remy
Department of Dermatology, Faculty of Medicine, Technical University, Munich, FRG

J. Rakoski
Department of Dermatology, Faculty of Medicine, Technical University, Munich, FRG

H.-U. Voigt
Department of Dermatology, Faculty of Medicine, Technical University, Munich, FRG

O. Mielcke
Department of Dermatology, Faculty of Medicine, Technical University, Munich, FRG

Noninvasive Techniques

Assessment of Erythema: A Comparison Between the Naked Eye and Laser Doppler Flowmetry

J. E. Wahlberg

Summary

Erythema is an essential part of the contact reaction and can be quantified by laser Doppler flowmetry, which records skin blood flow. Healthy subjects were exposed to solvents and nicotinates for different periods of time and the skin test sites were then assessed by laser Doppler flowmetry as well as by the naked eye. It is concluded that the naked eye cannot detect erythema until the skin blood flow has increased three to four times.

Key words:

Solvents - Erythema - Naked eye assessment - Skin blood flow - Laser Doppler flowmetry

Skin exposure to solvents is a common cause of irritant contact dermatitis. An inverse correlation exists between the boiling point of a solvent and its primary irritant effect [2]. Assessment of the irritant potential of chemicals is usually undertaken through examination of the exposed skin sites and with the use of different scores for the degree of erythema, edema, papules, etc. However, the subjectivity of the traditional visual scoring system has been criticized [8], and more objective methods are desirable. In recent years laser Doppler flowmetry has been applied for quantitative assessments of the erythema.

The aim of the present study was to visually and objectively (laser Doppler flowmetry) assess the response after topical application of solvents to human skin.

Materials and Methods

Test substances were as follows: Solvents included 1,2-propylene glycol, trichloroethylene, and 1-1-1-trichloroethane. Trafuril, based on nicotinates, was used as a positive control.

Laser Doppler flowmetry [3–7], which records skin blood flow, is noninvasive, without hazards and can be used in man as well as in experimental animals. Before application of the test substance, a premarked test site was measured (preapplication value). The test site was then measured intermittently or continuously and the kinetics and the duration of an increase in blood flow recorded and documented. The apparatus (Periflux, Perimed, Stockholm, Sweden) and the new integrating probe have been described in previous papers [3–7].

A glass ring with an inner diameter of 20 mm was fastened with rubber bands to the volar forearm of healthy subjects. The solvents were administered in excess (1.5 ml) so that the entire test site (3.1 cm^2) was covered. After various periods of time (1–9 min) the remaining solvents were removed with cotton and the test sites dabbed. They were examined for whitening [1] and erythema by independent observers. The recording started 1–7 min after removal of the solvents.

Results

The output signal from the laser Doppler flowmeter is expressed in relative and dimensionless blood flow values (BFV) [3].

Figure 1 shows a comparison between propylene glycol and lin. Trafuril. Propylene glycol caused no erythema and no increase in skin blood flow, compared with the pretreatment values.

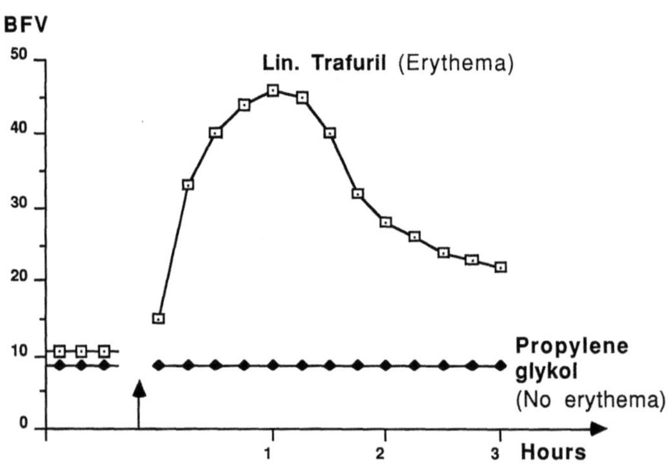

Fig. 1. Blood flow values (BFVs) after 5 min exposure to human volar forearms of lin. Trafuril (based on nicotinates; visible erythema) and propylene glycol (no erythema). Pretreatment BFVs are depicted to the left of the *arrow*

Figure 2 shows experiments with trichloroethylene, where the exposure time was varied. All exposures caused increase in blood flow compared with the preapplication values. Visual assessment demonstrated that the solvent caused an initial transient whitening [1], followed by erythema for the longer exposure times.

Figure 3 shows experiments with 1-1-1-trichloroethane, where the exposure time was varied. The recording started 1 or 7 min after removal of the solvent. The exposure caused increase in blood flow compared with the preapplication values. Slight erythema was observed at the test site exposed for 9 min.

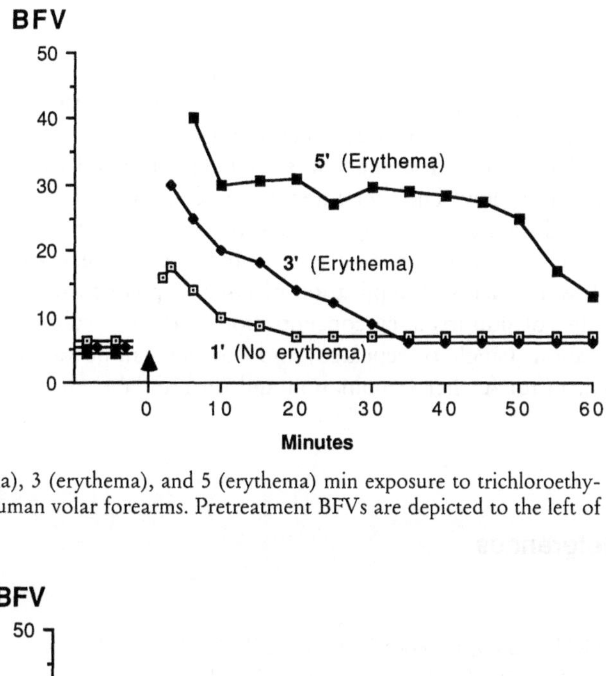

Fig. 2. BFVs after 1 (no erythema), 3 (erythema), and 5 (erythema) min exposure to trichloroethylene in excess (in glass ring) to human volar forearms. Pretreatment BFVs are depicted to the left of the *arrow*

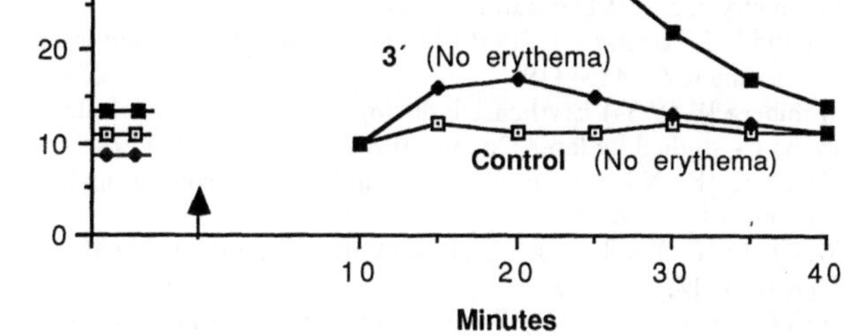

Fig. 3. BFVs after 3 (no erythema), and 9 (slight erythema) min exposure to 1,1,1-trichloroethane in excess (in glass ring) to human volar forearms. An unexposed control site (no erythema) is also shown. The recording started exactly at 10 min after application of the solvent. Pretreatment BFVs are depicted to the left of the *arrow*

Table 1. Laser Doppler flowmetry – fields of application

Predictive testing of irritancy:	Topical drugs, cosmetics, detergents, cleansing agents, products used in industry
Diagnostics:	Scleroderma, Raynaud's disease, patch-test reactions
Effects of drugs:	Vasodilators, minoxidil, sunscreens and UV, topical corticosteroids (blanching)
Skin physiology:	Regional variation

Discussion

It is demonstrated that skin blood flow, objectively assessed by laser Doppler flowmetry, must be raised three to four times until the naked eye can detect an erythema. Extended exposure times will give rise to erythema as well as an increase in skin blood flow. In no case was erythema observed without a corresponding rise in skin blood flow. The time interval between removal of solvent by dabbing with cotton and start of recording seems to be essential and it is suggested that the evaporation of any remaining solvent contributes to the decrease in blood flow values.

Possible fields of application of laser Doppler flowmetry are given in Table 1. In studies of skin irritancy concentration of the test substance, vehicle, number of applications (single or repeated) and skin site can be varied. The recorded curves can be kept for further examination and for interlaboratory comparisons [8].

References

1. Goldsmith LB, Friberg SE, Wahlberg JE (1988) The effect of solvent extraction on the lipids of the stratum corneum in relation to observed, immediate whitening of the skin. Contact Dermatitis 19: 348–350
2. Klauder JV, Brill FA (1947) Correlation of boiling ranges of some petroleum solvents with irritant action on skin. Arch Dermatol 56: 197–215
3. Nilsson GE, Otto U, Wahlberg JE (1982) Assessment of skin irritancy in man by laser Doppler flowmetry. Contact Dermatitis 8: 401–406
4. Salerud EG, Nilsson GE (1986) Integrating probe for tissue laser Doppler flowmeters. Med Biol Eng Comput 24: 415–419
5. Wahlberg JE (1984) Erythema-inducing effects of solvents following epicutaneous administration to man – studied by laser Doppler flowmetry. Scand J Work Environ Health 10: 159–162
6. Wahlberg JE, Nilsson GE (1984) Skin irritancy from propylene glycol. Acta Derm Venereol (Stockh) 64: 286–290
7. Wahlberg JE, Wahlberg ENG (1987) Quantification of skin blood flow at patch test sites. Contact Dermatitis 17: 229–233
8. Weil CS, Scala RA (1971) Study of intra- and interlaboratory variability in the results of rabbit eye and skin irritation tests. Toxicol Appl Pharmacol 19: 276–360

Addresses

J. E. Wahlberg
Department of Occupational Dermatology, National Institute of Occupational Health and Karolinska Hospital, S-10401 Stockholm, Sweden

Effect of Nonvisible Damage on the Water-Holding Capacity of the Stratum Corneum, Utilizing the Plastic Occlusion Stress Test (POST)

E. Berardesca, and H. I. Maibach

Summary

Skin surface water loss (SSWL) was studied after plastic occlusion stress test (POST) in visually non-damaged skin treated with sodium laurylsulfate for 3 days. SSWL decay curves and decay constants show striking differences between control and treated areas. The total amount of water trapped within the corneum and released at the 1st min is reduced in the treated site despite the higher transepidermal water loss noticeable in the terminal part of the curve reflecting the damage of the water barrier in irritated skin. The data suggest that clinically normal skin exposed to subliminal irritant stimuli is incapable of storing water within the stratum corneum, resulting in a decreased hydration.

Key words:

Sodium laurylsulfate - Nonvisible damage - Transepidermal water loss

Introduction

The water content of the stratum corneum is an equilibrium between the water reaching the horny layer from deeper tissues and the water evaporating at the skin surface in relation to the environmental relative humidity. The diffusion of water through the stratum corneum is a passive process, depending of the concentration gradient within the stratum corneum. The innermost horny layer is in equilibrium with the adjacent granular layer, while the outside cell layer, drier, is in equilibrium with the environment [1].

The water content of the stratum corneum can be monitored in vivo with several noninvasive techniques such as electrical measurements via skin impedance and resistance [2, 3]; microwave has been used in order to avoid the influences on the measures by ions or charges on the cell membranes [4]; photoacoustic methods are based on the recording of the photoacoustic signal arising in the tissue following pressure variations caused by periodic light radiation [5].

An indirect measure of the stratum corneum's water content can be achieved by means of transepidermal water loss (TEWL) assessment. Indeed, the greater the amount of water trapped within the stratum corneum, the higher is the evaporation rate at the surface [6]. Hydration achieved by occlusion results in an increased TEWL when the occluding film is removed [6] and until the water trapped within the stratum corneum evaporates and the corneum water content reaches the equilibrium with the environment. Skin surface water loss (SSWL) represents the evaporation of water from skin surface after occlusion. When all the excess water present in the corneum after occlusion has evaporated, SSWL equals TEWL. This technique can be utilized to quantitate the skin's water-holding capabilities and gives an indirect measurement of the in vivo water content.

The purpose of this study was to assess, in vivo, noninvasively, the effects of nonclinically detectable irritation induced by a surfactant on the water-holding capability of the stratum corneum. We utilize plastic occlusion stress test (POST) to discriminate subtle functional changes not previously discerned.

Materials and Methods

Six healthy white males entered the study (age range 29 ± 5 years). Once a day for 3 days consecutively 7% sodium laurylsulfate in distilled water was applied (open application) on the left forearm (0.03 ml/cm^2). The solution was allowed to dry without washing. On the 4th day, a 1-inch diameter plastic occlusive device (Hill Top chamber, Hill Top, Cincinnati, OH) was applied for 24 h both on the treated skin and on the adjacent control site. After removal, the skin surface water loss decay was recorded continuously on both sites with an evaporimeter (Servomed Ep-1, Servomed, Stockholm, Sweden). Skin temperature was recorded during the experiment with a telethermometer (Yellow Spring Instruments, CO, USA). The SSWL values were corrected and adjusted to the skin temperature of 30 °C [7]. The decay constants for each subject were calculated according to Wagner [8]. Statistical analysis was performed by means of the Wilcoxon rank test.

Results

Visible dermatitis was not discerned in any subject.

The SSWL decay with time reveals an exponential curve. When the values are transformed in log base 10, a linear relationship between SSWL decay versus time revealed (Fig. 1).

The SSWL decay constants of the six subjects are shown in Table 1. The mean decay constant of the untreated site is −log.0.050 (standard deviation ±0.018),

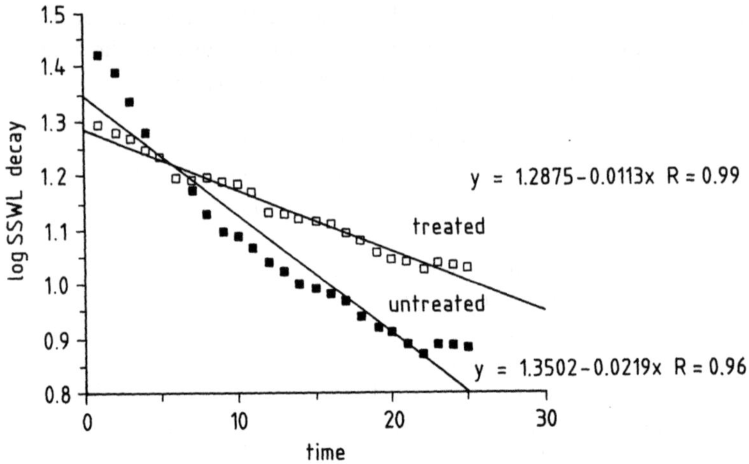

Fig. 1. Skin surface water loss decay in treated and untreated sites. Treatment was once daily application of 7% SLS *(open symbols)* for 3 days. Plastic occlusion was for 24 h. The decay values, transformed in log, show a linear pattern of decay vs time. Values at the 1st min are significantly different in the two groups ($P<0.05$)

Table 1. Skin surface water loss decay constants of treated and untreated sites; the mean decay constant is higher in untreated skin ($P<0.02$)

	Treated	Untreated
	−0.064	−0.067
	−0.012	−0.062
	−0.008	−0.058
	−0.029	−0.056
	−0.019	−0.021
	−0.022	−0.035
Mean ± SD	−0.026 ± 0.020	−0.050 ± 0.018

Table 2. Skin surface water loss values at 1st and 25th min in treated and untreated sites; the water content of the stratum corneum detected as skin surface water loss is significantly decreased in the treated site at the first min ($P<0.05$), but not at the 25th min

	1st min		25th min	
	Treated	Untreated	Treated	Untreated
	1.511	1.605	0.969	0.994
	1.298	1.392	1.162	0.757
	1.178	1.636	1.062	1.056
	1.377	1.406	0.991	0.758
	1.234	1.238	1.033	0.939
	1.166	1.261	0.969	0.791
Mean	1.29 ± 0.13	1.42 ± 0.16	1.03 ± 0.07	0.88 ± 0.13

while the treated is −log.0.026 (standard deviation ±0.020). The Wilcoxon signed-rank test for paired observations is statistically significant ($P<0.02$).

The linear regression in the untreated group is $y=1.3502–0.021$, with an r value of 0.96. The treated group has a y-intercept at 1.287 log SSWL and a slope of −0.011 with an r coefficient of 0.99. The treated site demonstrates a significantly decreased water content at the 1st min ($P<0.05$) as revealed by log SSWL (1.29±0.13) compared with the untreated (1.42±0.16). At the 25th min the water loss is higher in the treated site (1.03±0.07 vs 0.88±0.13). The difference is not significant.

Discussion

The plastic occlusion stress test (POST) was first utilized by Osmark et al. [9] to define the water-holding capacity of skin of the diaper area in infants. K. Roskos et al. (unpublished data) noted that the technique discriminated between old and white skin. The current data adds further support for the value of the POST in defining stratum corneum function after chemical exposures not demonstrating overt inflammation.

Skin occlusion with plastic film (Saran Wrap) was demonstrated to increase the water content (WC) of the stratum corneum and the transepidermal water loss (TEWL) [10]. This reflects the hydration of the stratum corneum. TEWL has a three fold increase within 24 h, but, when occlusion lasts several days, TEWL values dropped compared with the first day. Water content shows similar changes, but increases proportionally with prologed occlusion. Increased water binding within the corneum may have occurred after several days of occlusion, resulting in decreased surface evaporation rate [10]. Moreover, the effect of in vivo occlusion on human stratum corneum hydration-dehydration in vitro has been studied by Anderson et al. in 1973 [11]. The study showed that plastic occlusion for either 6 days or 14 days resulted in a production of stratum corneum that contained an increased mass per cm^2 of surface area of dry tissue. Since the increased mass did not alter the number of cell layers and the horny layer thickness, it should be stressed that this increase associated with occlusion treatment likely represents an increase of water-soluble materials. Indeed, the study reveals an increase both of energetically bound water to water-soluble materials and not energetically bound water (it can assume the ice structure at low temperatures, since bound water does not freeze), physically restricted to desorption. Previous workers have demonstrated that the ability of the corneum to bind water is related to hygroscopic water-soluble substances present in the horny layer (natural moisturizing factors). Since water-soluble substances are retained within the corneum by a lipid-containing semipermeable membrane system which allows these substances to take up water by osmosis, solvent extraction and consequent lipid removal reduce the ability of the corneum to bind water [12].

Our study reveals different SSWL patterns in untreated and SLS-treated skin. Although clinically detectable irritation was not elicited in the subjects, and treated skin did not show increased roughness or scaling, the water-holding capability of the stratum corneum is decreased in the treated site as shown by SSWL values at the 1st min.

The increase of water content subsequent to occlusion is significantly higher in control skin (1.42 vs 1.29; $P<0.05$). This could be related to the damage of the water barrier (lipids and natural moisturizing factors) produced by surfactants. Blank and Shappirio [13] reported increased dryness and less flexibility of cornified epithelium after soaking in soap and detergent solutions. There are water-soluble substances which can be extractable from calluses or from intact cornified epithelium by water alone or by aqueous solutions of soap or synthetic detergents. Recently, Fulmer and Kramer [14] described the effect of a surfactant on stratum corneum lipids. Daily application of 4% aqueous solution of sodium dodecylsulfate revealed increased skin dryness, as detected with an electrical impedance technique, and changes in stratum corneum lipid composition. While the total amount of lipids was not altered, the free cholesterol to cholesterol ratio was increased and the distribution of ceramides and free fatty acids modified. These results are interpreted in terms of a perturbation of keratinization and an altered desquamation. Furthermore, treatment with surfactants reduced the corneum's intercellular cohesion, dissolving the intercellular cement materials by low surface tension and the electrostatic effect [15].

Despite the lower water content at the 1st min after the removal of the occlusive device, the SSWL decay constant is higher in the surfactant-treated site because, after approximately 5 min, the surfactant-induced increase of TEWL biases the decay curve; TEWL becomes the prevalent constituent of the skin evaporation detected with the instrument. The decay constants of the two curves are significantly different ($P<0.02$) and the mean values at the 25th min, when the total amount of water held with occlusion has evaporated and the values express only TEWL, are higher in the treated site, representing the damage induced by the surfactant on skin water barrier.

Surfactant-induced skin damage, such as increased roughness, scaling, and dryness has been usually described after several days of treatment with in vitro experiments; moreover, the changes induced by the treatment have always been related to altered clinical appearance. Our study reveals that surfactant-induced changes are present just after a few nonocclusive applications of the irritant, even though the skin appears visually normal from a clinical and subjective viewpoint. Furthermore, this simple in vivo technique, may give useful information not only on skin TEWL, but also on water content and on the kinetics of dehydration after occlusion (SSWL).

The POST appears to be a simple but facile, robust and sophisticated method, to document nonvisible but putatively biologically relevant information on stratum corneum function. We suspect that this will not only be of biological interest but of clinical relevance as well when the clinical correlates are defined.

References

1. Blank HI, Moloney J, Emslie AG, Simon I, Apt C (1984) The diffusion of water through the stratum corneum as a function of its water content. J Invest Dermatol 82: 188–194
2. Salter DC (1979) Quantifying skin disease and healing in vivo using electrical impedance mea-

surements. In: Rolfe P (ed) Non invasive physiological measurements. Academic Press, London, pp 21–64
3. Borroni G, Berardesca E, Bellosta M (1982) Evidence for regional variation in water content of the stratum corneum in senile skin: an electrophysiological assessment. It Gen Rev Dermatol 19: 91–95
4. Jacques SL, Maibach HI, Suskind C (1981) Water content in the stratum corneum measured by a focus microwave probe: normal and psoriatic. Bioeng Skin 3: 118–119
5. Simon I, Emslie AG, Apt CM, Blank HI, Anderson RR (1981) Determination in vivo of the water concentration profile in human stratum corneum by a photoacoustic method. In: Marks R, Payne P (eds) Bioengineering and the skin. MTP Press, Lancaster, pp 187–195
6. Rietschel RL (1978) A method to evaluate skin moisturizers in vivo. J Invest Dermatol 70: 152–155
7. Mathias T, Wilson D, Maibach H (1981) Transepidermal water loss as a function of skin surface temperature. J Invest Dermatol 77: 219–220
8. Wagner J (1975) Linear compartment models. In: Wagner J (ed) Fundamentals of clinical pharmacokinetics. Drug Intelligence Publications, Hamilton, Illinois
9. Osmark K, Wilson D, Maibach H (1980) In vivo transepidermal water loss and epidermal occlusive hydration in newborn infants: anatomical region variation. Acta Derm Venereol (Stockh) 60: 403–407
10. Faegermann J, Aly R, Wilson DR, Maibach HI (1983) Skin occlusion: effect on pytirosporum orbiculare, skin PCO_2, pH, transepidermal water loss and water content. Arch Dermatol Res 275: 383–387
11. Anderson RL, Cassidy JM, Hansen JR, Yelling W (1973) The effect of in vivo occlusion on human stratum corneum hydration-dehydration in vitro. J Invest Dermatol 61: 375–379
12. Middleton JD (1968) The mechanism of water binding in stratum corneum. Br J Dermatol 80: 437–450
13. Blank I, Shappirio EB (1955) The water content of the stratum corneum. J Invest Dermatol 25: 391–401
14. Fulmer AW, Kramer GJ (1986) Stratum corneum lipid abnormalities in surfactant induced dry scaly skin. J Invest Dermatol 86: 598–602
15. Takahashi M, Aizawa M, Miyazawa K, Machida Y (1987) Effects of surface active agents on stratum corneum cell cohesion. J Soc Cosmet Chem 38: 21–28

Addresses

E. Berardesca
Department of Dermatology, University of Pavia, Pavia, Italy

H. I. Maibach
Department of Dermatology, University of California Medical School, San Francisco, USA

Comparability and Reproducibility of Results of Water Vapor Loss Measurements: A Study of Four Evaporimeters

J. Pinnagoda, R. A. Tupker, P. J. Coenraads, and J. P. Nater

Summary

A study was made of the comparability and reproducibility of the results of measurements of water loss both in vitro and in vivo using four ServoMed Evaporimeters (three single probe and one double probe). The optimum time for recording, after the application of the probe, was also determined. An evaporation device with a constant level of water loss was constructed for in vitro studies. These measurements showed that there were systematic differences among the results of four of the five probes. The fifth probe was distinctly out of range. For all probes, the reproducibility of results was high. The actual measurements of water loss depend on a gradient of water vapour pressure that creates a loss. The manufacturer's recommended calibration procedure, however, is based only on adjustments for the standard specified humidities and zero water loss. A calibration procedure which is based on an actual standard constant water loss should, therefore, also be included. In vivo, transepidermal water loss (TEWL) measurements on the human forearm of one individual showed the same probe as before to be distinctly out of range. Due to intraindividual variations in TEWL, comparative studies should best be conducted in vitro. TEWL values reached a stable constant state by 45 s. This is the optimum time for recording.

Key words:

Evaporimeter - Comparability - Reproducibility - Calibration - Standardization

Introduction

The methods used in the measurement of transepidermal water loss (TEWL) have varied over the years. The noninvasive method based on the estimation of the water vapour pressure gradient immediately adjacent to the surface of the skin, developed by Nilsson [2] has now replaced the invasive and more complicated methods of the past [2]. However, studies on the performance and accuracy of this method and inter- and intraindividual variations are few [1, 3, 4]. Moreover, studies on the calibration and comparative studies of the results obtained using different evaporimeters are totally lacking.

This study was conducted using four different Evaporimeters, to determine their comparability and the reproducibility of their results in:

1. In vitro water loss measurements (through an artificial membrane) in a constant evaporation environment

2a. In vivo transepidermal water loss (TEWL) measurements on the human forearm skin

b. The optimum time for recording after the application of the probe to the skin

Materials and Methods

Four ServoMed Evaporimeters (ServoMed, Vallingby, Sweden), three single-probe instruments (A, B, C) and one double-probe instrument (D), were used. All five probes (A, B, C, D_1, D_2) were simultaneously calibrated for the standard specified humidities as recommended[1] immediately before this investigation.

In Vitro. The measurements were performed in a closed cabinet at a controlled air temperature of 25 °C and controlled relative humidity of 40%.

A device with a constant level of evaporative water loss was constructed. A 5-cm diameter Petri dish filled with 10 ml water was used as the source of water loss. "Op-site" (Smith and Nephew, Hull, UK), a commercially available polyetherurethane wound-covering membrane, was stretched over the dish. Water evaporation through this membrane is constant under the controlled ambient conditions.

A retort stand was adjusted such that when the probes were attached, a distance of 3 mm between the probe surface and the membrane was achieved. An impermeable plastic shield, placed within this gap, was used to zero the Evaporimeters. The shield was pulled away by means of an attached string and the water loss was continuously recorded for a period of 6 min. The electronic filter for damping fluctuations was not used. Five successive measurements per probe were recorded.

In Vivo. The measurements on the forearm of one individual were performed in an air-conditioned room at 20 °C, within a transparent measuring box, designed to

[1] Operation Handbook (1981) ServoMed, Sweden

serve as a draught shield. TEWL was measured on the surface of the skin, at one location only, using the five different clamped probes. Three successive measurements per probe were recorded. TEWL was continuously recorded for a period of 4 min. The electronic filters, 10 and 20 s, were used after 2.5 min of the start of the recording.

Results

In Vitro. The measured water loss values reached a stable constant state (Fig. 1) after about 2 min from the start. The results of four of the probes (A, C, D_1 and D_2) show that there are certain systematic differences between them. The mean value for the final measured water loss in g/m²h in a decreasing order of magnitude is 7.5 (D_1), 7.0 (D_2), 6.9 (C) and 6.4 (A). Probe B measured a much lower value (3.7 g/m²h). This difference was outside the permissible range (±15% or ±2 g/m²h), specified by the manufacturer. Until stabilization (2 min), standard deviations (S.D.s) of the mean decreased from about 0.8 to 0.2 g/m²h. After stabilization they remained below 0.2 g/m²h.

In Vivo. The results for the TEWL from the forearm are given in Fig. 2. The mean value for the final measured water loss in g/m²h in a decreasing order of magnitude is 7.7 (C), 6.7 (D_1), 6.0 (D_2) and 5.4 (A). Probe B again measured a much lower level of water loss (2.8 g/m²h). This difference is again greater than 2 g/m²h. In addition, probes A and C show a difference of greater than 2 g/m²h, between them. In

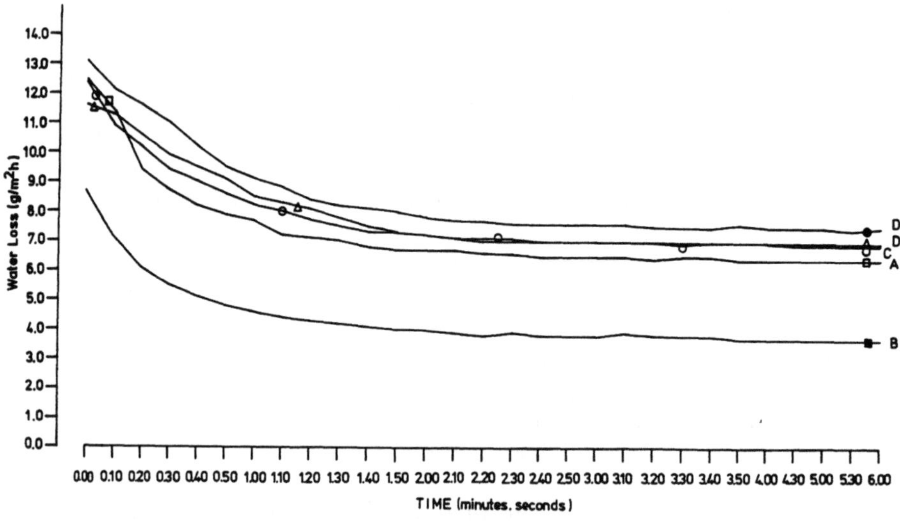

Fig. 1. The mean values of water loss (g/m²h) measured through a constantly evaporating artificial membrane with five different probes, in time. From the start of measuring until stabilization was reached (2 min), the SDs of the mean decreased from about 0.8 to 0.2 g/m²h. After stabilization they remained below 0.2 g/m²h. These SDs are too small to be represented graphically

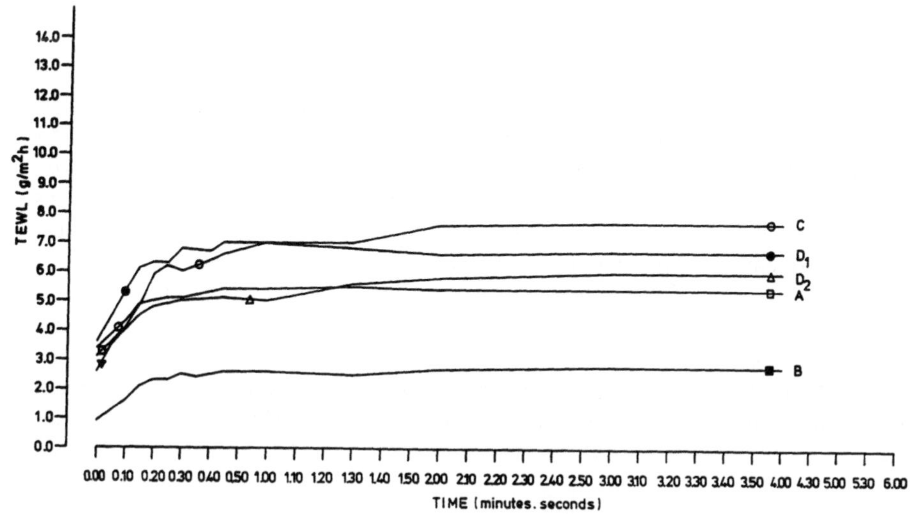

Fig. 2. The mean values of TEWL (g/m^2h) measured on the right forearm of one individual with five different probes, in time. From the start of measuring until stabilization was reached (45 s), the SDs of the mean decreased from about 0.4 to 0.2 g/m^2h. After stabilization they remained below 0.2 g/m^2h. For probes C and D_2, however, the SDs of the mean were somewhat different due to the fluctuations in TEWL. These SDs are too small to be represented graphically

contrast to in vitro, in vivo probe C measured at the highest level. This is due to sporadic fluctuations in TEWL.

The measured TEWL values reached a stable constant state after about 45 s from the start (Fig. 2). Until stabilization (45 s), the SDs of the mean decreased from about 0.4 to 0.2 g/m^2h. After stabilization it remained below 0.2 g/m^2h. For probes C and D_2, however, the SDs of the mean were somewhat different due to the fluctuations in TEWL.

Discussion

The in vitro measured water loss values are not always comparable among the instruments, although a constant level of water loss was measured in each case. Probe B records a much lower level than the other probes and beyond the permissible range. The small SDs of the mean values indicated the high reproducibility of the results for the individual Evaporimeters. In view of this, the manufacturer's stated permissible range becomes questionable. The differences arise only between the Evaporimeters and must be due to the limitations of the instruments. During calibration, one circuit is calibrated for humidity and the other is then adjusted until zero water loss is indicated.[1] This does not imply that the measured water loss values, us-

[1] Operation Handbook (1981) ServoMed, Sweden

ing different instruments, are always comparable. To enable successful and reliable interlaboratory comparison of results, it is recommended that an additional calibration procedure, to incorporate calibration for a measured water loss, be adopted. To this end, some form of a water evaporation device similar to the one used in our study should be agreed upon and a range of water loss values, measured at a standard height above the membrane, be specified as "standard". The water loss as measured by the evaporimeters may thus be checked and adjusted as required against this standard. The incorporation of a gain switch on the evaporimeters, or the sensitivity adjustment on all pen recorders, may be used to make such adjustments possible. TEWL, even in a single individual, varies in time due to sporadic fluctuations as result of intraindividual variations. Thus, comparability and reproducibility of results should be studied in vitro.

Stabilization of TEWL was reached between 30–45 s for all probes. The optimum time for recording, after the application of the probe to the skin, appears to be 45 s.

References

1. Blichmann CW, Serup J (1987) Reproducibility and variability of transepidermal water loss measurement. Acta Derm Venereol (Stockh) 67: 206–210
2. Nilsson GE (1977) Measurement of water exchange through skin. Med Biol Eng Comput 15: 209–218
3. Nilsson GE (1977) On the measurement of evaporative water loss. Methods and clinical applications. Linkoping University Medical Dissertation no 48, Linkoping, Sweden
4. Wheldon AE, Monteith JL (1980) Performance of a skin evaporimeter. Med Biol Eng Comp 18: 201–205

Addresses

J. Pinnagoda
Occupational Dermatology Unit, State University Hospital, Groningen, The Netherlands

R. A. Tupker
Occupational Dermatology Unit, State University Hospital, Groningen, The Netherlands

P. J. Coenraads
Occupational Dermatology Unit, State University Hospital, Groningen, The Netherlands

J. P. Nater
Occupational Dermatology Unit, State University Hospital, Groningen, The Netherlands

Nickel Content of Human Fingernails as a Measure of Occupational Exposure to Nickel

K. Peters, B. Gammelgaard, and T. Menné

Summary

The nickel concentration in the fingernails increases significantly with increasing exposure to nickel in the environment. It is proposed that this can serve as an objective measure of the degree of a patient's occupational exposure to nickel.

Key words:

Nickel exposure - Fingernails

Introduction

It is a common problem in occupational dermatology to decide whether or not a patient with an allergic nickel eczema has been exposed to nickel at his place of work. In many cases it is necessary to investigate the plant for possible exposure.

We studied the nickel concentration of the fingernails to determine whether this could serve as a useful and reliable indicator of occupational exposure to nickel.

Materials and Methods

The nickel concentration of the fingernails was determined using adsorbtion differential pulse voltammetry (ADPV), as described by Gammelgaard et al. [1], in three groups of persons representing different degrees of occupational exposure to nickel. **Group 0** ($n=95$) consisted of persons who were supposed not to be exposed to nickel (e.g. office workers, nurses, students, etc.). **Group 1** ($n=83$) consisted of persons who were moderately exposed to nickel in assembling nickel-plated components of locks and electrical switches. **Group 2** ($n = 51$) consisted of persons heavily exposed to nickel at their work in electroplating factories.

Results

The mean values and medians of the nickel concentration for the different grades of exposure were: **Group 0** (not exposed), $\bar{x} = 1.19 \pm 1.61$ ppm, $\tilde{x} = 0.49 \pm 0.13$ ppm; **Group 1** (assembling), $\bar{x} = 29.2 \pm 56.7$ ppm, $\tilde{x} = 13.8 \pm 5.6$ ppm; **Group 2** (electroplating), $\bar{x} = 123.5 \pm 288.8$ ppm, $\tilde{x} = 29.9 \pm 18.0$ ppm. The differences are statistically significant, $P\,0.001$ for mean values (Mann-Whitney rank sum test) and $P\,0.05$ for medians (median test).

The cumulative frequency distribution (Fig. 1) shows that 68% of the observations from the group of persons not exposed (group 0) are contained in the interval 0–1 ppm, whereas this is the case for only 1.2% of exposed persons. All observations from persons not exposed (group 0) are smaller than 8 ppm. This is true also for 35% of the group of moderately exposed persons (group 1) and for only 16% of the group of heavily exposed persons (group 2).

Discussion

The trial shows a significant increase of the nickel concentration in the fingernails in relation to exposure. Therefore, the nickel content of fingernail-clippings is a suitable measure of occupational nickel exposure.

The analysis of our data leads to the following conclusions, which may become of practical importance:

1. If the nickel content in the fingernails of a patient is less than 1 ppm, it is highly improbable that the patient is exposed to nickel.

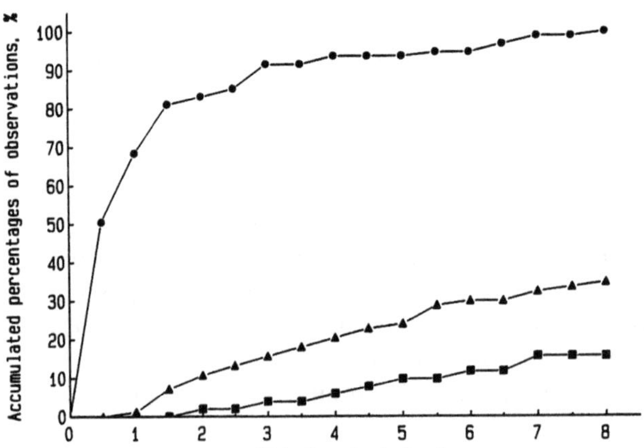

Fig. 1

2. At nickel contents greater than 8 ppm, it is highly probable that the patient is exposed to nickel.
3. With a nickel content between 1 and 8 ppm further investigations (e.g. inspection of the plant) are recommended. The probability of nickel exposure increases with increasing nickel content of the nails.

We believe that the use of this method will prove considerably more convenient than tests of nickel concentration in hair, blood, or urine [1, 2]. The test is inexpensive, easy to perform for the doctor and without any discomfort to the patient. In most cases use of this method would make it unnecessary to visit the plant.

References

1. Gammelgaard B, Andersen JR (1985) Determination of nickel in human nails by adsorption differential pulse voltammetry. Analyst 110: 1197–1199
2. Spruit D, Bongaarts PJM (1977) Nickel content of plasma, urine and hair in contact dermatitis. Dermatologica 154: 291–300
3. Peters K, Gammelgaard B, Menné T (1988) Nikkelindholdet i negle som indikator for erhvervsmæssig nikkelbelastning (With English summary). Arbejdsmiljøfondet, Copenhagen

Addresses

K. Peters
Department of Dermatology, KAS Gentofte, Copenhagen, Denmark

B. Gammelgaard
Royal Danish School of Pharmacy, Copenhagen, Denmark

T. Menné
Department of Dermatology, KAS Gentofte, Copenhagen, Denmark

In Vitro Diagnosis

Impact of 25 Years of In Vitro Testing in Allergic Contact Dermatitis

B. M. E. von Blomberg-van der Flier, D. P. Bruynzeel, and R. J. Scheper

Key words:

Allergic contact dermatitis - Lymphocytes - Lymphokines

Introduction

In allergic contact dermatitis (ACD), in vitro tests for T-cell immunity, based either on lymphocyte transformation or on lymphokine production, have now been performed for more than 20 years. In the beginning these tests were simply used as "black boxes", providing convenient in vitro parameters for ACD. During the past decade, all essential steps in the process of in vitro T-cell activation have been largely unravelled. Molecular requirements for efficient allergen presentation and T-cell triggering, as well as relevant culture conditions are now well defined.

The aim of this review is to evaluate in how far this tremendous increase in fundamental knowledge has contributed to the clinical applicability of in vitro tests in diagnosing ACD. For this purpose we listed published reports on in vitro tests in ACD and analyzed the relationship between diagnostic relevance of these in vitro studies and the year of performance, the technique and the allergen employed. In addition, we supplement our conclusions with results from an inquiry, held during the first European Contact Dermatitis Society meeting (Heidelberg, 1988) to record current dermatologists' opinion with regard to the clinical applicability of in vitro assays in diagnosing ACD.

Inventarization of In Vitro Tests in ACD

In Table 1, 25 years of diagnostic in vitro testing in ACD have been enumerated chronologically. All studies aiming at in vitro testing as a diagnostic tool have been included. The diagnostic value was evaluated by scoring the sensitivity and specificity of the test (for diagnosing patch-test reactivity), the capacity of a test to differentiate between patch-test positive patients and negative controls and, finally, the authors' opinion as to the clinical applicability of the test (for details see the legend to Table 1).

From Table 1 it is clear that positive reports have been published consistently since 1967. Neither the absolute numbers, nor the percentage of clinically applicable tests has increased during this period.

As to the assays used, the lymphocyte transformation test (LTT) has been performed most frequently, until 1972 by evaluating percentages of blastoid cells and since 1973 by measuring thymidine uptake. Both ways of evaluating lymphocyte transformation generally correlate well and have therefore been combined for the diagnostic scoring in Table 1. Lymphokine production was evaluated mostly with the leucocyte migration inhibition test (LMIT), i.e. by simultaneous assessment of both production and effect of LIF (leucocyte migration inhibition factor) in a buffy coat suspension. When lymphocyte transformation and lymphokine production were assessed in parallel, the LTT was generally more sensitive and the lymphokine assays more specific [14, 26, 61, 63]. Both LTT and lymphokine assays could be used diagnostically.

As to the allergens tested, clinically applicable tests have been recorded for a broad range of water-soluble and insoluble allergens. Surprisingly only a minority of the standard test battery allergens (ICDRG) have been employed in vitro. Positive in vitro responses were generally obtained by using non-toxic concentrations of free hapten in the cultures. Highly toxic allergens (urushiol, DNCB) have been successfully used after being conjugated to cells [10, 26, 32] or to soluble proteins [13]. In the leucocyte migration inhibition test also relatively non-toxic allergens, like nickel and chromium had to be conjugated beforehand [35, 56, 58]. Apparently, for each allergen as well as for each in vitro assay optimal stimulatory conditions have to be determined, thereby limiting routine clinical application of these tests.

Inquiry Results

In order to challenge our literature-based conclusions concerning the diagnostic value of in vitro tests in ACD, this survey was completed with an inquiry, held among 250 participants of the Heidelberg meeting in 1988. The majority of the 74 inquiry-responders had no experience with in vitro testing (Table 2), because they were insufficiently acquainted with such tests (41%) or considered these tests too laborious (32%), not yet reliable (7%) or unnecessary (25%). In Table 3 the in vitro experience of inquiry-responders has been specified. In vitro tests usually served research purposes; the LTT was the most frequently used assay, metals and drugs the most frequently tested allergens. It is clear from Table 3 that there is no consensus in the

Table 1. Diagnostic in vitro tests in ACD

Author	Year	Allergen	LTT-bl	LTT-thy	LMIT	MMIT	Other	Sensitivity	Specificity	Sign	Conclusion as to clinical use
Aspegren	1962	Nickel	*					+++	–	–	–
Nordquist	1967	Neomycin			*			+++	+++	+	+
Hanifin	1970	Beryllium		*				+++	+++	+	
Schöpf	1970	Gold	*					+++	+++	nt	
MacLeod	1970	Nickel		*				+++	+++	+	
Pappas	1970	Nickel	*	*				+++	–	–	–
Lenz	1971	Chromium	*					+++	nt	nt	++
Lenz	1971	Cobalt	*					+++	nt	nt	++
Lenz	1971	Formalin	*					+++	nt	nt	++
Lenz	1971	Mercury	*					+++	nt	nt	++
Lenz	1971	Nickel	*					+++	nt	nt	++
Lenz	1971	PPDA	*					+++	nt	nt	++
Lenz	1971	Procain	*					+++	nt	nt	++
Lischka	1971	Chromium	*					+	+++	+	–
Szilágyi	1971	Tuliposide		*				+++	+++	+	++
Forman	1972	Nickel				*		+	+++	nt	±
Forman	1972	Nickel	*	*				+++	+	+	±
Henderson	1972	Beryllium				*		+++	+++	nt	++
Hutchinson	1972	Nickel		*				++	+++	+	
Levene	1972	DNCB		*				+	+++	nt	
Thulin	1972	Chromium #			*			+++	+++	+	+
Yamada	1972	Chromium	*					++	++	+	–
Yamada	1972	Cobalt	*					+++	+++	nt	±
Yamada	1972	Formalin	*					–	nt	nt	–
Yamada	1972	Iodine	*					+++	+	nt	–
Yamada	1972	Mercury	*					+++	–	–	–
Yamada	1972	PPDA	*					+++	+	–	–
Yamada	1972	Urushiol	*					++	–	nt	–
Miller	1973	DNCB #		*				+++	+++	+	+
Millikan	1973	Nickel		*				+++	+++	+	+
Milner	1974	DNCB #		*				+++	++	+	±

Table 1. (continued)

Author	Year	Allergen	LTT-bl	LTT-thy	LMIT	MMIT	Other	Sensitivity	Specificity	Sign	Conclusion as to clinical use
Gimenez-Cam.	1975	Nickel		*				+++	+++	+	
Levis	1975	DNCB #		*				+++	nt	nt	
Levis	1975	DNCB #					*	+	nt	nt	
Mirza	1975	Nickel			*			+	+++	−	−
Mirza	1975	Nickel #			*			+++	++	+	+
Hamilton	1976	DNCB #			*			nt	nt	+	+
Jordan	1976	Nickel			*			+++	+++	+	+
Kim	1976	Nickel		*				+++	+++	+	±
Levis	1976	DNCB		*				+++	+++	+	
MacLeod	1976a	Nickel					*	++	+++	+	
MacLeod	1976b	Nickel			*			nt	nt	−	−
Nishioka	1976	DNCB #				*		+++	+++	+	±
Soeberg	1976	DNCB #		*				nt	+++	+	
Soeberg	1976	NDMA #		*				nt	nt	+	
Tio	1976	Chromium #			*			+++	+++	+	++
Thulin	1976	Nickel			*			+	+	−	−
Thulin	1976	Nickel #			*			++	++	+	−
Goering	1977	Div.		*				++	+++	+	
Goering	1977	DNCB		*				+++	nt	+	
Goering	1977	NDMA		*				+++	nt	nt	
Swoboda	1977	Nickel			*			+++	+++	+	+
Svejgaard	1978	Nickel		*				+++	+++	+	+
Adam	1979	Chloramf.	*					+++	nt	nt	+
Byers	1979	Urushiol #		*				++	+++	nt	
Dupuis	1979	Urushiol #		*				++	++	+	±
Veien	1979	Nickel		*				+++	++	+	
Silvennoinen	1980	Nickel		*				+++	++	+	+
Al-Tawil	1981	Nickel		*				+++	++	+	++
Nakano	1981	DNFB			*			++	+++	nt	
Oehling	1981	Chromium	*					−	+++	−	−
Oehling	1981	Nickel	*					−	+++	−	−

MacLeod	1982	Nickel					*	+ +	+ +	−	
MacLeod	1982	Nickel		*				+ +	+ +	−	
Rytter	1982	Chromium			*			+ + +	+ + +	+	+ +
Williams	1982 a	Beryllium		*				+ + +	nt	nt	+
Williams	1982 b	Beryllium				*		+ +	+ + +	+	−
Williams	1982 b	Beryllium		*				+ + +	+ + +	+	+ +
Al-Tawil	1983	Chromium		*				+ + +	+ + +	+	+ +
Nordlind	1983	Chromium			*			+ +	+ + +	+	±
Nordlind	1983	Nickel			*			−	+ + +	−	−
Al-Tawil	1984	Cobalt		*				+ +	+ + +	+	+ +
Camarasa	1984	Mercury		*				+ + +	+ + +	+	
Nordlind	1984 a	Nickel		*				+ + +	+	+	±
Nordlind	1984 b	Nickel		*				+ + +	+ +	+	±
Silvennoinen	1984	Gold		*				+ + +	nt	nt	+ +
Aldridge	1985	Nickel					*	+ +	+ + +	+	+ +
Al-Tawil	1985	Nickel		*				+ + +	+ +	+	±
Bruynzeel	1985	Penicill.		*				+ +	nt	nt	
Stejskal	1986	Alprenolol	*	*				+ + +	+ + +	+	+
Stejskal	1986	Bacampic.	*	*				+ + +	+ + +	+	+
Stejskal	1986	Quinidin	*	*				+ + +	+ + +	+	+
Tjernlund	1987	Nickel					*	+ +	+ + +	nt	
von Blomberg	1987	Nickel				*		+	±		
von Blomberg	1987	Nickel		*				+ + +	+ +	+	±
Botham	1988	Nickel		*				+ + +	+ + +	+	+
Prens	1988	Nickel		*				+ + +	+ + +	+	+

Evaluation of diagnostic relevance:
Sensitivity (sens) of tests was defined as the percentage of patch-test positive, allergic patients showing a positive in vitro response. In vitro responses were considered positive when stimulation indices exceeded 2 (in LTT) or migration inhibition exceeded 20% (LMIT and MMIT). Specificity (spec) of tests was defined as the percentage of negative in vitro tests in healthy controls. Both sensitivity and specificity were graded as follows: <20%, −; 20%–50%, +; 50%–80%, + +; and, >80%, + + +. The difference between patch-test positive patients and negative controls (sign) was recorded as – if not significant, and as + if $P<0.05$ (significance only tested when more than four patients per group). The authors' conclusion as to clinical use of the test was graded as: not applicable, −; dubious applicability, ±; restricted applicability, +; and, applicability stressed, + +
LTT-bl, Lymphocyte transformation test, evaluated by counting the percentages of blastoid cells; LTT-thy, lymphocyte transformation test, evaluated by measuring thymidine uptake; LMIT, leukocyte migration inhibition test (1-phase-system: production and effect of lymphokine measured simultaneously); MMIT, macrophage migration inhibition test (2-phase-system: production and effect of lymphokine measured separately); #, allergen pre-conjugated to cells or proteins; nt, not tested, or not evaluable because too few people were examined

Table 2. Details of inquiry-responders

	n	% of responders
Questionnaires distributed	250	
Total number of responders	74	100
Dermatologists	67	91
Involved in diagnosing ACD	71	96
Experience with in vitro tests	30	41

Table 3. Specification of in vitro experience ($n = 30$)

Purpose:		*Frequency:*			
Research	25	Occasionally			24
Case reports	5	Regularly			3
Diagnostics	9	Frequently			3
Assays:		*Allergens:*			
LTT	29	Nickel	12	Drugs	14
LMIT	5	Chromium	2	PPD	2
MMIT	5	Cobalt	2	Urushiol	1
Other	1	Mercury	1	DNCB	2
		Metals	4		
In vitro results:		*Opinion as to clinical use:*			
Supporting skin test data	12				
Supplementing skin test data	7	Applicable			8
Varying	6	Restricted applicability			5
Erratic	6	Not applicable			10
Interesting	2	No opinion			7
Negative	1				

For in vitro test abbreviations see legend to Table 1

group of experienced inquiry-responders with respect to clinical applicability of in vitro tests. Remarkably, only a minority of them (33%) considered in vitro tests not clinically applicable. The opinion on clinical applicability of the tests was not obviously related to the allergens tested.

Conclusions

Clinical application of in vitro tests in ACD have been propagated consistently since 1967. In the early 1970s it was generally expected that increase in the fundamental knowledge on T-cell activation would facilitate the use of diagnostic in vitro assays [47]. Most remarkably, however, the extensive current knowledge on cellular and molecular requirements for allergen presentation and T-cell activation did not obviously contribute to either methodology or success-rate of diagnostic in vitro tests in ACD.

The inquiry supported our view that, despite a consistent number of positive reports appearing yearly, in vitro tests have never really found a place in routine diagnostic procedures. An important obstacle is the fact that in vitro tests are labor-intensive compared with in vivo skin testing. Moreover frequent erratic results, inherent to bioassays, limit the test reliability. Although convenient alternatives for measuring lymphocyte growth in vitro are now being developed [12, 43], routine clinical application of a bioassay is not to be expected in the near future. Nevertheless, in vitro tests will remain extremely valuable for investigations on pathogenetic mechanisms in ACD.

In conclusion, 25 years of in vitro studies in ACD have taught us to appreciate in vitro testing as a delicacy rather than as daily food.

References

1. Adam H (1979) Zum Nachweis der chloramphenicol-Sensibilisierung mit Hilfe des auf morphologischen Auswertungskriterien basierenden Lymphozyten-Transformations-Tests. Dermatol Monatschr 165: 270–273
2. Al-Tawil NG, Marcusson JA, Möller E (1981) Lymphocyte transformation tests in patients with nickel sensitivity: an aid to diagnosis. Acta Derm Venereol (Stockh) 61: 511–515
3. Al-Tawil NG, Marcusson JA, Möller E (1983) Lymphocyte stimulation by trivalent and hexavalent chromium compounds in patients with chromium sensitivity. Acta Derm Venereol (Stockh) 63: 296–303
4. Al-Tawil NG, Marcusson JA, Möller E (1984) In vitro testing for cobalt sensitivity: an aid to diagnosis. Acta Derm Venereol (Stockh) 64: 203–208
5. Al-Tawil NG, Berggren G, Emtestam L, Fransson J, Jernselius R, Marcusson JA (1985) Correlation between quantitative in vivo and in vitro responses in nickel-allergic patients. Acta Derm Venereol (Stockh) 65: 385–389
6. Aldridge RD, Milton JI, Thomson AW (1985) Leukocyte procoagulant activity as an in vitro index of nickel contact hypersensitivity. Int Arch Allergy Appl Immunol 76: 350–353
7. Aspegren N, Rorsman H (1962) Short-term culture of leucocytes in nickel hypersensitivity. Acta Derm Venereol (Stockh) 42: 412–417
8. Botham PA, Everness KM, Gawkrodger DJ, Hunter JAA (1988) In vitro antigen presentation in nickel-induced contact sensitivity. (This volume)
9. Bruynzeel DP, Von Blomberg-van der Flier M, Scheper RJ, Van Ketel G, De Haan P (1985) Penicillin allergy and the relevance of epicutaneous tests. Dermatologica 171: 429–434
10. Byers VS, Epstein WL, Castagnoli N, Baer H (1979) In vitro studies of poison oak immunity. I. In vitro reaction of human lymphocytes to urushiol. J Clin Invest 64: 1437–1448
11. Camarasa JG, Calderon PG (1984) Lymphocyte transformation test in allergic contact dermatitis by mercury. In: MacDonald DM (ed) Immunodermatology. Butterworths, London, pp 37–39
12. Dotsika EN, Sanderson CJ (1987) A fluorometric assay determining cell growth in lymphocyte proliferation and lymphokine assays. J Immunol Methods 105: 55–62
13. Dupuis G (1979) Studies on poison ivy. In vitro lymphocyte transformation by urushiol-protein conjugates. Br J Dermatol 101: 617–624
14. Forman L, Alexander S (1972) Nickel antibodies. Br J Dermatol 87: 320–326
15. Gimenez-Camarasa JM, Garcia-Calderon P, Asensio J, De Moragas JM (1975) Lymphocyte transformation test in allergic contact nickel dermatitis. Br J Dermatol 92: 9–15
16. Göring HD, Schwalm I, Agatha G, Schubert H (1977) Die Antigen-Testung mit gefrierkonservierten Lymphozyten im LTT und LMHT. Dermatol Monatschr 163: 217–219
17. Hamilton DNH, Ledger V, Diamandopoulos A (1976) In vitro monitoring of cell mediated immunity to dinitrochlorobenzene. Lancet, 27 Nov: 1170–1171
18. Hanifin JM, Epstein WL, Cline MJ (1970) In vitro studies of granulomatous hypersensitivity to beryllium. J Invest Dermatol 55: 284–288

19. Henderson WR, Fukuyama K, Epstein WL, Spitler LE (1972) In vitro demonstration of delayed hypersensitivity in patients with berylliosis. J Invest Dermatol 58: 5–8
20. Hutchinson F, Raffle EJ, MacLeod TM (1972) The specificity of lymphocyte transformation in vitro by nickel salts in nickel sensitive subjects. J Invest Dermatol 58: 362–365
21. Jordan WP, Dvorak J (1976) Leukocyte migration inhibition assay (LIF) in nickel contact dermatitis. Arch Dermatol 112: 1741–1744
22. Kim CW, Schopf E (1976) A comparative study of nickel hypersensitivity by the lymphocyte transformation test in atopic and non-atopic dermatitis. Arch Dermatol Res 257: 57–65
23. Lenz U, Witkowski R (1971) Der Lymphozytentransformationstest als Hilfsmittel des Nachweises einer Kontaktallergie. Dermatol Monatsch 157: 68–72
24. Levene GM (1972) Lymphocyte transformation in contact sensitivity. Trans St Johns Hosp Dermatol Soc 58: 147–152
25. Levis WR, Whalen JJ, Powell JA (1976) Specific blastogenesis and lymphokine production in DNCB-sensitive human leucocyte cultures stimulated with soluble and particulate DNP-containing antigens. Clin Exp Immunol 23: 481–490
26. Levis WR, Whalen JJ, Powell JA (1975) Studies on the contact sensitization of man with simple chemicals. III. Quantitative relationships between specific lymphocyte transformation, skin sensitivity and lymphokine activity in response to dinitrochlorobenzene. J Invest Dermatol 64: 100–104
27. Lischka G (1971) Lymphocytentransformationstest bei Chromatallergie. Arch Dermatol Forsch 240: 212–218
28. MacLeod TM, Hutchinson F, Raffle EJ (1970) The uptake of labelled thymidine by leucocytes of nickel sensitive patients. Br J Dermatol 82: 487–492
29. MacLeod TM, Hutchinson F, Raffle EJ (1976a) Leucocyte aggregation in subjects with nickel dermatitis. Clin Exp Immunol 26: 528–530
30. MacLeod TM, Hutchinson F, Raffle EJ (1976b) The leukocyte migration inhibition test in allergic nickel contact dermatitis. Br J Dermatol 94: 63–64
31. MacLeod TM, Hutchinson F, Raffle EJ (1982) In vitro studies on blastogenic lymphokine activity in nickel allergy. Acta Derm Venereol (Stockh) 62: 249–250
32. Miller AE, Levis WR (1973) Studies on the contact sensitization of man with simple chemicals I. Specific lymphocyte transformation in response to dinitrochlorobenzene sensitization. J Invest Dermatol 61: 261–269
33. Millikan LE, Conway F, Foote JE (1973) In vitro studies of contact hypersensitivity: lymphocyte transformation in nickel sensitivity. J Invest Dermatol 60: 88–90
34. Milner JE (1974) In vitro lymphocyte responses in contact hypersensitivity. IV. J Invest Dermatol 62: 591–594
35. Mirza AM, Perera MG, Maccia CA, Dziubynski OG, Bernstein IL (1975) Leukocyte migration inhibition in nickel dermatitis. Int Arch Allergy Appl Immunol 49: 782–788
36. Nakano Y, Nakano K, Hara I (1981) Induction of leucocyte migration inhibitory factor (LIF) by stimulation with free hapten and water-insoluble epoxy resin. Clin Exp Immunol 45: 419–426
37. Nishioka K (1976) Detection of human contact sensitivity to dinitrochlorobenzene by the migration inhibition test. J Invest Dermatol 66: 351–354
38. Nordlind K (1986b) Further studies on the lymphocyte transformation test in diagnosis of nickel allergy. Int Arch Allergy Appl Immunol 75: 333–336
39. Nordlind K (1984a) Lymphocyte transformation test in diagnosis of nickel allergy. Int Arch Appl Immunol 73: 151–154
40. Nordlind K, Sandberg G (1983) Leukocytes from patients allergic to chromium and nickel examined by the sealed capillary migration technique. Int Arch Allergy Appl Immunol 70: 30–33
41. Nordquist B, Rorsman H (1967) Leucocyte migration in vitro as an indicator of allergy in eczematous contact dermatitis. Trans St Johns Hosp Dermatol Soc 53: 154–159
42. Oehling A, Diéguez, Lobera T (1981) Clinical aspects and cellular immunity in contact dermatitis due to chrome and nickel. Allergol Immunopathol 9: 233–240
43. Potter CD, Gotch IF, Warner GT, Oestrup J (1987) Lymphocyte proliferation and cytotoxic assays using flat-bed scintillation counting. J Immunol Methods 105: 171–177
44. Pappas A, Orfanos CE, Bertram R (1970) Non-specific lymphocyte transformation in vitro by nickel acetate. J Invest Dermatol 55: 198–200
45. Prens EP, Benne K, Van Joost T, Benner R (1988) In vitro nickel specific lymphocyte proliferation: methodological aspects. (This volume)

46. Rytter M, Hausten U-F (1982) Hapten conjugation in the leucocyte migration inhibition test in allergic chromate eczema. Br J Dermatol 106: 161–168
47. Scheper RJ, Oort J (1973) Some in vitro experimental methods in allergic contact dermatitis. Archs Belg Dermatol 28: 59–71
48. Schöpf E, Wex O, Schulz KH (1970) Allergische Kontaktstomatitis mit spezifischer Lymphocytenstimulation durch Gold. Hautarzt 21: 422–425
49. Silvennoinen-Kassinen S, Jakkula H, Karvonen J (1986) Helper cells carry the specificity of nickel sensitivity reaction in vitro in humans. J Invest Dermatol 86: 18–20
50. Silvennoinen-Kassinen S (1980) Lymphocyte transformation in nickel allergy: amplification of T lymphocyte responses to nickel sulphate by macrophages in vitro. Scand J Immunol 12: 61–65
51. Soeberg B, Andersen V (1976) Hapten-specific lymphocyte transformation in humans sensitized with NDMA or DNCB. Clin Exp Immunol 25: 490–492
52. Stejskal VDM, Olin RG, Forsbeck M (1986) The lymphocyte transformation test for diagnosis of drug-induced occupational allergy. J Allergy Clin Immunol 77: 411–426
53. Svejgaard E, Morling N, Svejgaard A, Veien NK (1978) Lymphocyte transformation induced by nickel sulphate: an in vitro study of subjects with and without a positive nickel patch test. Acta Derm Venereol (Stockh) 58: 245–250
54. Swoboda B, Fritz J, Ludvan M (1977) Nickelallergie und Leukozyten-Migrations-Hemmung. Dermatol Monatschr 163: 208–212
55. Szilagyi I, Dobozy A, Hunyadi J, Simon N (1971) Lymphozyten-Transformations-Test bei der Untersuchung der durch Tulpen verursachten Überempfindlichkeit. Berufsdermatosen 19: 14–22
56. Thulin H (1976) The leukocyte migration test in nickel contact dermatitis. Acta Derm Venereol (Stockh) 56: 377–380
57. Thulin H, Zachariae H (1972) The leukocyte migration test in chromium sensitivity. J Invest Dermatol 58: 55–58
58. Tio D (1976) A study on the clinical application of a direct leukocyte migration test in chromium contact allergy. Br J Dermatol 94: 65–70
59. Tjernlund U, Scheynius A, Strand A (1987) In vitro testing of contact sensitivity. Acta Derm Venereol (Stockh) 67: 417–421
60. Veien NK, Svejgaard E, Menné (1979) In vitro lymphocyte transformation to nickel: a study of nickel sensitive patients before and after epicutaneous and oral challenge with nickel. Acta Derm Venereol (Stockh) 59: 447–451
61. Von Blomberg-van der Flier M, Van der Burg CKH, Pos O, Van de Plassche-Boers EM, Bruynzeel DP, Garotta G, Scheper RJ (1987) In vitro studies in nickel allergy: diagnostic value of a dual parameter analysis. J Invest Dermatol 88: 362–368
62. Williams WR, Williams WJ (1982a) Development of beryllium lymphocyte transformation tests in chronic beryllium disease. Int Arch Allergy Appl Immunol 67: 175–180
63. Williams WR, Williams WJ (1982b) Comparison of lymphocyte transformation and macrophage migration inhibition tests in the detection of beryllium sensitivity. J Clin Pathol 35: 684–687
64. Yamada M, Niwa Y, Fujimoto F, Yoshinaga H (1972) Lymphocyte transformation in allergic contact dermatitis. Jpn J Dermatol 82: 94–97

Addresses

B. M. E. von Blomberg-van der Flier
Pathological Institute, Free University Hospital, Amsterdam

D. P. Bruynzeel
Department of Dermatology, Free University Hospital, Amsterdam

R. J. Scheper
Pathological Institute, Free University Hospital, Amsterdam

In Vitro Nickel-Specific T-Lymphocyte Proliferation: Methodological Aspects*

E. P. Prens, K. Benne, T. van Joost, and R. Benner

Summary

The conditions necessary for optimal and reproducible test results in the nickel specific in vitro T-lymphocyte proliferation assay (NiPA) were studied. For this purpose peripheral blood mononuclear cells (PBMCs) of nickel-allergic subjects were isolated by density-gradient centrifugation and, when necessary, further separated into T cells and non-T cells. The influence of basic variables such as the number of cells per well, culture medium, serum-type and the type of culture dishes (round- or flat-bottomed) on the result of this assay, were investigated in parallel experiments. Furthermore, in this study enhancement of Ni-specific T-lymphocyte proliferation was attempted by the addition of epidermal cells from normal or patch-tested skin areas, recombinant IL-2 after antigen priming or pre-treatment of the cells with neuraminidase. Optimal and reproducible proliferation was obtained in cultures set up with 2×10^5 PBMCs or with purified T cells in the presence of $4–8 \times 10^4$ epidermal cells from patch-tested skin, using RPMI 1640 with HEPES and 15% pooled human AB serum in round-bottomed wells. Under the established optimal conditions the NiPA showed a 100% sensitivity and a specificity of 93%. Pre-treatment of PBMCs with neuraminidase and the addition of epidermal cells or rIL-2 after nickel priming enhanced the proliferative response in low-grade sensitized individuals.

Key words:

In vitro nickel-proliferation assay - Nickel-contact dermatitis

* This study was supported by the Praeventiefonds, The Netherlands

Introduction

In vitro proliferation assays for detection of contact or drug hypersensitivity have often been judged as not correlating enough with in vivo exposure or as being too variable and thus unreliable for clinical use [1]. In vitro demonstration of nickel hypersensitivity was performed for the first time 20 years ago and since then has been described in several papers [2]. The nickel specific T-lymphocyte proliferation assay (NiPA) and the macrophage or leucocyte migration inhibition assay are used mostly for this purpose [2].

In this study the requirements for optimal in vitro nickel-specific T-lymphocyte proliferation were studied. Furthermore, enhancement of NiPA was attempted. Determination of the optimal conditions in the NiPA may lead to a reliable and sensitive in vitro assay for detection of other contact allergens.

Patients, Materials, and Methods

Sixty patients in total (54 females, 6 males) with patch-test proven nickel contact hypersensitivity were enrolled in this study. All oral and topical medication was stopped 1 week before venipuncture for the in vitro NiPA. Thirty persons (25 females, 5 males) with no history of contact hypersensitivity to nickel served as controls.

Peripheral blood mononuclear cells (PBMCs) were isolated from heparinized blood using the Ficoll-metrizoate (density 1.077 g/ml) density gradient centrifugation method. T cells were purified by rosetting with AET-treated sheep red blood cells. Cultures were set up in quadruplicate using 0.5×10^5 to 3×10^5 PBMCs or T cells (in 0.2 ml). In initial experiments optimal nickel concentrations were established. All further assays were performed using nickel ($NiSO_4$) concentrations in the optimal range, i.e. 5, 7.5 and 10 µg/ml.

Epidermal-cell suspensions were prepared from epidermal sheets from suction blisters. Suction blisters were also made in patch-tested skin areas at different time intervals, i.e. after 8, 48 or 72 h. Langerhans cell containing epidermal-cell suspensions were used as antigen-presenting cells (APCs), in concentrations ranging from 10^4 to 10^5 per well.

Proliferation was measured by adding 0.5 µCi or 1.0 µCi ^{3}H-thymidine to each culture 8 or 16 h before harvesting. This was initially done on days 3, 5, 6, 7 and 8 of culture, to study the kinetics in the NiPA. The proliferation values (expressed in disintegrations per minute, DPMs) were used to calculate the stimulation index (SI = Ni proliferation/background proliferation) and the specific proliferation or "delta" proliferation (SP = Ni proliferation minus background proliferation).

In the NiPA the following culture media were tested: RPMI 1640, DMEM, and IMDM (with and without HEPES), all supplemented with fresh L-glutamine, antibiotics (complete medium) and either with foetal calf serum or pooled human AB serum. IMDM was also used as a serum-free culture medium.

Recombinant IL-2 (rIL-2; a kind gift from Dr J. Besemer, Sandoz Vienna) was added on day 7 to nickel-stimulated and unstimulated (control) cultures and proliferation was measured 8, 24 and 48 h later. The maximal proliferation obtained by addition of rIL-2 was compared with the maximal proliferation of non-rIL-2 stimulated cultures.

PBMC, APC and/or T cells were incubated for 30 min at 37 °C with 0.01 to 0.2 U/ml neuraminidase (Sigma Chemical, St. Louis, MO). The cells were washed three times before further processing.

The statistical significance was calculated using the Wilcoxon rank-sum test.

Results

Under optimal conditions, all nickel-allergic patients tested ($n = 60$) showed significant proliferation in the NiPA when PBMCs were used. In the control group ($n = 30$) six persons showed significant proliferation and four showed positive reactions to nickel when patch-tested. Ninety percent of the patients showed peak proliferation on day 7. Under the established optimal conditions the NiPA showed a 100% sensitivity and a specificity of 93%.

The number of PBMCs per well and the well type were critical in patients with low grade nickel sensitization. In these patients significant proliferation only occurred with at least 2×10^5 PBMCs per round-bottomed well (Fig. 1). The use of HEPES buffered culture medium appeared critical in large and complex experiments of long duration. In our experiments the use of HEPES buffered complete RPMI 1640 culture medium supplemented with 15% human AB serum resulted in low background and high specific proliferation. Foetal calf serum induced high background proliferation in most patients, while nickel-specific proliferation was not markedly enhanced. Under serum-free conditions poor proliferation values were obtained.

If epidermal cells were used as APCs, the response was markedly enhanced. Epidermal cells from in vivo nickel-exposed skin induced T-cell proliferation without

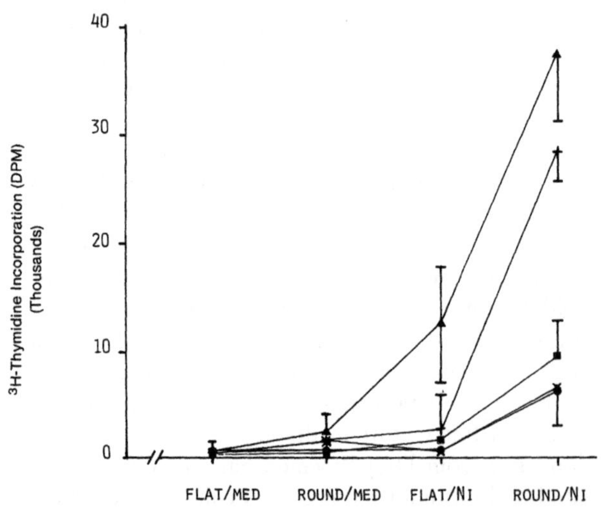

Fig. 1. Proliferative values obtained by culturing PBMCs of low grade nickel-sensitized patients in flat- and round-bottomed culture dishes

Table 1. The Effect of Addition of rIL-2 After Nickel Priming on 3H-Thymidine Incorporation

Patient	Patch test	PBMCs	PBMCs +IL-2	PBMCs +Ni	PBMCs +Ni+IL-2
CvD	+/++	1222±330	1394± 593	10220± 2360	22046± 7476
OV	+/++	959±117	6589±1815	3642± 1097	42497± 4357
CB	+/++	444±179	3681± 908	2325± 1272	20957± 6023
RT	++	609±200	1567± 373	2083± 112	6223± 1786
CM	++	1527±391	6580± 997	16146± 4940	20555± 6816
PP	++	573±281	4753±2215	6098± 2078	25062±12422
AS	+++	727±347	4601± 503	48612±10032	57223±14095
GK	+++	3714±683	3656±1235	58839± 8735	100913±17321
Controls					
WJ	neg.	2846±653	3486±1311	4313± 1721	4760± 2134
KI	neg.	656±378	3336±1188	955± 155	5572± 2539
JvD	neg.	1932±321	4494± 554	2636± 672	6260± 2552

Table 2. The Effect of Addition of rIL-2 After Nickel Priming on the Stimulation Index[a] and the Specific Proliferation[b]

Patient	Patch test	SI[a]-IL-2	SI+IL-2	SP[b]-IL-2	SP+IL-2
CvD	+/++	8.4	15.8	8998	20652
OV	+/++	3.8	6.4	2683	35908
CB	+/++	5.2	5.7	1881	17276
RT	++	3.4	4	1471	4656
CM	++	10.6	3.1	14619	13975
PP	++	10.6	5.3	5525	20309
AS	+++	66.9	12.4	47885	52622
GK	+++	15.8	27.6	55125	97257
Controls					
WJ	neg.	1.5	1.4	1467	1274
KI	neg.	1.5	1.7	299	2236
JvD	neg.	1.4	1.4	704	1766

further addition of nickel in vitro. This already occurred 8 h after nickel application to the skin; higher proliferation values were obtained with epidermal cells from day 3 positive patch tests.

Addition of rIL-2 to day 7 nickel-stimulated cultures resulted in higher specific proliferation values, especially in patients with low grade nickel allergy. The stimulation index was not dramatically increased due to higher background proliferation values induced by rIL-2 (Tables 1, 2).

Preincubation of PBMCs, APCs or T cells with neuraminidase enhanced the in vitro Ni-specific proliferative response by 30%–120%. The response to concanavalin A was also markedly enhanced. Background proliferation values of neuraminidase-treated control PBMCs, APCs or T cells were slightly higher.

Discussion

The great influence of the number of PBMCs on the proliferative response in the NiPA is not very remarkable. It is known that the log thymidine uptake is a linear function of the log cell dose [3]. From this one may conclude that either the number of nickel-specific T lymphocytes or the number of nickel-presenting cells in the circulation is limited. The ratio between these cells participating in the in vitro NiPA may also be of importance. This corresponds with our observation that the cell dose only forms a limiting factor in patients with low grade nickel hypersensitivity. Insufficient in vitro nickel-specific T-cell proliferation (i.e. a negative NiPA with $SI < 3$) due to a sub-optimal number of cells per well, can be overcome by the addition of exogenous rIL-2 (data not shown). At optimal cell concentrations addition of rIL-2 causes an enhancement of the proliferative response if expressed in specific or "delta" proliferation [4]. Since rIL-2 also causes increased background proliferation, the stimulation indexes are not increased after addition of rIL-2 (see Tables 1, 2).

The culture media and sera tested were found to have little effect on the sensitivity, but to have great influence on the signal-to-noise ratio in the NiPA. RPMI gives high specific proliferation and high stimulation indices. DMEM gives high specific proliferation but also high background proliferation and thus lower stimulation indices than RPMI. IMDM also gives high background proliferation, but this medium contains bovine serum albumin. Xenogeneic proteins (e.g. foetal calf serum or bovine serum albumin) are known to induce high background proliferation.

The use of round-bottomed wells is important because cell-to-cell contact (clustering) is facilitated in this type of well. The significance of cell to cell contact in antigen presentation has become clear recently. Adhesion molecules such as LFA-1a and -1b, ICAM-1, CD2 and LFA-3 are as important as the TcR, CD4, CD8 and HLA-DR [5]. The importance of LFA-3 and CD2 molecules appears from blocking experiments in the in vitro NiPa. Blocking with monoclonal anti LFA-3 (a kind gift of Dr T. Springer, Dana Farber, Boston), CD2 and anti HLA-DR antibodies resulted in almost comparable inhibition levels (data not shown).

Enhancement of the proliferative response in the NiPA by neuraminidase is also achieved by better cell-to-cell contact. Neuraminidase decreases cell-surface load, facilitating clustering between APCs and T lymphocytes. Furthermore, in animal experiments neuraminidase treatment has been shown to enhance MHC class II expression on APCs [6].

Certainly the most direct way to obtain strong in vitro responses to contact allergens is the use of epidermal cells as APCs. Epidermal cells have previously been shown to be potent APCs in the NiPA [7]. Also in our experiments epidermal cells consistently induced higher proliferation rates in the NiPA than did peripheral blood APCs, i.e. the T-cell depleted fraction of PBMCs. If epidermal cells from day 3 patch-test responses are used even higher proliferation rates are obtained, probably due to the presence of antigen-specific T cells in the epidermal-cell suspensions.

References

1. Baer RL (1986) The mechanism of allergic contact hypersensitivity. In: Fisher AA (ed) Contact dermatitis. Lea and Febiger, Philadelphia, pp 1–8
2. Von Blomberg vd Flier BME, Van den Burg CKH, Pos D, Van de Plassche-Boers EM, Bruynzeel DP, Garotta G, Scheper RJ (1987) In vitro studies in nickel allergy: diagnostic value of a dual parameter analysis. J Invest Dermatol 88: 362–368
3. Ross G, Dixon JB, Veevers A (1987) Variation in the lymphocyte transformation assay. Slope analysis of cell dose-response curves. J Immunol Methods 98: 189–193
4. Chain B, McCafferty I, Wallace G, Askenase Ph (1987) Improvement of the in vitro T cell proliferation assay by a modified method that separates the antigen recognition and IL-2 dependent steps. J Immunol Methods 99: 221–228
5. Springer TA, Dustin ML, Kishimoto TK, Marlin SD (1987) The lymphocyte function associated LFA-1, CD2 and LFA-3 molecules: cell adhesion receptors of the immune system. Annu Rev Immunol 5: 223–252
6. Boog CJP, Neefjes JJ, Boes J, Ploegh HL, Melief CJM (1988) Immune responses restored by alteration in carbohydrate chains of histocompatibility antigens on antigen presenting cells. In: Boog CJP (ed) Antigen presentation and restriction specificity in cytotoxic T lymphocyte responses. Thesis, University of Leiden, pp 71–79
7. Braathen LR (1980) Studies on human epidermal Langerhans cells. III. Induction of T lymphocyte response to nickel sulphate in sensitized individuals. Br J Dermatol 103: 517–526

Addresses

E. P. Prens

Departments of Dermatology and Immunology, University Hospital Rotterdam-Dijkzigt and Erasmus University, Rotterdam, The Netherlands

K. Benne

Departments of Dermatology and Immunology, University Hospital Rotterdam-Dijkzigt and Erasmus University, Rotterdam, The Netherlands

T. van Joost

Department of Dermatology, University Hospital Rotterdam-Dijkzigt and Erasmus University, Rotterdam, The Netherlands

R. Benner

Department of Dermatology, University Hospital Rotterdam-Dijkzigt and Erasmus University, Rotterdam, The Netherlands

The Role of MHC Class II Antigens in Mediating Accessory Cell Function In Vitro in Nickel-Induced Contact Sensitivity*

K. M. Everness, P. A. Botham, D. J. Gawkrodger, and J. A. A. Hunter

Summary

Mitogen- and antigen-driven T-cell proliferation is dependent upon the presence of MHC II$^+$ accessory cells. The ability of plastic-adherent blood cells and epidermal cells to act as accessory cells was assessed using a modified 6-day lymphocyte transformation test (LTT). Accessory cells from both the blood and epidermis of patients contact-sensitized to nickel were able to mediate antigen- (nickel sulphate) and mitogen-(concanavalin A) induced proliferation of purified autologous T cells. The requirements for MHC II molecules in accessory cell function were assessed by the addition of monoclonal antibodies to the LTT. Antibodies against HLA-DR markedly inhibited the antigen-specific response. In contrast, an antibody against HLA-DP only weakly inhibited cell proliferation and an antibody against HLA-DQ had no effect. These studies confirmed the importance of HLA-DR molecules in antigen-induced cell proliferation. Further work is needed to clarify the role of HLA-DP and HLA-DQ.

Key words:

MHC II antigens – Accessory cells – Nickel – Contact sensitivity

Introduction

In man a number of cell types, including macrophages [12], dendritic cells [15], epidermal cells [13], and B lymphocytes [1], have been shown to possess accessory cell function in vitro. Their functional capacity is dependent on the expression of cell-surface MHC class II antigens and the elaboration of interleukin-1 (IL-1).

* This work was supported by CASE studentship SERC

We have developed a lymphocyte transformation test (LTT) which discriminates reliably between individuals who are contact-sensitized to nickel and non-sensitized controls [7]. This method has been used to assess the accessory cell function of MHC class II antigen-bearing cells from both the blood and the epidermis in nickel-induced contact sensitivity, and to compare the role of three different MHC II molecules (HLA-DR, -DP, and -DQ) in mediating this process.

Materials and Methods

Subjects: Patients and Controls

Patients had positive allergic patch-test reactions against 5% $NiSO_4$ in petrolatum. Controls were volunteers who had no history of nickel-contact dermatitis.

Tissue Culture Medium

RPMI-1640, containing 100 µg ml^{-1} penicillin, 100 IU ml^{-1} streptomycin, 2×10^{-3} *M* L-glutamine and 2×10^{-5} *M* mercaptoethanol was used as tissue culture medium (TCM).

Preparation of Cell Populations

Peripheral blood mononuclear cells (PBMCs). PBMCs were obtained from the interface of heparinized blood centrifuged on lymphocyte separation medium.

Antigen-Presenting Cells (APCs): Plastic-Adherent Blood Cells. PBMCs were resuspended in TCM containing 15% autologous plasma (TCM-P) and incubated on plastic Petri dishes at 37 °C for 45 min. Non-adherent cells were removed using phosphate-buffered saline (PBS) and were the source of the enriched T-cell population (see below). Adherent cells were removed from the Petri dishes by gentle scraping, resuspended in TCM-P and irradiated (3000 rads).

Antigen-Presenting Cells (APCs): Epidermal Cells. Suction blisters were raised on the upper arms of volunteer patients and controls. Blister roofs were removed aseptically and placed in PBS containing 500 IU ml^{-1} penicillin, 500 µg ml^{-1} streptomycin, 250 µg ml^{-1} gentamycin and 12.5 µg ml^{-1} fungizone. A cell suspension was obtained by incubating the roofs with 0.3% trypsin for 45 min at 37 °C. Cells were then washed, resuspended in TCM-P and irradiated (3000 rads).

T-Cell Enrichment

Plastic non-adherent cells were incubated on a nylon wool column for 1 h at 37 °C, washed from the column, then incubated on glass for 2.5 h at 37 °C. The non-adherent cells were used as an enriched T-cell population.

Lymphocyte Transformation Test (LTT)

Stimulants used were 10 μg ml^{-1} con A and 5 μg ml^{-1} nickel sulphate ($NiSO_4.7H_2O$).

PBMCs (10^6 ml^{-1} in TCM-P) were placed in round-bottomed tissue culture plates (2×10^5 cells $well^{-1}$) and incubated at 37 °C in a humidified atmosphere containing 5% CO_2 for 6 or 7 days; 1 μCi ^{3}H-thymidine was added to the cells 18–20 h before they were harvested onto filter paper discs.

Radioactivity on the discs was assessed by liquid scintillation counting. Previous studies [7] had established that a stimulation index (SI = cells + stimulant cpm/cells alone cpm) ≥3 indicated nickel sensitivity.

Accessory Cell Function of Plastic-Adherent Blood Cells and Epidermal Cells

The 6-day LTT was carried out using PBMCs (10^6 ml^{-1}), T cells (10^6 ml^{-1}) and T cells + adherent cells (10^6 ml^{-1} T cells + 10^5 APCs) and T cells + epidermal cells (10^6 ml^{-1} T cells + $2–4 \times 10^5$ APCs).

Inhibition of LTT by Monoclonal Antibodies Against MHC II Molecules

The following monoclonal antibodies were used: DA6.231 (anti-HLA-DP, -DQ and -DR), L243 (anti-HLA-DR), B7/21 (anti-HLA-DP), Leu 10 (anti-HLA-DQ) and L368 (anti-beta-2-microglobulin). DA6.231 was a gift from Dr. K. Guy (MRC Cytogenetics Unit, Edinburgh) and L243 was a gift from Dr. S. Howie (University of Edinburgh). The remaining antibodies were purchased from Becton Dickinson. Cells were incubated with antibody for 1 h before adding mitogen (Con A) or antigen ($NiSO_4$) and carrying out a 6-day LTT, as described above.

Expression of MHC II Antigens by Cell Populations

To assess cell purity, expression of MHC II antigens was determined using the monoclonal antibody DA6.231 in a standard indirect immunofluorescence assay. The mean percentages of MHC II-positive cells were: 11% in PBMCs, <0.5% in nylon-wool purified T cells, 55% in plastic-adherent blood cells and 2% in epidermal cells.

Results

Accessory Cell Function of Plastic-Adherent Blood Cells

The ability of plastic-adherent blood cells to mediate mitogen- and antigen-induced T-cell proliferation was established in 18 experiments using cells from nickel-sensitive patients and in 16 experiments using cells from non-sensitized controls.

The SIs obtained using PBMCs, T cells alone and T cells reconstituted with plastic-adherent blood cells are shown in Table 1.

Stimulation of nylon-wool enriched T cells by Con A and/or $NiSO_4$ in five experiments (4, 10, 14, 17, 18) indicated that in these experiments the T cells were not fully enriched (i.e. the fraction contained some accessory cells).

Addition of 10^5 (10%) irradiated plastic-adherent blood cells to 10^6 T cells reconstituted or enhanced the T-cell response to Con A and $NiSO_4$ in 15/18 experiments using cells from nickel-sensitive patients and to Con A in 15/16 control experiments. There was no response by the control cells to 5 μg/ml $NiSO_4$.

Table 1. Stimulation indices obtained using 10 μg ml^{-1} Con A and 5 μg ml^{-1} nickel sulphate with PBMCs and nylon-wool enriched T cells with or without added plastic-adherent blood cells (Ads)

	10 μg/ml Con A			5 μg/ml $NiSO_4$		
	PBMCs	T	T + 10% Ads	PBMCs	T	T + 10% Ads
Patients						
1	6.0	1.2	3.6	4.1	N.T.	3.2
2	70.0	2.5	102.0	23.0	0.5	54.0
3	102.0	2.0	15.3	29.0	1.0	1.4
4	22.5	3.5	22.0	7.3	1.5	14.0
5	11.4	1.6	2.8	4.2	0.5	1.8
6	3.4	0.5	3.5	3.0	0.5	3.9
7	21.0	2.0	3.4	22.0	0.8	54.0
8	2.7	1.3	3.1	4.5	1.0	8.3
9	5.2	1.2	4.3	5.2	0.5	9.0
10	4.4	1.6	3.6	8.9	3.8	12.3
11	9.7	2.2	6.2	10.8	N.T.	16.6
12	3.3	1.3	2.1	3.2	N.T.	3.6
13	3.5	1.6	8.4	3.8	0.9	3.7
14	6.7	2.0	6.3	6.5	5.0	8.3
15	6.1	1.3	5.7	6.2	1.7	6.2
16	22.9	2.0	13.6	4.1	1.7	6.0
17	20.8	2.0	17.5	12.5	7.0	12.6
18	28.8	14.0	42.9	9.1	10.1	13.7
Controls						
A	88.0	1.3	9.6	1.0	N.T.	1.3
B	5.8	1.7	6.6	1.2	0.8	1.1
C	6.0	1.4	4.4	1.3	1.4	1.3
D	8.5	1.9	11.7	2.0	0.5	2.1
E	9.0	2.5	8.1	2.8	1.3	1.6
F	3.8	2.5	4.9	1.3	N.T.	1.1
G	7.4	1.4	5.4	2.7	N.T.	2.7
H	19.3	1.5	13.2	1.4	1.0	1.6
I	20.6	1.7	19.5	2.3	2.2	2.2
J	10.6	1.8	6.4	1.5	N.T.	1.1
K	76.0	1.1	9.1	1.0	0.8	0.7
L	5.6	1.6	9.4	0.9	N.T.	2.7
M	9.9	1.1	9.8	2.0	0.8	2.9
N	5.3	1.1	4.6	1.8	0.5	1.0
O	5.4	1.1	2.3	2.6	0.5	1.4
P	18.3	1.7	30.0	0.4	1.7	1.3

N.T., not tested

Using the paired *t*-test, SI differences for both unpurified PBMCs and for purified T cells, reconstituted with plastic-adherent blood cells and stimulated with either Con A or $NiSO_4$, were not significant.

Accessory-Cell Function of Epidermal Cells

Epidermal cells ($2–4 \times 10^5$) were added to 10^6 T cells in experiments using cells from five nickel-sensitive patients and from four controls. The SIs obtained are shown in Table 2. T cells from two of the patients (nos. 10, 18) were not fully enriched, but addition of epidermal cells did increase the responses of the T cells to both antigen and mitogen. Cells from the controls responded only to Con A. The addition of 4×10^5 (40%) epidermal cells to 10^6 T cells initiated the greatest proliferation against Con A; antigen-specific responses were similar when both 2×10^5 (20%) and 4×10^5 (40%) epidermal cells were used.

Role of MHC Class II Molecules In Accessory-Cell Function

The role of different MHC II molecules in accessory-cell function was assessed by adding to the LTT monoclonal antibodies against the class II molecules. Preliminary experiments had established that concentrations of antibody ≤ 260 ng ml^{-1} did not affect cellular proliferation non-specifically, for example by inducing cytotoxicity (data not shown). Antibodies L243 (anti-HLA-DR) and DA6.231 (anti-HLA-DR, -DP and -DQ) inhibited the antigen-specific proliferation of 10^6 T cells reconstituted with 10^5 (10%) plastic-adherent blood cells by $\geq 80\%$, using cells from five or six nickel-sensitive patients (Fig. 1). Inhibition of the response to Con A of the same cells was more variable, predominantly between 40% and 90%. Antibody B7/21 (anti-HLA-DP) caused some inhibition (32%–58%) of the nickel-induced response

Table 2. Stimulation indices obtained using 10 μg ml^{-1} Con A and 5 μg ml^{-1} nickel sulphate with PBMCs and T cells with or without added plastic-adherent blood cells (Ads) or epidermal cells (Eps)

	10 μg/ml Con A					5 μg/ml $NiSO_4$				
	PBMCs	T cells	T + 10% Ads	T + 20% Eps	T + 40% Eps	PBMCs	T cells	T + 10% Ads	T + 20% Eps	T + 40% Eps
Patients										
10	4.4	1.6	3.6	3.0	5.2	8.9	3.8	12.3	11.9	11.5
12	3.3	1.3	2.1	5.6	7.8	3.2	N.T.	3.6	5.6	6.5
13	3.5	1.6	8.4	22.7	28.3	3.8	0.9	3.7	5.9	6.9
14	6.1	1.3	5.7	23.8	29.3	6.2	1.7	6.2	12.0	11.0
18	28.8	14.0	42.9	72.2	102.0	9.1	10.1	13.7	23.0	28.4
Controls										
E	9.0	2.5	8.1	15.2	8.6	2.8	1.3	1.6	2.6	2.4
H	19.3	1.5	13.2	11.6	11.0	1.4	1.0	1.6	N.T.	1.5
M	9.9	1.1	9.8	14.4	28.3	2.0	0.8	2.3	1.8	2.8
P	18.3	1.7	30.0	42.2	72.5	0.4	1.7	1.3	1.0	0.5

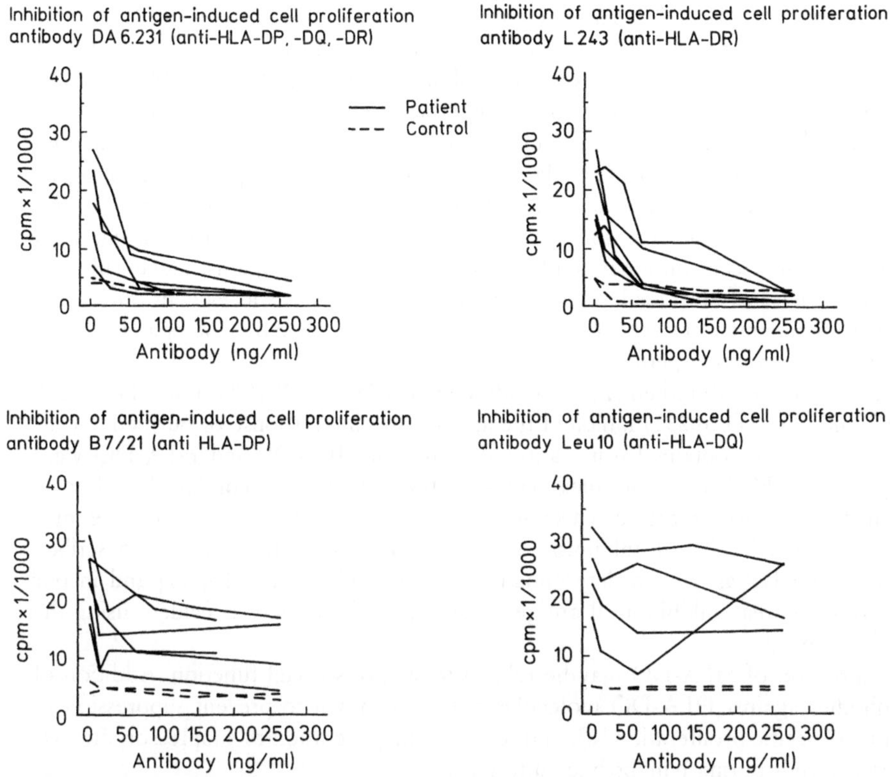

Fig. 1. Inhibition of antigen-specific proliferation by anti-MHC II antibodies. PBMCs (10^6 ml^{-1} in TCM-P) were incubated with monoclonal antibody for 1 h at room temperature before the addition of either Con A or $NiSO_4$. The 6-day LTT was then carried out. Results shown are mean cpm of quadruplicate cultures

(Fig. 1), but did not affect the response to Con A. Leu 10 (anti-HLA-DQ) and L368 (a control antibody against beta-2-microglobulin) did not affect either the antigen- or mitogen-induced cellular proliferation (the effect of the Leu 10 on antigen-specific proliferation is also shown in Fig. 1).

Discussion

In our laboratory the LTT, using 5 µg/ml nickel sulphate in a 6- or 7-day assay, is a highly sensitive and specific method for confirming a diagnosis of nickel-induced allergic contact dermatitis [7]. The studies reported in this communication have shown that the method can be adapted to study accessory-cell function in vitro.

We have shown that both plastic-adherent blood cells and epidermal cells possess accessory-cell function, as shown by their ability to mediate the proliferation of nylon-wool enriched T cells in response to the mitogen Con A and the antigen nickel sulphate. The epidermal cells contained approximately 2% MHC II^+ cells, in contrast to the 55% MHC II$^+$ cells present in the plastic-adherent blood cells. As epidermal cells were prepared from suction blisters obtained from clinically uninvolved skin, it is unlikely that there was any contribution to the number of MHC II$^+$ cells by the keratinocytes [14]. Therefore, Langerhans cells would be the only cells expected to act as accessory cells in our experiments. The finding that 20% epidermal cells are more effective than 10% plastic-adherent blood cells in permitting mitogen- or antigen-induced T-cell proliferation supports the finding of Braathen and Thorsby [3] that epidermal accessory cells (Langerhans cells) are more efficient than blood accessory cells on a per cell basis. T-cell proliferation against nickel sulphate in the presence of both epidermal and blood accessory cells was evident only when cells from patients were used. False-positive results, described by Chu et al. [5], were not obtained in our experiments.

As reported by Braathen [2], antibodies against HLA-DR (L243) and HLA-DP, -DQ and -DR (DA6.231) inhibited the antigen-specific response of purified T cells ($\geq$80%). Results obtained using antibodies against HLA-DP and HLA-DQ were more varied. HLA-DP molecules play an important role in secondary lymphocyte stimulation. However, they can also act as a restricting element for antigen presentation to cloned T cells [6]. Inhibition of DP-specific alloreactivity has been described by blocking DP-associated determinants with antibody TU39 [10, 11] and in our experiments weak inhibition of antigen-induced proliferation was evident using the antibody B7/21.

Expression of HLA-DQ may be related to suppressor-cell function. Addition of antibodies against HLA-DQ molecules has been shown to prevent suppression of antigen-specific proliferation [8], and to block the generation of suppressor and cytotoxic T cells during lymphocyte culture [9].

The relative inability of antibodies against HLA-DP and -DQ to affect accessory-cell function in our studies may result from the low levels of expression of these molecules on the accessory-cell surface. Dendritic cells, which are considered to be one of the most potent accessory cells [15], have been shown to express significant levels of HLA-DP and HLA-DQ only after several days in culture [4]. It is also possible, however, that the lack of inhibition of cellular proliferation seen with the antibodies against HLA-DP and -DQ may reflect the use of too low a concentration of the antibodies or a relatively lower affinity of these reagents for the relevant class II molecule.

Further studies are required therefore to elucidate the role of HLA-DP and -DQ molecules in antigen- and mitogen-driven responses in vitro.

References

1. Ashwell JD, Defranco AL, Paul WE, Schwartz RH (1984) Antigen presentation by resting B cells. Radiosensitivity of the antigen-presentation function and two distinct pathways of T cell activation. J Exp Med 159: 881–905
2. Braathen LR (1980) Studies on human epidermal Langerhans cells III. Induction of T Lymphocyte response to nickel sulphate in sensitised individuals. Br J Dermatol 103: 517–526

3. Braathen LR, Thorsby E (1983) Human epidermal Langerhans cells are more potent than blood monocytes in inducing some antigen-specific T-cell responses. Br J Dermatol 108: 139–146
4. Brooks CF, Moore M (1988) Differential MHC class II expression on human peripheral blood monocytes and dendritic cells. Immunology 63: 303–311
5. Chu AC, Shaw M, Elliot J (1987) In vitro stimulation of lymphocytes by nickel; reliability in detecting in vitro sensitivity and comparison of monocytes and Langerhans cells in antigen presentation. J Invest Dermatol 89: 322–323
6. Eckels DD, Lake P, Lamb JR, Johnson AH, Shaw S, Woody JN, Hartzman RJ (1983) SB-restricted presentation of influenza and herpes virus to human T-lymphocyte clones. Nature 301: 716–718
7. Everness KM, Gawkrodger DJ, Botham PA, Hunter JAA (1988) Nickel sensitivity and its detection by the in vitro stimulation of lymphocytes by nickel. Br J Dermatol 118: 274
8. Festenstein H, Ollier B (1987) Cellular typing and functional heterogeneity of MHC-encoded products. Br Med Bull 43: 122–155
9. Navarette C, Jaraquemada D, Fainbom L, Karr R, Hui K, Awad J, Bagnara M, Festenstein H (1985) Genetical and functional relationship of HLA-DR and HLA-DQ antigens. Immunogenetics 21: 97–101
10. Pawelec G, Schneider EM, Wernet P (1984) Cloned human T-lymphocytes with lymphostimulatory capacity preferentially activate suppressor cells. Eur J Immunol 14: 335–340
11. Pawelec G, Wernet P, Rosenlund R, Blaurock M, Schneider EM (1984) Strong lymphoproliferative suppressive function of PLT clones specific for SB-like antigens. Hum Immunol 9: 145–157
12. Seeger RC, Oppenheim JJ (1970) Synergistic interaction of macrophages and lymphocytes in antigen-induced transformation of lymphocytes. J Exp Med 132: 44–65
13. Stingl G, Katz SI, Clement L, Green I, Shevach EM (1978) Immunologic functions of Ia-bearing epidermal cells. J Immunol 121: 2005–2013
14. Tjernlund U, Scheynius A (1987) Amplification of T-cell response to PPD by epidermal cell suspensions containing HLA-DR expressing keratinocytes. Scand J Immunol 26: 1–6
15. Van Voorhis WC, Valinsky J, Hoffmann E, Luban J, Hair LS, Steinman RM (1983) Relative efficacy of human monocytes and dendritic cells as accessory cells for T cell replication. J Exp Med 158: 174–191

Addresses

K. M. Everness
ICI, Central Toxicology Laboratory, Alderley Park, Macclesfield, Cheshire SK10 4TJ, UK

P. A. Botham
ICI, Central Toxicology Laboratory, Alderley Park, Macclesfield, Cheshire SK10 4TJ, UK

D. J. Gawkrodger
University Department of Dermatology, Royal Hallanshire Hospital, Sheffield, S10 2JF, UK

J. A. A. Hunter
Department of Dermatology, University of Edinburgh, The Royal Infirmary, Edinburgh EH3 9YW, UK

A Modified Murine Local Lymph Node Assay for Identification of Contact Allergens

I. Kimber and C. Weisenberger

Summary

A modified murine local lymph node assay (LLNA) has been developed for the identification of contact allergens. Reactivity is measured as a function of T lymphocyte proliferation in the draining lymph node following topical exposure to the test chemical. Available data suggest that LLNA provides a rapid and cost-effective alternative to the currently available predictive test methods.

Key words:

Lymph node - T lymphocyte - Contact allergen

Introduction

There exist a variety of guinea pig test systems which may be used to predict the ability of a chemical to cause allergic contact dermatitis. Of those available the most widely employed are the Guinea Pig Maximization Test [3], the occluded patch test of Buehler [1] and the Optimization Test [4].

Although there is no doubt that such methods have played a valuable role in safety evaluation of chemicals, they are not without limitations. Thus, for instance, reactivity is invariably measured by the visual assessment of erythema and/or oedema following topical challenge; an end-point which is potentially subject to interpretive difficulties when coloured or irritant chemicals are examined.

Increased understanding of cellular immune responses in general, and of the mechanism and regulation of contact sensitivity in particular, provides an opportunity for the design of alternative, immunologically based predictive methods for the identification of skin allergens.

Contact sensitivity, an example of a delayed hypersensitivity reaction, is dependent upon the recognition of, and response to, topically applied chemicals by T lymphocytes. The current view is that, following exposure, epidermal dendritic cells, including Langerhans' cells, transport the allergen to the draining lymph node(s) where it is presented to T lymphocytes. Allergen-responsive T cells are induced to divide and differentiate; a process which results in systemic sensitisation.

It was our belief that the initiation of T lymphocyte activation in the draining node following topical exposure to the test chemical might provide an accurate means of evaluating the capacity of a compound to cause contact allergy. In preliminary studies various parameters of immune activation in the draining lymph nodes were examined in mice exposed to well-characterised contact allergens. Changes in lymph node weight, the frequency of large pyroninophilic cells and the initiation of T lymphocyte proliferation were recorded. Of these measurements T cell division proved to be the most sensitive marker of local immune activation. In initial experiments T lymphocyte proliferation was measured in vitro following culture of isolated lymph node cells with [^{3}H] thymidine in the presence or absence of interleukin-2 [2, 5]. A validation exercise was performed in which more than 80 chemicals were examined for which there existed historical data derived from the Magnusson and Kligman Guinea Pig Maximisation Test. The results of this study revealed that the Local Lymph Node Assay (LLNA) was both sensitive and selective. Thus, exposure to skin-sensitizing chemicals, but not to non-sensitizing agents, caused the induction of measurable hyperplasia in the drainage node. Furthermore, irritant concentrations of non-sensitising chemicals such as sodium dodecylsulphate failed to induce T lymphocyte proliferation.

As part of our continuing commitment to the development of the Local Lymph Node Assay we have recently evaluated a modified protocol in which after exposure of mice to the test agent, lymphocyte proliferation is measured following the intravenous injection of [^{3}H] thymidine. Representative results from this modified murine LLNA are described in this report.

Material and Methods

Mice. Young adult (6- to 8-week-old) CBA strain mice were used throughout these studies.

Chemicals. 4-Ethoxymethylene-2-phenyloxazol-5-one (oxazolone; Sigma Chemical Co., St Louis, Mo, USA), picryl chloride (BDH, Poole, Dorset, UK) and 2,4-dinitrochlorobenzene (DNCB; Sigma Chemical Co., St Louis, MO, USA) were used as commercial preparations dissolved in 4:1 acetone: olive oil (AOO).

Measurement of Lymph Node Cell Proliferation. Groups of mice ($n=4$) received 25 µl of test chemical in AOO or an equal volume of vehicle alone on the dorsum of both ears daily for 3 days. At various times thereafter exposed animals were injected intraveneously with 20 µCi of [^{3}H] methylthymidine (specific activity 2.5 Ci/mmol; Amersham International, Amersham, UK) in 0.25 ml of phosphate-buffered saline

(PBS). Mice were killed 5 h later and the draining auricular lymph nodes removed and pooled from each experimental group. The pooled lymph nodes were washed in 5% trichloracetic acid and processed for β-scintillation counting. Results were recorded as mean counts per minute per auricular lymph node.

Results

In preliminary experiments the capacity of oxazolone, picryl chloride and DNCB to induce proliferation in the draining auricular nodes was examined. The results recorded in Table 1 demonstrate that each of these well-characterised skin sensitizers caused a dose-dependent induction of lymph node cell proliferation. It will be apparent from these data that exposure of mice to vehicle (AOO) alone resulted in no such hyperplasia.

Subsequently, the kinetics of the proliferative response induced by exposure to oxazolone or DNCB were examined. Mice received 25 µl of the test chemical on three consecutive days and the proliferative activity in draining auricular nodes was measured 3, 4 and 5 days following the initiation of exposure. The maximum proliferative response induced by exposure to oxazolone was observed 3 days following the initiation of treatment. In contrast the peak proliferative response for DNCB-treated animals was recorded on day 5 (Table 2).

Table 1. The influence of repeated exposure to oxazolone, picryl chloride or DNCB on lymph node cell proliferation in CBA mice; response measured 3 days following initiation of treatment

Test concentration (%)	$[^3H]$ Thymidine incorporation (mean cpm/lymph node $\times 10^{-3}$)		
	Oxazolone	Picryl chloride	DNCB
1	7.92	5.83	2.14
0.5	6.31	4.92	1.24
0.25	5.13	3.73	0.82
0.1	3.71	2.02	ND
0.05	1.71	1.10	ND
0	0.04	0.02	0.03

ND, Not determined

Table 2. The influence of repeated exposure to oxazolone or DNCB on lymph node cell proliferation in CBA mice; kinetics of the response

Days following initiation of exposure	$[^3H]$ Thymidine incorporation (mean cpm/lymph node $\times 10^{-3}$)	
	0.5% Oxazolone	1.0% DNCB
3	5.91	1.87
4	4.82	2.12
5	3.61	2.46

Discussion

Topical exposure of mice to skin-sensitizing chemicals induces a dose- and time-dependent induction of T lymphocyte proliferation in the draining lymph note. Activity can be accurately and conveniently measured following the intravenous injection of [^{3}H] thymidine and the data recorded as mean isotope incorporation per lymph node.

The LLNA provides a cost-effective alternative to the currently available guinea pig tests and has the advantage of an objective end-point. Furthermore, the assay does not require the use of adjuvants and the test agent is applied via the relevant exposure route. Of some importance is the fact that activity in the LLNA is influenced neither by the irritancy of the test chemical nor by its colour.

Although formal inter-laboratory validation trials have yet to be completed it is tempting to suggest the available data indicate that the LLNA may provide a rapid and relatively inexpensive alternative predictive test method for use as an elective pre-screen in toxicology studies.

References

1. Buehler EV (1965) Delayed contact hypersensitivity in the guinea pig. Arch Dermatol 91: 171
2. Kimber I, Mitchell JA, Griffin AC (1986) Development of a murine local lymph node assay for the determination of sensitizing potential. Food Chem Toxicol 24: 585
3. Magnusson B, Kligmann AM (1969) The identification of contact allergens by animal assay. The guinea pig maximization test. J Invest Dermatol 52: 268
4. Maurer T, Weirich EG, Hess R (1980) The optimization test in the guinea pig in relation to other predictive sensitization methods. Toxicology 15: 163
5. Oliver GJA, Botham PA, Kimber I (1986) Models for contact sensitization – novel approaches and future developments. Br J Dermatol 115: 53

Addresses

I. Kimber

Immunology Group, Central Toxicology Laboratory, ICI plc, Alderley Park, Macclesfield, Cheshire SK10 4TJ, UK

C. Weisenberger

Immunology Group, Central Toxicology Laboratory, ICI plc, Alderley Park, Macclesfield, Cheshire SK10 4TJ, UK

Part 8

Preventive Measures

A Method for In Vitro Evaluation of Skin Protective Agents Against Epoxy Resin

N. Wiegersma, P. J. Coenraads, and J. P. Nater

Summary

Sensitization and subsequent allergic contact dermatitis due to contact with epoxy resin constitutes a major problem in epoxy workers. In search of ways to protect the skin against exposure to epoxy resin an in vitro method was used to evaluate the efficiency of a series of possible barriers. This method is based upon the determination of the breakthrough time of low molecular weight epoxy resin through a standardized layer of cream or polymer derived from an aerosol spray. Detection of the penetrated epoxy resin in the recipient medium, i. e. a test paper, was carried out by means of the naked eye and interferometric infrared spectroscopy. The method has been applied to a series of creams and aerosol-derived polymer films. Significant differences in breakthrough times were observed, indicating that the method can be used for the comparison of the barrier function of potential protective agents.

Key words:

Epoxy resin - Interferometric infrared spectroscopy - Skin protection

Introduction

The sensitizing capacity of the epoxy resin oligomer of the bisphenol A-type is a well-known phenomenon and constitutes an evident cause of occupational dermatitis [2–4]. In search of a barrier which can protect the skin of epoxy workers against contact with epoxy resin, a method was developed for the screening of such protective agents prior to clinical testing on patients with a proven hypersensitivity to epoxy.

The principle of this method is the determination of the breakthrough time through a layer of a potential barrier.

Materials and Methods

Preparation of a Cream Film

In principle the method consists in preparing a film of cream between sheets of filter paper with a confined spot area of 1 cm^2 (Schleicher and Schuell, no. Y211). The thickness of the film is controlled by placing between the papers, in addition to the cream, a 6 × 6 cm sheet of stainless steel 0.15 mm thick, having a central hole 2.5 cm in diameter with a 0.5-cm wide slit opening to one side [1].

All test papers were pressed at 340 technical atmospheres with a laboratory press. Using a syringe, 0.12 ml cream to be tested was placed in the confined spot of a test paper. The stainless steel sheet was placed over the filter paper with the central opening surrounding the cream. Two other test papers were centred and placed over the cream and the opening in the steel sheet. This assembly was then subjected to pressure (140 technical atmospheres). In this way the cream was forced into a circular film 2.5 cm in diameter and 0.15 mm thick. Any excess cream was extruded along the lateral slit in the stainless steel sheet.

Preparation of a Polymer Film

During a certain period of time, a polymer aerosol was sprayed on a piece of nylon shifting fabric (Scrynel NY100HC; Zuercher Beuteltuchfabrik), which had been stretched over a framework. The mesh aperture of this fabric is 100 µm; the open surface 46%. The spraying time was adjusted in such a way that a polymer film of approximately 1 mg/cm^2 was produced. After drying the fabric with the polymer it was cut into 3 × 3 cm fragments, which were weighed to determine the amount of polymer per square cm. A fragment of polymer/fabric was then pressed at 140 technical atmospheres together with a test paper.

Further Procedures

The assembly with the cream or the polymer layer was completed to a test sandwich using two stainless steel sheets (6 × 6 cm; 0.15 mm thick; with a 2.5 cm in diameter hole in the centre), one on either side, and the whole was held together by two letter clips. Immediately after assembly 0.02 ml low molecular weight epoxy resin (Shell, Epikote 828) was applied on top of the test sandwich within the confined spot area and the test sandwich was placed in an incubator at 28 °C. The breakthrough time was determined in the first instance with the naked eye; pinpoint leakage of epoxy in the bottom test paper can be easily detected as a transparent spot. These results were checked using Fourier transform infrared spectroscopy after extraction of the confined spot of the test paper with tetrahydrofuran.

With this method a series of nine commercially available creams and a series of eight polymer aerosols were tested.

Table 1. Breakthrough times of epoxy resin through cream and polymer films (eight tests per agent)

Cream	Breakthrough time	Polymer	Breakthrough time	Amount of polymer (mg/cm^2)
Kerodex 71	>5 days	1[a]	3–7 h	0.9–1.0
Kerodex 55	48–50 h	2	4–9 h	0.9–1.3
Dermotect 8	>5 days	3	5–6 h	0.9–1.1
Dermotect 10	3–5 h	4	1–5 h	0.5–1.2
Dermotect S5	40–48 h	5	>10 days	0.7–0.9
Chiron	25–30 h	6	>7 days	1.0–1.3
Calmurid	24–30 h	7	4–5 h	1.4–1.5
Cophasil	12–15 h	8	6–7 h	0.9–1.0
pH5-Eucerin	14–16 h			

[a] 1, Vinyl caprolactam based terpolymer; 2, copolymer, vinylacetate and vinylpyrrolidone; 3, polyvinyl pyrrolidone; 4, copolymer, vinylacetate and crotonic acid; 5, poly(methylvinylether/maleic acid); 6, acrylate protecting spray; 7, hairspray A; 8, hairspray B

Results

The results of this testing method are listed in Table 1. In a series of nine creams tested, two had a significantly higher breakthrough time than the other creams: Kerodex 71 and Dermotect 8, both with a breakthrough time of more than 5 days. The same applies to the series of polymer films tested; two polymers had much longer breakthrough times: more than 10 and 7 days for the polymers poly(methylvinylether/maleic acid) and an acrylate protecting spray, respectively. The breakthrough times for each of the other agents varied considerably, but were never more than 50 h.

Discussion

The results obtained indicate that our method can detect significant differences in breakthrough time for epoxy resin through potential skin barriers. Although there is a great variation in the results for the agents with relatively low breakthrough times, the differences with the four most effective barriers were significant and very well reproducible.

We therefore find the method useful, as an initial screening technique, prior to evaluation of the most promising agents on the skin of volunteers under circumstances which are closer to those in practice than laboratory conditions are.

References

1. Denton CR, Birmingham DJ, Perone VB (1955) A laboratory evaluation of silicone skin-protective preparations. Arch Dermatol 70: 7–12
2. Fregert S, Thorgeirrson A (1977) Patch testing with low molecular oligomers of epoxy resin in humans. Contact Dermatitis 3: 301–303
3. Heskel NS (1988) Epoxy resin dermatitis in a stained glass window maker. Contact Dermatitis 18: 182–183
4. Prens EP, De Jong G, Van Joost T (1986) Sensitization to epichlorohydrin and epoxy system components. Contact Dermatitis 15: 85–90

Addresses

N. Wiegersma
Occupational Dermatology Unit, University Hospital Groningen, The Netherlands

P. J. Coenraads
Occupational Dermatology Unit, University Hospital Groningen, The Netherlands

J. P. Nater
Occupational Dermatology Unit, University Hospital Groningen, The Netherlands

A New Glove Material Protective Against Epoxy and Acrylate Monomer

J. Roed-Petersen

Key words:

Glove material - Epoxy - Acrylate Monomer

More than 90% of the used epoxy resins are of the bisphenol-A type [1]. The monomer with a molecular weight of 340 is a strong sensitizer [12]. It is widely used in several branches of industry and may cause major dermatological problems and change of occupation among sensitized workers [11]. Also methyl-methacrylate monomer is a strong sensitizer [4] and appears to be the main cause of skin problems among dental technicians [3, 5]. Among orthopaedic surgeons several cases of sensitization from self-curing acrylate resins have been described [6, 10].

Both epoxy resin and methyl-methacrylate monomer readily penetrate plastic and rubber gloves [9, 10]. A new glove material, 4-H-glove, a laminate composed of five layers (Fig. 1), with a thickness of only 0.065 mm has in laboratory tests a breakthrough time >240 min for epoxy resin monomer, methyl-methacrylate monomer and a wide range of organic solvents [8].

The purpose of this study was to test the 4-H-glove material in vivo.

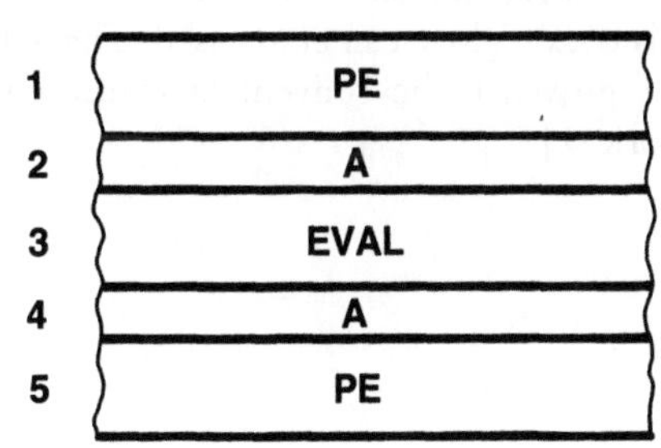

Fig. 1. 4-H-glove material, thickness 0.065 mm. *PE*, polyethylene; *A*, adhesive; *EVAL*, copolymer of ethylene and vinylalcohol

Materials and Methods

Patients with a proven allergy to epoxy of the bisphenol-a type or to methyl-methacrylate monomer volunteered for the study.

Samples of about 3 × 3 cm taken from a part of the 4-H-glove with and without a weld were used.

In the center of each sample a Finn chamber (Epitest, Helsinki, Finland) filled with epoxy resin 1% in pet. or methyl-methacrylate 1% in pet. was attached, fixed with Scanpore (Norgesplaster, Oslo). The samples was applied to the skin, fixed with Scanpore, for 48 h (epoxy resin) or 24 h (methyl-methacrylate). Readings were done after 48 h (epoxy resin) or 24 h (methyl-methacrylate) and on the following days for up to 4–7 days.

Results

No positive reactions were seen in eight patients sensitive to epoxy resin or four patients sensitive to methyl-methacrylate.

Discussion

Henriksen and Petersen have tested a wide range of common glove materials in vitro [8]. They found that only polyvinylalcohol (PVA), co-polymers of vinylalcohol and ethylene (E/VAL) and laminates of E/VAL and polyethylene (PE) had a breakthrough time > 240 min for epoxy resin monomer (DGEBA; Table 1). Blanken et al. [2] found that two of five samples of glove material gave total protection against epoxy resin during a test period of 48 h. These two materials, nitrile-butatoluene rubber and nitrile rubber, had a thickness of 0.56 mm and 0.50 mm respectively.

Generally, the thinner a glove material is, the lesser is the inconvenience in using gloves during work. The 4-H-glove is neither a usual disposable glove nor a glove for re-use. It is intended for industrial use for a maximum of 4 h, for example from starting a shift until lunch and from after lunch until the end of the shift. The manufacturer recommends wearing a cotton glove under the 4-H-glove to absorb sweat – this cotton glove can be re-used. The 4-H-glove will be distributed in eight sizes and has proven to be convenient in use-test among employees in industrial places of work [7].[1]

[1] It is distributed and manufactured by Safety 4 AS, Lundtoftegaardsvej 95, 2800 Lyngby, Denmark

Table 1. Breakthrough time for epoxy resin monomer of bisphenol-A type (DGEBA) through different membrane materials. (Modified from [8])

Material	Thickness (mm)	First trace of DGEBA (min)
Polyethylene (PE)	0.08	2.0
Butylrubber I (PIB, IIR)	0.22	2.5
Butylrubber II (PIB, IIR)	0.48	25
Polychloropropene (neopren, CR)	0.54	16
Ethylenpropylene-terpolymer (EPDM)	0.90	2.5
Chlorobutyl-EPDM-mix	1.32	11
Natural rubber (NR)	1.10	7.3
Polyisoprene (PIP)	1.10	6.5
Silicone rubber (VSi)	1.16	7.5
Polyvinylalcohol (PVA)	0.07	>240
PE//E/VAL-1//PE	0.056	>240
E/VAL-1//PE	0.095	>240
E/VAL-1	0.020	>240
E/VAL-2	0.016	>240

References

1. Adams RM (1983) (ed) Occupational skin disease, Grune and Stratton, New York, pp 241–250
2. Blanken R, Nater JP, Veenhoff E (1987) Protection against epoxy resins with glove materials. Contact Dermatitis 16: 46–47
3. Blichmann CW, Roed-Petersen J (1986) Erhvervsbetingede hudproblemer hos laboratorietandteknikere. Ugeskr Læger 148: 1370–1372
4. Chung CW, Giles AL (1977) Sensitization potentials of methyl, ethyl, and n-butyl methacrylates and mutual cross-sensitivity in guinea pigs. J Invest Dermatol 68: 187–190
5. Estlander T, Rajaniemi R, Jolanki R (1984) Hand dermatitis in dental technicians. Contact Dermatitis 10: 201–205
6. Fisher AA (1973) Acrylic bone cement sensitization and dermatitis. Cutis 12: 333–337
7. Henriksen HR, Madsen JØ, Petersen HJS (1987) Bedre prøvningscelle og vurdering af tæthed. Arbejdsmiljøfondets forskningsrapporter. Beskyttelsesklæder mod kemikalier II. Arbejdsmiljøfondet, Copenhagen
8. Henriksen HR, Petersen HJS (1986) Bedre handsker mod epoxy og andre kemikalier. Arbejdsmiljøfondets forskningsrapporter. Beskyttelsesklæder med kemikalier, Arbejdsmiljøfondet, Copenhagen
9. Pegum JS (1979) Penetration of protective gloves by epoxy resin. Contact Dermatitis 5: 281–283
10. Pegum JS, Medhurst FA (1971) Contact dermatitis from penetration of rubber gloves by acrylic monomer. Br Med J 2: 141–143
11. van Putten PB, Coenraads PJ, Nater JP (1984) Hand dermatoses and contact allergic reactions in construction workers exposed to epoxy resins. Contact Dermatitis 10: 146–150
12. Thorgeirsson A, Fregert S (1977) Allergenicity of epoxy resins in the guinea pig. Acta Derm Venereol (Stockh) 57: 253–256

Addresses

J. Roed-Petersen
Department of Dermatology, Gentofte Hospital, 2900 Hellerup, Denmark

Subject Index

Subject Index

A

B

C

Q

R

S

T

U

V

W

MIX
Papier aus verantwortungsvollen Quellen
Paper from responsible sources
FSC® C105338
FSC
www.fsc.org

If you have any concerns about our products,
you can contact us on
ProductSafety@springernature.com

In case Publisher is established outside the EU,
the EU authorized representative is:
Springer Nature Customer Service Center GmbH
Europaplatz 3, 69115 Heidelberg, Germany

Printed by Libri Plureos GmbH
in Hamburg, Germany